The nutrition handbook for food processors

Related titles from Woodhead's food science, technology and nutrition list:

Benders' dictionary of nutrition and food technology (ISBN 1 85573 475 3)
D. A. Bender and A. E. Bender

This classic dictionary remains an essential reference book for all those who need to know about nutrition, dietetics, food sciences and food technology. The Seventh edition provides succinct, authoritative definitions of over 5000 terms in nutrition and food technology (an increase of 25% from the previous edition). Definitions range from abalone and abscisic acid to zymogens and zymotachygraph. In addition, there is nutrient composition data for 287 foods.

'This valuable book continues to fulfil the purpose of explaining to specialists in other fields the technical terms in nutrition and food processing.'
Chemistry and Industry

'The book is certainly comprehensive and covers all aspects of food and nutrition sciences . . . Since obtaining a copy I have had occasion to use the dictionary on an almost daily basis.'
BNF Nutrition Bulletin

Functional foods: concept to product (ISBN 1 85573 503 2)
G. R. Gibson and C. M. Williams

Functional foods are widely predicted to become one of the biggest dietary trends of the next twenty-five years. The editors of this book have gathered together leading experts in the field in order to provide the food industry with a single authoritative resource. This book first defines and classifies the field of functional foods, paying particular attention to the legislative aspects in both the USA and EU. It then summarises the key work on functional foods and the prevention of disease. Finally, there is a series of chapters on developing functional products.

Antioxidants in food: practical applications (ISBN 1 85573 463 X)
J. Pokorný, N. Yanishlieva and M. Gordon

Antioxidants are an increasingly important ingredient in food processing, as they inhibit the development of oxidative rancidity in fat-based foods, particularly meat and dairy products and fried foods. Recent research suggests that they play a role in limiting cardiovascular disease and cancers. This new book provides a review of the functional role of antioxidants and discusses how they can be effectively exploited by the food industry, focusing on naturally occurring antioxidants in response to the increasing consumer scepticism over synthetic ingredients.

'An excellent reference book to have on the shelves.' *LWT Food Science and Technology*

Details of these books and a complete list of Woodhead's food science, technology and nutrition titles can be obtained by:

- visiting our web site at www.woodhead-publishing.com
- contacting Customer services (e-mail: sales@woodhead-publishing.com; fax: +44 (0) 1223 893694; tel.: +44 (0) 1223 891358 ext.30; address: Woodhead Publishing Ltd, Abington Hall, Abington, Cambridge CB1 6AH, England)

If you would like to receive information on forthcoming titles in this area, please send your address details to: Francis Dodds (address, tel. and fax as above; e-mail: francisd@woodhead-publishing.com). Please confirm which subject areas you are interested in.

The nutrition handbook for food processors

Edited by
C. J. K. Henry (Oxford Brookes University) and
C. Chapman (Unilever R & D Colworth)

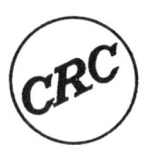

CRC Press
Boca Raton Boston New York Washington, DC

WOODHEAD PUBLISHING LIMITED
Cambridge England

Published by Woodhead Publishing Limited, Abington Hall, Abington
Cambridge CB1 6AH, England
www.woodhead-publishing.com

Published in North America by CRC Press LLC, 2000 Corporate Blvd, NW
Boca Raton FL 33431, USA

First published 2002, Woodhead Publishing Ltd and CRC Press LLC
© 2002, Woodhead Publishing Ltd
The authors have asserted their moral rights.

This book contains information obtained from authentic and highly regarded sources. Reprinted material is quoted with permission, and sources are indicated. Reasonable efforts have been made to publish reliable data and information, but the authors and the publishers cannot assume responsibility for the validity of all materials. Neither the authors nor the publishers, nor anyone else associated with this publication, shall be liable for any loss, damage or liability directly or indirectly caused or alleged to be caused by this book.

Neither this book nor any part may be reproduced or transmitted in any form or by any means, electronic or mechanical, including photocopying, microfilming and recording, or by any information storage or retrieval system, without permission in writing from the publishers.

The consent of Woodhead Publishing and CRC Press does not extend to copying for general distribution, for promotion, for creating new works, or for resale. Specific permission must be obtained in writing from Woodhead Publishing or CRC Press for such copying.

Trademark notice: Product corporate names may be trademarks or registered trademarks, and are used only for identification and explanation, without intent to infringe.

British Library Cataloguing in Publication Data
A catalogue record for this book is available from the British Library.

Library of Congress Cataloging in Publication Data
A catalog record for this book is available from the Library of Congress.

Woodhead Publishing ISBN 1 85573 464 8 (book) 1 85573 665 9 (e-book)
CRC Press ISBN 0-8493-1543-3
CRC Press order number: WP1543

Cover design by The ColourStudio
Typeset by SNP Best-set Typesetter Ltd., Hong Kong
Printed by TJ International, Padstow, Cornwall, England

Contents

List of contributors . . . . *xiii*

1 Introduction 1
 *Professor C. J. K. Henry, Oxford Brookes University;
 and Dr C. Chapman, Unilever R & D Colworth*

Part 1 Nutrition and consumers 5

2 What consumers eat 7
 A. Trichopoulou and A. Naska, University of Athens
 2.1 Introduction 7
 2.2 Dietary components and health 8
 2.3 Sources of dietary data 10
 2.4 Dietary data in Europe: national surveys 13
 2.5 Dietary data in Europe: European surveys 17
 2.6 Dietary patterns in Europe 22
 2.7 Future trends 28
 2.8 Sources of further information and advice 29
 2.9 References 29

3 Vitamins 34
 C. A. Northrop-Clewes and D. I. Thurnham, University of Ulster
 3.1 Introduction 34
 3.2 Vitamin A 35
 3.3 Vitamin A deficiency disorders (VADD) 35
 3.4 Bioavailability of provitamin carotenoids 38

3.5	Function	40
3.6	Health-related roles of β-carotene	42
3.7	Safety of vitamin A and β-carotene	44
3.8	Vitamin D	46
3.9	Specific nutritional deficiencies	47
3.10	Synthesis and actions of 1,25-OHD	48
3.11	Bone mineral density and fractures	50
3.12	Vitamin D and other aspects of health	51
3.13	Safety	52
3.14	Vitamin E	52
3.15	Biological activity	53
3.16	Coronary heart disease (CHD)	53
3.17	Other roles of vitamin E	55
3.18	Safety issues	57
3.19	Vitamin K	57
3.20	Biological activity	57
3.21	Vitamin K status and health	59
3.22	Safety	61
3.23	Vitamin C	62
3.24	Absorption and deficiency	62
3.25	Biochemical functions	63
3.26	Disease–nutrient interactions	63
3.27	Immune function	65
3.28	Toxicity	66
3.29	Vitamin B_1 (thiamin)	66
3.30	Functions and requirements	67
3.31	Clinical thiamin deficiency	68
3.32	Toxicity	70
3.33	Folate	70
3.34	Requirements	72
3.35	Folate, homocysteine and cardiovascular disease (CVD)	75
3.36	Causes of decreased folate status	76
3.37	Safety/toxicity	76
3.38	Cobalamin (vitamin B_{12})	77
3.39	Deficiency	78
3.40	Assessment and other issues	79
3.41	Safety/toxicity	80
3.42	Biotin	80
3.43	Pantothenic acid	81
3.44	Deficiency	81
3.45	Toxicity	82
3.46	Niacin	82
3.47	Vitamin B_6 (pyridoxine)	83
3.48	Deficiency	84
3.49	Safety/toxicity	85

3.50	Riboflavin	85
3.51	References	87

4 Minerals 97
C. Reilly, Oxford Brookes University
4.1	Introduction	97
4.2	Chemical characteristics	98
4.3	Impact on health, absorption and recommended intakes	98
4.4	Dietary sources, supplementation and fortification	100
4.5	Calcium	102
4.6	Iron	105
4.7	Zinc	107
4.8	Other minerals: iodine and selenium	110
4.9	Sources of further information and advice	113
4.10	References	114

5 Measuring intake of nutrients and their effects: the case of copper 117
L. B. McAnena and J. M. O'Connor, University of Ulster
5.1	Introduction	117
5.2	The nutritional role of copper	118
5.3	Dietary copper requirements	120
5.4	Sources of copper	120
5.5	Copper deficiency	121
5.6	Copper toxicity	122
5.7	General limitations in assessing nutrient intake	124
5.8	Putative copper indicators	125
5.9	Functional copper status	127
5.10	Mechanisms of copper absorption	127
5.11	Copper distribution in the body	131
5.12	Assessment of copper absorption	132
5.13	Current research and future trends	133
5.14	Sources of further information and advice	135
5.15	References	136

6 Consumers and nutrition labelling 142
L. Insall, Food and Drink Federation, London
6.1	Introduction: the problem of providing nutrition information	142
6.2	Current EU nutrition legislation	144
6.3	Consumer expectations and understanding of nutrition labelling	149
6.4	The use of nutrition panels	151
6.5	Improved nutrition labelling	157
6.6	Future trends	161

viii Contents

    6.7   Sources of further information and advice 163
    6.8   References 163

7 New approaches to providing nutritional information 165
J. A. Monro, New Zealand Institute for Crop & Food Research
    7.1   Introduction 165
    7.2   Why food processors need new types of nutritional
           information 165
    7.3   Limitations of food composition data in food processing 168
    7.4   Foundations for practical nutritional information 170
    7.5   Limitations of food composition data: the case of
           carbohydrates 173
    7.6   Relative glycaemic potency and glycaemic-glucose
           equivalents 174
    7.7   Faecal bulking index and wheat bran equivalents 180
    7.8   Conclusion and future trends 186
    7.9   Sources of further information and advice 188
    7.10   References 188

Part 2 Processing and nutritional quality 193

8 The nutritional enhancement of plant foods 195
D. Lindsay, CEBAS-CSIC, Spain
    8.1   Introduction 195
    8.2   The nutritional importance of plants 196
    8.3   Strategies for nutritional enhancement 196
    8.4   The priorities for nutritional enhancement 198
    8.5   Relationship of structure to nutritional quality
           (bioavailability) 201
    8.6   Nutritional enhancement versus food fortification 202
    8.7   Constraints on innovation 204
    8.8   Future trends 206
    8.9   Further information 206
    8.10   References 206

9 Enhancing the nutritional value of meat 209
J. D. Higgs, Food To Fit; and B. Mulvihill, Consultant
    9.1   Introduction 209
    9.2   Meat consumption trends 210
    9.3   Cancer 211
    9.4   Concerns about fat 214
    9.5   Reductions in the fat content of red meat 215
    9.6   Fatty acids in meat 217
    9.7   Protein 223
    9.8   The functionality of meat 224
    9.9   Meat, Palaeolithic diets and health 226

	9.10	Meat and satiety	227
	9.11	Meat and micronutrients	228
	9.12	Future trends	234
	9.13	Conclusion	237
	9.14	References	237

10 The stability of vitamins during food processing 247
P. Berry Ottaway, Berry Ottaway and Associates Ltd

	10.1	Introduction	247
	10.2	The vitamins	247
	10.3	Factors affecting vitamin stability	248
	10.4	Fat-soluble vitamins	249
	10.5	Water-soluble vitamins	253
	10.6	Vitamin–vitamin interactions	259
	10.7	Vitamin loss during processing	260
	10.8	Vitamins and food product shelf-life	262
	10.9	Protection of vitamins in food	263
	10.10	References	264

11 Thermal processing and nutritional quality 265
A. Arnoldi, University of Milan

	11.1	Introduction	265
	11.2	The Maillard reaction	266
	11.3	Nutritional consequences and molecular markers of the Maillard reaction in food	273
	11.4	Melanoidins	275
	11.5	Transformations not involving sugars: cross-linked amino acids	277
	11.6	Metabolic transit and *in vivo* effects of Maillard reaction products	280
	11.7	Formation of toxic compounds	282
	11.8	Future trends	285
	11.9	Sources of further information and advice	285
	11.10	References	286

12 Frying 293
J. Pokorný, Prague Institute of Chemical Technology

	12.1	Introduction	293
	12.2	Changes in frying oil	294
	12.3	Impact of deep frying on nutrients	296
	12.4	Future trends	298
	12.5	Sources of further information and advice	299
	12.6	References	299

13 The processing of cereal foods 301
A. J. Alldrick, Campden and Chorleywood Food Research Association; and M. Hajšelová, Consultant

Contents

13.1 Introduction ... 301
13.2 The nutritional significance of cereals and cereal processing ... 302
13.3 Mechanical processing ... 303
13.4 Thermal processing ... 305
13.5 Developing nutritionally-enhanced cereal-based foods ... 308
13.6 Conclusions ... 311
13.7 Sources of further information and advice ... 311
13.8 References ... 312

14 Extrusion cooking ... 314
M. E. Camire, University of Maine
14.1 Introduction ... 314
14.2 Impact on key nutrients: carbohydrates ... 317
14.3 Proteins ... 320
14.4 Lipids ... 321
14.5 Vitamins ... 321
14.6 Minerals ... 323
14.7 Other nutritional changes ... 324
14.8 Future trends ... 325
14.9 Sources of further information and advice ... 326
14.10 References ... 326

15 Freezing ... 331
J. M. Fletcher, Unilever R & D Colworth
15.1 Introduction ... 331
15.2 Change and stability in frozen foods ... 332
15.3 Vegetables and fruits ... 333
15.4 Meat and fish ... 336
15.5 Nutritional implications of new developments in freezing ... 337
15.6 Sources of further information and advice ... 339
15.7 References ... 340

16 Modified atmosphere packaging (MAP) ... 342
F. Devlieghere, Ghent University; M. I. Gil, CEBAS-CSIC, Spain; and J. Debevere, Ghent University
16.1 Introduction ... 342
16.2 Principles of MAP ... 342
16.3 The use of oxygen in MAP ... 345
16.4 Applications of MAP in the food industry ... 346
16.5 The microbial safety of MAP ... 350
16.6 The effect of MAP on the nutritional quality of non-respiring food products ... 354
16.7 The effect of MAP on the nutritional quality of fresh fruit and vegetables ... 356
16.8 References ... 362

| 17 | **Irradiation** | 371 |

D. A. E. Ehlermann, *Federal Research Centre for Nutrition, Germany*

- 17.1 Introduction ... 371
- 17.2 The history of food irradiation ... 372
- 17.3 The principles of irradiation ... 373
- 17.4 The effects of irradiation on food ... 377
- 17.5 The safety of irradiated food ... 378
- 17.6 The nutritional adequacy of irradiated food ... 379
- 17.7 Vitamins ... 380
- 17.8 Carbohydrates ... 383
- 17.9 Lipids ... 383
- 17.10 Proteins ... 384
- 17.11 The wholesomeness of irradiated food ... 384
- 17.12 Current and potential applications ... 385
- 17.13 Consumer attitudes and government regulations ... 386
- 17.14 World Trade Organization, Codex Alimentarius and international trade ... 389
- 17.15 Future trends ... 390
- 17.16 Sources of further information and advice ... 391
- 17.17 References ... 392

| 18 | **Microwave processing** | 396 |

D. A. E. Ehlermann, *Federal Research Centre for Nutrition, Germany*

- 18.1 Introduction ... 396
- 18.2 The principles of microwave heating ... 398
- 18.3 The effects of microwave radiation on food ... 401
- 18.4 The safety of microwave-heated food ... 403
- 18.5 The nutritional adequacy of microwave heated food ... 405
- 18.6 Future trends ... 405
- 18.7 References ... 406

| 19 | **Ohmic heating** | 407 |

R. Ruan, X. Ye and P. Chen, *University of Minnesota*;
C. Doona and I. Taub, *US Army Natick Soldier Center*

- 19.1 Introduction ... 407
- 19.2 The principles of ohmic heating ... 407
- 19.3 The advantages of ohmic heating ... 409
- 19.4 The effect of ohmic heating on nutrient loss: thermal destruction ... 413
- 19.5 The effect of ohmic heating on nutrient loss: diffusion ... 415
- 19.6 Electrolysis and contamination ... 416
- 19.7 Future trends ... 416

xii   Contents

    19.8 Sources of further information and advice 419
    19.9 References 420

20 Infrared processing 423
    C. Skjöldebrand, ABB and Lund University, Sweden
    20.1 Introduction: the principles of infrared heating 423
    20.2 Infrared processing in the food industry 425
    20.3 Infrared processing and food quality 428
    20.4 Infrared processing and nutritional quality 430
    20.5 Future trends 430
    20.6 References 431

21 High pressure processing 433
    Indrawati, A. Van Loey and M. Hendrickx, Katholieke
    Universiteit, Leuven
    21.1 Introduction 433
    21.2 High pressure processing in relation to food quality
           and safety 433
    21.3 High pressure technology and equipment for the
           food industry 435
    21.4 Commercial high pressure treated food products 436
    21.5 Effect of high pressure on vitamins 437
    21.6 Effect of high pressure on lipids 442
    21.7 Effect of high pressure on other health-related
           food compounds 445
    21.8 Future trends in high pressure research 448
    21.9 Sources of further information and advice 448
    21.10 Acknowledgements 449
    21.11 References 449
    21.12 Appendices 453

22 Continuous-flow heat processing 462
    N. J. Heppell, Oxford Brookes University
    22.1 Introduction: definition of the process 462
    22.2 Principles of thermal processing 463
    22.3 Process equipment and product quality 464
    22.4 Processing and key nutrients: proteins 468
    22.5 Carbohydrates and fats 469
    22.6 Vitamins 470
    22.7 Future trends 471
    22.8 Sources of further information and advice 472
    22.9 References 473

Index 474

Contributors

(* indicates the main point of contact)

Chapter 1

Professor C. J. K. Henry
School of Biological and Molecular Sciences
Oxford Brookes University
Oxford
OX3 0BP
UK

Tel: +44 (0) 1865 483818
Fax: +44 (0) 1865 483242
Email: jhenry@brookes.ac.uk

Dr. C. Chapman
Unilever R & D
Colworth House
Sharnbrook
Bedfordshire
MK44 1LQ
UK

Tel: +44 (0) 1234 222005
Fax: +44 (0) 1234 222539
Email: clare.chapman@unilever.com

Chapter 2

A. Trichopoulou & A. Naska*
School of Medicine
Department of Hygiene and Epidemiology
University of Athens
75 M.Asias St.
GR-115 27
Athens
Greece

Tel: +30 10 74 62 073
Fax: +30 10 74 62 079
Email: anaska@nut.uoa.gr
Email: antonia@nut.uoa.gr

Chapter 3

Dr C. A. Northrop-Clewes* &
Professor D. I. Thurnham
Northern Ireland Centre for Diet &
Health (NICHE)
School of Biomedical Sciences
University of Ulster
Coleraine
BT52 1SA
Northern Ireland

Tel: +44 (0) 2870 324473
Fax: +44 (0) 2870 324965
Email: di.thurnham@ulster.ac.uk
Email: c.clewes@ulster.ac.uk

Chapter 4

C. Reilly
School of Biological and Molecular
Sciences
Oxford Brookes University
Oxford
OX3 0BP
UK

Tel: +44 (0) 1608 677245
Email: reiyan99@aol.com

Chapter 5

L. B. McAnena *& J. M. O'Connor
Northern Ireland Centre for Diet and
Health (NICHE)
University of Ulster
Cromore Road
Coleraine
BT52 1SA
Northern Ireland

Tel: +44 (0) 208 7032 4883
Fax: +44 (0) 870 1367 653
Email: l.mcanena@ulst.ac.uk
Email: jm.oconnor@ulst.ac.uk

Chapter 6

L. Insall
Scientific and Regulatory Affairs
Division
Food and Drink Federation
6 Catherine Street
London
WC2 5JJ
UK

Tel: +44 (0) 207 836 2460
Fax: +44 (0) 207 836 0580
Email: lynn.insall@fdf.org.uk

Chapter 7

J. A. Monro
Crop & Food Research
Private Bag 11-600
Palmerston North
New Zealand

Tel: +64 6 356 8300
Fax: +64 6 351 7050
Email: monroj@crop.cri.nz

Chapter 8

D. Lindsay
Food Science and Technology
Department
CEBAS (CSIC)
Murcia 30800
Spain

Tel: +34 968 27 45 87
Fax: +34 968 27 47 93
Email: dlindsay@terra.es

Contributors xv

Chapter 9

J. D. Higgs*
Food To Fit
PO Box 6057
Greens Norton
Towcester
Northamptonshire
NN12 8GG
UK

Email: jennette@foodtofit.co.uk

B. Mulvihill

Chapter 10

P. Berry Ottaway
Berry Ottaway & Associates Ltd.
1a Fields Yard
Plough Lane
Hereford
HR4 0EL
UK

Tel: +44 (0) 1432 270886
Fax: +44 (0) 1432 270808
Email: berry.ottaway@dial.pipex.com

Chapter 11

A. Arnoldi
DISMA
University of Milan
Via Celoria 2
20133- Milano
Italy

Tel: +39 02 5031 6806
Fax: +39 02 5031 3062
Email: anna.arnoldi@unimi.it

Chapter 12

J. Pokorný
Department of Food Chemistry and
Analysis
Faculty of Food and Biochemical
Technologies
Prague Institute of Chemical
Technology
Technická 5
CZ-166 28 Prague 6
Czech Republic

Tel: +4202 2435 3264
Fax: +4202 333 9990
Email: jan.pokorny@vscht.cz

Chapter 13

A. J. Alldrick*
Campden & Chorleywood Food
Research Association
Chipping Campden
Gloucestershire
GL55 6LD
UK

Tel: +44 (0) 1386 842127
Fax: +44 (0) 1386 842150
Email: a.alldrick@campden.co.uk

M. Hajšelová
Pump Cottage
Blacksmiths Lane
Beckford
Tewkesbury
Gloucestershire
GL20 7AH
UK

Tel: +44 (0) 1386 882105
Email: anton.mirka@hron.fsnet.co.uk

Chapter 14

M. E. Camire
Department of Food Science &
Human Nutrition
University of Maine
5735 Hitchner Hall
Room 105
Orono
ME 04469-5735
USA

Tel: +1 207 581 1627
Fax: +1 207 581 1636
Email: mary_camire@umit.maine.edu

Chapter 15

J. M. Fletcher
Unilever R & D
Colworth House
Sharnbrook
MK44 1LQ
Bedfordshire
UK

Tel: +44 (0) 1234 222550
Fax: +44 (0) 1234 222409
Email: john.fletcher@unilever.com

Chapter 16

F. Devlieghere* & J. Debevere
Department of Food Technology and
Nutrition
Ghent University
Coupure Links, 653
9000 Ghent
Belgium

Tel: +32 9 264 61 78
Fax: +32 9 225 55 10
Email: frank.devlieghere@rug.ac.be

M. I. Gil
Food Science and Technology
Department
CEBAS (CSIC)
Apartado de Correas 4195
Murcia 30800
Spain

Tel: +34 968 39 63 15
Fax: +34 968 39 62 13
Email: migil@cebas.csic.es

Chapters 17 & 18

D. A. E. Ehlermann
Institute of Process Engineering
Federal Research Centre for Nutrition
Haid-und-Neu-Str. 9
D-76131 Karlsruhe
Germany

Tel: +49 721 6625-0
Fax: +49 721 6625-303
Email:
dieter.ehlermann@bfe.unikarlsruhe.de

Chapter 19

R. Ruan*, X. Ye & P. Chen
Department of Biosystems &
Agricultural Engineering
Department of Food Science and
Nutrition
University of Minnesota
1390 Eckles Avenue
St. Paul
Minnesota 55108
USA

Tel: +1 (612) 625 1710
Fax: +1 (612) 624 3005
Email: ruanx001@tc.umn.edu

C. Doona and I. Taub
US Army Natick Soldier Center
Natick
Massachusetts 01760
USA

Chapter 20

C. Skjöldebrand
ABB
SE-11396 Stockholm
Sweden

Tel: +46 8 458 5151
Fax: +46 8 458 5989
Email:
christina.skjoldebrand@se.abb.com

Chapter 21

Indrawati*, A. Van Loey &
M. Hendrickx
Faculty of Agriculture and Applied
Biological Sciences
Department of Food and Microbial
Technology
Laboratory of Food Technology
Katholieke Universiteit, Leuven
Kasteelpark Arenberg 22
B-3001 Leuven
Belgium

Tel: (016) 32 15 85
Fax: (016) 32 19 60
Email: indrawati@agr.kuleuven.ac.be
Email:
marc.hendrickx@agr.kuleuven.ac.be

Chapter 22

N. J. Heppell
School of Biological and Molecular
Sciences
Oxford Brookes University
Oxford
OX3 0BP
UK

Tel: +44 (0)1865 483956
Fax: +44 (0)1865 484017
Email: njheppell@brookes.ac.uk

1

Introduction

C. J. K. Henry, Oxford Brookes University; and C. Chapman, Unilever R & D Colworth

Improving the nutritional quality of food is a key requirement for the food industry. There are a number of factors which have made this area one of growing importance, including:

- Increasing health consciousness among consumers and concern about their dietary intake;
- New research on the links between diet and health, including the prevention of chronic disease;
- Ageing populations in many developed countries prone to degenerative disorders such as cancer, heart disease, osteoporosis, diabetes and stroke;
- Growing pressure on public health spending, leading to a greater emphasis on prevention and more individual responsibility for health;
- Changes in the regulatory framework.

Since Professor Arnold Bender's *Food processing and nutrition* (Bender, 1978), there have been relatively few comprehensive reviews of the impact of food processing on the nutritional quality of food. In the intervening period there has been continuing research on the contribution of key nutrients to health and on how these are affected by individual food processing operations. New technologies have emerged which also need to be taken into consideration. Building on Professor Bender's work and that of others in the field (for example, Henry and Heppell (1998)), *The nutrition handbook for food processors* seeks to summarise current research on key nutrients, their contribution to health and, in particular, how they are affected by both established and emerging food processing technologies.

Part 1 provides a context for the rest of the book. Chapter 2 discusses current evidence on what consumers eat. It compares the wide range of European surveys, their respective strengths and weaknesses, to establish an up-to-date picture of dietary patterns in Europe. Against this background of food intake, Chapter 3 provides an authoritative and comprehensive review of the latest research on the role of vitamins in health, considering such issues as function and bioavailability, sources, requirements, the impact of deficiency, safety and toxicity. The next chapter reviews the impact of minerals such as calcium, iron and zinc on health together with dietary sources, intake, supplementation and fortification. Chapter 5, which concentrates on copper, also considers in detail the methodological problems in accurately measuring nutrient intake and effects.

It is consumers who make the final decision on what they eat based on a range of factors including, amongst many others, convenience and accessibility, price and brand image, perceived sensory quality and nutritional value. In assessing the latter they need appropriate information. Chapters 6 and 7 discuss how this information is best supplied. Chapter 6 considers the current regulatory regime in the EU and manufacturers' responsibilities in labelling. In particular, it discusses research on how well consumers actually understand and use nutritional information together with ways in which such information can be improved so that consumers can make more informed choices in achieving the right diet. With the advent of so-called functional foods, nutritional science has moved from the objective of defining and achieving a balanced diet to the concept of 'optimised' nutrition actively preventing disease (Roberfroid, 2000). Against this background, Chapter 7 looks at current limitations in the accuracy of nutritional information, both from the point of view of food composition and the impact of nutrients on health. Using the example of carbohydrates, it suggests new ways of measuring and presenting information on the health impact of food components.

Against this background of research on nutrients and the way consumers assess nutritional quality, the major part of this handbook is devoted to assessing the impact of food processing on key nutrients. The first two chapters in Part 2 look at raw materials. Chapter 8 discusses the strategies available for the nutritional enhancement of plant foods, most notably genetic modification. Meat is an important food in its own right and a component in many food products. Its contribution to health is both significant and controversial. Chapter 9 discusses health concerns about meat, how meat production has adapted to meet these concerns, and the latest research on the nutritional and broader functional benefits of meat consumption. The following chapters then look at individual processes and their impact on the nutritional quality of food. They are preceded by an introductory chapter which reviews more broadly the stability of vitamins during processing and how vitamin losses can be avoided. The remaining chapters follow a broadly similar pattern, describing an individual process and its applications, and then looking at the range of research on its impact on key nutrients from vitamins and minerals to lipids, carbohydrates and proteins. Chapters cover both traditional operations such as frying (Chapter 12) and freezing (Chapter 15) and newer technologies such as modified atmosphere packaging (Chapter 16), ohmic heating (Chapter 19) and high pressure processing (Chapter 21). A number of chapters look at thermal processing which has a particularly significant impact on nutritional as well as sensory quality. Chapter 11 looks more broadly at the impact of thermal processing on food composition, with a particular focus on the Maillard reaction. As well as frying and ohmic heating, there are chapters on continuous-flow heat processing (Chapter 22), extrusion cooking (Chapter 14), microwave and infrared heating (Chapters 18 and 20). Chapter 13 looks at baking and other processes used particularly in the preparation of cereal foods.

References

BENDER A E (1978), *Food processing and nutrition*. Academic Press, London.
HENRY C K J and HEPPELL N J (1998), *Nutritional aspects of food processing*. Aspen Publishers, Gaithersburg.
ROBERFROID M (2000), 'Defining functional foods' in Gibson G R and Williams C M, *Functional foods: concept to product*. Woodhead Publishing Ltd, Cambridge.

Part 1

Nutrition and consumers

2

What consumers eat

A. Trichopoulou and A. Naska, University of Athens

2.1 Introduction

Documenting and monitoring dietary patterns are priorities in nutritional epidemiology, in the planning of national food and nutrition policies and in the evaluation of nutrition education strategies. Early efforts in documenting dietary patterns were focused on identifying the specific nutrients that may be responsible for effects on people's health, but recently research has expanded towards studying patterns of food intake. Food data are often derived from:

- Food Balance Sheets, providing information on food supply at the population level.
- Household Budget Surveys, which collect data on food availability in the household, based on nationally representative samples of households.
- specifically designed Individual Dietary Surveys, providing information on the food intake of free-living individuals.

In section 2.1 of the present chapter, food data sources are presented and commented upon, with emphasis on the dietary information collected. Section 2.2 provides an overview of individual dietary surveys undertaken in Europe, during the last 20 years, and discusses the factors that need to be taken into consideration before data from varied sources are combined and compared. European studies (DAFNE, EPIC, MONICA and SENECA) that allow for international comparisons are also presented and the section concludes with examples of European studies designed to address specific, nutrition-related research questions. Based on currently available data, the last section of the chapter describes dietary patterns in Europe and attempts to identify socio-demographic factors responsible for the disparities observed.

2.2 Dietary components and health

The availability of food in Europe has never been as good as in recent decades. Affluent though European countries are, sub-groups of populations experience the deficiency of minerals and micronutrients that play a vital role in health and development (Serra-Majem, 2001). A significant proportion of European infants and children are today experiencing a low dietary intake of iodine and iron (Trichopoulou and Lagiou, 1997a; WHO, 1998). The iodine deficiency leads to several disorders collectively referred to as Iodine Deficiency Disorders (IDD), with goitre (hyperplasia of thyroid cells), cretinism (mental deficiency) and severe brain damage being the most common. It is estimated that IDD may affect approximately 16% of the European population. Furthermore, inadequate levels of folate have been implicated with a rise in the blood homocysteine levels, leading possibly to increased risk of cardiovascular disease (CVD). European policies address such deficiencies either by recommending the consumption of foods rich in the implicated micronutrients or with supplementation policies (e.g. iodised salt, flour supplemented with folic acid).

The general increase, however, in the quantity and variety of food available has mostly been accompanied by the emergence of degenerative conditions such as CVD, various types of cancer, non-insulin dependent diabetes mellitus, obesity, osteoporosis and hypertension. Documenting and monitoring dietary patterns has therefore become a priority in the formulation of dietary recommendations and the planning of national food, nutrition and agricultural policies (Société Française de Santé Publique. Health and Human Nutrition, 2000).

However, there are questions that emerge early in the formulation of a nutrition and food policy: these concern the nature of the best diet and the objectives of an ideal diet. With respect to chronic nutrition-related conditions, most of our existing knowledge relies on evidence accumulated mainly in relation to the two most common categories of disease, cardiovascular disease and cancer.

With respect to CVD, there is strong evidence that the intake of vegetables, fruits and pulses reduces the risk, although there is no agreement to what extent the apparent protection is conveyed by fibre, homocysteine-reducing folic acid, antioxidant compounds in vegetables and fruits, the high quantities of olive oil that usually accompany high intake of vegetables and legumes, or the complementary reduced consumption of red meat and lipids of animal origin (Willett, 1994, 1998).

The mainstream view on the effects of macronutrients on CVD is that dietary lipids high in saturated fatty acids and especially trans-fatty acids increase the risk. On the contrary, polyunsaturated fatty acids and some long chain n-3 fatty acids have beneficial effects. Monounsaturated lipids, overwhelmingly present in olive oil, also act beneficially by reducing the disadvantageous low density lipoprotein cholesterol (LDL-C) and increasing the protective high density lipoprotein cholesterol (HDL-C) (Mattson and Grundy, 1985; Mensink and Katan, 1987). Complex carbohydrates do not adversely affect the risk for CVD and their effect on HDL-C is less favourable than that of monounsaturated lipids

(Mensink and Katan, 1987). Refined carbohydrates substantially affect postprandial hyperglycemia and they appear to accentuate insulin resistance. With respect to other nutrients, there is converging, but not yet conclusive, evidence that moderate alcohol intake, vitamin E and folic acid are inversely associated with the risk of coronary heart disease (CHD) (Gaziano et al, 1993; Stampfer et al, 1993; Robinson et al, 1998). Salt intake, on the contrary, contributes to the elevation of blood pressure levels in susceptible individuals and thus to the increase of CVD risk (Beilin et al, 1999).

The evidence on the role of specific dietary factors in cancer aetiology has been critically summarised in recent reviews (Willett and Trichopoulos, 1996; Willett, 2000). With respect to food groups, vegetable consumption, and perhaps less definitely fruit consumption, have a beneficial effect on a broad spectrum of human cancer types. Among macronutrients, animal protein intake has been reported to increase the risk for colorectal cancer, while intake of saturated fat is positively associated with endometrial, prostate, colorectal, lung and kidney cancer. Although the percentage of calories from dietary lipids does not appear related to colon cancer, greater risks have been seen with higher consumption of red meat, possibly suggesting that factors other than dietary lipids *per se* may be important. Fibre intake, on the contrary, appears to protect against cancer of the pancreas and the large bowel. There are also indications of a protective role of monounsaturated lipids against breast cancer (Trichopoulou, 1995). Concerning micronutrients the evidence is largely insufficient. Recent studies indicate an inverse association of lycopene (Gann et al, 1999), selenium (Yoshizawa et al, 1998) and vitamin E (Tzonou et al, 1999) with prostate cancer, folic acid in relation to colon and breast cancers (Giovannucci et al, 1998); while beta-carotene supplements have been found to be ineffective against lung cancer risk (Hennekens et al, 1996).

Consumption of large quantities of alcoholic beverages, particularly in conjunction with tobacco smoking, has been reported to increase the risk of cancer in the upper respiratory and digestive tract, whereas alcoholic cirrhosis frequently leads to liver cancer. There are also data suggesting that intake of smaller quantities of alcohol may be linked to the occurrence of breast and colorectal cancer. Among added substances, only salt appears to be an important contributor to stomach cancer. Moreover, intake of salty fish very early in life has been linked to the occurrence of nasopharyngeal cancer in Southern Asia. Finally, in Central Asia and Southern America the intake of very hot drinks has been found to increase the risk of esophageal cancer (Kinjo et al, 1998).

Many of the early efforts have been focused on identifying specific dietary components that may be responsible for effects on people's health. Evaluating the effects of specific foods and nutrients, rather than integral dietary patterns, on disease illustrates how shifting from the empirical evidence may increase uncertainty. Dietary exposures are unusually complex and strongly intercorrelated. Current data suggest that apparently favourable effects cannot be exclusively attributed to specific components and in several instances these components may act synergistically (Gerber et al, 2000). Consequently, instead of focusing only on nutrients within foods, research has expanded towards studying patterns of food intake (Trichopoulos et al, 2000).

2.3 Sources of dietary data

As mentioned earlier, food data are often derived from:

- Food Balance Sheets that provide information on food supply at the population level.
- Household Budget Surveys that collect data on food availability in the household, based on nationally representative samples of households.
- specifically designed Individual Dietary Surveys that provide information on the food intake of free-living individuals, over a specified time period.

2.3.1 Food balance sheets

The food balance sheets (FBSs) assembled by the Food and Agriculture Organisation (FAO) describe the current and developing structure of the national dietary patterns, in terms of the major food commodities that disappear from the national markets (*www.fao.org*). A food balance sheet is completed at national level, on the basis of the annual food production, imports and exports, changes in stocks and the agricultural and industrial uses within a country. When these have been taken into account, the remaining quantities represent the food that can be assumed to have been available for human consumption in that country (Kelly et al, 1991).

Since 1949, FBSs are regularly collected on a world-wide basis and, in spite of their limitations, countries with no routine information on the food consumption of their population and those interested in comparing their national dietary patterns with those of other populations have traditionally used them (Helsing, 1995).

International comparisons based on the time series FBS data, in conjunction with information from other sources, can help to indicate trends in the food available to the overall population of one country in relation to others, and have thus been used for ecological correlations of food patterns with the morbidity and mortality of nutrition-related diseases. The user of these data, however, should bear in mind their constraints and interpret comparisons with due caution (Southgate, 1991). The accuracy of recording differs considerably between countries and commodities. Although data on their own food production are collected in some countries, these sources of information can be largely under-recorded. Waste and food given to pets may also be sources of error, since they are considerably dependent on time, cultures and type of commodities. Lastly, the conversion of foodstuffs into nutrient equivalents by the application of factors derived from various sources must be prudently treated.

2.3.2 Household budget surveys

The household budget surveys (HBSs) are periodically conducted by the National Statistical Offices of most European countries in nationally representative samples of households. By recording the values and quantities of household food purchases, the HBSs can adequately depict the dietary patterns prevailing in representative population samples. Moreover, the concurrent recording of demographic and socio-economic characteristics of the household members may allow exploratory analyses on the evaluation of their effects on dietary choices. One of the main advantages of the multi-purpose HBSs is their periodic undertaking by Governmental Services, making them a readily available and thus an affordable source of dietary information in developed and developing countries (Trichopoulou, 1992).

The HBSs can be thought of as occupying a position between the FBSs and the specially designed individual food consumption surveys. Like food balance sheets, the HBSs allow intercountry comparisons on a regular basis but, moving from total population to household level, they further allow the calculation of both the mean and the distribution of food availability within the population and specific subgroups (Trichopoulou et al, 1999).

Issues of comparability can be raised when using HBS data for international comparisons. The data collection methodology is uniform enough to allow such comparisons, but the food information recorded in the various countries may be of different forms and levels of detail. The methodology, however, for addressing these discrepancies has been developed in the context of the **DA**ta Food **NE**tworking (DAFNE) project (Lagiou et al, 2001; Friel et al, 2001). However, since HBSs are not primarily designed to collect nutritional information, the food data bear limitations, which need to be considered when they are used for nutritional purposes (van Staveren et al, 1991; Southgate, 1991; Trichopoulou, 1992). The following points should be borne in mind:

- In most cases, no records are collected on the type and quantity of food items and beverages consumed outside the home.
- Information on food losses and waste, food given to pets, meals offered to guests, use of vitamin and mineral supplements and the presence of pregnant or lactating women is not consistently collected.
- Data are collected at household level and estimation of the individuals' intake requires the application of stochastic statistical models.
- Information on nutrient intake is not readily available. Nevertheless, appropriate conversion factors based on food composition tables are developed for converting quantity data into nutrients.

Despite their limitations, the HBSs provide a resource for the conduct of a wide range of nutritional analyses. They also constitute a reasonable alternative to specially designed individual-based nutrition surveys for most Mediterranean and central/eastern European countries. HBS data could help highlight issues such as differences in dietary patterns (Byrd-Bredbenner et al, 2000), high risk population groups on account of their nutritional habits, relationships between diet and morbidity/mortality data (Lagiou et al, 1999) and dietary intakes of additives and contaminants.

2.3.3 Individual dietary surveys

The specially designed individual dietary surveys (IDSs) primarily aim at the collection of information on the food intake of free-living individuals over a specified period. The individual surveys, when intakes of the subject are recorded as adequately as possible, are expected to provide evidence on the food quantities consumed and to allow the calculation of both the mean and the distribution of food and nutrient intake among the whole or segments of the population.

The methods used to assess individual intake can be broadly divided into two generic categories (Willett, 1998):

- *Recall methods of sporadic or habitual diet.* They can be limited to the previous 24 hours (24-hour dietary recall), where subjects are asked to recall everything they consumed the previous day, or to a diet history referring to a broader and less precisely defined time period using food frequency methods.
- *Record methods of daily* intake, where subjects are required to keep records of everything they eat and drink for one (24-hour food record) or more days. The 7-day weighed record is the one commonly used.

The quantification of foods consumed and the selection of items to be included in the food list, in the case of closed lists, are critical components of data collection. Standard, natural and household units, three-dimensional food models, photographs, drawings of foods and geometric shapes are often used for documenting portion sizes.

Recall methods, in comparison to the record ones, do not require literacy; they are not expected to cause alterations in the eating behaviour of the subject, since the information is collected after the fact; and they have minimal respondent burden. Nevertheless, recall methods are subject to respondents' memory, a limitation not present in food records. In recent surveys, dietary recalls are collected using computer software programmes that allow data to be uniformly collected, by prompting interviewers to ask all the necessary questions, and may further reduce the cost of data collection and processing.

The food records and the 24-hour recall may be used to estimate the absolute intake of energy, macronutrients and some vitamins and minerals that are commonly found in the food supply. Both methods are frequently used in describing the mean intake of aggregated food groups and in validating food frequency questionnaires. These short-term methods are completely open ended, they accommodate any food or food combination reported by the subject and they allow recording information at various levels of detail including the type of food, the food source, the food processing and preparation methods. They are therefore particularly useful for estimating intakes of culturally diverse populations. One single day of intake, however, is highly unlikely to be representative of usual intake. For this reason the collection of multiple days of intake is required in order to estimate as adequately as possible the subjects' usual intake.

Food frequency questionnaires are food lists of differing length and the information collected can refer either to the frequency of consuming certain foods and beverages, or to both the frequency and estimates of the portions consumed. The underlying principle of the food frequency method is that the average long-term diet reflects the conceptually important exposure, and therefore makes the food frequency questionnaires the method of choice for measuring dietary exposures in epidemiological studies. In constructing a food frequency questionnaire, careful attention must be given to the format of the food frequency section, the selection of foods that will be included in the food list and the clarity of the questions. Food frequency questionnaires can be administered to large population groups; they can be applied as interviews or in a self-administered form and are relatively easy and less time consuming to complete when compared to other dietary assessment methods. It should, however, be borne in mind that food frequency questionnaires including a restricted food list may result in reducing the true variance of intake.

For most investigations of nutritional epidemiology, the relative ranking of individuals according to their food and nutrient intakes is adequate for determining correlations of relative risks. In such cases, food frequency questionnaires constitute the primarily selected dietary assessment method. In situations, however, when the aim is to compare the nutrient intakes of various populations or to evaluate compliance with dietary recommendations, estimates of the absolute energy and macronutrient intakes may be required. In such instances, records or 24-hour recalls are generally the methods of choice (Willett, 1998).

2.4 Dietary data in Europe: national surveys

A number of European countries have carried out national dietary surveys. Table 2.1 summarises basic information on the various IDSs that have been undertaken in 20 European countries during the last 20 years.

The surveys are often designed to document the dietary patterns of the general population or segments of it and possibly to identify groups at nutritional risk. In other instances, the primary aim is to address country-specific objectives. The selection of the dietary survey method depends on a number of different factors and investigators may frequently have to compromise according to the specific objectives of the survey and the inherent cost of setting it up.

When the option of running international comparisons using these data is raised, a number of methodological constraints emerge. It can directly be noted that a variety of dietary assessment methods are used, making it difficult to accomplish comparability at the international level (Friedenreich, 1994). The differences in the data collection methodology are reflected in the type and accuracy of the data collected. Some dietary surveys, usually those conducted with food frequency questionnaires, collect data on the intake of particular foods,

Table 2.1 Specially designed dietary surveys undertaken in the general population of 20 European countries during the last 20 years.

Country	Name of the survey	Years of data collection	Sample size (number of individuals)	Survey Population Gender	Age (yrs)	Dietary assessment method
Austria	Austrian Study on Nutritional Status (ASNS)	1991–1994 1993–1997	2 173 2 065	F + M F + M	6–18 19–65	7 day record 24 hour recall, diet history
Belgium	Belgian Interuniversity Research on Nutrition and Health (BIRNH)	1995, 1998 1980–1985	78 10971	F + M F + M	Elderly 25–74	7 day record 1 day record
Croatia	Croatian Study on Schoolchildren's Nutrition	1997–1998	348	F + M	12–14	24 hour recall and food frequency questionnaire
Denmark	Dietary Habits in Denmark National Dietary Survey National Continuous Dietary Survey	1985 1995 2000–2002	2 242 3 098 1 500 (2000)	F + M F + M F + M	15–80 1–80 4–75	diet history 7 day record 7 day record
Finland	Dietary Survey of Finnish Adults (FINDIET)	1992 1997	1861 2862 290	F + M F + M F + M	25–64 25–64 65–74	3 day record 24 hour recall
France	National Food Consumption Survey (ASPCC) Individual National Food Consumption Surveys (INCA)	1985–1995 1993–1994 1993–1994 1998–1999	1778 1229 1500 1018 1985	F + M F + M F + M F + M F + M	18–62 18+ 2–85 3–14 15+	diet history 7 day record 7 day record 7 day record

Country	Survey	Year	N	Sex	Age	Method
Germany	National Nutrition Survey in former West Germany	1985–1989	24632	F + M	4–70+	7 day record
	National Health Survey in former East Germany	1991–1992	1897	F + M	18–79	diet history
	German Nutrition Survey	1998	4030	F + M	18–79	diet history
Hungary	First Hungarian Representative Nutrition Survey	1985–1988	16641	F + M	15–60+	Two 24 hour recalls and food frequency questionnaire
	Hungarian Randomised Nutrition Survey	1992–1994	2559	F + M	18–60+	Three 24 hour recalls and food frequency questionnaire
Iceland	Icelandic National Nutrition Survey	1990	1240	F + M	15–80	diet history
Ireland	Irish National Nutrition Survey	1990	1214	F + M	8–18+	diet history
	North-South Food Consumption Survey	1998	1379	F + M	18–64	7 day record
Italy	INN-CA	1994–1996	3600	F + M	0–94	7 day record
Lithuania	Baltic Nutrition and Health Survey	1997	2183	F + M	20–65	24 hour recall and food frequency questionnaire
Netherlands	Dutch National Food Consumption Survey	1987–1988	5898	F + M	1–79	2 day record
		1992	6218	F + M	1–92	2 day record
		1997–1998	6250	F + M	1–97	2 day record
Norway	National Dietary Survey among Adults (NORKOST)	1993–1994	3144	F + M	16–79	food frequency questionnaire
		1997	2672	F + M	16–79	food frequency questionnaire
	National Dietary Survey	1993	1705	F + M	13	food frequency questionnaire
			1564		18	food frequency questionnaire
		1999	2400	F + M	6 and 12 months	food frequency questionnaire
		1999	2010	F + M	2	food frequency questionnaire

Table 2.1 Continued

Country	Name of the survey	Years of data collection	Sample size (number of individuals)	Survey Population Gender	Survey Population Age (yrs)	Dietary assessment method
Poland	Dietary Habits and Nutritional Status of selected populations	1991–1994	1126 2193 4945	F + M	11–14 18 20–65	24 hour recall
Portugal	National Dietary Survey	1980	13080	F + M	1–65+	24 hour record
Slovak Republic	Assessment of food habits and nutritional status	1991–1999	3337 4556 4807	F + M	11–14 15–18 19–88	24 hour recall and food frequency questionnaire
Sweden	HULK	1989	2036	F + M	1–74	7 day record
	Riksmaten	1997–1998	1215	F + M	18–74	7 day record
Switzerland	Swiss Health Survey	1992–1993	26000	F + M	15–74	food frequency questionnaire
United Kingdom	The Dietary and Nutritional Survey of British Adults (NDNS)	1986–1987	2197	F + M	16–64	7 day record
	National Diet and Nutrition Survey: Children aged 1½–4½ yrs	1992–1993	1675	F + M	1½–4½	4 day record
	National Diet and Nutrition Survey: people aged 65 yrs and over	1994–1995	1687	F + M	65+	4 day record
	National Diet and Nutrition Survey: young people aged 4–18 yrs	1997	1701	F + M	4–18	7 day record

Adapted from Verger et al, 2002.

selected for their relevance to the objectives of the survey. Therefore, the results' efficacy for calculating the energy and nutrient intake is limited. Methods such as 24-hour recalls and food records, on the other hand, do not necessarily reflect habitual intake. In highly demanding surveys, such as those requiring weighed diaries of multiple days, a significant proportion of subjects may drop out, introducing bias in the sample.

The representativeness of the survey population, the potential of the data (e.g. suitability for energy and nutrient calculations), the elements that may affect the reliability of the collected data and the accuracy of the results (e.g. participation rate), are all factors affecting the suitability of a dietary survey to be used for international comparisons (Haraldsdóttir, 1991). The error possibly introduced by the application of various food composition databases for estimating nutrient intakes should also be considered. The documented lack of compatibility of food composition data from various countries (Deharveng et al, 1999) may compromise the validity of the observed relationships.

It is generally acknowledged that dietary intake cannot be estimated without error and each method has its strengths and weaknesses. The knowledge of the method's limitations and of the nature and the magnitude of the errors will lead to a more scientific and sensible interpretation of the results. Although dietary surveys differ widely in the accuracy of their estimates of quantities of food eaten, these differences are usually not listed when the results are presented. These differences are seldom obvious and must be borne in mind when various surveys are compared.

The often prohibitive cost of special dietary surveys may limit the European coverage of data collection. Being expensive and labour intensive, such surveys are regularly undertaken only in a limited number of countries, usually those with robust economies and years of experience in the field. In the modern world of rapid changes, however, nutrition surveillance and intervention programmes should make use of dietary surveys that have built-in mechanisms of continuity over time and extensive coverage.

2.5   Dietary data in Europe: European surveys

In Europe, there is a need for sources of dietary data that would provide a regular and comparable flow of information. A limited number of studies on documenting and monitoring the dietary intake in Europe have been conducted. The EPIC and SENECA projects are examples of studies that developed procedures to allow the collection of harmonised data across countries. DAFNE is an example of a European project that aimed at achieving post-harmonisation of data already collected.

2.5.1   The DAta Food NEtworking (DAFNE) initiative

The DAFNE initiative aims at exploiting the HBS-derived data for nutritional purposes and developing a cost-effective food databank, based on data collected in the European HBSs. The project has been successful in developing the methodology for harmonising food, demographic and socio-economic data collected in the HBSs of fourteen European countries (Belgium, Croatia, France, Germany, Greece, Hungary, Italy, Luxembourg, Norway, Poland, Portugal, the Republic of Ireland, Spain and the United Kingdom). The project is coordinated by the Department of Hygiene and Epidemiology of the Medical School, University of Athens, Greece.

The initial objective of the DAFNE project was the creation of comparable categories of food and socio-demographic information, allowing intra- and inter-country comparisons of nutritional habits and the identification of socio-demographic variables affecting them. Although several socio-demographic characteristics are recorded in the HBSs and many of them are included in the final roster of variables to be studied, the DAFNE team is currently focusing on locality (degree of urbanisation of the area where the household was situated), education and occupation of household head, as well as on household composition. These variables are used for the characterisation of the socio-demographic status of the household.

The development of a food classification system that would allow international comparisons of dietary patterns was a central element in the development of an HBS-based European food databank One of the intermediate results of the harmonisation procedure is the development of the DAFNE food classification system, which allows the categorisation of HBS-collected food data into 56 detailed subgroups. These subgroups can be aggregated at various levels ending up at 15 main food groups (Lagiou et al, 2001). The feasibility studies undertaken in the context of the DAFNE project demonstrated that the prospect of using HBSs for the assessment of dietary information is realistic and the potential considerable, assuming political will, administrative support and a minimal adjustment in infrastructure (Trichopoulou and Lagiou, 1997b, 1998).

In order to evaluate the nutritional information available in the DAFNE databank, a comparison of individualised HBS data with food consumption values derived from specially designed IDSs has recently been undertaken (Naska et al, 2001a, 2001b; Vasdekis et al, 2001). Preliminary results of this analysis show that there is considerable scope in using the DAFNE databank to achieve an average estimate of the populations' food habits, to run international comparisons and to complement with regular information the data collected in the specially designed individual dietary surveys.

2.5.2 The European Prospective Investigation into Cancer and Nutrition (the EPIC study)

The EPIC is a multi-centre prospective cohort study with the aim of investigating the complex relation between nutrition and other lifestyle and environmental factors in relation to the incidence of and mortality from cancer and other diseases (Riboli, 1992). The study is being undertaken in ten European countries (Denmark, France, Germany, Greece, Italy, the Netherlands, Norway, Spain,

Sweden and the United Kingdom) and is co-ordinated by the International Agency for Research on Cancer (IARC) in Lyon, France.

EPIC was initiated in 1990 with pilot and methodological studies to test the validity and feasibility of drawing, determining representative portions and storing biological samples, of taking anthropometric measurements and of collecting data through different types of questionnaires and from variable European populations (Riboli and Kaaks, 1997). Upon the finalisation and the standardisation of the study protocol, the fieldwork was undertaken from 1993 to 1998 and more than 480 000 subjects were included in the cohort.

Eligible subjects were generally drawn from the general population, residing in a given geographical area. In some countries different sampling frames were used in order to ensure a good participation rate and complete follow-up; this did not seriously violate the sampling scheme of a cohort study. According to the study protocol, men over 40 years and women over 35 years of age were recruited. The lower age limit for women was selected to ensure a sufficient number of subjects for investigating risk factors for premenopausal cancers. The upper age limit of the cohort is less precisely defined and varies between 60 and 74 years, depending on the study centre.

Standardised protocols have been developed to collect data on the subjects' medical history, current medication, several lifestyle factors, anthropometry, diet and collection of blood samples. Sections of optional questions were added in some cases to address country-specific objectives. The questionnaire on physical activity was the same in the majority of the countries. A standard common protocol was used for the anthropometric measurements, allowing for tests of within- and between-observer variability.

For the dietary assessment, study subjects were requested to complete a centre-specific dietary questionnaire on their habitual food habits. In most countries a semi-quantitative, interviewer- or self-administered food frequency questionnaire was used. Preliminary analyses of the data colleted through the baseline questionnaire were undertaken in the coordinating center and included the estimation of the energy and selected nutrient intake and the daily consumption of major food groups.

Additionally, a random sample from each cohort selected on the basis of the number and age-gender distribution of expected cancer cases was interviewed by trained interviewers using a computerised software programme (the EPIC-SOFT) specially designed to collect standardised 24-hour recalls of foods consumed during the preceding day (Slimani et al, 1999).

In the field of collecting dietary data at a European level, the EPIC project contributed by developing methods for collecting comparable individual dietary intake data in culturally diverse populations. Although EPIC was not primarily aiming at documenting dietary patterns in Europe, the central database includes information on the habitual (using the food frequency method) and the sporadic (using one 24-hour recall) diet of more than 480 000 Europeans with heterogeneous dietary habits, covering the diet of Mediterranean regions, the central European food patterns and the dietary habits of the Nordic populations.

2.5.3 MONItor trends in CArdiovascular diseases (the WHO-MONICA study)

The WHO-MONICA (The WHO MONICA Project, 1989; Tunstall-Pedoe et al, 2000) is a collaborative project designed to study the relationship between trends:

1. In the main cardiovascular risk factors and CVD morbidity and mortality.
2. In the acute medical care for CHD and the lethality of the disease.
3. In the incidence of CHD and stroke.

To address the above research questions, data were collected in thirty nine centres in twenty six countries of four continents. Although the MONICA study was not solely undertaken in Europe, the majority of the MONICA populations were Europeans. Two types of databases were set up in each population, within a time period of ten years:

- One, including cross-sectional data on the prevalence of cardiovascular risk factors in the general adult population, aged 35–64 years. The data collection was undertaken at least twice (one at the beginning and one at the end of the period) and preferably three times within the ten-year period.
- The second, including longitudinal data on the incidence of CVD through a continuous registration of fatal and non-fatal coronary and/or stroke events.

The project started in the early 1980s and was concluded in the mid-1990s. The most essential criteria and procedures for recruitment and the standardisation of measurements, fieldwork, quality control and data storage are thoroughly described in the MONICA Manual (The WHO-MONICA Project, 1989–1999). A number of quality assessment reports and MONICA-related publications are available at the MONICA website (*www.ktl.fi/monica*).

The fieldwork for the core study included standardised questionnaires, anthropometric and biological measurements and study of medical records. Quality assurance in MONICA was based on several procedures described in the MONICA Manual, such as international training sessions, continuous internal and external quality control procedures, regular communication with the quality control and reference centres, and the elaboration and publication of several retrospective quality assessment reports. The core data were centralised in the MONICA Data Centre in Helsinki, Finland.

2.5.4 Nutrition and the elderly in Europe – the Euronut-SENECA study

In 1986 the Management Group of the Concerted Action on Nutrition and Health in the European Community (Euronut), decided to embark on a study of nutrition in the elderly. An international longitudinal study was thus initiated to study the effective use of food and food resources to enhance the quality of life in older persons, both in social and biological terms (de Groot et al, 1991). The first phase of the study was carried out in 19 centres of 12 European countries in 1988 and 1989. The follow-up study took place in 1993 in 9 out of the 19 centres. The first part was a cross-sectional study aiming at exploring the dietary patterns of elderly populations living in different European communities and at running international comparisons. The follow-up study provided the opportunity to analyse the effect of ageing and the relation of nutrition and health parameters with age.

Approximately 2600 individuals born between 1913 and 1918 were studied using strictly standardised methodology. The basic protocol was standardised and common to all participating groups. Data were collected on the dietary intake of the subjects, on their nutritional status (by collecting and analysing blood samples), on their anthropometric characteristics, physical activity, life-style, health and performance.

Food consumption data were collected during a personal interview, using a modified version of the dietary history method consisting of two parts: first, an estimated 3-day record including two weekdays and one weekend day, and secondly a checklist of foods. The food record was collected to assist the interviewer in having an idea of the subjects' eating pattern. In order to assess the habitual pattern of intake, subjects were questioned about their usual intake using the preceding month as the reference period. Portion sizes were recorded either by weighing, or were based on standardised household measures. Food consumption data were converted into energy and nutrients by using country-specific food composition tables (Euronut SENECA investigators, 1991).

2.5.5 International studies to address specific objectives

Apart from the four international projects described above, there are numerous other studies with European coverage, designed to address specific, nutrition-related research questions. Although some dietary information is recorded in these surveys, the data collected cannot be informative on the dietary patterns of the populations. Two European studies, with specific nutrition-related objectives, are indicatively presented below.

The calcium intake and peak bone mass (CALEUR) study is a European multi-centre study undertaken from 1994 to 1997 in six European countries (Denmark, Finland, France, Italy, the Netherlands and Poland) and coordinated by the TNO-Nutrition and Food Research Institute (Zeist, the Netherlands). CALEUR was a cross-sectional study aiming at evaluating the association between the dietary calcium intake and the radial bone density in two age groups: adolescent girls aged 11–15 years and young women of 20–23 years of age (Kardinaal et al, 1999).

Another international study with specific objectives was the TRANSFAIR study, also coordinated by the TNO-Nutrition and Food Research Institute in the Netherlands. The TRANSFAIR study aimed at determining the *trans*-fatty acid content of 1299 food samples in fourteen European countries (Belgium, Denmark, Finland, France, Germany, Greece, Iceland, Italy, the Netherlands, Norway, Portugal, Spain, Sweden and the United Kingdom) (Van Poppel et al, 1998), at calculating the *trans*-fatty acid intake of the fourteen European populations, using data from representative food consumption surveys (Hulshof et al, 1999) and at studying in a cross-sectional design the relationship of

2.6 Dietary patterns in Europe

During the second half of the twentieth century, there have been significant changes in the foods Europeans choose to eat, their eating occasions and how much they spend on food. The development of new production methods in the crop and livestock sectors of agriculture and the advancement of food science have significantly increased the quantity and variety of food available. Progress in food technology has facilitated the production of foods preserved in new ways and the formulation of entirely new or fundamentally modified products. The rising number of meals eaten outside the home; the shift away from traditional dishes prepared from raw ingredients; the tendency towards the consumption of products, which are considered to be 'healthy'; and the interest in new, foreign foods are the results of alterations in the Europeans' perceptions and lifestyle.

Data from the FBSs show that over the last few decades, European eating patterns have been quite labile and subject to various changes. Bearing in mind the caveats of using FBSs for nutritional purposes, data for the 15 member states of the European Union (Fig. 2.1) show a constant increase in the meat supply from 185 g/person/day in 1970 to 236/g/p/d in the late 1990s. Cereal availability has been generally static. The trend for the supply of vegetables is unclear, as no

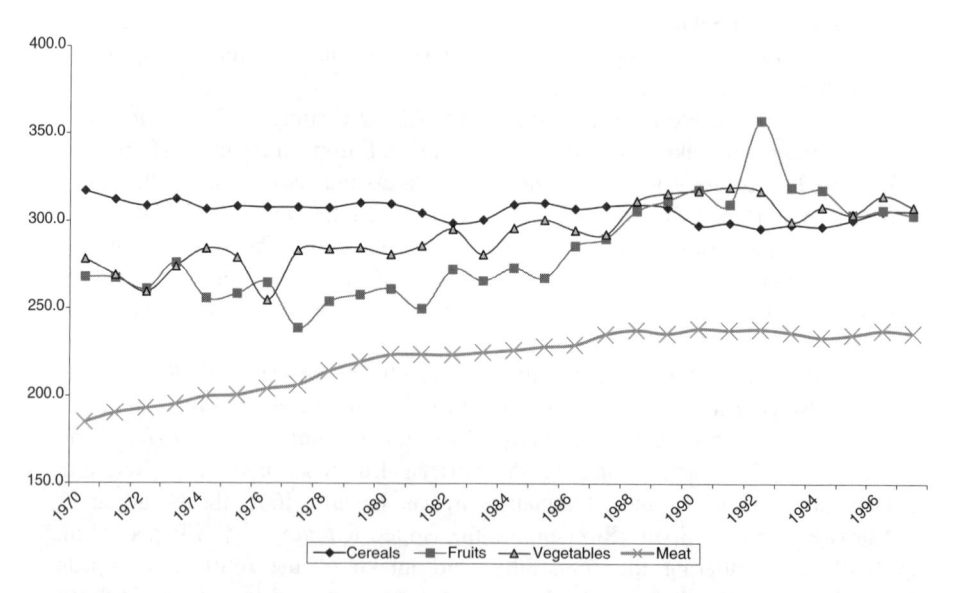

Fig. 2.1 Supply (g/person/day) of 4 food groups (cereals, meat, fruits and vegetables) in the 15 EU member states. Data from the 1970–1997 Food Balance Sheets. (www.fao.org)

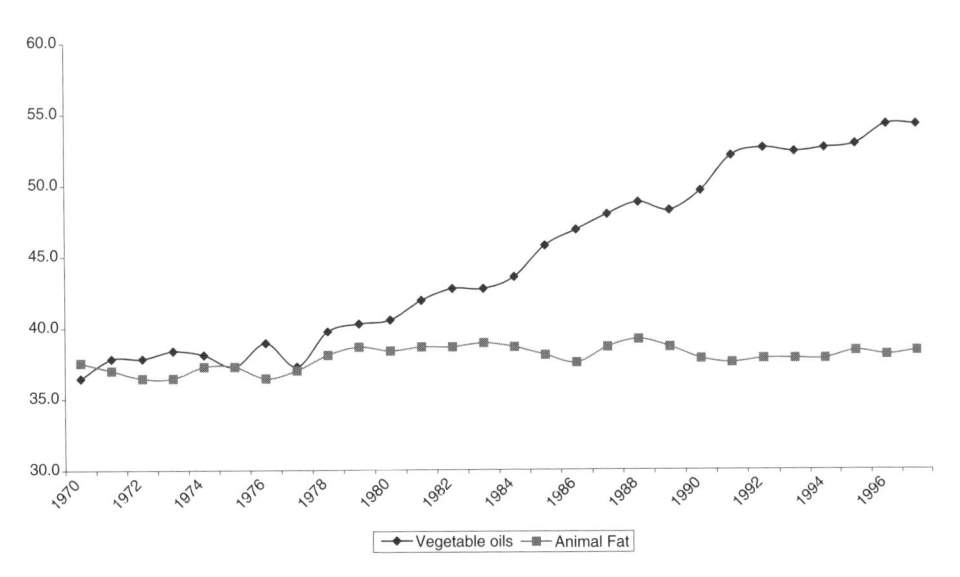

Fig. 2.2 Supply (g/person/day) of vegetable oils and animal fat in the 15 EU member states. Data from the 1970–1997 Food Balance Sheets. (www.fao.org)

Total added lipids (g/prs/day)

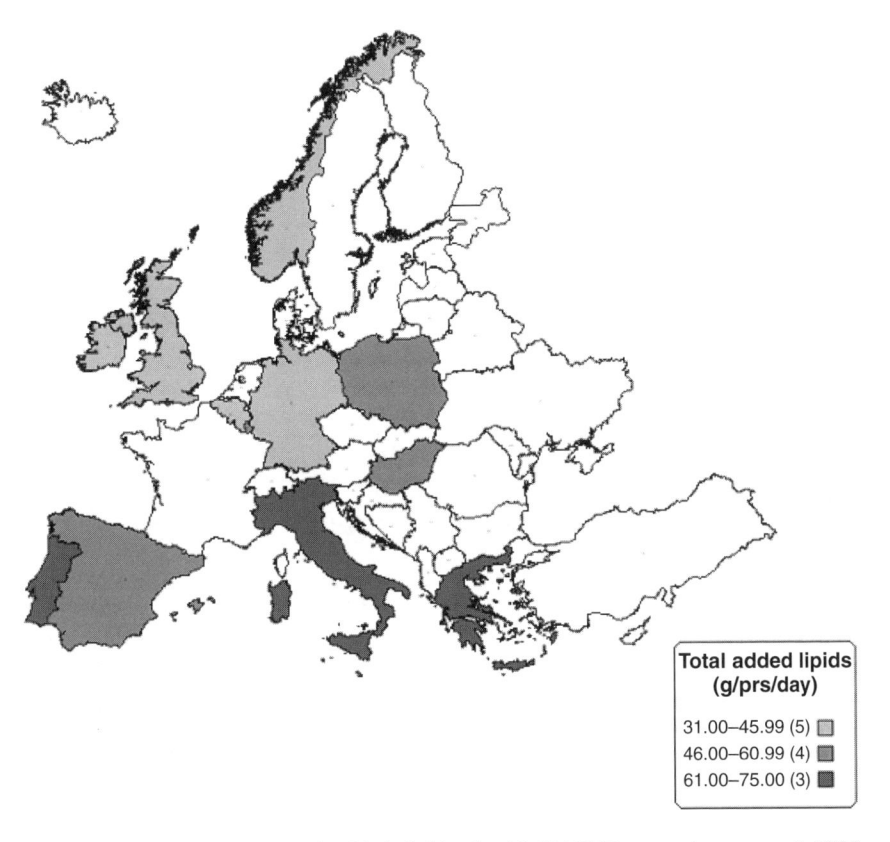

31.00–45.99 (5)
46.00–60.99 (4)
61.00–75.00 (3)

Fig. 2.3 Availability of total added lipids, in 12 DAFNE countries, around 1990 (g/person/day). (Trichopoulou, 2001)

24   The nutrition handbook for food processors

constant pattern can be identified. Fruit supply, on the other hand, is continuously increasing in the 15 member states since 1978, probably reflecting the documented consumers' preference to increase their fruit rather than vegetable intake, as well as the availability of fruit regardless of season (Naska et al, 2000).

The availability of vegetable oils has always been higher than that of animal fat (Fig. 2.2). It is worth noting, however, that in the 1970s, the supply of both vegetable oils and animal fats was estimated to be approximately 37 g/p/d, but since 1978 a remarkable increase in the vegetable oil availability started, which was not followed by a similar trend in the availability of animal fat.

Between countries data clearly show that the European region is characterised by a divergence in eating behaviours. Results from the DAFNE databank collected around 1990 in 12 European countries reveal considerable variations in food availability of different European populations (Trichopoulou, 2001).

Total added lipids (Fig. 2.3) cover both oils, generally of vegetable origin, and solid or semi-solid fat, either from animal sources, or following industrial processing mainly of vegetable oils (margarine). Total added lipid availability varies between 75 g/p/d in Italy to 32 g/p/d in the UK. When the type of lipid is exam-

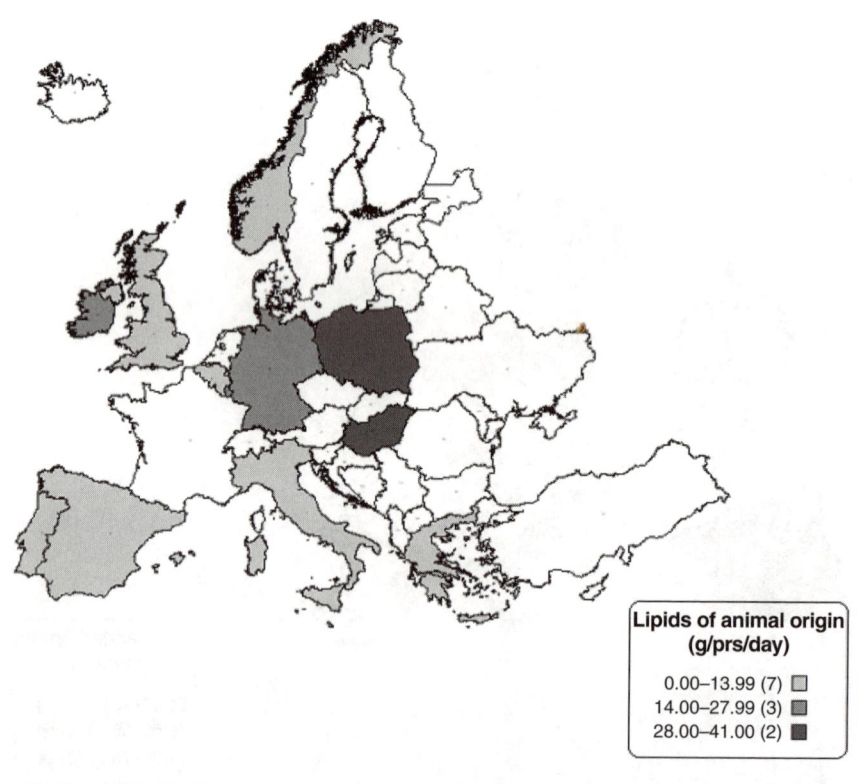

Fig. 2.4   Availability of added lipids of animal origin, in 12 DAFNE countries, around 1990 (g/person/day). (Trichopoulou, 2001)

ined, however, butter and animal fat (Fig. 2.4) account for less than 10% of the total added lipid availability in the Mediterranean countries, while they exceed 30% in the majority of northern and central European countries. Margarine is gradually becoming the lipid of preference in northern Europe, with its availability rising as high as 75% of total added lipids in Norway. In the Mediterranean countries, vegetable oils (Fig. 2.5) represent the lipid of preference; 62% of the vegetable oil availability in Italy and 83% in Greece is olive oil.

The north-south dietary pattern may also be noted when the availability of fresh vegetables (Fig. 2.6) and fruits (Fig. 2.7) is estimated. Two Mediterranean countries, Greece and Spain, lead in the availability of vegetable and fruit availability respectively. The proportion of fresh vegetables consumed varies between countries, from 58% in Germany to 97% in Portugal. Again, fruit is mainly consumed fresh in the Mediterranean countries. In Ireland, availability of fruit barely exceeds 100 g/p/d; 79% of the total fruit is purchased fresh.

Figure 2.8 presents the meat (red meat, poultry and meat products) availability by the educational status of the household head. The mean daily availability has been estimated to exceed 180 g/p/d in Hungary, Poland and Luxembourg and

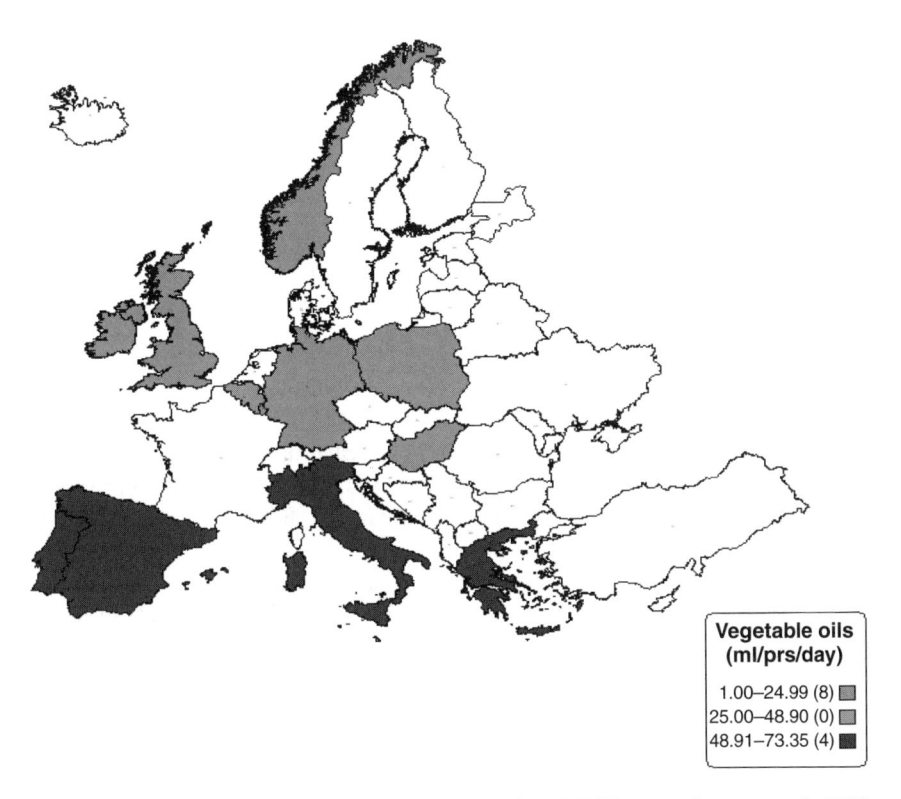

Fig. 2.5 Availability of vegetable oils, in 12 DAFNE countries, around 1990 (ml/person/day). (Trichopoulou, 2001)

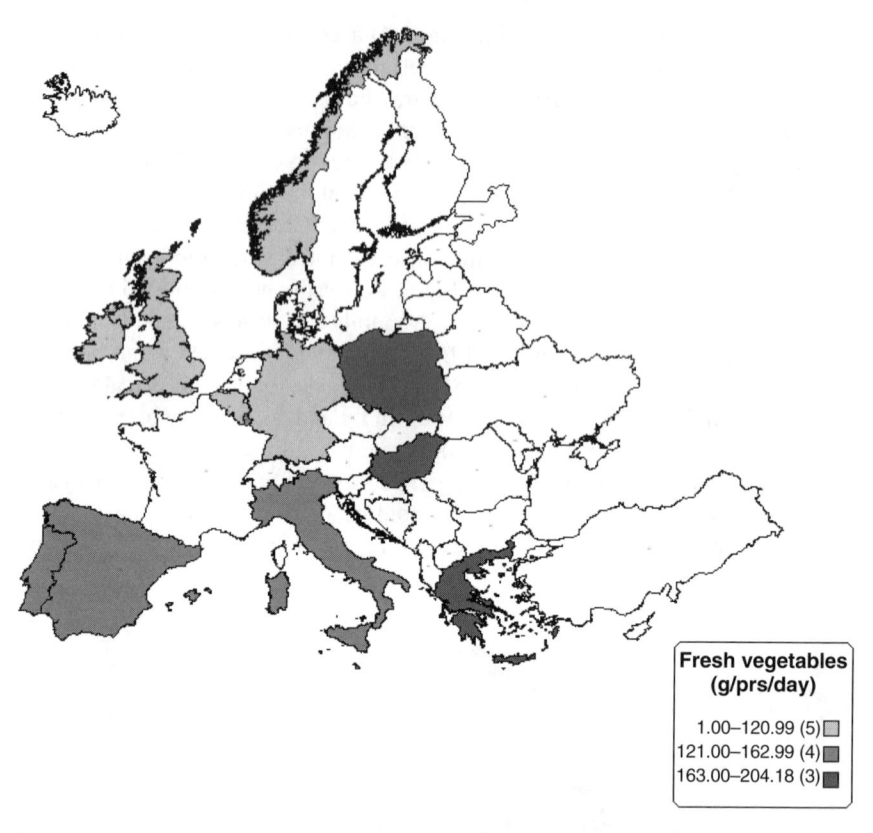

Fig. 2.6 Availability of fresh vegetables, in 12 DAFNE countries, around 1990 (g/person/day). (Trichopoulou, 2001)

it is around 130 g/p/d in Norway, Portugal and Greece. Data presented in Fig. 2.8 further reveals a tendency for lower consumption among the more educated households. It is further worth noting that the Mediterranean countries have become important meat consumers which is not what they were in the past. The availability of different meat types varies among the participating countries. For example, while Greeks seem to prefer beef, Spaniards show a preference towards poultry and processed meat.

Interesting patterns are also revealed when food availability is studied according to the degree of urbanisation of the permanent residence (household locality). A general trend is noticed: the availability of added lipids decreases as one moves from the rural to the urban areas (the DafneSoft, *www.nut.uoa.gr*). This is also true for the availability of vegetable oils. Norway is an exception; here vegetable oil availability increases in the urban areas, whereas the opposite is true for total added lipids. This pattern could be interpreted in terms of easier access to information on health issues and current nutrition advice among urban populations; People living in the urban areas have a lower overall consumption of lipids, and a higher consumption of vegetable oils.

Fresh Fruits (g/prs/day)

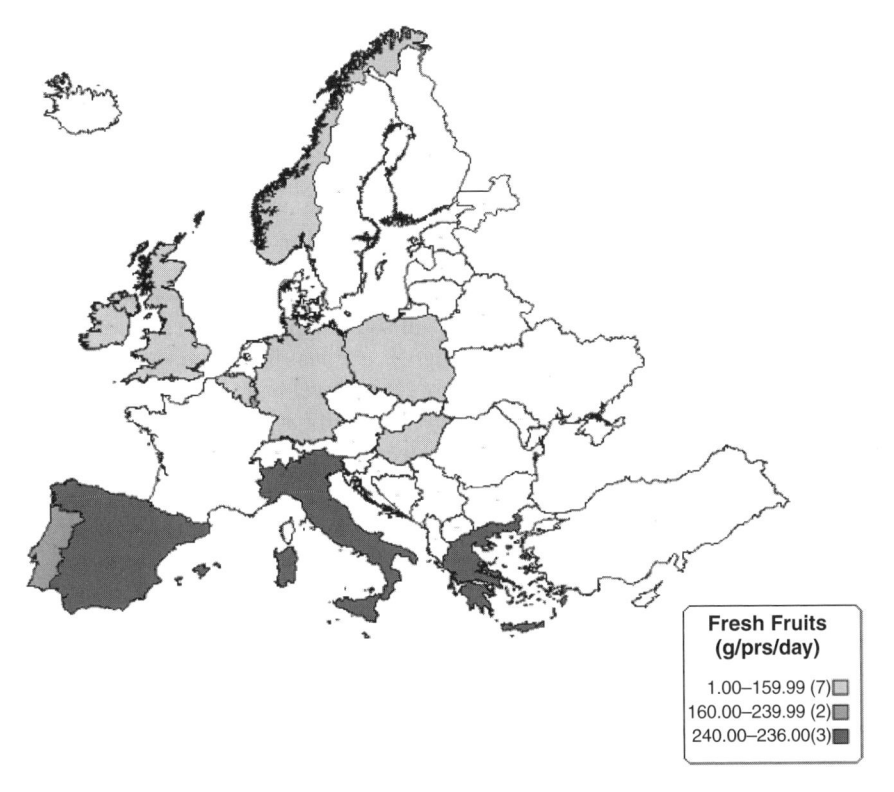

1.00–159.99 (7)
160.00–239.99 (2)
240.00–236.00(3)

Fig. 2.7 Availability of fresh fruits, in 12 DAFNE countries, around 1990 (g/person/day). (Trichopoulou, 2001)

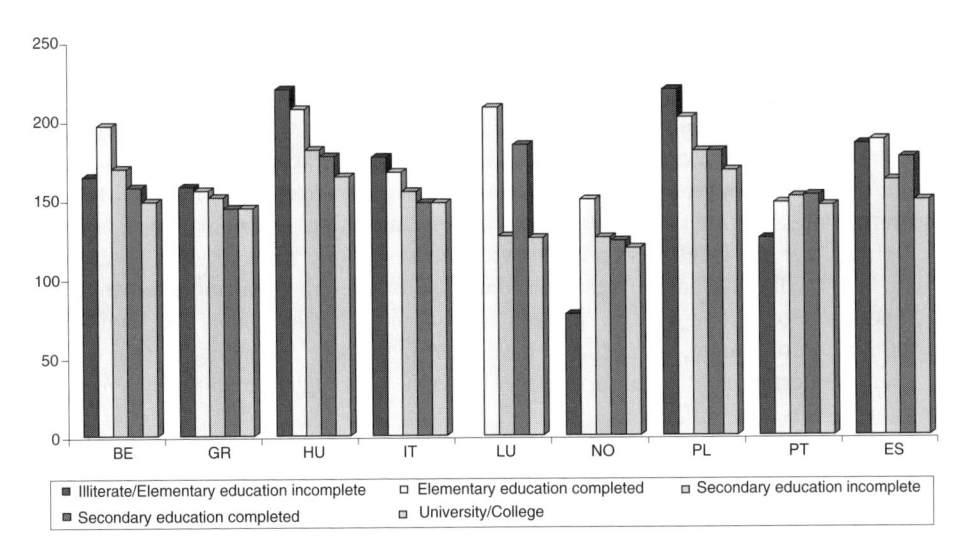

Fig. 2.8 Average availability of meat (red meat, poultry and meat products) by educational level of household head, around 1990 (g/person/day). (Trichopoulou, 2001)

(BE = Belgium; GR = Greece; HU = Hungary; IT = Italy; LU = Luxembourg; NO = Norway; PL = Poland; PT = Portugal; ES = Spain)

Data collected in the context of national surveys presented in Table 2.1 have been included in numerous reports and scientific papers, readily accessible in the international literature. Information on food consumption patterns of selected European populations can also be retrieved from publications referring to country-specific cohorts of the EPIC study (Kesse et al, 2001; Schulze et al, 2001; Fraser et al, 2000; Agudo and Pera, 1999). The large volume of nutritional data collected in EPIC is now being analysed and results on the dietary pattern of the EPIC cohort of ten European countries will soon be published. Furthermore, to overcome possible inconsistencies among the national food composition tables, the EPIC investigators are now in the process of developing standardised tables, which will serve for harmonised estimations of nutrient intake.

Information on the dietary patterns of selected European populations may also be retrieved from publications of the Euronut-SENECA study on the nutrition of an elderly population. Examination of the SENECA data reveals considerable variability in dietary intake within and between countries (De Groot et al, 1992). The SENECA data further pinpoints groups of elderly with inappropriate meal frequency, persons not having regular cooked meals, persons eating alone and those with food-budgeting problems (de Groot and van Staveren, 2000).

2.7 Future trends

The majority of sources of dietary data clearly suggest that there remains considerable room for improvement in the Europeans' diet. As we enter a new millennium weighted with much information, priorities could be set to clarify the objectives of a prudent diet. Are they to prolong life as much as possible, or to maximise quality-adjusted life expectancy? We must also consider externalities that should take into account our cultural heritage, protection of the environment and macroeconomic considerations.

The factors influencing consumer choice are many and varied. It is thus naïve to assume that in order to promote healthy eating it is sufficient to tell consumers what constitutes a healthy diet. An effective strategy to improve nutritional health must address a wide range of conceptions, misconceptions and perceptions, concerning diet and its effects on health and disease.

The Mediterranean diet has been identified as 'the most realistic alternative, open to people long-used to Western type of diet' (Trichopoulou and Lagiou, 1997a). Furthermore, four studies have been published, evaluating the role of the Mediterranean diet, as operationally defined through the following eight components:

- high monounsaturated-to-saturated lipid ratio (mainly olive oil),
- moderate ethanol consumption,
- high consumption of legumes,
- high consumption of cereals (including bread),
- high consumption of fruits,
- high consumption of vegetables,

- low consumption of meat and meat products,
- moderate consumption of milk and dairy products.

The first of these studies was conducted in Greece (Trichopoulou et al, 1995), the second in Denmark (Osler and Schroll, 1997), the third in Australia (Kouris-Blazos et al, 1999) and the fourth in Spain (Lasheras et al, 2000). All have shown that the Mediterranean diet has beneficial, substantial and statistically significant effects on longevity.

2.8 Sources of further information and advice

Data on dietary patterns of European citizens can be retrieved from:

1. The World Health Organisation, Regional Office for Europe, available at *www.who.dk*
2. WHO Regional Office for Europe. Program for Nutrition and Food Security (2001). Urban and peri-urban food and nutrition action plan. Elements for community action to promote social cohesion and reduce inequalities through local production and local consumption.
3. The Food and Agriculture Organisation, available at *www.fao.org*
4. The DAFNE Software Program (DafneSoft v1.0), which can be freely downloaded at *www.nut.uoa.gr*
5. *Dietary Patterns in Europe in 10 Countries Participating in the EPIC Study.* Public Health Nutrition Special Issue (to be published in August 2002)

2.9 References

AGUDO A and PERA G (1999), 'Vegetable and fruit consumption associated with anthropometric, dietary and lifestyle factors in Spain. EPIC Group of Spain. European Prospective Investigation into Cancer', *Public Health Nutrition*, Sep, **2**(3), 263–71

BEILIN L J, PUDDEY I B and BURKE V (1999), 'Lifestyle and hypertension', *Am J Hypertens*, **12**, 934–5

BYRD-BREDBENNER C, LAGIOU P and TRICHOPOULOU A (2000), 'A comparison of household food availability in 11 countries', *J Hum Nutr Dietet*, **13**, 197–204

DE GROOT L C, HAUTVAST J G and VAN STAVEREN W A (1992), 'Nutrition and health of elderly people in Europe, the EURONUT-SENECA Study', *Nutr Rev*, Jul, **50**(7), 185–94

DE GROOT L C, VAN STAVEREN W A and HAUTVAST J G (eds) (1991), 'EURONUT-SENECA Nutrition and the elderly in Europe', *Eur J Clin Nutr*, Dec, **45**, Supplement 3

DE GROOT L C and VAN STAVEREN W A (2000), 'SENECA's accomplishments and challenges', *Nutrition*, Jul–Aug, **16**(7–8), 541–3

DEHARVENG G, CHARRONDIERE U R, SLIMANI N, SOUTHGATE D A T and RIBOLI E (1999), 'Comparison of nutrients in the food composition tables available in the nine European countries participating in EPIC', *Eur J Clin Nutr*, **53**, 60–79

Euronut SENECA investigators (1991), 'Design, methods and participation', *Eur J Clin Nutr*, Dec, **45**, Supplement 3, 5–22

FRASER G E, WELCH A, LUBEN R, BINGHAM S A and DAY N E (2000), 'The effect of age, sex, and education on food consumption of a middle-aged English cohort-EPIC in East Anglia', *Prev Med*, Jan, **30**(1), 26–34

FRIEDENREICH C M (1994), 'Methodologic issues for pooling dietary data' *Am J Clin Nutr*, Jan, **59** (1 Suppl), 251–2S

FRIEL S, NELSON M, MCCORMACK K, KELLEHER C and THRISKOS P (2001), 'Methodological issues using Household Budget Survey expenditure data for individual food availability estimation, Irish experience in the DAFNE pan-European project', *Public Health Nutrition*, **4**(5B), 1143–8

GANN P H, MA J, GIOVANNUCCI E, WILLETT W, SACKS F M, HENNEKENS C H and STAMPFER M J (1999), 'Lower prostate cancer risk in men with elevated plasma lycopene levels, results of a prospective analysis', *Cancer Res*, **59**, 1225–30

GAZIANO J M, BURING J E, BRESLOW J L, GOLDHABER S Z, ROSNER B, VANDENBURGH M, WILLETT W and HENNEKENS C H (1993), 'Moderate alcohol intake, increased levels of high density lipoprotein and its subfractions and decreased risk of myocardial infarction', *N Engl J Med*, **329**, 1829–34

GERBER M J, SCALI J D, MICHAUD A, DURand M D, ASTRE C M, DALLONGEVILLE J and ROMON M M (2000), 'Profiles of a healthful diet and its relationship to biomarkers in a population sample from Mediterranean southern France', *J Am Diet Assoc*, **100**(10), 1164–71

GIOVANNUCCI E, STAMPFER M J, COLDITZ G A, HUNTER D J, FUCHS C, ROSNER B A, SPEIZER F E and WILLETT W C (1998), 'Multivitamin use, folate and colon cancer in women in the Nurses' Health Study', *Ann Intern Med*, **129**, 517–24

HARALDSDÓTTIR J (1991), 'Dietary surveys and the use of the results' in WHO Regional Publications, *Food and Health Data, their use in Nutrition Policy-making*, European Series No **34**, Denmark

HELSING E (1995), 'Traditional diets and disease patterns of the Mediterranean, circa 1960', *Am J Clin Nutr*, **61** (6 Suppl), 1329–37S

HENNEKENS C H, BURING J E, MANSON J E, STAMPFER M, ROSNER B, COOK N R, BELANGER C, LAMOTTE F, GAZIANO J M, RIDKER P M, WILLETT W and PETO R (1996), 'Lack of effect of long-term supplementation with beta carotene on the incidence of malignant neoplasms and cardiovascular disease' *N Engl J Med*, **334**, 1145–9

HULSHOF K F, VAN ERP-BAART M A, ANTTOLAINEN M, BECKER W, CHURCH S M, COUET C, HERMANN-KUNZ E, KESTELOOT H, LETH T, MARTINS I, MOREIRAS O, MOSCHANDREAS J, PIZZOFERRATO L, RIMESTAD A H, THORGEIRSDOTTIR H, VAN AMELSVOORT J M, ARO A, KAFATOS A G, LANZMANN-PETITHORY D and VAN POPPEL G (1999), 'Intake of fatty acids in western Europe with emphasis on trans fatty acids, the TRANSFAIR Study' *Eur J Clin Nutr*, Feb, **53**(2), 143–57

KARDINAAL A F M, ANDO S, CHARLES P, CHARZEWSKA J, ROTILY M, VAANANEN K, VAN ERP-BAART A M, HEIKKINEN J, THOMSEN J, MAGGIOLINI M, DELORAINE A, CHABROS E, JUVIN R and SCHAAFSMA G (1999), 'Dietary calcium and bone density in adolescent girls and young women in Europe', *J Bone Miner Res*, **14**, 583–92

KELLY A, BECKER W and HELSING E (1991), 'Food Balance Sheets', in WHO Regional Publications, *Food and Health Data, their use in Nutrition Policy-making*, European Series No **34**, Denmark

KESSE E, CLAVEL-CHAPELON F, SLIMANI N, VAN LIERE M and E3N GROUP (2001), 'Do eating habits differ according to alcohol consumption? Results of a study of the French cohort of the European Prospective Investigation into Cancer and Nutrition (E3N-EPIC)', *Am J Clin Nutr*, Sep, **74**(3), 322–7

KINJO Y, CUI Y, AKIBA S, WATANABE S, YAMAGUCHI N, SOBUE T, MIZUNO S and BERAL V (1998), 'Mortality risks of oesophageal cancer associated with hot tea, alcohol, tobacco and diet in Japan', *J Epidemiol*, **8**, 235–43

KOURIS-BLAZOS A, GNARDELLIS C, WAHLQVIST M L, TRICHOPOULOS D, LUKITO W and TRICHOPOULOU A (1999), 'Are the advantages of the Mediterranean diet transferable to other populations? A cohort study in Melbourne, Australia', *Br J Nutr*, **82**, 57–61

LAGIOU P, TRICHOPOULOU A, HENDERICKX H K, KELLEHER C, LEONHAUSER I U, MOREIRAS O, NELSON M, SCHMITT A, SEKULA W, TRYGG K and ZAJKAS G for the DAFNE I and II projects of the European Commission (1999), 'Household budget survey nutritional data in relation to mortality from coronary heart disease, colorectal cancer and female breast cancer in European countries. Data Food Networking', *Eur J Clin Nutr*, **53**, 328–32

LAGIOU P, TRICHOPOULOU A and the DAFNE contributors (2001), 'The DAFNE initiative, The methodology for assessing dietary patterns across Europe using household budget survey data', *Public Health Nutrition*, **4**(5B), 1135–42

LASHERAS C, FERNANDEZ S and PATTERSON A M (2000), 'Mediterranean diet and age with respect to overall survival in institutionalised, non-smoking elderly people', *Am J Clin Nutr*, **71**, 987–92

MATTSON F H and GRUNDY S M (1985), 'Comparison of effects of dietary saturated, monounsaturated and polyunsaturated fatty acids on plasma lipids and lipoproteins in man', *J Lipid Res*, **26**, 194–202

MENSINK R P and KATAN M B (1987), 'Effect of monounsaturated fatty acids versus complex carbohydrates on high-density lipoproteins in healthy men and women', *Lancet*, Jan, 17, **I**(8525), 122–5

NASKA A, VASDEKIS V G, TRICHOPOULOU A, FRIEL S, LEONHAUSER I U, MOREIRAS O, NELSON M, REMAUT A M, SCHMITT A, SEKULA W, TRYGG K U and ZAJKAS G (2000), 'Fruit and vegetable availability among ten European countries, how does it compare with the 'five-a-day' recommendation? DAFNE I and II projects of the European Commission', *Br J Nutr*, Oct, **84**(4), 549–56

NASKA A, PATERAKIS S, EECKMAN H, REMAUT A M and TRYGG K (2001a), 'Methodology for rendering household budget and individual nutrition surveys comparable, at the level of the dietary information collected', *Public Health Nutrition*, **4**(5B), 1153–8

NASKA A, VASDEKIS V G S and TRICHOPOULOU A (2001b), 'A preliminary assessment of the use of household budget survey data for the prediction of individual food consumption', *Public Health Nutrition*, **4**(5B), 1159–68

OSLER M and SCHROLL M (1997), 'Diet and mortality in a cohort of elderly people in a north European community', *Int J Epidemiol*, **26**, 155–9

RIBOLI E (1992), 'Nutrition and cancer, background and rationale of the European Prospective Investigation into Cancer and Nutrition (EPIC)', *Ann Oncol*, Dec, **3**(10), 783–91

RIBOLI E and KAAKS R (1997), 'The EPIC Project, rationale and study design. European Prospective Investigation into Cancer and Nutrition', *Int J Epidemiol*, **26**, Suppl 1, S6–14

RIMM E B, GIOVANUCCI E L, WILLETT W C, COLDITZ G A, ASCHERIO A and ROSNER B (1991), 'Prospective study of alcohol consumption and risk of coronary disease in men', *Lancet*, **331**, 464–8

ROBINSON K, ARHEART K, REFSUM H, BRATTSTROM L, BOERS G, UELAND P, RUBBA P, PALMA-REIS R, MELEADY R, DALY L, WITTERMAN J and GRAHAM I (1998), 'Low circulating folate and vitamin B_6 concentrations, risk factors for stroke, peripheral vascular disease, and coronary artery disease. European COMAC Group', *Circulation*, **97**, 437–43

SCHULZE M B, HOFFMANN K, KROKE A and BOEING H (2001), 'Dietary patterns and their association with food and nutrient intake in the European Prospective Investigation into Cancer and Nutrition (EPIC)-Potsdam study', *Br J Nutr*, Mar, **85**(3), 363–73

SERRA-MAJEM L (2001), 'Vitamin and mineral intakes in European children. Is food fortification needed?' *Public Health Nutrition*, Feb, **4**(1A), 101–7

SLIMANI N, DEHARVENG G, CHARRONDIERE R U, VAN KAPPEL A L, OCKE M C, WELCH A, LAGIOU A, VAN LIERE M, AGUDO A, PALA V, BRANDSTETTER B, ANDREN C, STRIPP C, VAN STAVEREN W A and RIBOLI E (1999), 'Structure of the standardized computerized 24-h diet recall interview used as reference method in the 22 centers participating in the EPIC project. European Prospective Investigation into Cancer and Nutrition', *Comput Methods Programs Biomed*, Mar, **58**(3), 251–66

Société Française de Santé Publique. Health and Human Nutrition (2000), 'Element for European Action', *Collection Santé et Société No 10*. French Presidency of the European Community

SOUTHGATE D A T (1991), 'Database requirements for calculations from food balance sheet data and household budget surveys' in WHO Regional Publications, *Food and Health data, their use in nutrition policy-making,* European Series No 34, Denmark

STAMPFER M J, HENNEKENS C H, MANSON J E, COLDITZ G A, ROSNER B and WILLETT W C (1993), 'Vitamin E consumption and the risk of coronary disease in women', *N Engl J Med,* **328**, 1444–9

TRICHOPOULOS D, LAGIOU P and TRICHOPOULOU A (2000), 'Evidence-based nutrition', *Asia Pacific J Clin Nutr,* **9** (suppl.), S4–S9

TRICHOPOULOU A (ed.) (1992), 'Methodology and Public Health Aspects of Dietary Surveillance in Europe, The Use of Household Budget Surveys', *Eur J Clin Nutr,* **46**, Supplement 5

TRICHOPOULOU A (1995), 'Olive oil and breast cancer' (editorial), *Cancer Causes and Control,* **6**, 475–6

TRICHOPOULOU A and LAGIOU P (1997a), 'Options for dietary development based on science and reason' in Scientific and Technological Options Assessment (STOA) Report to the European Parliament *Nutrition in Europe, Nutrition Policy and Public Health in the European Union and models for European eating habits on the threshold of the 21st century,* PE Number 166.481. European Union. Luxembourg, Directorate General for Research pp. 39–51

TRICHOPOULOU A and LAGIOU P (eds) (1997b), 'DAFNE I – Methodology for the exploitation of HBS data and results on food availability in 5 European countries' Luxembourg, Office for Official Publications of the European Communities

TRICHOPOULOU A and LAGIOU P (eds) (1998), 'DAFNE II – Methodology for the exploitation of HBS data and results on food availability in 6 European countries' Luxembourg, Office for Official Publications of the European Communities

TRICHOPOULOU A and the DAFNE contributors (2001), 'The DAFNE databank as a simple tool for nutrition policy', *Public Health Nutrition,* **4**(5B), 1187–90

TRICHOPOULOU A, KOURIS-BLAZOS A, VASSILAKOU T, GNARDELLIS C, POLYCHRONOPOULOS E, VENIZELOS M, LAGIOU P, WAHLQVIST M L and TRICHOPOULOS D (1995), 'Diet and survival of elderly Greeks, a link to the past', *Am J Clin Nutr,* **61**, 1346–50S

TRICHOPOULOU A, LAGIOU P, NELSON M, REMAUT-DE WINTER A M, KELLEHER C, LEONHAUSER I U, MOREIRAS O, SCHMITT A, SEKULA W, TRYGG K and ZAJKAS G for the DAFNE I and II projects of the European Commission. (1999), 'Food disparities in 10 European countries, their detection using Household Budget Survey data – The DAta Food NEtworking (DAFNE) initiative', *Nutr Today,* **34**(3), 129–39

TUNSTALL-PEDOE H, VANUZZO D, HOBBS M, MÄHÖNEN M, CEPAITIS Z, KUULASMAA K and KEIL U for the WHO MONICA Project (2000), 'Estimation of contribution of changes in coronary care to improving survival, event rates, and coronary heart disease mortality across the WHO MONICA Project populations', *Lancet,* 355, 688–700

TZONOU A, SIGNORELLO L B, LAGIOU P, WUU J, TRICHOPOULOS D and TRICHOPOULOU A (1999), 'Diet and cancer of the prostate, a case-control study in Greece', *Int J Cancer,* **80**, 704–8

VAN POPPEL G, VAN ERP-BAART M A, LETH T, GEVERS E, VAN AMELSVOORT J, LANZMANN-PETITHORY D, KAFATOS A and ARO A (1998), '*trans*-fatty acids in foods in Europe, the TRANSFAIR study', *J Food Comps Analysis,* **11**, 161–9

VAN STAVEREN W A, VAN BEEM I and HELSING E (1991), 'Household budget surveys' in WHO Regional Publications, *Food and Health Data, their use in Nutrition Policy-making,* European Series No **34**, Denmark

VASDEKIS V G S, STYLIANOU S and NASKA A (2001), 'Estimation of age and gender-specific food availability from household budget survey data', *Public Health Nutrition,* **4**(5B), 1149–52

VERGER P, IRELAND J, MØLLER A, ABRAVICIUS J A, DE HENAUW S and NASKA A (2002) 'Improvement of comparability of dietary intake assessment using currently available individual food consumption surveys', *Eur J Clin Nutr,* **56** (suppl. 2), 518–24

The WHO MONICA Project (1989), 'A worldwide monitoring system for cardiovascular diseases, Cardiovascular mortality and risk factors in selected communities', *World Health Stat*, **A**, 27–149

WILLETT W C (1994), 'Diet and health, what should we eat?' *Science*, **264**, 523–7

WILLETT W C (1998), *Nutritional Epidemiology*, 2nd ed Oxford University Press, New York

WILLETT W C (2000), 'Diet and cancer', *The Oncologist*, **5**, 393–404

WILLETT W C and TRICHOPOULOS D (1996), 'Nutrition and cancer, a summary of the evidence', *Cancer Causes and Control*, **7**, 178–80

World Health Organisation, Regional Office for Europe (1998), *Comparative analysis of nutrition policies in WHO European Member States*, WHO Publications

YOSHIZAWA K, WILLETT W C, MORRIS S J, STAMPFER M J, SPIEGELMAN D, RIMM E B and GIOVANNUCCI E (1998), 'Study of prediagnostic selenium level in toenails and the risk of advanced prostate cancer', *J Natl Cancer Inst*, **90**, 1219–24

3
Vitamins

C. A. Northrop-Clewes and D. I. Thurnham, University of Ulster

3.1 Introduction

Vitamins are classically defined as a group of organic compounds required in very small amounts for the normal development and functioning of the body. They are not synthesised by the body, or only in insufficient amounts, and are mainly obtained through food (Machlin and Huni, 1994).

There are thirteen vitamins: four are fat-soluble, namely vitamins A (retinol), D (calciferols), E (tocopherols) and K (phylloquinone and menaquinones) and nine are water-soluble, vitamin C (ascorbate) and the B-complex made up of vitamins B_1 (thiamin), B_2 (riboflavin), B_6 (pyridoxal, pyridoxamine and pyridoxine), B_{12} (cobalamin), folic acid, biotin, niacin and pantothenic acid. No single food contains all of the vitamins and therefore a balanced and varied diet is necessary for an adequate intake.

3.1.1 Dietary reference values

Prior to 1991 relatively few micro-nutrients were covered in official British government publications on energy, protein, vitamin and mineral requirements (Whitehead, 1991). The 1979 definition of the Recommended Dietary Allowance (RDA) was 'the average amount of the nutrient which should be provided per head in a group of people if the needs of practically all members of the group are to be met.' However, the RDA values have always been derived differently depending on whether energy or nutrients were being considered.

In 1987 the Committee on Medical Aspects of Food Policy (COMA) convened a panel to review the old RDAs of energy, fat, non-starch polysaccharides, sugars, starches, protein, vitamins and minerals for groups of people in the United

Kingdom (Department of Health and Social Security, 1979). The panel changed the 'requirements' nomenclature, and whereas most sets of RDAs provided only a single value for the micronutrients, the new Dietary Reference Values (DRVs) set three levels of values for each age and sex grouping. The aim was to describe the range of requirements in different individuals more adequately. The estimated average requirement (EAR) represents the mean requirement of the average individual, the reference nutrient intake (RNI) is nominally set at the mean plus two standard deviations (2 SD), and the lower reference nutrient intake (LRNI) is nominally the mean minus an estimated 2 SD. The three parameters describe the spread of requirements.

It was thought that the EAR might be increasingly used in food labelling thus providing all dietary constituents in food with a common baseline for comparison but the RNI is the key value for clinical and health purposes. Table 3.1 is the summary table of the RNI for six B vitamins, plus vitamins A, C and D. Within the context of the UK, the reason for considering only 9 out of the 13 vitamins was that the panel thought only those micronutrients for which some possibility of deficiency existed needed to be dealt with in such detail. In addition, there was insufficient information for pantothenic acid, biotin and vitamins E and K to provide a complete data set of recommendations, hence only single safe intake recommendations were considered (Whitehead, 1992).

Table 3.2 gives a summary of the principal food sources and major functions of each vitamin.

3.2 Vitamin A

Vitamin A can be obtained in two forms: pre-formed retinol, usually as retinyl esters, or as provitamin A carotenoids, such as α- and β-carotene and α- and β-cryptoxanthin. In the UK about a quarter to a third of dietary vitamin A is obtained from fruits and vegetables, the majority of this as β-carotene. In many developing countries up to 100% of dietary intake can be from plant sources and in these communities, where exposure to infection is usually high, it is most likely to find vitamin A deficiency disorders (VADD). One of the earliest clinical signs of vitamin A deficiency (VAD) is night blindness (XN), an impaired ability to see in dim light. Severe deficiency produces partial or total blindness. The most vulnerable groups to VADD are infants and young children and pregnant and lactating women.

3.3 Vitamin A deficiency disorders (VADD)

Vitamin A deficiency disorders may be defined as a level of depletion of total body stores of retinol and of its active metabolites such that normal physiologic function is impaired. Dietary intake does not accurately reflect status since intake may fluctuate considerably in different seasons and the body only stores vitamin

Table 3.1 Reference nutrient intakes (RNI) for vitamins

Age	Thiamin mg/d	Riboflavin mg/d	Niacin mg/d	Vitamin B_6 mg/d#	Vitamin B_{12} µg/d	Folate µg/d	Vitamin C mg/d	Vitamin A µg/d	Vitamin D µg/d
0–6 months	0.2	0.4	3.0	0.2	0.3	50	25	350	8.5
7–9 months	0.2	0.4	4.0	0.3	0.4	50	25	350	7
10–12 months	0.3	0.4	5.0	0.4	0.4	50	25	350	7
1–3 years	0.5	0.6	8.0	0.7	0.5	70	30	400	7
4–6 years	0.7	0.8	11	0.9	0.8	100	30	500	–
7–10 years	0.7	1.0	12	1.0	1.0	150	30	500	–
Males									
11–14 years	0.9	1.2	15	1.2	1.2	200	35	600	–
15–18 years	1.1	1.3	18	1.5	1.5	200	40	700	–
19–50 years	1.0	1.3	17	1.4	1.5	200	40	700	–
50 + years	0.9	1.3	16	1.4	1.5	200	40	700	***
Females									
11–14 years	0.7	1.1	12	1.0	1.2	200	35	600	–
15–18 years	0.8	1.1	14	1.2	1.5	200	40	600	–
19–50 years	0.8	1.1	13	1.2	1.5	200	40	600	–
50 + years	0.8	1.1	12	1.2	1.5	200	40	600	***
Pregnancy/Lactation	+0.1*	+0.3	**	**	**	+100	+10	+100	10
0–4 months	+0.2	+0.5	+2	**	+0.5	+60	+30	+350	10
4 + months	+0.2	+0.5	+2	**	+0.5	+60	+30	+350	10

\# Based on protein providing 14.7% of EAR for energy.
* For last trimester only.
** No increment.
*** After age 65 the RNI is 10.0µg/d for men and women.
DEPARTMENT OF HEALTH 1991.

Vitamins 37

Table 3.2 Food sources and major functions of principal vitamins

Vitamin	Principal food sources	Major functions in the body
Vitamin A	Animal sources: liver, egg yolk, fish, whole milk, butter, cheese. Plant sources (as provitamin A): carrots, yellow and dark green leafy vegetables, pumpkin, apricots, melon, red palm oil.	Helps to keep mucosal membranes healthy, thus increasing resistance to infections; essential for vision; promotes bones and tooth development. Vegetable consumption may be protective against certain cancers.
Vitamin D	Fish-liver oils (sardine, herring, salmon, mackerel), eggs, meat, milk.	Promotes hardening of bones and teeth, increases the absorption of calcium.
Vitamin E	Vegetable oils (peanut, soya, palm, corn, sunflower etc). Other sources: nuts, seeds, whole grains, leafy green vegetables.	Protects vitamins A and C and fatty acids; prevents damage to cell membranes. Antioxidant.
Vitamin K	Green leafy vegetables, soybeans, beef liver, green tea, egg yolks, potatoes, oats, asparagus, cheese.	Helps blood to clot. May play a role in bone health.
Vitamin C	Citrus fruits, sweet peppers, parsley, cauliflower, potatoes, strawberries, broccoli, mango, Brussels sprouts.	Formation of collagen, wound healing; maintaining blood vessels, bones, teeth; absorption of iron, calcium, folate; production of brain hormones, immune factors; antioxidant
Thiamin (B_1)	Dried brewers yeast, animal products, whole grains, nuts, pulses, dried legumes.	Helps release energy from foods; promotes normal appetite; important in function of nervous system.
Folate	Main sources: liver, dark green leafy vegetables, beans, wheat germ and yeast. Other sources: egg yolk, beet, orange juice, whole wheat bread.	Aids in protein metabolism; promotes red blood cell formation; prevents birth defects of spine, brain; lowers homocysteine levels and thus coronary heart disease risk.
Cobalamins (B12)	Animal products (particularly liver, kidneys, heart, brain) fish, eggs, dairy products.	Aids in building of genetic material; aids in development of normal red blood cells; maintenance of nervous system.
Vitamin B_6	Chicken, liver of beef, pork, fish (tuna, trout, salmon, herring), peanuts and walnuts, bread, whole-grain cereals.	Aids in protein metabolism, absorption; aids in red blood cell formation; helps body use fats
Biotin	Yeast, liver, kidney, egg yolk, soybeans, nuts and cereals.	Helps release energy from carbohydrates; aids in fat synthesis.
Pantothenic acid	Yeast, liver, heart, brain, kidney, eggs, milk, vegetables, legumes, whole grain cereals.	Involved in energy production; aids in formation of hormones.
Niacin	Yeast, liver, poultry, lean meats, nuts and legumes. Less in milk and green leafy vegetables.	Energy production from foods; aids digestion, promotes normal appetite; promotes healthy skin, nerves.
Riboflavin (B_2)	Yeast, liver, milk and milk products, meat, eggs, and green leafy vegetables.	Helps release energy from foods; promotes healthy skin and mucous membranes; possible role in preventing cataracts.

A when the intake exceeds requirements. Tissue concentrations may be assessed by measuring serum or breast milk retinol, or by using the retinol dose response (RDR), modified retinol dose response (MRDR), or by dilution with stable isotopes. Functional indicators include pupillary dark adaptometry (PDA), conjunctival impression cytology (CIC), and xerophthalmia.

3.4 Bioavailability of provitamin carotenoids

De Pee and West (1996) proposed that control of VADD depends to a large extent on an adequate supply of vitamin A and the vitamin A supply is determined by:

Food intake × (pro)-vitamin A content × bioavailability/bioefficacy, where
Bioavailability = fraction of ingested nutrient available for normal physiological functions and storage (Jackson, 1997)
Bioefficacy = efficiency of absorption and conversion of ingested nutrient to the active form e.g. β-carotene to retinol (van Lieshout et al, 2001).

3.4.1 Relationship between bioefficacy and vitamin A requirements

The RNI for children up to 5 years of age is 400μg retinol equivalents (RE)/day, which can easily be met from the diet if animal foods are available e.g. 1 egg (50g) contains about 100μg RE, 25g chicken liver contains 3000μg RE. Plants also contribute to vitamin A intake e.g. 1 raw carrot (20g) contains 400μg β-carotene, a 70g portion of spinach contains 600μg β-carotene and with a bioefficacy of 100% would supply 400 and 600μg RE respectively. But the pro-vitamin A carotenoids are absorbed less efficiently than retinol, that is, their bioefficacy is less than 100%. Therefore the effective supply of vitamin A from fruits and vegetables is much lower than that from retinol in animal foods (van Lieshout et al, 2001). If 1 mole β-carotene (Fig. 3.1) yields 2 moles retinol then, using 100% bioefficacy, 1μmol (0.537μg) β-carotene would be absorbed and converted totally to 2μmol (0.572μg) retinol, i.e. 0.537/0.572 = 0.94μg β-carotene is equivalent to 1μg retinol. The results of the 'Sheffield' studies carried out by the Medical Research Council (MRC) during the Second World War provided important information to establish the relative equivalency of carotenoids and retinol (Hume and Krebs, 1949). These and other studies suggested that 6μg β-carotene or 12μg of other pro-vitamin A carotenoids in a mixed diet had the same activity as 1μg retinol (FAO/WHO 1967). Therefore, according to FAO/WHO the bioefficacy of β-carotene in food is (100%*0.94)/6 = 16%. But in the 1990s evidence was accumulating that the bioefficacy of provitamin A carotenoids in fruit and vegetables was only 20–30% of the FAO/WHO estimates of 16%. The efficiency with which β-carotene in dark green leafy vegetables (DGLV) is metabolised to vitamin A was re-examined and various bioconversion factors have been put forward:

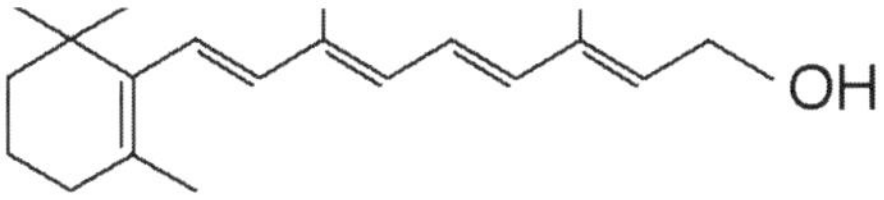

Fig. 3.1 Structures of all-*trans*-retinol and β-carotene.

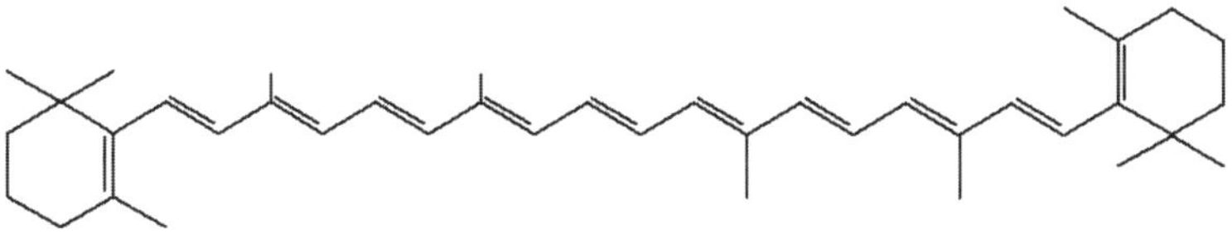

- 4:1 (Gopalan et al, 1989)
- 6:1 (Report of a Joint FAO/WHO expert consultation 1988)
- 12:1 (Report of the Institute of Medicine 2001)
- 21:1 and 26:1 (de Pee et al, 1998; Khan et al, 1998; van het Hof et al, 1999)

Assuming that 100 g DGLV contains 3000 μg β-carotene and a child of 4 years needs an RNI of 400 μg RE/day then using bioconversion factors of 12:1, 21:1 or 26:1, the child would need 160 g, 280 g or 360 g of DGLV each day to meet requirements.

3.4.2 Equivalence factor as calculated by IOM

In January 2001, the US National Academy of Sciences/Institute of Medicine (IOM) announced a new equivalence factor (12:1) for the conversion of β-carotene to retinol. The basis for formulating the equivalency factor was to relate the absorption of β-carotene in a principally mixed vegetable diet to that from oil in healthy and nutritionally-adequate individuals. The recommendations were based on a product of relative absorption of β-carotene in mixed vegetable diet (1:6) (van het Hof et al, 1999) to the amount of retinol formed (1 μg) when 2 μg β-carotene was fed in oil (Sauberlich et al, 1974). In the van het Hof study, the increase in serum β-carotene concentration after consumption of β-carotene-rich vegetables was 1/7 or 14% of the increase after consumption of β-carotene in oil. The Institute of Medicine (IOM) (2001) adjusted the value to 1/6 or 17%, because of the low fruit content in the diet used. From these two studies, the IOM concluded that the bioefficacy of β-carotene in oil was $(100\% * 0.94)/2 = 47\%$ (Sauberlich et al, 1974) and 17% from mixed vegetables (van het Hof et al, 1999). Thus bioefficacy from vegetables in a mixed diet was $17\% * 0.47 = 8\%$, that is 12 μg β-carotene in food has the same vitamin A activity as 1 μg retinol. The

12:1 ratio is referred to as the retinol activity equivalence (RAE) (Northrop-Clewes, 2001a).

In the calculation, the IOM used the mean ratio from only one 'oil study'. There were in fact 5 'oil' studies (Booher et al, 1939; Wagner, 1940; Hume and Krebs, 1949; Sauberlich et al, 1974; Tang et al, 2000) and if the data from all the studies had been used a bioconversion value of 3.5 µg β-carotene to 1 µg retinol would have been calculated giving an RAE of 21 instead of 12 as quoted. The IOM are at present reconsidering the published data (van Lieshout, 2001). How we interpret the bioconversion factors for β-carotene proposed by IOM or by others still needs much more thought before any of them can be put to practical use. However, even if the RAE is only 12:1, there are probably not sufficient vegetables in developing countries to meet that required, therefore, there must be other, as yet undiscovered factors, that influence bioefficacy. Despite this, intake of fruit and vegetable-sources of provitamin A should be encouraged, for although the bioefficacy of β-carotene is apparently so poor, it has to be remembered that the majority of the world's children are not VAD.

3.5 Function

Vitamin A, its analogues and metabolites function in vision, cell differentiation, embryogenesis, the immune response, reproduction and growth.

3.5.1 Vision

In vision, vitamin A is required in two forms for two processes:

1. As 11-*cis*-retinal in rhodopsin which on exposure to light in the retina isomerises to a transoid intermediate, triggering a series of conformational changes in membrane potential which is transmitted to the brain.
2. As retinoic acid to maintain normal differentiation of the cells of the conjunctival membranes, cornea and other ocular structures hence preventing xerophthalmia (Ross, 1999).

3.5.2 Cell differentiation

The role of vitamin A in cell differentiation has been clarified since the identification of two sets of nuclear receptors, RXR and RAR, which are activated by retinoic acid isomers (Olson et al, 2000). Each of the receptors has three distinct forms α, β and γ and six domains involved in transcription of genes. RAR binds either all-*trans* or 9-*cis* retinoic acid, while RXR binds only 9-*cis* retinoic acid. Both receptors are dimers, however, the RXR receptors form homodimers with themselves as well as heterodimers with RAR, the vitamin D receptor, the triiodothyronine receptor and several other nuclear transcription receptors (see also sections 3.12.3, 3.20.2 and 3.21.3). These interactions usually activate gene expression but RAR can also be inhibitory.

3.5.3 Embryogenesis

Both retinoic acid and retinol are essential for embryonic development, however, retinoic acid does not seem to be involved in vertebrate embryogenesis before gastrulation. After gastrulation specific genes of the Hox family are expressed in a wave starting about 7.5 days postcoitus in the mouse. The presence of retinoids together with their binding proteins and receptors in a temporally precise manner provides strong circumstantial evidence that retinoic acid-activated RARs regulate Hox gene expression (Ross, 1999). The Hox family consists of 38 genes arranged in four chromosomal clusters, which code for transcription factors that regulate development along the posterior axis. Retinoic acid is also thought to act in limb development and formation of the heart, eyes and ears. Experimental VAD has demonstrated that major target tissues of retinoic acid include the heart, central nervous system and structures derived from it, the circulatory, urogenital and respiratory systems and the development of skull, skeleton and limbs. Homeostasis of retinoic acid is maintained by enzyme systems, which are developmentally regulated by vitamin A. Inadequate vitamin A nutrition during early pregnancy may account for some paediatric congenital abnormalities (Zile, 2001). However, the study of this aspect of vitamin A is in its 'infancy' and much more work is still to be done. A high incidence of spontaneous abortions and birth defects has been observed in the foetuses of women taking therapeutic doses of 13-*cis* retinoic acid. The drugs Accutane (13-*cis* retinoic acid) and etretinate, an aromatic analogue of all-*trans* retinoic acid have been most implicated in such effects (Armstrong et al, 1994). The dysmorphogenic effects caused by retinoids depend on dosage (exposure), the form of the retinoid, its rate of metabolism and stage of foetal development at the time the retinoid is taken. Retinoids are teratogenic during the period of foetal organogenesis (first trimester) (Ross, 1999).

3.5.4 Immunity

One of the first names for vitamin A was 'the anti-infective vitamin', which was based on the increased number of infections noted in VAD animals and humans (Ross, 1996). In VAD the humoral response to bacterial, parasitic and viral infections, cell-mediated immunity, mucosal immunity, natural killer cell activity and phagocytosis are all impaired. The primary immune response to protein antigens is markedly reduced but the response to bacterial lipopolysaccharides or the process of immunological memory essential for secondary response does not seem to be affected (Ross and Hammerling, 1994).

A major site for vitamin A action in the immune response is the T-helper cell and studies have shown that the activity of T-helper cells variety 1 (Th1) precedes that of Th variety 2 (Th2) and that vitamin A supports Th2 development (Cantorna et al, 1994). Hence, in the presence of VAD the ratio of Th1 : Th2 may become elevated during an immune response. Retinol, probably in the form of 14-hydroxy-retroretinol (HRR), is thought to be involved in the proliferation of normal B- and T-cells, an action which can be modulated by some cytokines. Retinoic acid, the usual active form of vitamin A, appears to be inactive in these systems (Olson et al, 2000). The enzyme responsible for the conversion of retinol to HRR has not been characterised.

3.6 Health-related roles of β-carotene

3.6.1 β-Carotene as an antioxidant

The ability of carotenoids to act as antioxidants can be measured *in vitro*, *ex vivo*, or *in vivo*. LDL isolated from an individual who has been supplemented with carotenoids and then evaluated for its antioxidant activity is an extension of an *in vivo* study, i.e. *ex vivo*. However, when carotenoids are added to plasma and then the oxidisable value of the LDL is measured it is more like an *in vitro* model (Krinsky, 2001). Many studies report using the *ex vivo* method of measuring the oxidisability of the LDL particles after feeding increased amounts of carotene-containing foods. However, when using fruits and vegetables the outcome is variable and difficult to interpret because they also contain vitamin C, polyphenols and flavonoids, which are also potential antioxidants. One study which gave additional dietary fruits and vegetables to subjects reported an increase in the resistance of LDL to oxidation (Hininger et al, 1997) while two other studies found no effect (Chopra et al, 1996; van het Hof et al, 1999). The differing results obtained may be due to different time periods on the diets, different degrees of change in the plasma carotenoids or to different study populations (Krinsky, 2001).

3.6.2 β-Carotene and protection from cancer

The strongest epidemiological evidence suggesting high intake of fruits and vegetables might give protection against lung cancer came from prospective studies in which low plasma β-carotene was associated with a higher incidence of lung cancer. Carotenoid intake was associated with reduced cancer risk in 8 prospective studies and 18 out of 20 retrospective studies (Zeigler et al, 1996). Based on the results of these studies, three major intervention studies investigated the protective effect of β-carotene in the prevention of lung cancer:

(a) The alpha-tocopherol, beta-carotene (ATBC) Cancer Prevention study, was a randomised-controlled trial that tested the effects of daily doses of 50 mg (50 IU) vitamin E (all-racemic α-tocopherol acetate), 20 mg of β-carotene, both or placebo in a population of more than 29 000 male smokers for 5–8 years. No reduction in lung cancer or major coronary events was observed with any of the treatments. What was more startling was the unexpected increases in risk of death from lung cancer and ischemic heart disease with β-carotene supplementation (ATBC Cancer Prevention Study Group, 1994).

(b) Increases in risk of both lung cancer and cardiovascular disease mortality were also observed in the beta-Carotene and Retinol Efficacy Trial (CARET), which tested the effects of combined treatment with 30 mg/d β-carotene and retinyl palmitate (25 000 IU/d) in 18 000 men and women with a history of cigarette smoking or occupational exposure to asbestos (Hennekens et al, 1996).

(c) The third study was the Physicians Health Study, in which 22 071 US male physicians were randomised to get 50 mg β-carotene or aspirin (325 mg), or both or neither every other day for 12 years. There was no evidence of a significant beneficial or harmful effect on cancer or cardiovascular disease, but the number of smokers in the study was too small to be certain whether β-carotene was harmful in the group or not (Hennekens et al, 1996).

One other study should also be mentioned. The Cancer Prevention Study II, a prospective study on more than one million US adults investigated the effect of commercially available multivitamins and/or vitamins A, C, and/or E on mortality during a 7 year follow-up. The use of multivitamins plus A, C and/or E significantly reduced the risk of lung cancer in former smokers and in those who never smoked, but increased the risk in men who smoked and used vitamins A, C and/or E compared with men who reported no supplement use. Thus the 'antioxidant' vitamins A, C and E only appear to benefit male non-smokers. No association with smoking was seen in women (Watkins et al, 2000).

3.6.3 Reasons for increased cancer risk associated with β-carotene supplementation

The mechanism for the increased risk associated with β-carotene supplementation in smokers is unclear. One suggestion is that the subjects of the studies already had a 'high risk' of developing lung cancer and many might have had undetected tumours at the start. The stage of carcinogenesis that β-carotene might affect is not known but if mediated by the immune system the effect might be at the promotional stages preceding the formation of a malignant tumour (Hughes, 2001). The immune system appears to be particularly sensitive to oxidative stress. Immune cells rely heavily on cell-to-cell communication, particularly via membrane bound receptors, to work effectively. Cell membranes are rich in polyunsaturated fatty acids and if peroxidised, can lead to a loss of membrane integrity, altered membrane fluidity and result in alterations in intracellular signalling and cell function. It has been shown that exposure to reactive oxygen species (ROS) can lead to a reduction in cell-membrane expression (Hughes, 2001). In addition, the production of ROS by phagocytic immune cells can damage the cells themselves if not adequately protected by antioxidants such as β-carotene, lycopene and lutein.

One of the major unresolved dilemmas of β-carotene research is the intake required to optimise immune function and provide other health benefits (Hughes, 2001). Most studies have been done using pharmacological doses of β-carotene and it is not clear whether different intakes are associated with different outcomes. It is also possible that supplemental β-carotene might be interfering with intestinal absorption of other possible chemopreventive nutrients e.g. β-carotene can inhibit absorption of lutein, α-carotene and canthaxanthin, all of which show good antioxidant properties (Olson, 1999). Another explanation might be that β-carotene is acting as a pro-oxidant in the presence of high oxygen tension in the lung.

The apparent protection of a diet high in fruit and vegetables is likely to be the result of a multifactorial effect from a number of components in those foods. Two recent prospective studies found that subjects entering the studies with higher plasma β-carotene concentrations from dietary intake had a lower risk of lung cancer (McDermott, 2000). This finding perhaps suggests more studies using dietary enrichment with carotenoids rather than pharmacological supplements should be carried out.

3.7 Safety of vitamin A and β-carotene

3.7.1 Safety of retinol

Symptoms of hypervitaminosis A may occur in the skin, nervous system, musculoskeletal, circulatory systems or in internal organs. Toxicity varies with the dose, body mass, age, sex, disease conditions, concurrent drugs being taken and environmental chemical exposure (Blomhoff, 2001). Toxicity is rare from natural diets, the exception is from high intakes of liver (3–5 mg/100 g) (Northrop-Clewes, 2001b). Fortified foods are used in industrialised countries and can be consumed excessively (e.g. children may consume several bowls of breakfast cereal a day). Supplements, i.e. multiple micro-nutrients containing vitamin A, are readily available in industrialised countries and the usual content is:

- 1500 µg RE non-pregnant, non-lactating women.
- 1000 µg RE pregnant/lactating women.
- 750 µg RE for children < 5 years.

However, in general, healthy individuals in industrialised countries should not need supplements, as eating a balanced diet should provide all the nutrients required. In contrast, VAD is common among women of reproductive age living in deprived conditions and may be associated with a substantial increase in maternal mortality. The immediate postpartum period represents an opportunity to provide such women with a large dose of vitamin A, which benefits both mother and child. Since 1982 WHO/UNICEF/IVACG have recommended supplementing postpartum women and their infants, where VADD are a public health problem, with:

- Mothers: 200 000 IU < 6 weeks post partum.
- Infants: 25 000 IU at 6, 10, 14 weeks and 100 000 IU at 9 months.

However, theoretical calculations and recent data suggest the dose is too small and so in 2001, new WHO supplement recommendations were proposed:

- Mothers: 200 000 IU at delivery + 200 000 IU < 6–8 weeks after delivery
- Infants: 50 000 IU at 6, 10, 14 weeks + 100 000 IU 6–11 months + 200 000 IU every 4–6 months after 12 months.

Acute toxicity

Acute hypervitaminosis A can be defined as any toxicity manifested following a single very high dose or several very high doses over a few days (Blomhoff,

2001). Symptoms of acute toxicity include: increased cerebrospinal fluid pressure, bulging fontanelle in infants, headache and blurred vision in adolescents and adults, loss of appetite, nausea, vomiting lassitude and abdominal pain.

An acceptable dose for mothers is 400 000 IU vitamin A (120 mg retinyl palmitate i.e. 1 IU = 0.3 μg retinol) post partum while 50 000 IU is assumed safe for 0–6 month infants, 100 000 IU for infants > 6 months and 200 000 IU for those > 12 months old. However, in infants and children 25 000–50 000 IU occasionally leads to bulging fontanel. In about 6% of infants 300 000 IU can lead to nausea and vomiting and to diarrhoea in about 16% and although this is transient, it is unacceptable (IOM, 2001).

Retinyl esters in plasma are indicators of high or recent vitamin A intake i.e. they transiently increase after a vitamin A-rich meal, 1–2 × RNI and particularly with supplementation. Plasma retinoic acid will also go up after eating liver or taking high doses of vitamin A, and in lactating women the retinoic acid may go into the breast milk although this has not been measured. Breast milk retinyl palmitate is a useful indicator to monitor total maternal vitamin A intake, that is, milk retinol concentration will be very similar to plasma retinol. There is no evidence of an upper concentration of breast milk vitamin A that is harmful to infants.

Chronic toxicity from retinol
Definitions of upper limits of toxicity (IOM, 2001)

No observed adverse effect level (NOAEL) or the highest dose which has no adverse effect.

Tolerable upper intake level (UL) is the highest level of intake that is likely to pose no risk for almost all members of the population, where UL = NOAEL/uncertainty factor (UF).

Chronic hypervitaminosis A can be defined as any symptom resulting from continued ingestion of high doses of vitamin A for months or years (Blomhoff, 2001). In adults, there are many reports of chronic toxicity where the intake of vitamin A exceeds 15 mg/d, characterised by headache, fatigue, anorexia, itchy skin, liver damage, desquamation of mucous membranes and of skin.

The NOAEL for adults is set 15 mg/d and the UL is 3 mg/d, where the UF = 5 because of severe irreversible effect and inter-individual variability in sensitivity. If the UL was <3 mg, 50% of adults in the US would exceed the UL, yet few cases of liver toxicity are seen. The mean normal US liver concentration is 100 μg/g (range 10–1400 μg/g).

In infants and young children toxicity produces bulging fontanelle. The NOAEL is 6 mg/d and the UL is 0.6 mg/d, where the UF = 10 because of uncertainty and inter-individual variability in sensitivity.

In women of child-bearing age, toxicity can lead to teratogenicity, therefore the NOAEL is set at 4.5 mg and the UL at 3 mg/d (10 000 IU). The most serious effects of vitamin A toxicity include foetal resorption, birth defects, abortion and permanent learning difficulties in the offspring (IOM, 2001) (see section 3.3.3).

3.7.2 Safety of β-carotene

Experimental studies with animals have shown that β-carotene is not mutagenic or teratogenic. In addition, doses of 180 mg/day have been used over many years to treat patients with erythropoietic protoporphyria, with no evidence of vitamin A toxicity (Blomhoff, 2001). β-Carotene is considered not to be toxic because absorption becomes inefficient at high intakes, possibly because conversion of β-carotene and other provitamin A carotenoids is regulated by the vitamin A status of the individual. In two studies in which very different large intakes of β-carotene were given (15 and 40 mg), the mean absorption of β-carotene was <2 mg suggesting the human intestine possess only a limited capacity to absorb β-carotene (van Vliet et al, 1995; O'Neill and Thurnham, 1998).

3.8 Vitamin D

Recognition of the antirichitic effect of meat fat in the 1920s, as well as the protective effects of sunlight led to the discovery of vitamin D. Vitamin D is the name given to a group of fat-soluble compounds essential for maintaining the mineral balance of the body. Vitamin D is also known as calciferol and the antirachitic vitamin and its principal function is to regulate calcium and phosphate metabolism. It has two main forms: ergocalciferol, vitamin D_2 (plant origin) and cholecalciferol, vitamin D_3 (animal origin).

Vitamin D is produced from endogenous sources, synthesised in the skin from 7-dehydrocholesterol (7DHC) in a reaction catalysed by the ultra-violet (UV) light, and exogenous sources from the diet. There are only a few natural food sources, egg yolk, oily fish, butter and milk (Table 3.2). Margarines and spreads are fortified with vitamin D. Vitamin D, either natural or added, is stable in foods, and storage, processing and cooking do not affect its activity. The normal human diet is, however, a trivial source of vitamin D, since the biggest source results from exposure to sunlight. However, vitamin D production by the skin is strongly related to latitude and season, because short UV wavelengths of light are necessary for photoconversion. This means that in the UK and other countries in the northern latitudes, sunlight during the winter months is ineffective for the production of vitamin D because the sun is so low in the sky, the absorption by ozone too great and UV-B radiation too scattered (Maxwell, 2001).

There are at least 37 metabolites of vitamin D (Norman, 1990) but only three: 25 hydroxyvitamin D (25-OHD), 1,25 dihydroxvitamin D_3 (1,25-OHD) and 24, 25 dihydroxyvitamin D (24,25-OHD) have any important biological activity. Plasma 25-OHD is an index of availability of vitamin D and the normal range is 20–150 nmol/L (8–60 ng/ml). Values below 25 nmol/L (10 ng/ml) indicate risk of deficiency and toxicity occurs at levels above 150 nmol/L (60 ng/ml). The average intake within the UK ranges from 0.5 to 8 µg/day, dependent on season, with a mean around 3 µg/day. Table 3.1 shows no DRV for those aged between 4 and 65 years as usual daily activity of able-bodied persons should provide sufficient exposure to UV light. The elderly and those confined indoors are recommended

Vitamins   47

Table 3.3 Main causes of rickets and osteomalacia

Cause	Clinical features
Lack of sunlight	vitamin D deficiency e.g. in Asian immigrants and the elderly
Malabsorption	coeliac disease postgastrectomy intestinal bypass surgery
Renal disease: tubular	inherited hypophosphataemia Fanconi syndrome
Renal disease: glomerular	Osteodystrophy Dialysis bone disease

to take 10μg/day. Vitamin D is stored in various fat depots throughout the body and, because of its lipid nature, it is carried by a specific transport protein, α_2-globulin, within the circulation.

3.9 Specific nutritional deficiencies

3.9.1 Asian communities in the UK
Osteomalacia in adults and rickets in children occur as a result of vitamin D deficiency or from a disturbance in its metabolism (see Table 3.3). The frequency of occurrence depends on the distribution of the populations affected. In the nineteenth century nutritional rickets were endemic in industrial cities of Britain due to the poor diet and environmental conditions of children. As a result of effective public health measures privational rickets virtually disappeared from the UK by 1940 (Maxwell, 2001). However, in the 1960s low vitamin D status was found to be common among immigrant Asian children, adolescents and women living in the UK due to a combination of factors including the type of vegetarian diet, which was high in phytate from unleavened breads (see section 3.11), low calcium intake and limited exposure to sunlight. A striking reduction in Asian rickets occurred in Glasgow when free vitamin D supplements were introduced for children up to 18 years old (Smith, 2000).

3.9.2 Elderly
The elderly, especially those over 75 years, may have 25-OHD levels less than 12 nmol/L during the winter months because they expose insufficient skin to the sun during the summer months. Fifteen elderly people, living at 37° latitude who formerly went outside infrequently, were studied over a 4 week period while spending 0, 15 and 30 minutes on a veranda exposing the face and legs to sunlight. At the end of the study period, plasma 25-OHD levels increased by

18.5 nmol/L (7.4 µg/ml) in the group spending 30 minutes/day and there was a small but insignificant rise in those who spent 15 minutes outside (Reid et al, 1986). Reid and his co-workers thought this a safe inexpensive method for the prevention of osteomalacia in frail elderly subjects. Histologically proven osteomalacia occurs in 2–5% of the elderly in hospitals (Campbell et al, 1994) and low plasma 25-OHD in up to 40% of elderly living in homes and hospitals. Dietary or supplementary vitamin D may be the only effective way of maintaining or improving status in this group when it is not possible to expose them to sunlight.

3.9.3 Other diseases linked to vitamin D deficiency

After nutritional vitamin D deficiency, coeliac and renal diseases are the most important causes of osteomalacia and rickets. In coeliac disease there is a patchy enteropathy of the gut which can potentially lead to fat malabsorption. The efficient absorption of fat is essential for the absorption of fat-soluble vitamins, thus in patients with inadequate sunlight exposure, vitamin D deficiency can occur. Patients with kidney diseases are also susceptible to vitamin D deficiency as the enzyme necessary to convert 25-OHD to the metabolically active vitamin D metabolite, 1,25-OHD, is located in the kidney.

3.9.4 Vitamin D and type 1 diabetes

A follow-up study in Finland of 10 821 people born in Oulu and Lapland in 1966 showed that those who received recommended supplements of vitamin D during their first year of life were 80% less likely to develop type 1 diabetes over the next 30 years. Type 1 diabetes is thought to be an autoimmune disease caused when immune system cells attack insulin-producing cells in the pancreas. Vitamin D is known to be an immune system suppressant and the authors believe that vitamin D might somehow inhibit this autoimmune reaction (Hyppönen et al, 2001). Finnish children are less exposed to sunlight than those in more southerly countries, hence most receive vitamin D supplements. It is also suggested that mothers' worries over UV exposure and skin cancer may also be contributing to world-wide increases in type I diabetes. There is evidence that parents are restricting children's exposure to sunlight by using more sun-screen than previously and this might have played a part. Early infections with enterovirus and childhood obesity were also associated with increased risks of type 1 diabetes (Hyppönen et al, 2001). Nevertheless, none of the above explains the molecular role in the pathogenesis of type 1 diabetes and more work is needed in the area.

3.10 Synthesis and actions of 1,25-OHD

The most biologically active form of calciferol is 1,25-OHD and its synthesis is tightly controlled (Loveridge, 2000). The kidney produces both dihydroxylated forms of vitamin D (1,25 and 24,25-OHD); the dominant form is determined by

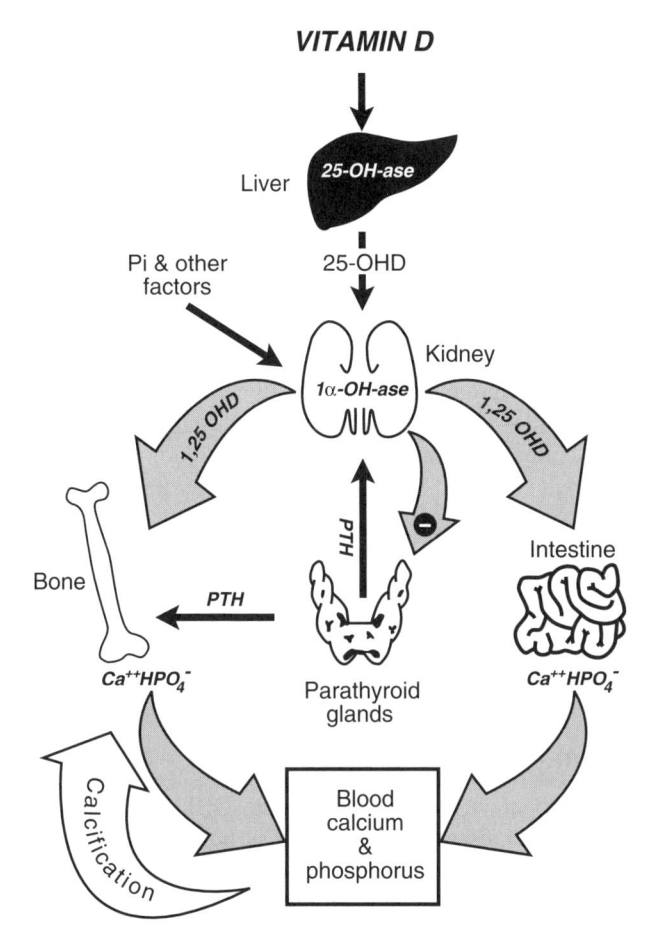

Fig. 3.2 Metabolism of vitamin D and the biological actions of 1,25 dihydroxyvitamin D (1,25-OHD) in raising blood calcium from bone resorption and/or the intestinal absorption. The figure shows the stimulatory role of parathyroid hormone (PTH) on kidney synthesis of 1,25-OHD and the feedback inhibition. (From Holick MF, 'McCollum Award Lecture, 1994: vitamin D – new horizons for the 21st century', *Am J Clin Nutr*, 1994, **60**, 619–30) (Reproduced with permission by the *American Journal of Clinical Nutrition*. © Am J Clin Nutr. American Society for Clinical Nutrition.)

the circulating level of parathyroid hormone (PTH), plasma calcium concentrations and the current vitamin D status of the body. In response to PTH in the vitamin D-deficient state, 1,25-OHD production is high (and this directly induces feedback inhibition of PTH production within the parathyroid gland) and 24,25 OHD is low. In the vitamin D-adequate state, 1α-hydroxylase activity in the kidney is increased and more 24,25-OHD is produced. Again, 1,25-OHD directly reduces PTH production in the parathyroid gland (Fig. 3.2). Under most circumstances the principal site for 1,25-OHD production is the kidney; however, during pregnancy the placenta also seems to have a role in producing it at the time of increased calcium requirements by the foetus (Loveridge, 2000).

Vitamin D maintains plasma calcium concentrations by stimulating intestinal calcium absorption by the small intestine and/or the resorption of calcium from bone. Calcium transport across intestinal cells is stimulated by 1,25-OHD by inducing the production of calcium binding protein (CBP) within the villous cells, and inducing an extremely low concentration of cystolic calcium within the enterocyte. 1,25-OHD also promotes cell maturation within the intestine (Suda et al, 1990) and in studies using vitamin D-deficient rats, villous length is only 70% of that of normal rats. Serum calcium is tightly controlled but a number of studies suggest it peaks in the summer perhaps because of improved vitamin D status, growth stimulation in children and higher intestinal calcium absorption (McCance and Widdowson, 1943). More recent studies, using radio-isotopes, have shown fractional calcium absorption was significantly higher in post-menopausal women evaluated from August to October than from March to May (Krall and Dawson-Hughes, 1991). In addition, increased intestinal calcium retention was associated with a lower rate of bone loss from the radius. The changes in calcium absorption and excretion could be accounted for by small seasonal increases in 1,25 OHD during the summer months found in some of the studies (Sherman et al, 1990).

3.11 Bone mineral density and fractures

In the presence of adequate dietary calcium, 1,25-OHD increases bone formation and growth plate mineralisation by providing sufficient calcium to allow calcification to occur. In contrast, prolonged vitamin D deficiency results in a poorly mineralised skeleton. When calcium is limited the skeleton is sacrificed because appropriate concentrations of calcium are required for vital nerve and muscle activity. Seasonal increases in PTH may have an adverse effect on bone loss. It is known that accelerated bone loss occurs in hyperparathyroidism (Maxwell, 2001) and increased PTH activity is a determinant in vertebral osteoporosis. However, studies by Krall and Dawson-Hughes (1991) showed that serum concentrations of 25-OHD >95 nmol/L prevent a seasonal increase in PTH. This suggests that when vitamin D status is poor, PTH stimulates 1,25-OHD production, which acts primarily on the bone to release calcium for essential activities. When vitamin D status is good, sufficient 1,25-OHD is produced to stimulate intestinal absorption of calcium so the bone is spared.

In the UK and the USA, seasonal changes in hip fractures have been recognised with peak fracture rates occurring during the winter months. The role of vitamin D deficiency in the pathogenesis of osteoporotic fractures is controversial and the inverse association with hip fracture rates could just be coincidence. However, seasonal changes in bone mineral density (Krolner, 1983) and the inverse seasonal changes in PTH, could be related to the accelerated bone loss. In addition, vitamin D is known to regulate the synthesis of osteocalcin (Reichel et al, 1989), the matrix protein in bone, thus a causal association between low 25-OHD levels and osteoporosis in postmenopausal women (Villareal et al, 1991) is possible (see also sections 3.20.2 and 3.21.3).

3.12 Vitamin D and other aspects of health

3.12.1 Behaviour

Specific vitamin D receptors are found in parts of the brain and spinal cord (Maxwell, 2001). Seasonal changes in 25-OHD and 1,25-OHD could have an effect on hormonal function, mood and behaviour. For example, seasonal affective disorders (SAD) appear to have a latitude gradient, with mood changes due to a reduction in daylight hours and altered circadian secretion of melatonin. Whether seasonal changes in UV light and vitamin D contribute is unknown.

3.12.2 Colon cancer

Mortality rates from colon cancer are highest in those areas that receive the least amount of sunlight. A prospective study of 26 000 volunteers investigated the association between 25-OHD and the risk of colon cancer. In those with 25-OHD concentrations of 50 nmol/L (20 ng/ml) or more, the risk of colon cancer was decreased threefold. However, confounding factors such as consumption of milk, meat or fat in the diet were not considered but these observations and previous epidemiological and laboratory studies suggest good vitamin D status in conjunction with calcium nutrition might lower the risk of colon cancer (Garland et al, 1989).

3.12.3 The immune system

Experimental evidence from animals, both *in vitro* and *in vivo*, has shown an immunological role for 1,25 OHD_3 in both lymphocytes and monocytes (Yang et al, 1993). Strict lactovegetarians, particularly in immigrant Asians, have an 8.5-fold increased risk of tuberculosis compared with those who ate meat or fish daily. Since vitamin D deficiency is more common among vegetarian Asians and it is known to have effects on immunological function in animals, vitamin D deficiency may be responsible for reduced immunocompetence (Maxwell, 2001).

The mechanism for the immunological role of vitamin D is not known, but the hormone receptor for 1,25-OHD is now recognised as one of a superfamily, the so-called 'Steroid-Thyroid-Retinoid-Superfamily'. It is understood that if these nuclear receptors and their activating substances are to recognise response elements within responsive genes, they must act in pairs and a member of the retinoid family must serve as a partner if the dimer is to function. Thus vitamin A, usually in the form of retinoic acid, is a regulator for several hormone response systems including vitamin D (Kliewer et al, 1994) (see section 3.5.2). The anti-infection properties of vitamin A are widely recognised and interactions between vitamins A and D status may therefore be important in regulating immune function.

3.13 Safety

Infants are most at risk of developing hypervitaminosis D. There are some reports of hypercalcaemia in infants given 50μg vitamin D/day and mild hypercalcaemia at doses of 15mg orally every 3–5 months (Department of Health, 1991).

3.14 Vitamin E

In 1922, a factor X, an antisterility factor, was found to be a fat-soluble component and essential for prevention of foetal death and sterility in rats. Vitamin E, as it became known, was isolated from wheat germ in 1936 and given its present name, tocopherol from the Greek words 'tokos' and 'pherein' which means 'to bring forth children'. It is now known that there are several forms of tocopherol and the term vitamin E is used to denote any mixture of biologically active tocopherols. Vitamin E activity is currently defined in mg α-tocopherol equivalents (α-TE) where 1 mg α-TE equals the activity of 1 mg RRR-α-tocopherol. Formerly international units (IU) were used and vitamin E is still occasionally quoted in this way in clinical trials. Where DL-α-tocopherol acetate is used, 1 IU equals 0.67 mg α-TE (Duthie, 2000).

There are eight naturally-occurring vitamin E compounds, four tocopherols and four tocotrienols, all synthesised by plants. The tocopherols are quantitatively and physiologically the more important. The most active of these compounds is α-tocopherol, which accounts for 90% of the vitamin E present in human tissues. Vegetable oils are the major sources of tocopherols. Sunflower and olive oil contain mainly α-tocopherol while in soya oil, the γ form accounts for 60% of total tocopherol. Other food groups provide substantial amounts of α-tocopherol including meat, fruit, nuts, cereals and eggs (Table 3.2). There is a widely available synthetic form of vitamin E, DL-α-tocopherol that consists of eight stereoisomers in approximately equal amounts. The synthetic form is used in animal feeds and is available in capsule form as a supplement for humans. Tocopherols and tocotrienols are readily oxidised to quinones, dimers and trimers by light, heat, alkali and divalent metals such as copper and iron so synthetic preparations are often protected by acetylation and succinylation (Duthie, 2000).

The assessment of vitamin E status is difficult because clinical signs of deficiency are not often seen, except occasionally in premature babies or in persons with fat malabsorption. This suggests that modern diets, which provide approximately 10mg vitamin E/d in the UK are adequate (Gregory et al, 1990). However, epidemiological evidence that intakes of vitamin E and other antioxidants are inversely correlated with the risk of some cancers and heart disease have led to some suggestions that optimal intake should be more than DRVs.

Vitamin E status can be measured as plasma tocopherol concentration but increased concentration of serum lipids appears to cause tocopherol to leave cell membranes and go into the circulation hence increasing blood levels. Because of this, plasma tocopherol is usually expressed in relation to circulating lipids, the most commonly used ratio being serum tocopherol:cholesterol. Values for serum α-tocopherol ≤11.6 µmol/L or of the α-tocopherol:cholesterol ratio ≤2.2 µmol/mmol indicate a risk of vitamin E inadequacy (Thurnham et al, 1986).

3.15 Biological activity

The biological activity of vitamin E is almost entirely due to its antioxidant properties. *In vivo* vitamin E appears to be the major lipid-soluble antioxidant component in membranes and is particularly effective in preventing lipid peroxidation, which is a series of chemical reactions involving the oxidative deterioration of polyunsaturated fatty acids (PUFA). Lipid peroxidation may cause the disruption of cell structure and function and may play an important role in the aetiology of many diseases e.g. heart disease and cancer. In biological systems the peroxidative cascade is likely to be terminated by vitamin E:

$$\text{PUFA}:\text{H} + \text{R}\bullet = \text{PUFA}\bullet + \text{RH} \quad [3.1]$$
Non-radical PUFA + Free radical = PUFA Radical + Non-radical product

$$\text{PUFA}\bullet + \text{O}_2 = \text{PUFAOO}\bullet \quad [3.2]$$
PUFA Radical + oxygen = peroxyl PUFA Radical

$$\text{tocopherol-OH} + \text{PUFAOO}\bullet = \text{tocopherol-O}\bullet + \text{PUFAOOH} \quad [3.3]$$
$$= \text{tocopheroxy radical} + \text{lipid hydroperoxide}$$

When vitamin E donates hydrogen it becomes a free radical but is relatively unreactive and the chain reaction is halted because the unpaired electron on the oxygen atom becomes delocalised within the aromatic ring structure. The concentration of vitamin E in cell membranes is low, about 1 molecule for every 2000 phospholipid molecules, therefore in order for vitamin E to continue to protect the membranes, it must be reduced to its original structure by vitamin C or other reducing compounds in the immediate environment. Likewise, lipid hydroperoxide has to be removed from the membrane for although it is semi-stable, its structure is altered by oxidation and it is potentially pro-oxidative in the presence of transition metals. Lipid hydroperoxides can be released from the phospholipid structure in membranes by phospholipase A2 and then degraded by selenium-dependent glutathione peroxidase in the cytoplasm or associated with the cell membrane (Chaudiere and Ferrari-Iliou, 1999).

3.16 Coronary heart disease (CHD)

Epidemiological studies have reported an inverse relationship between the incidence of CHD and vitamin E status using a variety of methods. A descriptive correlation study of 24 developed countries showed that the supply of α-tocopherol was strongly related to CHD and explained the low rates of heart disease in some European countries (Bellizzi et al, 1994). For example, Spain, with low rates of CHD, has estimated intakes of 18–25 mg/day vitamin E, whereas in the UK, where the number of deaths from CHD is one of the highest, the intake of vitamin E is only 4.7–11.9 mg/day. Biochemical evidence to support the epidemiological data suggests that the susceptibility of LDL-cholesterol to oxidative modification to an atherogenic form is key in the development of atherosclerosis. Oxidised LDL is taken up by monocytes, which are attracted to a site of injury on an arterial wall. Monocytes are transformed to macrophages and oxidised LDL appears to decrease the ability of macrophages to leave the arterial wall. The enhanced uptake of oxidised LDL may then convert macrophages into foam cells, the precursors of plaque, which block the artery. Studies *in vitro* have shown that oxidation of LDL can be inhibited by addition of antioxidants to the LDL. If LDL is exposed to a copper-mediated oxidation system, vitamin E in the outer phospholipid layer of the LDL is depleted first, followed by the carotenoids, lycopene and β-carotene. LDL oxidation is further delayed if vitamin C is present in the external medium, probably because vitamin C can regenerate vitamin E. In addition, studies by Esterbauer et al (1992) suggest that increasing the vitamin E or ubiquinone content of LDL by dietary supplementation also inhibits oxidation of LDL to the atherogenic form.

There is also some biochemical evidence which supports the hypothesis that low dietary vitamin E is correlated with less vitamin E in blood and higher risks of heart disease (Gey, 1993). However, more recent studies suggest that plasma α-tocopherol concentrations are very similar in several European countries in spite of widely differing vitamin E intakes (Howard et al, 1996; Olmedilla et al, 2001). Furthermore, the susceptibility of LDL to oxidation does not differ in people living in different countries with very different vitamin E intakes (Wright et al, 2002).

3.16.1 Randomised trials

Although observational studies have provided support for the potential health benefits of antioxidants, there remains a deficiency of direct experimental evidence from randomised trials. In the ATBC study, mentioned earlier (see section 3.6), there was not only no reduction in lung cancer or major coronary events, there was in fact an increase in lung cancer (ATBC Cancer Prevention Study Group, 1994). What was more startling was an unexpected increase in death from haemorrhagic stroke associated with vitamin E supplementation (50 mg/day). Some more positive results emerged from a study carried out in China where 130 000 adults from Linxian Province, who did not have cardiovascular disease at entry, were randomly assigned to receive daily vitamin E (30 mg), β-carotene and selenium supplements or placebo. During the 5.2 years of follow-up, there was a 9% decrease in 'deaths from any cause' without any significant reduction in cardiovascular events. However, the dose of vitamin E was smaller than the ATBC study, other supplements were included, nutritional status was poorer and cardiovascular risk of this population very much lower than that of the industrial west. Therefore the beneficial effect cannot be attributed to vitamin E alone (Blot et al, 1993). Lastly, treatment with vitamin E alone had no apparent benefit on cardiovascular outcomes in The Heart Outcomes Prevention Evaluation (HOPE) study. The HOPE study was a double-blind randomised trial with a 2 × 2 factorial design, to evaluate the effect of either 400 IU vitamin E daily from natural sources or matching placebo, and either ramiprol (an angiotensin-converting-enzyme inhibitor) or placebo for 4.5 years on 2545 women and 6996 men at high risk for cardiovascular events (Heart Outcomes Prevention Evaluation Study, HOPE, 2000).

Secondary prevention trials have been a little more supportive of the idea that vitamin E provides protection against heart disease. The Cambridge Heart Antioxidant Study (CHAOS) in patients with angiographic evidence of coronary atherosclerosis found high doses of α-tocopherol (400 or 800 IU/d) reduced risks of myocardial infarction (MI) and all cardiovascular events by 77% and 47% respectively (Stephens et al, 1996). Furthermore, secondary analysis of the ATBC study showed individuals with a history of MI at the start of the study had a reduced risk of subsequent nonfatal MI of 38%; however, risk of fatal coronary end points was not reduced (ATBC Prevention Study Group, 1994).

In conclusion, the apparent benefits of vitamin E in individuals with existing coronary disease were not consistent with the proposed role of antioxidants to prevent initiation or block propagation of lesions (HOPE, 2000). However, Steinberg hypothesised that unlike agents that lower cholesterol or blood pressure which have an immediate benefit, antioxidants may have to be used for more than 5 years to have demonstrable benefits, since the primary mechanism of these agents may be in the prevention of new lesions (Stephens et al, 1996). Further work on the possible effects of vitamin E on the clinical aspects of cardiovascular disease is needed. At present possibly the best advice to give is to recommend a balanced diet with emphasis on antioxidant-rich fruits, vegetables and whole grains.

3.17 Other roles of vitamin E

Vitamin E is the most effective chain-breaking lipid-soluble antioxidant in biological membranes, where it contributes to membrane stability and protects critical cellular structures against damage from free radicals and reactive products of lipid oxidation (Burton and Ingold, 1981). There are suggestions however that it has a variety of other effects, for example on immune function, platelet and vascular functions, prevention of oxidative damage to DNA and DNA repair and modulation of signal transduction pathways (Morrissey and Sheehy, 1999).

3.17.1 Immuno-enhancement
Immune function in the elderly is often the focus of vitamin-supplementation studies but, while some workers, e.g. Meydani et al (1997), were able to demon-

strate improvements in both cellular and humoral responses from vitamin E supplements, others who used less vitamin E (67 mg αTE/d) were unable to do so (de Waart et al, 1997). Meydani and colleagues suggested that a consumption of at least 147 mg α-TE/d (ie 5–10 times a normal dietary intake) was needed to benefit the immune response. Dose may play a critical role in the effects of vitamin E on immune function and high doses may enhance the immune system of the aged by suppression of prostaglandin E_2 (PGE_2) production and/or decreasing free radical formation. An increase in oxidant stress associated with an inadequacy of vitamin E will stimulate nuclear factor κB (NFκB) formation, stimulating inflammation and the formation of PGE_2 (Grimble, 1997). At low concentrations PGE_2 is believed to be necessary for certain aspects of cellular immunity. However, at higher concentrations, it suppresses several indices of cellular and humoral immunity such as antibody formation, delayed-type hypersensitivity (DTH) skin tests, lymphocyte proliferation and cytokine production (Meydani and Beharka, 2001). Tocopherols decrease the release of arachidonic acid from membrane phospholipids, resulting in a decreased production of PGE_2, hence mega-doses of vitamin E may stimulate immune function reducing the risk of free radical formation and reducing the substrate for PGE_2 formation, but such doses can have adverse effects. Mega-dose amounts of vitamin E have been reported to antagonise the pro-coagulant effects of vitamin K and this can have serious consequences in elderly people on warfarin therapy (Corrigan and Marcus, 1974).

3.17.2 Vascular effects of vitamin E
In addition to the protection provided by vitamin E against LDL oxidation, several studies have consistently reported that platelet aggregation is reduced by vitamin E supplements but amounts used to demonstrate these effects are generally in excess of 250 mg α-TE/d (Morrissey and Sheehy, 1999). However, a reduction in reactive oxygen species (ROS) that is promoted by vitamin E can protect against vascular cell dysfunction, preventing adhesion molecule expression and recruitment of monocytes and the production and release of nitric oxide (Baeuerle and Henkel, 1994; Goldring et al, 1995). α-Tocopherol has also been shown specifically to inhibit the proliferation of smooth muscle cells through modulation of protein kinase C and not a mechanism related to its antioxidant properties (Azzi et al, 2001).

3.17.3 Oxidative damage to DNA and DNA repair
Despite the use of high doses of vitamin E, large changes in the vitamin content of blood and liver and extended periods of study in animals and humans (smokers and non-smokers), vitamin E does not appear to have affected repair products of oxidative DNA damage, sister-chromatid exchanges in peripheral lymphocytes or DNA adducts in lymphocytes (Morrissey and Sheehy, 1999).

3.18 Safety issues

Although the intake from dietary sources is usually not greater than 20 mg/d, few adverse effects have been reported even from doses up to 3200 mg/d (Bendich and Machlin, 1988).

3.19 Vitamin K

The parent structure of the vitamin K group is 2-methyl-1,4-napthoquinone, also known as menadione. Menadione is not a natural constituent of foods but does possess biological activity in vertebrates (Shearer, 2000). Constituents of the naturally occurring vitamin K group all possess the napthoquinone ring structure but differ in the structure of the side chain at the 3 position. There are two main groups according to whether plants or bacteria produce them. In plants, the major form of vitamin K is phylloquinone (vitamin K_1), which has the same phytyl side chain as chlorophyll. Bacteria synthesise menaquinones (vitamin K_2) with side chains based on a number of repeating prenyl units (MKn). The primary functions of vitamin K are in blood coagulation and in bone metabolism.

The major dietary sources of vitamin K are shown in Table 3.2; however, green vegetables contain the highest concentrations and are the largest contributors to dietary intakes (Booth et al, 1996). The relative phylloquinone content of vegetables reflects its association with photosynthetic tissues, with highest values being found in dark green leafy vegetables, e.g. spinach and cabbage (300–600 µg/100 g). Fermented cheeses contain two major menaquinones MK-8 and MK-9 at concentrations of 50–100 and 10–20 µg/100 g respectively. Moulds do not normally synthesise menaquinones so MK-8 and 9 are thought to be derived from the starter fermentation bacteria.

Many bacteria present in the human intestine synthesise menaquinones, the major forms being MK-10 and -11 produced by *Bacteroides*, MK-8 by *Enterobacteria*, MK-7 by *Veillonella* and MK-6 by *Eubacterium lentum*. Most are found in the distal colon where the menaquinone content is about 20 µg/100 g dry weight, but there is no direct evidence that this pool is bioavailable. However, the widespread presence of very long-chain forms in the liver, e.g. MK10–13, does require explanation because these forms are not detected in commonly eaten foods but are typical of those produced by *Bacteroides* (Conly, 1992). There is, therefore, some debate as to the contribution of intestinal-derived K_2 to vitamin K status (Lipsky, 1994; Suttie, 1995).

3.20 Biological activity

3.20.1 Blood clotting

Vitamin K is required for the biological activity of several coagulation factors including four procoagulants, factors II (prothrombin), VII, IX and X and two feedback anticoagulants, proteins C and S. A seventh plasma protein (Z) may have a haemostatic role but its function is currently unknown (Shearer, 2000). Specifically, vitamin K functions as a cofactor for vitamin K-dependent carboxylase, a microsomal enzyme that facilitates the post-translational conversion of glutamyl (Glu) residues in the protein precursor to γ-carboxyglutamic acid (Gla). The biological relevance of the Gla structure is that it forms a cage structure to which divalent metal ions such as calcium may be bound (Berkner, 2000).

The synthesis of clotting factors occurs in the hepatic tissue. In its severest form, vitamin K deficiency results in bleeding syndrome due to lowering of circulating levels of the procoagulant factors and their replacement by undercarboxylated species.

3.20.2 Bone

Two vitamin K-dependent bone proteins were identified towards the end of the twentieth century. In 1975, it was found that bone tissue contains the Gla protein osteocalcin (BGP), which is one of the most abundant proteins in the body (Hauschka et al, 1975). In 1985 the matrix Gla protein, MGP, was discovered in bone, dentine and cartilage (Price, 1988). Osteocalcin is a water-soluble 49-residue protein and accounts for up to 80% of the total γ-carboxyglutamyl content of mature bone (Olson, 1999). Its discovery changed the thinking about the role of vitamin K. Although the exact role of osteocalcin in bone metabolism is still not understood, the available data suggest a regulatory function of osteocalcin in bone mineral maturation (Weber, 2001). Osteocalcin is synthesised by osteoblasts and since its concentration in blood reflects osteoblast activity, measurement of total osteocalcin in blood has become accepted as a marker of bone turnover (Khosla and Kleerekoper, 1999). In addition, the extent to which osteocalcin is carboxylated is believed to be a more sensitive measure of vitamin K status than the conventional tests involving blood coagulation. High serum concentrations of undercarboxylated osteocalcin (ucOC) are indicators of low vitamin K status and vice versa (Weber, 2001).

Work during the 1980s using cultured osteosarcoma cells showed that osteocalcin and MGP are regulated by 1,25-OHD (Olson, 1999). However, more recent studies have demonstrated that retinoic acid receptors and vitamin D hormone receptors may form heterodimers that bind to the osteocalcin promoter in the cells allowing retinoic acid and 1,25-OHD to work synergistically in the cultured cells, i.e. osteocalcin and MGP may mediate some of the actions of vitamin D on bone. It has been shown that a deficiency of osteocalcin does not appear to affect repair of bone structure but in bone disease, plasma osteocalcin is elevated (Price, 1988). The author concluded that osteocalcin may stimulate bone remodelling and calcium mobilisation while MGP may be associated with the inhibition of growth-plate mineralisation.

There is evidence that vitamin K positively influences calcium balance, a key mineral in bone metabolism. Humans given a diet rich in vitamin K showed an increase in calcium retention within the body (Sakamoto et al, 1999). There is some evidence to suggest that proteins located in the kidney are responsive to vitamin K and that γ-carboxy-glutamic acid may be involved in calcium retention and contribute to the effect.

3.21 Vitamin K status and health

3.21.1 Adults
Vitamin K deficiency in adults leading to clinical bleeding is almost unheard of, except as a consequence of hepato-intestinal disorders which disturb the absorption or utilisation of the vitamin. Use of warfarin or other anti-coagulant drugs, i.e. vitamin K antagonists, in the management of thromboembolic disease, reduces circulating concentrations of vitamin K-dependent clotting factors. The anticoagulants inhibit the biosynthesis of prothrombin and other vitamin K-dependent factors in the liver and others factors in extrahepatic tissues, leading to clotting factor deficiencies in the body (Olson, 1999). Studies investigating the effect of anticoagulants on bone health have shown mixed results but the participants were severely ill with chronic vascular disease which would have affected physical activity, a very important factor in bone health and may be the reason why vitamin K status did not appear to be important (Weber, 2001).

3.21.2 Infants
Newborn infants are a special case in vitamin K nutrition for several reasons: lipids are not easily transferred across the placenta, the neonatal liver is immature with respect to prothrombin synthesis, breast milk is low in vitamin K and the infant gut is sterile at birth. As a result of this unique combination of factors infants can develop a condition known as haemorrhagic disease of the newborn (HDN). The term HDN was first used in 1894 by Townsend who described it as a self-limiting bleeding disorder of newborns of unknown origin (Shearer, 2000). Until the late 1960s HDN was thought to be a problem of the first week of life; however, two other forms have now been identified: late HDN, a more serious condition, that occurs between weeks 3 and 6 of life and early HDN occurring in the first 24 hours, probably caused by antagonistic drugs taken during pregnancy. Late HDN is rare, about 4–70 cases per 100 000 births but world-wide is a significant cause of infant morbidity and mortality. Late HDN has a high incidence of intercranial haemorrhage resulting in death or severe and permanent brain damage in 50% of cases. One risk factor for both the late and classical forms of HDN is exclusive breast-feeding, which may be aggravated by the low concentrations of vitamin K in breast milk 1–10 µg/L (cf. formula milk ~50 µg/L). A second risk factor might be the 'precarious' hepatic stores of vitamin K found in newborns possibly due to poor placental transfer (Shearer, 2000). As a result of this phenomenon the COMA panel recommended all babies should be given prophylactic vitamin K at birth (Whitehead, 1991). Recent interest in late HDN has come from a reported increase in the syndrome since the early 1980s. In many

developed countries the increased incidence followed a decline in vitamin K prophylaxis since its introduction in the 1940s and an increase in exclusive breast-feeding. Prophylaxis was often given as an intramuscular dose at birth but since 1992 concerns about an epidemiological association between the intramuscular route and later childhood cancer has seen a shift towards the oral route of administration (Shearer, 2000). Work published by Autret-Leca and Jonville-Bera (2001) suggest oral administration of a single dose of vitamin K protects against classical and early vitamin K deficiency bleeding but that intramuscular prophalylaxis is needed for late HDN. Although the risk of solid tumours associated with vitamin K administration is unlikely there remains a low potential risk of lymphoblastic leukaemia in childhood. Autret-Leca and Jonville-Bera suggest formula-fed neonates without risk of haemorrhage should receive 2 mg oral dose of vitamin K followed by a second 2 mg dose between days 2 and 7. Infants exclusively or nearly exclusively breast-fed should receive weekly oral administration of 2 mg (25 μg/day) vitamin K, after the first two doses of the vitamin, until completion of breast-feeding. High-risk neonates (premature, neonatal disease, hepatic disease, maternal drugs inhibiting vitamin K activity) should receive the first dose intramuscularly or by a slow intravenous route. Subsequent doses should be administrated according to the clotting factor profile specific to each infant.

3.21.3 Bone health

Despite gaps in knowledge it appears that sub-optimal vitamin K status may play a role in osteoporosis. Patients with osteoporotic fractures tend to have very low plasma levels of vitamin K. Much of this evidence is circumstantial based on associations of measures of vitamin K status with fractures or biomarkers of bone metabolism and some of the evidence is conflicting (Binkley and Suttie, 1995; Shearer, 1995; Vermeer et al, 1995). French workers have shown an age-dependent impairment of γ-carboxylation of osteocalcin and strong associations of ucOC with hip fracture risk (Szulc et al, 1993) and bone mineral density (BMD) (Szulc et al, 1994). The work also showed a potential influence of vitamin D on γ-carboxylation, which may indicate interactions between vitamins D and K, an area requiring further investigation. It has also been shown that 'matrix Gla protein' which is an important regulator of bone strength and growth is determined by a vitamin A response gene (Gudas et al, 1991). To what extent vitamins A and K interact at the gene level is not known.

3.21.4 Intervention studies

A number of adult intervention studies have been carried out, particularly on postmenopausal women, which have shown vitamin K to be effective in reducing ucOC in serum. Takahashi et al (2001) used 89 osteoporotic patients with vertebral fractures, 24 patients with hip fractures, 43 pre- and 48 post-menopausal

Japanese women. They gave either a daily dose of 45 mg vitamin K_2 alone or vitamin K_2 plus 1 µg 1-α hydroxyvitamin D_3 or vitamin D alone. After four weeks of treatment with vitamin K alone or vitamin K plus D, ucOC was significantly decreased, but was not changed in those who received vitamin D alone. There was a disproportion of ucOC/intact OC in postmenopausal women and those with hip or vertebral fractures, vitamin K and vitamins K plus D markedly decreased the ratio of ucOC/intact OC to approximately 80%, but vitamin D did not decrease the ratio. This work confirmed previous studies (Plantalech et al, 1990; Douglas et al, 1995; Schaafsma et al, 2000).

The first intervention study to look at the influence of vitamin K on bone strength was published by Akjba et al (1991) who recruited 17 dialysis patients losing bone mass due to renal insufficiency. They supplemented the patients with 45 mg vitamin K_2 for 1 year and measured bone mass at different points on the skeleton. They found loss of bone was reduced in the vitamin K group. The findings were confirmed in subsequent studies by Orimo et al (1992) who carried out a placebo-controlled trial studying 546 patients with osteoporosis to whom they gave either 45 mg vitamin K_2 or 1 µg 1-α-hydroxy vitamin D_3 for 48 weeks. Arm BMD increased by 2.1% in the vitamin K group but decreased by 2.4% in the vitamin D group ($P < 0.001$); no difference in vertebral BMD was found. A more recent study reported that 45 mg vitamin K_2 or placebo given for 2 years to 241 osteoporotic women increased BMD and significantly reduced occurrence of new fractures (14 in the vitamin K vs. 35 in the placebo group) (Shiraki et al, 2000). Finally, preliminary data from a placebo-controlled, randomised, clinical trial on 244 post-menopausal women aged 60–85 years, after a 2 year intervention period, showed a significant increase in the BMD of the distal radius in a group receiving 200 µg vitamin K_1 plus 10 µg vitamin D and 1 g calcium (Bolton-Smith et al, 2001).

3.22 Safety

There have been no adverse effects associated with the ingestion of natural sources of vitamin K. One clinical intervention study used up to 90 mg of vitamin K_2 daily over 2 years without any relevant adverse side-effects (Orimo et al, 1998). The COMA report states that 'natural vitamin K vitamins seem remarkably free from toxic effects when taken orally even in milligram quantities' (Department of Health, 1991). Guidelines issued by the Institute of Medicine state, 'A search of the literature revealed no evidence of toxicity associated with the intake of either phylloquinone (vitamin K_1) or menaquinone (vitamin K_2) form of vitamin K' (IOM, 2001). The only studies reporting an adverse effect of vitamin K were retrospective analyses for factors associated with childhood cancer that suggested an increased risk in those infants receiving vitamin K at birth (Golding et al, 1990, 1992). Subsequent studies conducted in both Europe and the USA, however, failed to confirm the reports (IOM, 2001).

3.23 Vitamin C

Humans, other primates and guinea pigs depend on external sources of vitamin C for their requirements; most other animals synthesise ascorbic acid within the body. The vitamin C content in body tissues varies widely with highest concentrations in the pituitary, adrenals, leukocytes, eye lens and brain and the lowest levels in plasma and saliva (Thurnham, 2000). The ascorbic acid (AA) body pool in adults has been determined using isotope labelled AA as a tracer. Pharmacokinetic data was obtained from healthy men given doses of $1\text{-}^{14}C$ labelled AA with steady-state intakes of 30 to 180 mg/d AA. The data showed the body half-life of AA was inversely related to intake up to a maximum of 20 mg/kg body weight, corresponding to a plasma AA concentration of 57 μmol/L, and an AA intake of 100 mg/d (Kallner et al, 1981). In normal adults about 2.7% of the exchangeable body pool of ascorbate is degraded each day, which is independent of body pool size (Baker et al, 1971; Kallner et al, 1979).

3.24 Absorption and deficiency

Vitamin C intakes are usually similar in men and women and absorption of the water-soluble vitamin causes few problems, however plasma and leukocyte AA concentrations tend to be higher in women than men (Thurnham, 1994). AA is absorbed in the intestine via an energy/sodium dependent carrier-mediated transport mechanism (Stevenson, 1974). AA is converted into dehydroacorbic acid (DHAA) which is transported across the cell membrane more quickly than AA and, once in the epithelial cells, DHAA is reduced back to AA. At high intakes the process is saturated. Up to 180 mg there is an average absorption of 70%, but absorption decreases to 50% with intakes up to 1.5 g and further decreases to 16% with intakes of 12 g (Kubler and Gehler, 1970).

When the body pool falls below 300 mg vitamin C there is evidence of impaired function (Hodges et al, 1969). Plasma vitamin C levels are sensitive to recent dietary intake with values <11 μmol/L indicating biochemical depletion (Sauberlich, 1975). The early symptoms of vitamin C deficiency are fatigue, lassitude, loss of appetite, drowsiness, insomnia, feeling run-down, low resistance to infection and petechiae (minor capillary bleeding). Those most at risk of vitamin C deficiency are cigarette smokers, alcohol users, institutionalised elderly and people on certain drugs. Deprivation of vitamin C for long periods leads to scurvy, characterised by weakening of collagenous structures, resulting in widespread bleeding. Scurvy in infants results in bone malformations. The earliest clinical signs of deficiency are bleeding gums and loosening of teeth. Today, scurvy is relatively rare. An LNRI of 10 mg/d for adults has been shown to prevent scurvy in the UK and elsewhere but this level has little margin of safety (Bartley et al, 1953).

3.25 Biochemical functions

Vitamin C can act both as an antioxidant and a pro-oxidant. AA can readily donate electrons to quench a variety of reactive free radicals and oxidant species and is easily returned to its reduced form by electron donors such as glutathione, flavonoids, tocopherol and NADPH (Zeigler et al, 1996; Xu and Wells, 1996). Vitamin C can scavenge hydroxyl, peroxyl and superoxide radicals as well as reactive peroxide, singlet oxygen and hypochlorite species (Bendich et al, 1986; Sies and Stahl, 1995). Vitamin C is believed to be of fundamental importance as an antioxidant in tissues. The evidence suggests that it protects against plasma lipid and low density lipoprotein peroxidation by scavenging peroxyl radicals from the aqueous phase before they can initiate lipid peroxidation, which it does by regenerating oxidised vitamin E to the active reduced form (Thurnham, 1994). *In vitro* vitamin C is rapidly lost when plasma is exposed to peroxyl radicals, cigarette smoke or activated neutrophils and its disappearance is accompanied by the onset of lipid peroxidation (Halliwell, 1994). In the eye, high levels of AA provide antioxidant protection against photolytically-generated free radicals in the lens, cornea, vitreous humour and retina. High concentrations of AA, 8–10 times higher than plasma levels, are found in seminal fluid to protect sperm proteins. Oxidative stress has been associated with sperm agglutination and decreased male fertility (Jacob, 1999).

Vitamin C can also be violently pro-oxidant, as *in vitro,* it has been shown to release iron from ferritin and stimulate lipid peroxidation (Halliwell, 1994). The reducing properties of vitamin C are responsible for the conversion of Fe^{3+} to Fe^{2+} which is extremely important in the absorption of iron, but within the tissues could be potentially harmful because Fe^{2+} is a potent free-radical catalyst able to produce hydroxyl radicals (Stadtman, 1991). Stadtman and colleagues have argued that much ongoing protein damage involves metal ion-dependent $OH^{\bullet}$ generation, hence a small rise in $OH^{\bullet}$ generation over a lifetime could increase the incidence of age-related cancer (Tanner, 1976). In the healthy human body, most transition metal ions are safely sequestered and are not available to catalyse free radical reactions, but metals are always in transit within and between cells, hence it is possible that interactions of metal ions with ascorbate could contribute to oxidative damage (Halliwell, 1994). However, it is probable that the antioxidant properties of ascorbate predominate in healthy people most of the time.

3.26 Disease–nutrient interactions

Disease and stress lower both plasma and leukocyte ascorbate concentrations (Thurnham, 1994, 1997). It has been recognised for many years that smokers have lower plasma ascorbate concentrations than non-smokers, even when dietary intake is taken into account. The effect is similar to that seen during surgical stress or infection but the stress of smoking is more easily studied (Thurnham, 2000).

It has been argued that smokers have an increased turnover of vitamin C, so in order to maintain their body pool and circulating levels at similar levels to those of non-smokers, intake would need to be higher, 80 mg/d (Kallner et al, 1981; Smith and Hodges, 1987). However, an alternative explanation might be that vitamin C can act as a pro-oxidant in plasma, hence the body may be lowering concentrations to minimise the potential pro-oxidant damage caused by smoking and other stresses (Thurnham, 1994). The mechanism which reduces plasma vitamin C is also linked to the processes activated by the onset of disease. One of the earliest features of the body's response to trauma is a release of neutrophils from the bone marrow (Sipe, 1985). Such neutrophils are able to actively accumulate vitamin C (Moser and Weber, 1984) and rapid falls in plasma and leucocyte vitamin C following trauma have been reported (Vallance et al, 1978).

The need to lower circulating vitamin C concentrations in the presence of trauma may be linked to an increased risk of reaction between vitamin C and iron (Thurnham, 1994). During infection, the capacity to bind iron in plasma does not diminish and in fact several acute phase proteins with the capacity to bind iron increase (eg ferritin and lactoferrin). Nevertheless there is increased likelihood that iron and other transition metals are released in the immediate locality surrounding damaged tissues (Chevion et al, 1993), and therefore vitamin C concentrations may be reduced to minimise the risk of aggravating the damage still more. Reactions between iron and vitamin C are known to occur in situations where tissue integrity is reduced. So amounts of dietary vitamin C that would normally be tolerated easily can cause acute haemolysis and coma in persons with conditions where their red cells are more susceptible to oxidative stress such as glucose-6-phosphate dehydrogenase deficiency or nocturnal haematuria (Thurnham, 1994).

There are also other groups within industrialised countries where there may be risks associated with elevated intakes of vitamin C. In North European communities, genetic haemochromatosis has a gene frequency of 1 in 20, such that approximately 1 in every 300 individuals are at risk of iron overload. Although they appear apparently healthy, giving vitamin C without an iron-chelating agent to such people can potentially produce serious clinical effects (Halliwell, 1994). As indicated above, iron is usually bound to transport, storage or tissue proteins and the body is therefore protected from its damaging reactions. If localised or more general breakdown of tissue integrity should occur during infection, inflammation, strenuous exercise or other traumas resulting in an acute phase response, then metal ions are potentially released into the circulation. In addition as we get older, we get sicker and in humans with advanced atherosclerotic lesions, catalytic metal ions capable of free radical reactions can be measured. In fact, the contents of such a lesion will stimulate OH˙ formation in the presence of peroxide and ascorbate *in vitro*. Should older people take large doses of antioxidant vitamins? The Finnish study suggests that people who have been smokers for many years and may well be on their way to developing cancer and/or cardiovascular disease, are harmed by high dose β-carotene treatment (ATBC Cancer

Prevention Study Group, 1994). Furthermore, there are controversial suggestions that high body copper and/or iron stores are associated with increased risk of cancer and cardiovascular disease. This could mean that in the event of injury or trauma, more iron and copper would be available to catalyse free radical reactions (Halliwell, 1994). As stated earlier, a decline in plasma ascorbate at the onset of oxidative stress is probably beneficial, for although vitamin C is helping to scavenge radicals and recycle vitamin E, its reduction in plasma may prevent any problems if metal ions are released. Furthermore, it must be remembered that oxidised vitamin C can be regenerated within erythrocytes and other tissues (Chaudiere and Ferrari-Iliou, 1999), and if the radical scavenging properties of vitamin C are to be maintained, regeneration of reduced vitamin C has to be increased if plasma concentrations are lower. Hence, giving high doses of vitamin C to sick people may not be a good idea.

Fruits and vegetables are associated with a decreased risk of cardiovascular disease and many types of cancer and neurodegenerative disease, but the role of vitamin C in this effect is uncertain (Halliwell, 2001). Supplementation trials with vitamin C using biomarkers of oxidative damage to DNA bases to measure levels of oxidative DNA damage *in vivo* showed little evidence of a beneficial effect, except where vitamin C intakes were low. In addition, no conclusive evidence of a protective effect of vitamin C in studies on strand breaks, micronuclei or chromosomal aberrations were found (Halliwell, 2001). There is some evidence that diet-derived vitamin C may decrease gastric cancer in some populations but whether this is due to its antioxidant or other properties is uncertain.

3.27 Immune function

Phagocytes and lymphocytes can concentrate vitamin C up to 100 times higher than the plasma and this may indicate a physiological role for AA in these immune cells (Thurnham, 2000). The vitamin also affects many immune modulators like blood histamine, serum complement, prostacyclin, prostaglandins and B- and T-cell cyclic nucleotides (Jariwalla and Harakeh, 1996; Siegal, 1993). Results from studies on the effects of supplementation on the immune functions have been inconsistent. Many studies show the vitamin has beneficial effects while others show no effect. For example, a double blind study giving 1 or 4g AA daily to 24 free-living women produced increases in serum AA concentrations but no difference in leukocyte AA concentrations or function (Ludvigsson et al, 1979). AA inactivates or inhibits a wide range of viruses *in vitro* including human immunodeficiency virus (HIV), yet no clinical efficacy has been demonstrated (Jariwalla and Harakeh, 1996). A review of 21 controlled human trials of megadose ascorbate intake in those exposed to the common cold showed no consistent effect on reducing the incidence of colds although the duration of episodes and the severity of symptoms were reduced by an average of 23% (Jariwalla and Harakeh, 1996). The vitamin may have acted by reducing inflammation associated with reactive oxidants produced by phagocytic leukocytes or by antihistaminic action.

It has been suggested that concentrations of plasma AA of 40–50 μmol/L, from an intake of 50–60 mg/day, are optimal for protection against heart disease (Gey, 1993). However, it is clear that plasma vitamin C is influenced by many factors other than diet, therefore it is difficult to suggest that any particular plasma concentration is optimal for all situations (Thurnham, 2000).

3.28 Toxicity

Claims that intakes of vitamin C above those recommended can protect or cure various diseases are debatable. Mega-doses of vitamin C (10 g/d or more) were said to protect against the common cold and could be used in the treatment of advanced cancer. Neither has been substantiated and in fact, four cancer patients died of haemorrhagic tumour necrosis soon after vitamin C treatment was started (Halliwell, 1994). Possible risks associated with high intakes include diarrhoea (at intakes of ≥4 g/d) and increased production of oxalate leading to kidney stones in a small number of individuals with a high propensity for synthesising oxalate (Balcke et al, 1984). 'Systemic conditioning' where a sudden cessation of high intakes may precipitate scurvy due to high turnover were not confirmed following studies in guinea pigs and humans.

3.29 Vitamin B_1 (thiamin)

The thiamin molecule consists of a pyrimidine ring with an amine group joined to a sulphur-containing thiazole ring. In the tissues thiamin occurs most commonly as thiamin diphosphate (TDP), a coenzyme important in carbohydrate metabolism and as thiamin triphosphate (TTP) which is located in nervous tissues (Thurnham, 2000). Thiamin is also important in fat and alcohol metabolism to be discussed later (section 3.31). Diets high in carbohydrate require more thiamin than diets high in fat so symptoms of the deficiency disease beriberi occur where there is dietary deficiency of thiamin and where energy from the diet is provided mainly from carbohydrate sources.

Beriberi occurred in Japan, China and South-east Asia in epidemic proportions during the nineteenth and early twentieth centuries and dated from the introduction of steam-powered, rice-milling machines which made polished rice more widely available. At the end of the nineteenth century Takaki, Director General of the Medical Department of the Japanese navy, found that by supplementing rice with fish, vegetables, meat and barley, beriberi was almost eradicated (Sinclair, 1982). However, ordinary people in the poor social conditions prevailing at that time were not able to supplement their diets and the problem of beriberi became a difficult one for the colonial powers of the day as the death toll rose. The Dutch government set up an expert committee and a man named Eijkman was appointed to tackle the problem. Within six years Eijkman had shown beriberi to be a nutritional problem (Eijkman, 1897). Eijkman fed both stale and freshly-cooked polished rice to chickens and produced a paralytic condition closely resembling beriberi (Luyken, 1990). Subsequently, Funk (1911) isolated the anti-beriberi factor from the rice polishings and first used the word 'vitamine' to describe the vital amine essential for life.

Thiamin is present in all natural foods (Table 3.2). However, in many parts of the developing world thiamin is obtained either from unrefined cereal grains or starchy roots and tubers. The milling process of cereals removes most of the thiamin and polished rice is particularly low in thiamin (80 μg/100 kg). Rice which is parboiled before milling retains a lot of its thiamin (190 μg/100 kg) because water-soluble vitamins diffuse inward during the process (Padua and Juliano, 1974). Thiamin is water-soluble and is stable in slightly acidic water up to boiling point. Thiamin is unstable in alkaline solution and is, therefore, lost during the distillation process to produce alcohol.

In the British diet 45% of thiamin is obtained from fortified white flour products (fortified at 2.4 mg thiamin/kg white flour). Human milk is low in thiamin. The mean range reported by The Committee on Medical Aspects of Food Policy (CMAFP) for analyses from five centres in Great Britain was 0.59 μmol/L (0.49–0.79) which is equivalent to 0.23 μg/4.2 MJ (1000 kcal) (CMAFP, 1977). Thiamin concentration in mothers' milk is not increased by giving supplements, but the concentration does increase naturally over the first 6 weeks of lactation from 0.41 to 0.65 μmol/L (Thurnham, 2000).

3.30 Functions and requirements

Thiamin has two distinct functions:

1. TDP is the co-enzyme for pyruvate dehydrogenase (EC 1.2.4.1) and transketolase (EC 2.2.1.1.) in carbohydrate metabolism, α-ketoglutarate dehydrogenase (EC1.2.4.2.) in the citric acid cycle and branched chain keto-acid dehydrogenase (EC 1.2.4.4.) in the metabolism of branched chain amino acids.
2. TTP acts in nerves (and maybe muscles) to activate a chloride ion channel (Bender, 1999). In addition, TTP may play a fundamental role in the control of conductance of axonal membranes as well as in other neurological processes.

Estimations of thiamin requirements have been based on a variety of biochemical methods. The finding that urinary thiamin output falls below 15 μg/d in people with beriberi provided the reference point against which other methods such as thiamin loading, glucose loading and transketolase (TKL) activation are all compared (Department of Health and Social Security, 1979). Early studies in men suggested that thiamin intakes of 0.4 mg/d were near to the minimum at low energy intakes (Williams, 1961). Epidemiological evidence suggested beriberi occurred when the intake of thiamin was 0.2 mg/1000 kcal or less (Williams et al, 1943). Later studies found that at a thiamin intake of 0.16 mg/1000 kcal both urinary and TKL measurements were abnormal and thiamin intakes of 0.3 mg/1000 kcal were needed to get these values into the normal range (Sauberlich et al, 1979). From these and other studies the COMA panel accepted that thiamin requirements were linked to energy metabolism, and therefore to energy intake, and hence set the RNI at 0.4 mg/4.2 MJ for men (Table 3.1) (Department of Health and Social Security, 1979).

Women are less frequently affected by beriberi than men even when eating the same food (Platt, 1958; Tang, 1989), but there is no consistent data that the needs of women are different. Bamji (1970) suggested that 0.21–0.26 mg thiamin/1000 kcal would normalise measurements of TKL and thiamin excretion in young women. Others reported urinary thiamin excretion only reached normal values at intakes of 0.51 mg/1000 kcal. The COMA panel set the same RNI for women as for men.

3.30.1 Thiaminase enzymes

The thermolabile anti-thiamin factors (ATFs) include thiaminase I (EC 2.5.1.2.) and II (EC 3.5.99.2). Thiaminase I is found in the viscera of freshwater fish, in shellfish, ferns, a limited number of seafish, plants and several micro-organisms. Destruction of thiamin occurs either by base-exchange between thiazole and other bases or hydrolytic cleavage of the methylene bridge between the pyrimidine and thiazole moieties. Thiaminase II is found in several micro-organisms e.g. *Clostridium thiaminolyticus, Candida aneurolytic.* It hydrolyses thiamin to 2-methyl-4-amono-5-hydroxymethyl pyrimidine and 4-methyl-5-(2-hydroxyethyl) thiazole. Cooking food destroys these heat-labile enzymes, but food which is not generally cooked i.e. is eaten raw or fermented, may lose thiamin during its preparation or in the gastrointestinal tract. Thermostable ATFs have been shown to be in ferns, tea, betel nuts, some vegetables and some animal tissues (Tanphaichitr, 1999).

3.31 Clinical thiamin deficiency

Cardiac failure, muscle weakness, peripheral and central neuropathy and gastrointestinal malfunction have been seen in animals and humans on diets deficient in thiamin. The circulatory effects of thiamin deficiency are no doubt linked to attempts by the body to increase metabolism of energy-forming substances. Other effects may well be due to impaired nerve transmission and/or the energy deficiency; the precise biochemical reasons have not been established.

3.31.1 Beriberi

Children and adults may present with dry (paralytic or nervous) or wet (cardiac), or cerebral (Wernicke-Korsakoff syndrome) forms of beriberi.

a. Wet beriberi
In addition to peripheral neuropathy, common signs in wet beriberi include: oedema, tachycardia, wide pulse pressure, cardiomegaly and congestive heart failure. Patients with wet beriberi respond dramatically to intramuscular doses of 25 mg for 7–14 days, followed by oral doses of 10 mg three times a day until the patient fully recovers (Tanphaichitr, 1999).

b. Dry beriberi
A peripheral neuropathy, dry beriberi is characterised by a symmetric impairment of sensory, motor and reflex functions affecting the distal segments of the limbs more severely than the proximal ones (Thurnham, 2000). Dry beriberi can be more resistant to treatment. Disappearance of impaired sensation occurs between 7 and 120 days, and recovery of motor weakness within 60 days of the start of treatment (Tanphaichtir, 1999).

c. Wernicke-Korsakoff syndrome
In Wernicke's disease, failure of energy metabolism predominantly affects neurons and their functions in selected areas of the central nervous system. Biochemical lesions that affect TKL and nucleic acid metabolism may cause glial changes. Membranous structures are visibly altered and secondary demyelination follows (Tanphaichitr, 1999). Prolonged alcohol consumption is associated with a variety of neuropsychiatric conditions, including the dense amnesic disorder known as Korsakoff's syndrome. Korsakoff's syndrome is frequently diagnosed in alcoholics after an episode of acute thiamin deficiency. The accepted view within the medical literature is that the etiology of this disorder lies in thiamin deficiency or Wernicke's encephalopathy. However, examination of the published reports of pure thiamin deficiency unaccompanied by chronic and excessive consumption of alcohol shows that, in this group of patients, the rate of progression to Korsakoff's syndrome is low. This result suggests that the memory impairments associated with alcohol-related brain damage cannot be attributed to thiamin deficiency alone. The etiology of alcohol-related cognitive impairments such as Korsakoff's syndrome is still poorly understood, but several lines of evidence suggest multiple causal factors interact to produce deficits in performance (Homewood and Bond, 1999).

d. Early, less well-recognised thiamin deficiency
What are less widely recognised are the lesser degrees of thiamine deficiency that can be caused by situations of hypermetabolism, for example, by burns, trauma, surgery and acute febrile illness. These situations are most likely to be seen in patients who are given additional carbohydrate loading via glucose-containing intravenous fluids and in those who already had marginal thiamin status to begin with. This includes alcohol abusers, the homeless and others on inadequate diets.

Part of the reason for this lack of recognition is the speed with which biochemical evidence of thiamin deficiency can occur on such diets (Brin, 1964) and also because there is no clearly recognised clinical syndrome corresponding to marginal (biochemical) thiamin status. Another reason is that clinicians simply do not think of thiamin status often enough. It is relatively easy to test for thiamin status using activity levels of the thiamin-dependent enzyme erythrocyte TKL; however, the test is not commonly available in clinical laboratories.

3.32 Toxicity

Chronic intakes in excess of 50 mg/kg or more than 3 g/day are toxic to adults with a wide variety of clinical signs including headache, irritability, insomnia, rapid pulse, weakness, contact dermatitis, pruritus (Ibner et al, 1982).

3.33 Folate

The folate molecule is a double aromatic ring of a pteridine attached to *para*-aminobenzoate and glutamate. Folic acid (pteroyl glutamic acid) is the parent molecule of a large number of derivatives known as folates. Folic acid is physiologically inactive until it has been enzymatically reduced to dihydrofolate when it can enter the body's folate pool (Fig. 3.3). The main naturally occurring forms are tetrahydrofolate (THF), 5-methylTHF and 10-formylTHF. The characteristic sign of folate deficiency is megablastosis, with abnormal, multi-lobed neutrophil nuclei and giant platelets in peripheral blood. Other rapidly regenerating tissues like intestinal mucosa might also be affected by folate deficiency (Department of Health, 1991).

In 1872 Biemer described a severe, rapidly progressive and sometimes fatal anaemia of pregnancy (McNulty, 1997). However, this condition was not linked to a dietary deficiency until 1931 when it was established that cases of macrocytic anaemia in poor, pregnant women in India responded to treatment with crude liver or yeast extract (Wills, 1931). The new nutritional factor was called 'vitamin M', 'vitamin Bc' and 'factor U', but isolating and successful chemical synthesis of folic acid, as it became known, was not achieved until the 1940s. Subsequently, neural tube defects (NTD) and anencephaly were linked to poor folate status during pregnancy (Smithells et al, 1976) and, following a randomised double-blind trial, folate supplements were found to lower significantly the recurrence of NTD (MRC Vitamin Study Research Group, 1991) (section 3.34.1). Currently, the greatest interest in folate metabolism is centred around its role in lowering plasma homocysteine concentrations and links to cardiovascular disease (section 3.35). Stockstad (1990) describes the history of folic acid in a book which reviews the key advances in the biochemistry and physiology of folates.

A diet that is rich in other B vitamins and vitamin C is usually rich in folate (Whitehead, 1991). Rich food sources of folate include liver, yeast extract and green leafy vegetables (Table 3.2). However, liver is not eaten by a sufficiently large proportion of the population to make a significant contribution to intake, but beer (90 µg/L folate) may account for 10% of dietary folate intake in British

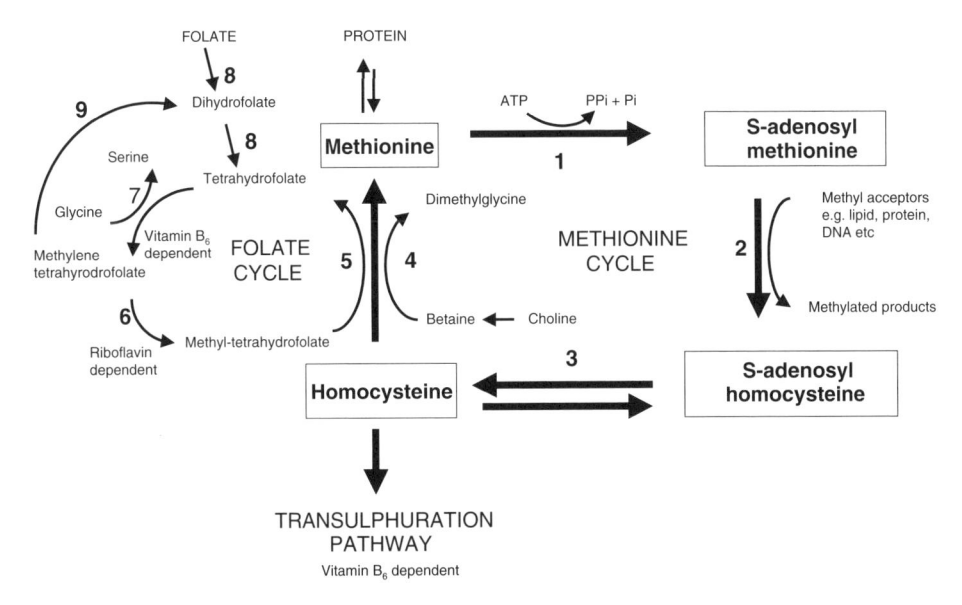

Fig. 3.3 Interrelationships between methionine and folate metabolic cycles.

Key:
1. Methionine adenosyl transferase EC 2.5.1.6
2. S-adenosylmethionine-dependent methyltransferase EC 2.1.1
3. S-adenosylhomocysteine hydrolase EC 3.3.1.1
4. Betaine:homocysteine methyltransferase EC 2.1.1.5
5. 5-Methyltetrahydrofolate:homocysteine methyl transferase (vitamin B_{12} dependent) EC 2.1.1.13
7. 5,10-Methyltetrahydrofolate reductase (vitamin B_2 dependent) EC 1.1.99.15
7. Serine hydroxymethyl transferase (vitamin B_6 dependent) EC 2.1.2.1.
8. Tetrahydrofolate dehydrogenase 1.5.1.3.
9. Thymidylate synthase EC 2.1.1.45

adults (McNulty, 1997)! There are concerns about the bioavailability of dietary folate (Gregory, 1995). Food folates are present mainly as polyglutamate derivatives which have to be converted to a monoglutamyl form by folate conjugase to be absorbed by the jejunum. Changes in the pH of the lumen contents, or the presence of folate conjugase inhibitors, folate binders or other specific food components can all adversely affect the rate of hydrolysis and uptake of the vitamin (McNulty, 1997). These factors account for the wide range of folate bioavailability of the naturally occurring folate polyglutamates in all foods.

Stable isotope studies have found 50% relative bioavailability of polyglutamyl compared to monoglutamyl forms of folate (Gregory et al, 1991). Hence the relative bioavailability of folates from a mixed diet is difficult to predict and is considerably less than when the vitamin is eaten as a supplement or in a fortified food.

Folates are involved in a number of single carbon transfer reactions, especially in the synthesis of purines, pyrimidines, glycine and methionine. THF can have one-carbon units added, for example formyl, methyl or methylene and these are attached to either the N5 or N10 nitrogen or both (Scott, 2000). The principal source of the one-carbon units is serine. The one-carbon units are donated once to change uracil to a thymine-type base during the biosynthesis of pyrimidine, and twice during the biosynthesis of purines. Pyrimidine biosynthesis generates dihydrofolate from 5,10 THF, which is then reduced back to THF. In the two reactions of purine biosynthesis 5,10 formyl THF is the donor of carbon and THF is generated by both reactions. In all three reactions the cofactor THF is then available to attach another one-carbon unit and repeat the process. Only a small amount of the cofactor is required in cells because of the continuous regeneration back to the THF form. These cycles could be called the DNA and/or RNA biosynthetic cycles since they provide the *de novo* synthesis of the bases used to make these structures (Scott, 2000).

In addition to the role described above, folates also participate in the methylation cycle (Fig. 3.3). Enzymes called methyl transferases exist in all mammalian cells and transfer methyl groups to a wide range of acceptors. In all cases the source of the methyl groups is the methyl group of methionine, which is passed on after it has been activated with ATP to form S-adenosylmethionine (SAM). Donations of the methyl groups from SAM produce S-adenosylhomocysteine (SAH) which is rapidly hydrolysed to homocysteine. Homocysteine is remethylated either from choline or by the folate cofactor 5-methylTHF. The methylation cycle is essential in intermediary metabolism requiring a continuous supply of methyl groups and for which a major source is the folate cofactor.

3.34 Requirements

Biochemical evidence of folate status can be obtained in a variety of ways. The lower limit of normal serum folate is accepted as 6.8 nmol/L (3 µg/L). Tissue levels are better indicated by the concentration of folate in red cells, which is buffered against short-term changes (Department of Health, 1991) and concentrations below 0.23 µmol/L (100 µg/L) are considered to be severely deficient. Values between 0.23 and 0.34 µmol/L (100–150 µg/L) indicate marginal stores. Liver values greater than 6.8 nmol/g (3 µg/g) indicate adequate reserves (Department of Health, 1991). The RNI for folate for different age groups are summarised in Table 3.1. However, in recent years new evidence suggests that the RNI should possibly be increased in some groups.

3.34.1 Folate requirements in women
Conventional views on folate deficiency and its role in the aetiology of NTD suggested that the sole adverse outcome was the arrest of cell division because of inadequate folate-dependent DNA biosynthesis (section 3.39). Recently this was revised because, although those women whose babies' NTDs such as spina bifida (Fig. 3.4) had low folate status, the blood concentrations were often within the

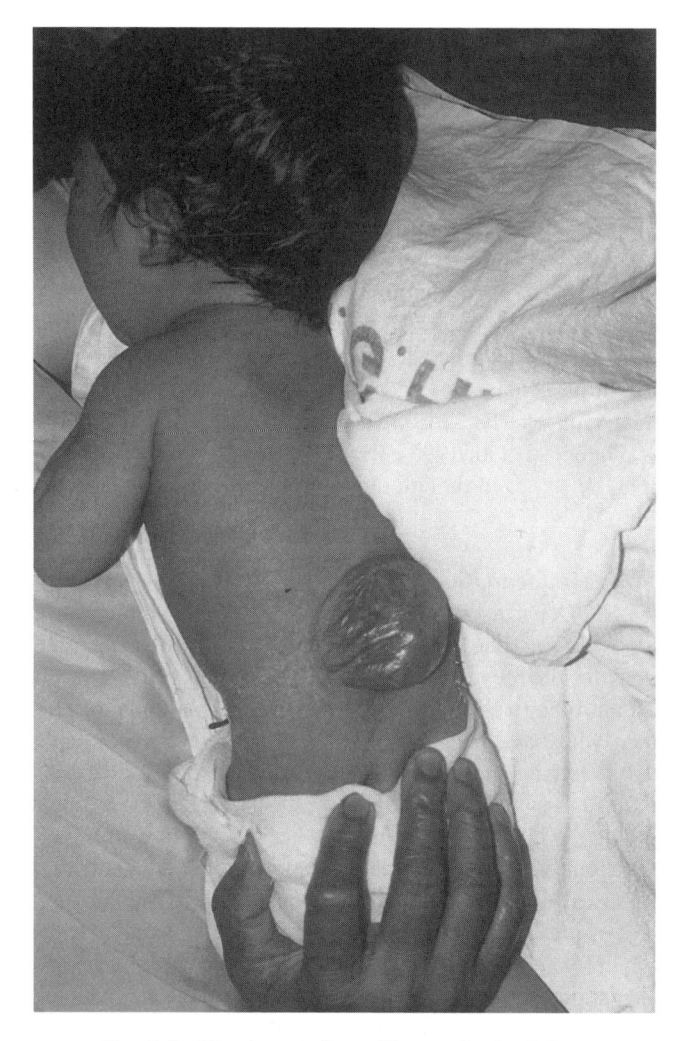

Fig. 3.4 New-born infant with neural tube defect.

accepted normal range. In addition an increased risk of cardiovascular disease and stroke has been associated with low folate status (see section 3.41) (Scott, 2000).

NTDs are major malformations in which there is a failure of the developing neural tube to close properly during the fourth week of embryonic life. Incomplete closure of the spinal cord results in spina bifida while incomplete closure of the cranium results in anencephaly (McNulty, 1997). The latter condition means the babies will either die *in utero* or shortly after birth.

The MRC trial provided the first unambiguous confirmation of the effectiveness of periconceptional folic acid in the prevention of NTDs (MRC Vitamin

Study Research Group, 1991). The study was a randomised double-blind trial conducted in 33 centres in 7 countries over 8 years and showed that folic acid had a 72% protective effect in preventing the recurrence of NTD in nearly 1200 women who had a previously-affected pregnancy. A subsequent study by Czeizel and Dudas (1992) confirmed the MRC study and added that folic acid also prevented first occurrence NTD (Czeizel and Dudas, 1992).

A possible mechanism for folate and/or folic acid protection against NTDs was put forward by Whitehead et al (1995) to explain why folate was effective against NTDs, even though folate status was not noticeably poor. They suggested that genetic polymorphisms existed within a population where the metabolism of folate was disturbed and higher concentrations were needed for full functionality. In particular, they identified a variant form of the gene for 5,10-methyleneTHF reductase (E.C. 1.7.99.5) present in approximately 10% of the UK population (Whitehead et al, 1995). Possession of this variant gene may increase the risk of NTDs, etc. even though dietary folate might be marginally adequate.

3.34.2 New recommendations

In 1992, The UK Department of Health revised their recommendations for folic acid and proposed 5 mg folic acid/day in tablet form to stop the recurrence of NTD and 400 μg/day for the prevention of NTD, to be started before conception and to be continued until the twelfth week of pregnancy (Department of Health, 1992). Those women who have had a previously affected pregnancy have a 10-fold increased risk of having another NTD baby; however, 95% of cases are first time occurrences and these women are causing the most concern (Department of Health, 1992). Targeting the latter group is difficult because of the number of unplanned pregnancies (about 50%) and the malformations of NTD occurring so early in pregnancy. To deal with the problem the Department of Health proposed three possible ways of preventing first occurrence NTD: (1) increased intake of foods naturally rich in folate, (2) folic acid supplementation, (3) folic acid fortification.

Supplementation is effective if taken but a study of 411 pregnancies in London in 1994 indicated only 3% of women had taken folic acid before conception (Clark and Fisk, 1994). Increasing food folate would require women to eat three times their current intake, however, even when this is achieved experimentally it does not appear to optimise folate status (McNulty, 1997). Although food fortification is the most promising there are worries that too high a folate intake might mask a vitamin B_{12} deficiency in the elderly. Extra dietary folic acid might reduce the erythrocyte effects of vitamin B_{12} deficiency (i.e. megablastosis) and delay the diagnosis. An undiagnosed vitamin B_{12} deficiency can progress to a neuropathy following the remission of the anaemia (Cuskelly et al, 1996).

3.34.3 Fortification

In 1998 folic acid fortification of grain foods in the USA was made mandatory. The Food and Drug Administration opted for a low level of fortification of

1400 µg/kg product because of some concerns over safety issues (United States Department of Health and Human Services, 1996). It was expected that this level of fortification would result in a mean additional intake of 100 µg/day in the US population which would be low enough to carry no risk of masking vitamin B_{12} deficiency, but others argued it would be ineffective in preventing NTD (McNulty, 2001). Recent data published indicates that the incidence of NTD in the US has fallen by almost 20% following the introduction of the fortification policy (Honein et al, 2001).

COMA recommended mandatory food fortification to the UK government in 2000 (Department of Health, 2000). The main conclusion of the report was 'universal folic acid fortification at 2400 µg/kg in food products as consumed would have a significant effect in preventing NTD-affected conceptions and births without resulting in unacceptably high intakes in any group of the population'. This level of fortification has been estimated to increase mean folic acid intakes by 200 µg/day which is predicted to reduce NTD pregnancies by 41%.

In the COMA report, estimates of exposure of different sections of the poulation were made by modelling dietary intake data from 4 National Diet and Nutrition Surveys for each age group at 5 possible levels of fortification of flour: 1400 µg/kg, 2000 µg/kg, 2400 µg/kg, 2800 µg/kg and 4800 µg/kg. At each level of fortification the number of NTD-affected births per year prevented, as well as the percentage of people over 50 years who would be exposed to a folic acid intake greater than 1 mg/day (upper tolerable limit), was calculated. If white flour were fortified with 2400 µg/kg, the results predict all subjects would have total folate intake above the LRNI and mean intakes would increase to 343 and 365 from 153 and 165 µg/day for girls and boys aged 11–12 years respectively, 10% of whom currently do not meet the LRNI (Moynihan et al, 2001).

The report is currently undergoing consultation by the four UK Health Departments and the Food Standards Agency (McNulty, 2001).

3.35 Folate, homocysteine and cardiovascular disease (CVD)

Cardiovascular disease remains one of the main causes of mortality in the western world and approximately two-thirds of cases are attributable to traditional environmental and genetic factors. However, in the last decade it has emerged that a moderate rise in the amino acid homocysteine in plasma constitutes a risk factor for atherosclerotic vascular disease in the coronary and peripheral blood vessels (Ward, 2001). The B vitamins folate, B_{12} and B_6 all play a key role in homocysteine metabolism and deficiencies of any one of the three B vitamins can result in homocysteinaemia. However, folate appears to be the most important and has been shown to lower plasma homocysteine concentrations at doses of 0.2–10 mg/day in both healthy and hyper-homocysteinaemic subjects (Ward, 2001) (see Fig. 3.3).

There is considerable variation throughout Europe in the rate of CVD mortality. In southern Europe more fruit and vegetables are eaten and this appears to be associated with lower incidence of CVD. The consumption of fruit and vegetables has traditionally been associated with increased antioxidant intake (see sections 3.6, 3.15, 3.25) but green vegetables are also one of the main sources of folate, contributing more than 30% of total dietary folate intake.

A recent meta-analysis of 12 randomised controlled trials, which included 1114 subjects, demonstrated that folic acid in the range of 0.5–5 mg/day lowers plasma homocysteine by approximately 25% with 0.5 mg/day as effective as 5 mg/day (Clark and Homocysteine Lowering Trials Collaboration 1998). Furthermore, the greatest lowering was in those with the highest baseline homocysteine concentrations (Ward, 2001). Doses as high as 0.5 mg/day can only be achieved using supplementation. It was of interest, therefore, to investigate whether dietary modification or fortification with lower levels of folic acid could also be effective. Results indicated that homocysteine concentrations were significantly lowered in response to doses of 100 and 200 µg/day but no additional lowering was found with 400 µg/day (Ward, 2001). When the fall in homocysteine was expressed in tertiles, only the top two tertiles showed lowering. Homocysteine and folate (serum or red cell) showed no response with any of the doses in the bottom tertile. It was concluded that 200 µg/day folic acid was the optimal homocysteine-lowering dose: interestingly the same dose had previously been predicted to be optimal in reducing the risk of NTD (Daly et al, 1997).

3.36 Causes of decreased folate status

Dietary folate deficiency has been previously associated with poor socio-economic groups but now is thought to exist in 5–10% of the population of most communities. Intestinal absorption is impaired in those with coeliac disease or tropical sprue which if left untreated can lead to folate deficiency (Scott, 2000) (see also section 3.33). Pregnancy is associated with increased folate catabolism, particularly in the second and third trimesters, when it exceeds intake. Women who enter pregnancy with adequate stores or receive prophylaxis during pregnancy will avoid deficiency. Haemolytic anaemia, a condition with increased cell division, can also lead to folate deficiency (Scott, 2000). Anticonvulsant drug therapy is associated with folate deficiency but the mechanism is not known (Scott, 2000). It was suggested that the drugs cause folate malabsorption or excretion of folate through hepatic enzyme induction but this theory has now been discarded. Chronic alcoholics usually have folate deficiency. The aetiology is unclear. Suggestions are that alcohol causes decreased intestinal absorption, increased renal excretion and is directly toxic to bone marrow and other cells (Scott, 2000).

3.37 Safety/toxicity

Claims have been made that very high folate intakes may result in mood changes but this work has received little or no subsequent support (Hunter et al, 1970). The most important aspect of folate toxicity has occurred as a result of efforts to raise folate status, not by dietary means, but by using supplements and fortification, to protect against NTDs and/or cardiovascular disease. Supplements containing 400µg/day, an adequate amount to give protection, are probably safe. However, because only a minority of those at risk, particularly in the poorer socio-economic groups, can be persuaded to take the supplements, fortification is being considered as an alternative method (Scott et al, 1994). Fortification is associated with some difficulties, because in order to deliver the target dose to those who need it, others who already have a high intake may get up to 10 times that amount. In addition, high amounts of folate will mask vitamin B_{12} deficiency thus allowing the associated neuropathy to develop. High amounts of folate have also been implicated in destabilising epilepsy, which is being controlled with anticonvulsants and accelerating the growth of certain tumours (Scott, 2000). In these effects, toxicity may be dependent on the sustained appearance of folate, instead of 5-methylTHF normally presented to cells. The dose of folate at which any of the above adverse reactions can occur is not known but in calculating safe levels for fortification, 1 mg/d was taken as the upper tolerable intake level to prevent masking of vitamin B_{12} deficiency in the elderly (McNulty, 2001). The recent work by Ward et al (1997) to determine the minimum dose to lower homocysteine concentrations suggests a supplement of 200µg/day to be effective. Hence the proposed level of fortification (2.4 mg/kg flour) should provide the extra 200µg folate/day for both the homocysteine-lowering effects and for reducing risk of NTDs (see section 3.35) and should not exceed safe levels of intake.

3.38 Cobalamin (vitamin B_{12})

Compounds with vitamin B_{12} activity consist of a corrinoid ring surrounding an atom of cobalt, the only known function of cobalt in the human body (Department of Health, 1991). Vitamin B_{12} is involved in recycling folate coenzymes in methionine synthesis (see section 3.33) and degradation of valine via methylmalonyl CoA. Interaction with the folate group of coenzymes is responsible for the condition, megaloblastic anaemia, in which vitamin B_{12} deficiency results in the same syndrome as folate deficiency (see section 3.34) as it is needed to regenerate THF (Fig. 3.3).

Only microorganisms synthesise vitamin B_{12} and the vitamin gets into the food chain from the bacteria present in the digestive system of herbivores. Herbivores are then eaten by animals higher in the food chain. For humans, food sources of vitamin B_{12} include almost all animal products, certain algae and bacteria. Vitamin B_{12} is not present in vegetables or fruits. The dietary intake of vitamin B_{12} is about 5µg/day (Weir and Scott, 1998). The current RDA for B_{12} in most countries is between 1 and 20µg/day; the British RNI are given in Table 3.1. Since food sources of vitamin B_{12} are limited to those of animal origin, vegetarians and especially vegans are at risk of becoming deficient and should take an oral supplement. Studies on these groups have shown evidence of biochemical deficiency such as raised concentrations of homocysteine and methylmalonic acid but no clinical evidence of anaemia or neuropathy. The exception is breastfed infants of vegans, who have developed neuropathy.

3.39 Deficiency

Deficiency of vitamin B_{12} produces two diseases in humans, megoblastic anaemia and a specific neuropathy or subacute combined degeneration of the spinal cord. These complications are seen mainly in pernicious anaemia, first described by James Coombe in 1824 (Wickramasinghe, 1995). The disease is usually fatal in 1–3 years and was first understood by George Minot and William Murphy (1926) who demonstrated that feeding a daily diet of lightly cooked beef liver induced a remission of the anaemia. Subsequently, the beef was shown to have an extrinsic factor (vitamin B_{12}) which required an intrinsic factor (IF) for its normal absorption. IF was produced by normal stomachs but not by those with pernicious anaemia. IF was shown to complex with vitamin B_{12} for uptake and transport by a specific receptor on the ileal enterocytes in the terminal ileum of humans (Weir and Scott, 1995).

The body has no mechanism to control the effects of vitamin B_{12} deficiency. It may be associated with clinical complications such as atheroma, causing coronary thrombosis, stroke, and peripheral vascular disease, neural tube defects or hepatic drain on the stores by steatosis.

The most important causes of B_{12} deficiency are the various forms of intestinal malabsorption of which the autoimmune disease, pernicious anaemia, is the most common. Autoantibodies are produced against the parietal cells of the stomach so the cells can no longer produce IF or hydrochloric acid (HCl). Patients with hypochlorhydria, such as the elderly and postgastrectomy patients, may exhibit malabsorption of dietary cobalamin and a lack of IF prevents absorption of vitamin B_{12}.

Reduced secretion of pancreatic enzymes and bicarbonate leads to impaired digestion of haptocorrins (Hc) (also called R binders, TC I and III or cobalaphilin) and elevation of intestinal pH. Haptocorrins are glycoproteins which bind to vitamin B_{12} in the terminal ileal cells and transport it in the plasma to the cells of the body. Raised pH and low pancreatic enzymes result in cobalamin malabsorption because the transfer of cobalamin from dietary haptocorrins binders to IF is impaired.

Grasbeck-Immerslund syndrome (Weir and Scott, 1999) is a rare congenital disorder where the ileal receptor is either missing or malfunctioning.

Bacterial overgrowth (Weir and Scott, 1999) of the small intestine by colonic bacteria at concentrations greater than 10^8 organisms/L can result in B_{12} deficiency caused by competitive uptake of vitamin B_{12} by the micro-organisms.

Patients with AIDS are known to develop plasma vitamin B_{12} deficiency (Weir and Scott, 1999); however, the pathogenic significance of this still needs to be determined. The condition is thought to be due to failure of the IF-B_{12} complex uptake by the ileal intrinsic factor enterocyte cell wall receptor.

The condition, transcobalamin II (TC II) deficiency (Weir and Scott, 1999), usually presents within the first or second month of life. TC II transports cobalamin from the ileum to the liver where it can be stored or to the tissues where it can be used. Deficiency results in a potentially lethal effect. Early symptoms are vomiting, weakness, failure to thrive and megaloblastic anaemia. The TC defect can be due to TC II being absent or it may be immunologically normal but fail to bind cobalamin, or it may bind cobalamin but fail to be taken up by the cell wall receptor.

Several drugs, such as colchicine, neomycin, *p*-aminosalicylate and alcohol cause vitamin B_{12} malabsorption (Halsted and McIntyre, 1972). In addition, commonly used antacid drugs, such as cimetidine, ranitidine and omeprazole, decrease gastric acid essential for the absorption of vitamin B_{12} from food. The anaesthetic nitrous oxide is known to inactivate methionine synthesis by oxidising vitamin B_{12} to an inactive form. Prolonged exposure to nitrous oxide has been shown to cause neuropathy and subacute combined degeneration of the spinal cord in humans (Layzer et al, 1978).

3.40 Assessment and other issues

The determination of serum vitamin B_{12} concentrations has been the method of choice to assess status for many years. Acceptable concentrations are 147 pmol/L (200 µg/L) and a risk of deficiency is indicated by concentrations <74 pmol/L (100 µg/L). Most circulating vitamin B_{12} is carried on TC I, which is biologically inactive, but representative of the status of the individual. Conventially TC I was measured by a microbiological assay which has been the 'gold standard'. Recently a radiometric assay based on competitive binding between endogenous vitamin B_{12} and an exogenous radioactive form of vitamin B_{12} for a binder has been used. It has been suggested that measuring holo TC II might be a better way of assessing cobalamin deficiency. However, a recently introduced indirect measurement of intra-cellular cobalamin deficiency may be a more functional measure of B_{12} status (Green, 1995). It is the measurement of the substrates of two cobalamin-dependent enzymes, methylmalonic acid (MMA) and homocysteine.

3.40.1 Plasma and urinary methylmalonic acid

Normal variations in dietary intake of MMA do not affect plasma levels. MMA is excreted in the urine and is closely correlated with plasma concentrations. Plasma MMA levels rise in renal failure and in cobalamin deficiency but not in folate deficiency. Plasma concentrations rise from normal values of 0.1–0.4 µmol/L to 50–100 µmol/L in vitamin B_{12} deficiency. MMA in urine or plasma is a sensitive measure of absolute and/or functional vitamin B_{12} deficiency, and is especially useful in the diagnosis of sub-clinical vitamin B_{12} deficiency in the elderly.

3.40.2 Homocysteine

Plasma homocysteine comes predominantly from dietary methionine, although concentrations are sensitive to dietary vitamin B_{12}, folate and pyridoxine, the vitamin co-factors associated with its metabolism (Fig. 3.3). Normal homocysteine concentrations are higher in men than in premenopausal women, but increase with age especially after age 60.

Plasma homocysteine concentrations rise in deficiency states of folate, vitamin B_{12} and pyridoxine, in persons with inborn errors of the enzymes of homocysteine metabolism and in those with defects associated with the synthesis of vitamin B_{12} coenzymes required for normal function of methionine synthetase. However, plasma MMA concentrations seem to be more specific and sensitive indicators of vitamin B_{12} status than homocysteine concentrations and are significantly better than plasma vitamin B_{12}. It is not unknown for normal individuals with normal plasma vitamin B_{12} concentrations to have had elevated levels of MMA that fell after a single injection of vitamin B_{12}. In vitamin B_{12} deficiency, elevated levels of both MMA and homocysteine seem to occur before a fall in plasma vitamin B_{12} (Green, 1995).

3.41 Safety/toxicity

Vitamin B_{12} has extremely low toxicity. It has been found to be toxic in animals only at g/kg levels and no toxic effects have been seen in humans (Department of Health, 1991).

3.42 Biotin

Biotin is a bi-cyclic compound consisting of an imidazole ring fused to a tetrahydrothiophene ring with a valeric acid side-chain. Biotin acts as a co-factor for several carboxylases used in fatty acid synthesis and metabolism and gluconeogenesis and branched-chain amino acid metabolism (Halsted and McIntyre, 1972).

Biotin is widely distributed in food sources (Table 3.2) but the bioavailability of biotin is governed by binding substances in food. For example, biotin is tightly bound by the imidazole ring to avidin in egg white which is released on cooking and in an unavailably-bound form in wheat (Halsted, 2000). Biotin is also synthesised by intestinal flora and *in vivo* studies suggest there is significant absorption of biotin from the proximal and transverse colon which may be from intestinal bacteria. The extent to which biotin is available is not known. Biotin and its metabolites are excreted at a rate of 6–50 µg/day in urine and faecal excretion of biotin is 3–6 times the intake (Department of Health, 1991).

Signs of biotin deficiency have been recorded in in-patients receiving total pareneral nutrition for prolonged periods. Biotin supplements (60–200 µg) appeared to resolve the deficiency. The COMA panel did not set DRVs but the average intake by British men is 39 µg/day (range 15–70 µg) and by women 26 µg/day (10–58 µg), hence the average requirement is thought to lie within this range (Department of Health, 1991), but if microbial biotin is utilised by humans, requirements may be much higher.

Three of the four biotin-dependent carboxylases are mitochondrial: propionyl-CoA carboxylase, methylcrotonyl-CoA carboxylase and pyruvate carboxylase; the fourth, acetyl-CoA carboxylase, is found in the mitochondria and the cytosol. Pyruvate carboxylase is a key enzyme in gluconeogenesis, so impairment as a result of biotin deficiency may lead to fasting hypoglycaemia. Work with chicks showed a fatal hypoglycaemia called 'fatty liver-kidney syndrome' was due to impaired gluconeogenesis caused by deficient activity of pyruvate carboxylase. Several workers have suggested that biotin deficiency may cause sudden infant death syndrome (SIDS) by an analogous pathogenic mechanism (Mock, 1999). The hypothesis was supported by demonstrating that hepatic biotin concentrations were significantly lower in infants who died from SIDS than those dying from other causes. Further work is needed to confirm this finding.

There are no reports of biotin toxicity in amounts up to 10 mg/day.

3.43 Pantothenic acid

Pantothenic acid is a dimethyl derivative of butyric acid linked to alanine. The vitamin is linked through phosphate to form $4'$-phosphopantetheine and coenzyme A (CoA), the primary active form. As a constituent of CoA and its esters, the vitamin is essential for numerous reactions involved in lipid and carbohydrate metabolism including fatty acid synthesis and degradation, steroid hormone synthesis and gluconeogenesis (Halsted, 2000).

Rich dietary sources of pantothenic acid are listed in Table 3.2. Especially high levels of pantothenate are found in royal bee jelly (511 µg/g) and in ovaries of tuna and cod (2.3 mg/g). Human breast milk pantothenate content increases five-fold within 4 days of the birth of the baby from 2.2 to 11.2 µmol/L, similar to that found in cow's milk.

No biochemical method has been accepted for determining pantothenate concentrations in humans. Measurements have been made on blood levels and urine excretion but it has not been possible to interpret the results in terms of dietary needs. The COMA panel derived no DRVs for pantothenate and as there are no signs of pantothenic acid deficiency in the UK, intakes of between 3 and 7 mg/day were deemed adequate even during pregnancy and lactation (Department of Health, 1991).

3.44 Deficiency

3.44.1 Nutritional melalgia

Deficiency in humans is rare and has only been detected in conditions of severe malnutrition. In World War II prisoners of war in the Philippines, Japan and

Burma experienced numbness of their toes and painful burning sensations in their feet (nutritional melalgia). They were treated with yeast extract as a source of all B vitamins.

3.44.2 Hair colour
Early studies showed a loss of fur colour in black and brown rats fed a pantothenic acid-deficient diet; as a consequence pantothenate became known as the anti-grey hair factor. Even though there is no evidence to support the idea that loss of hair colour with age is related to pantothenic acid deficiency, it is still added to shampoos (Bender, 1999).

3.44.3 Alzheimer's disease
In Japan, homopantothenate (pantoyl γ-aminobutyrate), the next highest homologue of pantothenic acid, is used to enhance cognitive function, especially in Alzheimer's disease. It acts via γ-aminobutyrate receptors to increase acetyl choline release and cholinergic function in the cerebral cortex and hippocampus (Bender, 1999). A rare side-effect of the treatment is hepatic encephalopathy and the excretion of a variety of dicarboxylates, both effects being reversed by pantothenate, suggesting homopantothenate may cause pantothenate deficiency. If this is verified dicarboxylic aciduria may provide a marker of pantothenate status. However, the alternative theory might be that the adverse effects are due to toxicity of homopantothenate which is antagonised by pantothenate.

3.45 Toxicity
There are no reports of toxicity with intakes up to 10 g/day.

3.46 Niacin
Niacin is a generic term for nicotinic acid and nicotinamide, both of which are substrates for the synthesis of nicotinamide nucleotide coenzymes, NAD and the phosphorylated derivative of NADP (Powers, 1999). The major metabolic role of NAD(P) is as a coenzyme in oxidation and reduction reactions. Niacin is therefore of crucial importance in intermediary metabolism and requirement is related to energy expenditure (Department of Health, 1991). Deficiency of niacin results in pellagra, which is fatal if untreated.

Quantitation of dietary niacin must take into account the dual source of the vitamin, the vitamin nicotinic acid and the amino acid tryptophan. Niacin in food is quantified as niacin equivalents (NE). Dietary sources are listed in Table 3.2 but meat is a rich source of both tryptophan and niacin.

High intake of tryptophan results in greater efficiency of conversion to niacin.

Oestrogens reduce the rate of tryptophan metabolism, so where pellagra is common, twice as many women as men are affected. However, before puberty and after menopause there are no sex differences. It is generally believed that 1 NE is equivalent to 60 mg of tryptophan or 1 mg dietary niacin.

The mean observed requirement for niacin to prevent or cure pellagra, or to normalise the urinary excretion of N-methyl nicotinamide (NMN) and its onward metabolite methyl pyridone carboxamide (MPCX), in experimental subjects maintained on niacin-deficient diets and in energy balance, is 5.5 mg/4.2 MJ (1000 kcal). A coefficient of variation of 10% gives an RNI of 6.6 mg/4.2 MJ (i.e. plus 2 SD) and an LNRI of 4.4 mg/4.2 MJ. A summary of niacin requirements is given in Table 3.1.

Niacin deficiency causes pellagra and occurs in parts of India and the African continent. Pellagra is frequently associated with the 'hungry season', strong sunshine and with diets of mainly maize and millet. The clinical features of pellagra are dermatitis, diarrhoea and dementia. Pellagra is occasionally found in malnourished alcoholic patients and it has been found associated with the intake of mycotoxins from the mould *Fusarium*. Pellagra occurs in Hartnup's disease, an autosomal recessive disorder with impaired absorption of several amino acids including tryptophan (Thurnham, 2000).

Classic pellagra responds dramatically to nicotinamide or niacin given at a dose of 100–300 mg/day in three doses. In addition to niacin, it is usual to give riboflavin and pyridoxine and a diet high in calories and protein. Mental changes disappear within 24–48 hours but dermal lesions may take 3–4 weeks. A dose of 40–200 mg niacin/day can be used to treat the symptoms of Hartnup's disease. Doses of 1–2 g/day of niacin are used to manage patients with hypertriglyceridaemia and/or hypercholesterolaemia. However, nicotinic acid, but not nicotinamide, in excess of 200 mg causes vasodilation of cutaneous blood vessels. Higher doses cause vasodilation of other blood vessels and a transient drop in blood pressure (Thurnham, 2000).

3.47 Vitamin B$_6$ (pyridoxine)

The term vitamin B$_6$ includes three pyridines: pyridoxine, pyridoxal and pyridoxamine and their 5′-phosphorylated derivatives, which are metabolically interconvertible. The liver is the main tissue responsible for converting pyridoxine and pyridoxamine phosphates into pyridoxal 5′-phosphate (PLP). PLP is the main coenzyme form of the vitamin and the co-factor for a large number of enzymes catalysing reactions of amino acids (Department of Health, 1991). PLP is also the main extra-cellular form of the vitamin, being transported in plasma bound to albumin. PLP, which is not enzyme-bound, is oxidised to pyridoxic acid and excreted in urine (Powers, 1999).

The vitamin is widely distributed in foods (Table 3.2), although much of the vitamin B$_6$ in some vegetables may be present as glycosides, which are unavailable. The intestinal bacteria are also able to synthesise relatively large amounts of pyridoxine (Department of Health, 1991). Intestinal absorption takes place mainly in the jejunum by non-saturable, passive diffusion of the non-phosphorylated forms of the vitamin. Post-absorptive phosphorylation of all three forms is catalysed by pyridoxal kinase and the phosphorylation constitutes a form of cellular trapping in intestinal cells and other tissues (liver, muscles and brain) as the charge on the phosphate hinders efflux through the cell membrane. Pyridoxine exhibits greater stability than other forms of the vitamin. As the hydrochloride salt, it is used in dietary supplements and food fortification because of its stability, comparative ease of manufacture and low cost (Gregory, 2001).

The total body pool of vitamin B_6 is about 15 µmol/kg body weight. Isotope tracer studies have indicated a turnover of about 0.13%/day hence the estimated minimum requirement for replacement is 0.02 µmol (5 µg)/kg body weight or 350 µg/day for a 70 kg adult. Vitamin B_6 is extensively required in protein metabolism hence depletion studies have shown that deficiency develops more quickly on high protein intakes (80–160 g/day) and repletion is faster at lower intakes of protein (30–50 g/day). Therefore RNIs are based on protein intakes and estimated at 15–16 µg/g protein (Department of Health, 1991). At average intakes of about 100 g protein/day, this gives an RNI of 1.5–1.6 mg vitamin B_6 (Table 3.1). Average intakes in Britain are between 20 and 30 µg/g protein (Thurnham, 2000).

3.48 Deficiency

Clinical deficiencies in vitamin B_6 are rare. However, severe deficiency of vitamin B_6 was reported in 1954 when infants were fed formula, which had been severely heated during manufacture. The heating caused the formation of pyridoxyllysine, which has anti-vitamin metabolic activity. The affected infants suffered seizures, which responded to B_6 supplements (Coursin, 1954).

Other groups vulnerable to vitamin B_6 deficiency and deficiency of other water-soluble vitamins, are those suffering from malabsorption, coeliac disease, chronic alcoholics and those undergoing dialysis for renal failure.

Clinical signs of deficiency are inflammation of the tongue, lesions of the lips and corners of the mouth; however, these symptoms are also seen in riboflavin deficiency. Peripheral neuropathy is found in thiamin as well as in pyridoxine deficiency. Finally, microcytic hypochromic (sideroblastic) anaemia associated with pyridoxine deficiency is caused by impaired synthesis of haem (Thurnham, 2000).

3.48.1 Vitamin B_6 and plasma homocysteine

Evidence suggests that elevated homocysteine concentrations are a risk factor for cardiovascular disease. As several steps in the metabolism of homocysteine are vitamin B_6-dependent, several workers have investigated the effects of vitamin

B_6 nutrition on plasma homocysteine concentrations and its metabolites. However, fasting homocysteine concentrations are only weakly related to vitamin B_6 status. It appears that reduced efficiency of the vitamin B_6 dependent trans-sulphuration reactions are adequately countered by cellular remethylation capacity, and the steady state of plasma homocysteine is unaffected. That is, plasma homocysteine is much more strongly influenced by folate and vitamin B_{12} status than vitamin B_6 status (Gregory, 2001).

3.49 Safety/toxicity

Sensory neuropathy developed in 7 patients taking 2–7 g/day pyridoxine and although there was residual damage in some patients, withdrawal of these extremely high doses resulted in considerable recovery of sensory nerve function (Schaumburg et al, 1983). Dalton and Dalton (1987) reported peripheral sensory neuropathy in 60% of 172 women taking 50–500 mg B_6/day for between 6 and 60 months, and even in women taking only 50 mg B_6/day, 40% reported symptoms of peripheral sensory neuropathy. Within 6 months of stopping the supplements all the women recovered.

3.50 Riboflavin

The concept of 'accessory growth factors' in biological fluids such as milk which enabled rats to grow on a purified carbohydrate diet led to the characterisation of a flavin component in 1932 (Bates, 1987). It was given a number of names, usually indicating the food of extraction e.g. lactoflavin (milk), ovoflavin (egg); later it was called vitamin G in the USA and finally vitamin B_2 or riboflavin (Thurnham, 2000). Riboflavin is an isoalloxazine ring linked to a ribityl side-chain. Modifications of the ribityl side-chain include an ester phosphate linkage to form flavin mononucleotide (FMN), and the latter can then be linked with adenine monophosphate to form flavin adenine dinucleotide (FAD). FMN and FAD are the two coenzyme forms of riboflavin in tissues (Thurnham, 2000).

Principal dietary sources are dairy products, meat and in some countries beer, and a small amount from green vegetables (see Table 3.2). Cereals are often a poor source of riboflavin, but because of the amount consumed, they often make a significant contribution to meeting requirements in developing countries. For example, in The Gambia the staple food is rice made with a sauce of stewed groundnuts and both are poor sources of riboflavin (Bates, 1987). In developed countries cereals are often fortified with riboflavin and eaten with milk; in this way they make a significant contribution to the dietary intake (Thurnham, 2000). Riboflavin is heat-stable, so losses through cooking are only about 10%, but it is easily destroyed by sunlight in such products as milk.

Riboflavin coenzymes are required in the Krebs cycle, hence requirements for riboflavin are often linked to energy requirements. One particularly important enzyme which requires riboflavin is glutathione reductase (EC 1.6.4.2). This enzyme is needed to maintain glutathione in the reduced state (GSH). The enzyme occurs in all aerobic tissues and GSH is an important constituent to maintain the cellular redox potential and cellular integrity. Riboflavin coenzymes are also required in the metabolism of other nutrients. Riboflavin is required to convert pyridoxine phosphate to pyridoxal phosphate, therefore a deficiency in riboflavin may impair the conversion of tryptophan to niacin (section 3.46). Anaemia is sometimes associated with riboflavin deficiency but this may be partly related to impaired conversion of folic acid to 5N-methyl-tetrahydrofolic acid (see Fig. 3.3).

There are few epidemiological studies which can be used to determine minimum requirements, because classical signs of deficiency are not completely specific and respond only moderately to riboflavin supplements (Department of Health, 1991). Requirements are also dependent on the status of other nutrients and precipitating factors (Thurnham et al, 1971). In 1990, a survey of British adults showed the median intake of riboflavin for men was 2.03 mg/day and for women it was 1.56 mg/day. Erythrocyte glutathione reductase activation coefficient (EGRAC) values below 1.3 represent adequate tissue saturation and satisfactory long-term riboflavin status. EGRAC values of 1.3 or above were found in ~2% of British adults on normal diets. Mean dietary intakes in the latter persons corresponded to intakes of 1.3 mg/day for men and 1.1 mg/day for women. The COMA panel decided to base their RNIs on those intakes (Table 3.1, Department of Health, 1991).

The widespread consumption of dairy products and use of fortified foods in industrialised countries provides a high dietary intake for most people, hence the very small proportion of poor EGRAC values in the UK National Survey (Gregory et al, 1990). Furthermore, there were only ~15% with raised EGRAC results in the Pre-School Child Survey (Gregory et al, 1995). These results contrast markedly with values found in developing countries where availability of dairy foods and animal food in general is restricted. Status is at best marginal and often influenced by seasonal availability of food.

Clinical signs of deficiency are often associated with damage to the epithelium but are non-specific. For example, cracks in the corners of the mouth (angular stomatitis) are frequently linked to riboflavin deficiency but can also occur in other water-soluble, vitamin-deficient states e.g. niacin, pyridoxine and folate. Cracked lips (cheilosis), swollen red beefy tongue (glossitis) and scrotal dermatitis are also associated with the deficiency. In experimental studies, growth inhibition is a typical sign of severe deficiency. In developing countries, poor growth is characteristic in many infants and children and riboflavin deficiency undoubtedly contributes to the problem.

The low solubility of riboflavin prevents its absorption from the gastrointestinal tract in amounts sufficient to produce toxic effects. When 120 mg/day were used for 10 months to treat congenital methaemoglobinaemia, no adverse effects were reported (Department of Health, 1991).

3.51 References

AKJBA T, KURIHARA S and TACHIBANA K (1991), 'Vitamin K (K) increased bone mass (BM) in hemo-dialysis patients (pts) with low-turnover bone disease (LTOBD)', *J Am Soc Nephrol*, **608**, 42–9

Alpha-tocopherol Beta-Carotene (ATBC) Cancer Prevention Study Group (1994), 'The effect of vitamin E and beta carotene on the incidence of lung cancer and other cancers in male smokers', *New Engl J Med*, **330**, 1029

ARMSTRONG R B, ASHENFELTER K O, ECKHOFF C, LEVIN A A and SHAPIRO S S (1994), 'General and reproductive toxicology of retinoids', in *The retinoids: Biology, Chemistry and Medicine*, 2 ed, M B Sporn, A B Roberts and D S Goodman (eds), New York, Raven Press, 545–72

AUTRET-LECA E and JONVILLE-BERA A P (2001), 'Vitamin K in neonates: how to administer, when and to whom', *Pediatric Drugs*, **3**, 1–8

AZZI A, ARATRI E, BOSCOBOINIK D, CLEMENT S, OZER N, RICCIARELLI R, SPYCHER, S and STOCKER, A (2001), 'Vitamins and regulation of gene expression', in *Functions of Vitamins beyond Recommended Dietary Allowances*. Bibl Nutr Dieta, No 55, P Walter, D Hornig and U Moser (eds), Basel, Karger, 177–88

BAEUERLE P A and HENKEL T (1994), 'Function and activation of NFκB in the immune system', *Ann Rev Immunol*, **12**, 141–79

BAKER E M, HODGES R E, HOOD J, SAUBERLICH H E, MARCH S C and CANHAM J E (1971), 'Metabolism of ^{14}C- and ^{3}H-labeled L-ascorbic acid in human scurvy', *Am J Clin Nutr*, **24**, 444–54

BALCKE P, SCHMIDT P, ZAZGARNIK J, KOPSA H and HAUBENSTOCK A (1984), 'Ascorbic acid aggravates secondary hyperoxalemia in patients on chronic hemodialysis', *Ann Intern Med*, **100**, 344–5

BAMJI M S (1970), 'Transketolase activity and urinary excretion of thiamin in the assessment of thiamin-nutrition status of Indians', *Am J Clin Nutr*, **23**, 52–8

BARTLEY W, KREBS H A and O'BRIEN J R P (1953), *Vitamin C Requirements of Human Adults*, London, HMSO, 280

BATES C J (1987), 'Human riboflavin requirements and metabolic consequences of deficiency in man and animals', in *World Review of Nutrition and Dietetics* 50, G H Bourne (ed), Basel, Karger, 215–65

BELLIZZI M C, FRANKLIN M F, DUTHIE G G and JAMES W P T (1994), 'Vitamin E and coronary heart disease: the European paradox', *Eur J Clin Nutr*, **48**, 822–31

BENDER D A (1999), 'Optimum nutrition: thiamin, biotin and pantothenate', *Proc Nutr Soc*, **58**, 427–33

BENDICH A and MACHLIN L J (1988), 'Safety of oral intake of vitamin E', *Am J Clin Nutr*, **48**, 612–19

BENDICH A, MACHLIN L J, SCANDURRA O, BURTON G W and WAYNER D D M (1986), 'The antioxidant role of vitamin C', *Adv Free Rad Biol Med*, **2**, 419–44

BERKNER K L (2000), 'The vitamin K-dependent carboxylase', *J Nutr*, **130**, 1877

BINKLEY N C and SUTTIE J W (1995), 'Vitamin K nutrition and osteoporosis', *J Nutr*, **125**, 1812–21

BLOMHOFF R (2001), 'Vitamin A and carotenoid toxicity.' *Food Nutr Bull*, **22**, 320–34

BLOT W J, LI J Y, TAYLOR P R, GUO W, DAWSEY S, WANG G Q, YANG C S, ZENG S F, GAIL M and LI G Y (1993), 'Nutrition intervention trials in Linxian, China: supplementation with specific vitamin/mineral combinations, cancer incidence and disease specific mortality in the general population', *J Natl Cancer Inst*, **85**, 1483–93

BOLTON-SMITH C, MOLE P A, MCMURDO M E T, PATERSON C R and SHEARER M J (2001), 'Two-year intervention with phylloquinone (vitamin K_1), vitamin D and calcium effect on bone mineral content of older women', *Ann Nutr Metabol*, **45**(Suppl I), 46

BOOHER L, CALLISON E and HEWSTON E (1939), 'An experimental determination of the minimum vitamin requirements of normal adults', *J Nutr*, **17**, 317–31

BOOTH S L, PENNINGTON J A T and SADOWSKI J A (1996), 'Food sources and dietary intakes of vitamin K_1 (phylloquinone) in the American diet: data from FDA Total Diet Study', *J Am Dietetic Soc*, **96**, 149–54

BRIN M (1964), 'Erythrocyte as a biopsy tissue for functional evaluation of thiamin adequacy', *J. Am Med Assoc*, **187**, 762–6

BURTON G W and INGOLD K U (1981), 'Autoxidation of biological molecules. 1. The antioxidant activity of vitamin E and related chain-breaking phenolic antioxidants in vitro', *J Am Chem Soc*, **103**, 6472–7

CAMPBELL G A, KEMM J R, HOSKING D J and BOYD R V (1994), 'How common is osteomalacia in the elderly?' *Lancet*, **2**, 386–8

CANTORNA M T, NASHOLD F E and HAYES C E (1994), 'In vitamin A deficiency multiple mechanisms establish a regulatory T helper cell imbalance with excess Th1 and insufficient Th2 function', *J Immunol*, **152**, 1515–22

CASTENMILLAR J J A and WEST C E (1998), 'Bioavailability and bioconversion of carotenoids', *Ann Rev Nutr*, **18**, 19–38

CHAUDIERE J and FERRARI-ILIOU R (1999), 'Intracellular antioxidants from chemical to biochemical mechanisms', *Food Chem Toxicol*, **37**, 949–62

CHEVION M, JIANG Y, HAR-EL R, BERENSHTEIN E, URETZKY G and KITROSSKY N (1993), 'Copper and iron are mobilized following myocardial ischaemia: possible predictive criteria for tissue injury', *Proc Natl Acad Sci*, **90**, 1102–6

CHOPRA M, MCLOONE U J, O'NEILL M, WILLIAMS N and THURNHAM D I (1996), 'Fruit and vegetable supplementation – effect on *ex vivo* LDL oxidation in humans', in *Natural Antioxidants and Food Quality in Atherosclerosis and Cancer Prevention*, J T Kumpulainen and J T Saonen (eds), Cambridge, Royal Society of Chemistry, 150–5

CLARK M A and FISK N M (1994), 'Minimal compliance with the Department of Health recommendation for routine folate prophylaxis to prevent neural tube defects', *Br J Obs Gynaecol*, **101**, 709–10

CLARK R and Homocysteine Lowering Trials Collaboration (1998), 'Lowering blood homocysteine with folic acid based supplements: meta-analysis of randomised trials', *Br Med J*, **316**, 894

CMAFP (Committee on Medical Aspects of Food Policy) (1977), *The composition of mature human milk*, Report on health and social subjects, no. 12, Department of Health and Social Security, London, HMSO

CONLY J M S K (1992), 'Quantitative and qualitative measurements of K vitamins in human intestinal contents', *Am J Gastroenterol*, **87**, 311–16

CORRIGAN J J and MARCUS S (1974), 'Coagulopathy associated with vitamin E ingestion' *J Am Med Assoc*, **230**, 1300–1

COURSIN D B (1954), 'Convulsive seizures in infants with pyridoxine-deficient diet', *J Am Med Assoc*, **154**, 406–8

CUSKELLY G J, MCNULTY H and SCOTT J M (1996), 'Effect of increasing dietary folate on red-cell folate: implications for the prevention of neural tube defects', *Lancet*, **347**, 657–9

CZEIZEL A E and DUDAS I (1992), 'Prevention of the first occurrence of neural-tube defects by periconceptual vitamin supplementation', *New Engl J Med*, **327**, 1832–5

DALTON K and DALTON M J T (1987), 'Characteristics of pyridoxine overdose neuropathy syndrome', *Acta Neurol Scand*, **76**, 8–11

DALY S, MILLS J, MOLLOY A, CONLEY M, LEE Y, KIRKE P, WEIR D and SCOTT J (1997), 'Minimum effective dose of folic acid for food fortification to prevent neural tube defects', *Lancet*, **350**, 105

DE PEE S and WEST C E (1996), 'Dietary carotenoids and their role in combating vitamin A deficiency: a review of the literature', *Eur J Clin Nutr*, **50**, Suppl 3, S38–S53

DE PEE S, WEST C E, PERMAESIH D, MARUUTI S, MUHILAL and HAUTVAST J G A J (1998), 'Orange fruit is more effective than are dark green, leafy vegetables in increasing serum

concentrations of retinol and β-carotene in school children in Indonesia', *Am J Clin Nutr*, **68**, 1058–67
DE WAART F G, PORTENGEN L, GOEKES G, VERWAAL C J and KOK F J (1997), 'Effect of 3 months vitamin E supplementation on indices of the cellular and humoral immune response in elderly subjects', *Br J Nutr*, **78**, 761–74
Department of Health (1991), *Dietary Reference Values for Food Energy and Nutrients for the United Kingdom*, Report of the Panel on Dietary Reference Values of the Committee on Medical aspects of Food Policy, London, HMSO 41
Department of Health (1992), *Folic Acid and the Prevention of Neural Tube Defects*. Report from an Expert Advisory Group, London, HMSO
Department of Health (2000), *Folic acid and the Prevention of Disease*. Report on Health and Social Subjects, London, The Stationery Office
Department of Health and Social Security (1979), *Recommended Daily Amounts of Food and Energy and Nutrients for Groups of People in the United Kingdom*, London, HMSO
DOUGLAS A S, ROBINE S P and HUTCHISON J D (1995), 'Carboxylation of osteocalcin in post-menopausal osteoporotic women following vitamin K and vitamin D supplementation', *Bone*, **17**, 15
DUTHIE G G (2000), 'Fat-soluble vitamins: vitamin E and its antioxidant role in relation to other dietary components', in *Human Nutrition and Dietetics*, 10 ed, J S Garrow, W P T James and A Ralph (eds), London, Churchill Livingstone, 226–36
EIJKMAN C (1897), 'Ein Versuchnzur Bekampfung der Beri-Beri', *Virchows Archiv fur Pathologisch anatomie und Physiologie und fur klinische Medizin*, **149**, 187–94
ESTERBAUER H, GEBICKI J, PUHL H and JURGENS G (1992), 'The role of lipid peroxidation and antioxidants in the oxidative modification of LDL', *Free Rad Biol Med*, **13**, 341–9
FAO/WHO Expert Consultation (1988), Joint report, *Requirements of vitamin A, iron, folate and vitamin B_{12}*, Rome, Food and Agriculture Organization of the United Nations/World Health Organisation
FAO/WHO (1967), 'Requirements of vitamin A, thiamine, riboflavin and niacin', *FAO Food and Nutrition Series* 8, Rome, FAO
FUNK C (1911), 'The chemical nature of the substance which cures polyneuritis in birds induced by a diet of polished rice', *J Physiol*, **43**, 395–400
GARLAND C F, COMSTOCK G W, GARLAND F C, HELSING K J, SHAW E K and GORHAM E D (1989), 'Serum 25-hydroxyvitamin D and colon cancer: eight-year prospective study', *Lancet* **2**, 1176–8
GEY K F (1993), 'Prospects for the prevention of free radical disease, regarding cancer and cardiovascular disease', *Br Med Bull*, **49**, 679–99
GOLDING J, PATERSON M, KINLEN L J (1990), 'Factors associated with childhood cancer. A national cohort study', *Br J Cancer*, **62**, 304–8
GOLDING J, GREENWOOD R, BIRMINGHAM K and MOTT M (1992), 'Childhood cancer, intramuscular vitamin K and pethidine given during labour', *Br Med J*, **305**, 341–6
GOLDRING C E P, NARAYANAN R, LAGADEC P and JEANNIN J-F (1995), 'Transcriptional inhibition of the inducible nitric oxide synthase gene by competitive binding of the NF-κB/rel proteins', *Biochem Biophys Res Comm*, **209**, 73–9
GOPALAN C, RAMA SASTR B V, BALASUBRAMANIAN S C, NARASINGA RAO B S, DEOSTHALE Y G and PANT K C (1989), *Nutritive Value of Indian Foods*, New Delhi, ICMR Offset Press
GREEN R (1995), 'Metabolite assays in cobalamin and folate deficiencies', in *Megaloblastic Anaemia, Clinical Haematology*, S N Wickramasinghe (ed), London, Bailliere Tindall, 533–66
GREGORY J F (1995), 'The bioavailability of folate', in *Folate in Health and Disease*, L B Bailey (ed), New York, Marcel Dekker 195–235
GREGORY J F (2001), 'Vitamin B_6 deficiency', in *Homocysteine in Health and Disease*, R Carmel and D W Jocobsen (eds), Cambridge University Press, Cambridge, UK 307–20
GREGORY J R, FOSTER K, TYLER H and WISEMAN M (1990), *The Dietary and Nutritional Survey of British Adults*, London, HMSO

GREGORY J F, BHANDARI S D, BAILEY L B, TOTH J P and CERDA J J (1991), 'Relative bioavailability of deuterium-labelled monoglutamyl and hexaglutamyl folates in human subjects', *Am J Clin Nutr*, **53**, 736–40

GREGORY J R, COLLINS D L, DAVIES P S W, HUGHES J M and CLARKE P C (1995), *National Diet and Nutrition Survey: Children aged 1 1/2 to 4 1/2 years*, London, HMSO

GRIMBLE R F (1997), 'Effect of antioxidant vitamins on immune function with clinical applications', *Int J Vit Nutr Res*, **67**, 312–20

GUDAS L J, SPORN M B and ROBERTS A B (1991), 'Cellular biology and biochemistry of the retinoids', in *The Retinoids: Biology, Chemistry and Medicine*, 2 ed, MB Sporn, AB Roberts and DS Goodman, New York, Raven Press

HALLIWELL B (1994), 'Vitamin C: the key to health or a slow acting carcinogen?', *Redox Reports*, **1**, 5–9

HALLIWELL B (2001), 'Vitamin C and genomic stability', *Mutation Research*, **475**, 29–35

HALSTED C H (2000), 'Biotin and pantothenic acid', in *Human Nutrition and Dietetics*, 10 ed, J S Garrow, W P T James and A Ralph (eds), London, Churchill Livingstone, 281–2

HALSTED C H and MCINTYRE P A (1972), 'Intestinal malabsorption caused by aminosalicylic acid therapy', *Arch Int Med*, **130**, 935–9

HAUSCHKA P V, LAIN J B and GALLOP P M (1975), 'Direct indentification of the calcium-binding amino acid, gamma carboxyglutamate, in mineralised tissue', *Proc Nat Acad Sci*, **72**, 3925–9

Heart Outcomes Prevention Evaluation (HOPE) Study (2000), 'Vitamin E supplementation and cardiovascular events in high-risk patients', *New Engl J Med*, **342**, 154–60

HENNEKENS C H, BURNING J E, MANSON J E and STAMPFER M (1996), 'Lack of effect of long-term supplementation with beta-carotene on the incidence of malignant neoplasms and cardiovascular disease', *New Engl J Med*, **334**, 1145

HININGER I, CHOPRA M, THURNHAM D I, LAPORTE F, RICHARD M J, FAVIER A and ROUSSEL A-M (1997), 'Effect of increased fruit and vegetable intake on the susceptibility of lipoprotein to oxidation in smokers', *Eur J Clin Nutr*, **51**, 601–6

HODGES R E, BAKER E M, HOOD J, SAUBERLICH H E and MARCH S C (1969), 'Experimental scurvy in man', *Am J Clin Nutr*, **22**, 535–48

HOLICK M F (1994), 'McCollum Award Lecture, 1994: vitamin D – new horizons for the 21st century', *Am J Clin Nutr*, **60**, 619–30

HOMEWOOD J and BOND N W (1999), 'Thiamin Deficiency and Korsakoff's Syndrome – Possible role of thiamine', *Alcohol*, **19**, 75–84

HONEIN M A, PAULOZZI L J, MATHEWS T J, ERICKSON J D and WONG L-Y (2001), 'Impact of folic acid fortification of the US food supply on the occurrence of neural tube defects', *J Am Med Assoc*, **285**, 2981–6

HOWARD A N, WILLIAMS N R and PALMER C R (1996), 'Do hydroxy carotenoids prevent coronary heart disease? A comparison between Belfast and Toulouse', *Int J Vit Nutr Res* **66**, 113–18

HUGHES D A (2001), 'Dietary carotenoids and human immune function', *Nutrition*, **17**, 823–7

HUME E M and KREBS H A (1949), *Vitamin A Requirement of Human Adults: an Experimental Study of Vitamin A deprivation in man*, London, Medical Research Council

HUNTER R, BARNES J, OAKLEY H F and MATTHEWS, D M (1970), 'Toxicity of folic acid given in pharmacological doses to healthy volunteers', *Lancet*, **1**, 61–2

HYPPÖNEN E, LÄÄRÄ E, REUNANEN A, JÄRVELIN M-R and VIRTANEN S M (2001), 'Intake of vitamin D and risk of type 1 diabetes: a birth-cohort study', *Lancet*, **358**, 1500

IBNER F L, BLASS J P and BRIN M (1982), 'Thiamin in the elderly, relation to alcoholism and to neurological degenerative disease', *Am J Clin Nutr*, **36**, 1067–82

Institute of Medicine (2001), 'A report of the panel on micronutrients, subcommittees on upper reference levels of nutrients and of interpretation and use of dietary reference intakes, and the standing committee on the scientific evaluation of dietary reference intakes,' *Dietary Reference Intakes for vitamin A, vitamin K, arsenic, boron, chromium, copper, iodine, iron, manganese, molybdenum, nickel, silicon, vanadium, zinc*, Washington DC, Food and Nutrition Board, National Academy Press

JACKSON M J (1997), 'The assessment of bioavailability of micronutrients: introduction', *Eur J Clin Nutr*, **51**, Suppl 1, S1–S2

JACOB R A (1999), 'Vitamin C', in *Modern Nutrition in Health & Disease*, 9 ed, M E Shils, J A Olson, M Shihe and A C Ross (eds), Baltimore, Lippincott, Williams & Wilkins, 467–83

JARIWALLA R J and HARAKEH S (1996), 'Antiviral and immunodilatory activities of ascorbic acid', in *Subcellular biochemistry, Ascorbic acid: Biochemistry and Biomedical Cell Biology*, J R Harris (ed), New York, Plenum Press, 215–31

KALLNER A B, HARTMANN D and HORNIG D H (1979), 'Steady state turnover and body pool of ascorbic acid in man', *Am J Clin Nutr*, **32**, 530–9

KALLNER A B, HARTMANN D and HORNIG D H (1981), 'On the requirements of ascorbic acid in man: steady-state turnover and body pool in smokers', *Am J Clin Nutr*, **34**, 1347–55

KHAN N C, WEST C E, DE PEE S and KHOI H H (1998), 'Comparison of effectiveness of carotenoids from dark green leafy vegetables and yellow and orange fruits in improving vitamin A status of breastfeeding women in Vietnam', Washington, DC, ILSI

KHOSLA S and KLEEREKOPER M (1999), 'Biochemical markers of bone turnover', in *Primer on the Metabolic Bone Diseases and Disorders of Mineral Metabolism*, M J Favus (ed), Philadelphia, Lippincott Williams & Wilkins, 128

KLIEWER S A, UMESONO K, EVANS R M and MANGLESDORF D T (1994), 'The retinoid X receptors. Modulators of multiple hormonal signalling pathways', in *Vitamin A in Health and Disease*, R Blumhoff (ed), New York, Marcel Dekker, 239–55

KRALL E A and DAWSON-HUGHES B (1991), 'Relation of fractional 47Ca retention to season and rates of bone loss in healthy postmenopausal women', *J Bone Mineral Res* **6**, 1323–9, Abstract

KRINSKY N I (2001), 'Carotenoids as antioxidants', *Nutrition*, **17**, 815–17

KROLNER B (1983), 'Seasonal variation of lumbar spine bone mineral content in normal women', *Calcified Tissue Int*, **35**, 145–7

KUBLER W and GEHLER J (1970), 'On the kinetics of the intestinal absorption of ascorbic acid: a contribution to the calculation of an absorption process that is not proportional to the dose', *Int J Vit Nutr Res*, **40**, 442–53

LAYZER R B, FISHMAN R A and SCHAFER J A (1978), 'Neuropathy following abuse of nitrous oxide', *Neurology*, **28**, 485

LIPSKY J J (1994), 'Nutritional sources of vitamin K', *Mayo Clin Proc*, **69**, 462

LOVERIDGE N (2000), 'Vitamin D (calciferols)', in *Human Nutrition and Dietetics*, 10 ed, J S Garrow, W P T James and A Ralph (eds), London, Churchill Livingstone, 221–6

LUDVIGSSON J, HANSSON LO and STENDAHL O (1979), 'The effect of large doses of vitamin C on leucocyte function and some laboratory parameters', *Int J Vitamin Nutr Res*, **49**, 160–5

LUYKEN R (1990), '*Polyneuritis in Chickens, or the Origin of Vitamin Research*' (first English edition of papers by Christian Eijkman published 1860–1896, lying at the root of international vitamin research), Basel, Roche

MACHLIN L J and HUNI, J E S (1994), 'Introduction', in *Vitamins*, Basel, Hoffmann-La Roche, i–iv

MAXWELL J D (2001), 'Seasonal variation in vitamin D', *Proc Nutr Soc*, **53**, 533–43

MCCANCE R A and WIDDOWSON E M (1943), 'Seasonal and annual changes in the calcium metabolism of man', *J Physiol*, **102**, 42–9

MCDERMOTT J H (2000), 'Antioxidant nutrients: current dietary recommendations and research update', *J Am Pharm Assoc*, **40**, 785

MCNULTY H (1997), 'Folate requirements for health in women', *Proc Nutr Soc*, **56**, 91–303

MCNULTY H (2001), 'Increasing evidence in favour of mandatory fortification with folic acid', *Br J Nutr*, **86**, 425–6
MEYDANI S N, MEYDANI M, BLUMBERG J B, LEKA L S, SIBER G, LOSZEWSKI R, THOPMSON C, PEDROSA M C, DIAMOND R D and STOLLER B D (1997), 'Vitamin E supplementation enhances immune response in healthy elderly: A dose response study', *J Am Med Assoc*, **277**, 1380–6
MEYDANI S N and BEHARKA A A (2001), 'Vitamin E and immune response in the aged', in *Functions of Vitamins beyond recommended Dietary Allowances*, P Walter et al (eds), Basle, Karger, 148–58
MINOT G R and MURPHY W P (1926), 'Treatment of pernicious anaemia by a special diet', *J Am Med Assoc*, **87**, 470–6
MOCK D C (1999), 'Biotin', in *Modern Nutrition in Health and Disease*, 9 ed, M E Shils, et al (eds), Baltimore, Lippincott, Williams & Wilkins, 459–66
MORRISSEY P A and SHEEHY P J A (1999), 'Optimal nutrition: vitamin E', *Proc Nutr Soc*, **58**, 459–68
MOSER H and WEBER F (1984), 'Uptake of ascorbic acid by human granulocytes', *Int J Vit Nutr Res*, **54**, 47–53
MOYNIHAN P J, RUGG-GUNN A J, BUTLER T J and ADAMSON A J (2001), 'Dietary intakes of folate by adolescents and the potential effect of flour fortification with folic acid', *Br J Nutr*, **86**, 529–34
MRC Vitamin Study Research Group (1991), 'Prevention of neural tube defects: results of the Medical Research Council vitamin study', *Lancet*, **338**, 131–7
NORMAN A W (1990), 'The vitamin D endocrine system in bone', in *Bone Regulatory Factors: Morphology, Biochemistry, Physiology and Pharmacology*, Nata ASI series vol 184, A Pecile and B de Bernard (eds), New York, Plenum Press, 93–109
NORTHROP-CLEWES C A (2001a), *Report of XX International Vitamin A Consultative Group Meeting Hanoi 2001* 'Recommendations for food-base interventions: why is VAD not a problem in developed countries?' Task Force SIGHT AND LIFE, 1, Basel 24–5
NORTHROP-CLEWES C A (2001b) *Report of XX International Vitamin A Consultative Group Meeting Hanoi 2001*, 'Safety issues with vitamin A,' Task Force SIGHT AND LIFE, 1, Basel 23–4
OLMEDILLA B, GRANADO F and SOUTHON S (2001), 'Serum concentrations of carotenoids and vitamins A, E, and C in control subjects from five European countries', *Brit J Nutr*, **85**, 227–38
OLSON, J A, LOVERIDGE N, DUTHIE G G and SHEARER M J Y (2000), 'Fat-soluble vitamins: vitamin A (retinol)', in *Human Nutrition and Dietetics*, 10 ed, J S Garrow, W P T James and A Ralph (eds), London, Churchill Livingstone, 211–20
OLSON R E (1999), 'Vitamin K', in *Modern Nutrition in Health and disease*, 9 ed, M E Shils, et al (eds), Baltimore, Lippincott, Williams & Wilkins, 363–80
O'NEILL M E and THURNHAM D I (1998), 'Intestinal absorption of β-carotene, lycopene and lutein in men and women following a standard meal: response curves in the triacyl-glycerol-rich lipoprotein fraction', *Br J Nutr*, **79**, 149–59
ORIMO H, SHIRAKI M and FUJITA T (1992), 'Clinical evaluation of menatetrenone in the treatment of involutional osteoporosis – a double blind multicenter comparative study with 1-α-hydroxyvitamin D_3 (abstract)', *J Bone Mineral Res*, **7**(Suppl I), S122
ORIMO H, SHIRAKI M and TOMITA A (1998), 'Effects of menatetrenone on the bone and calcium in osteoporosis: a double-blind placebo-controlled study', *J Bone Mineral Res*, **16**, 106
PADUA A B and JULIANO B O (1974), 'Effect of parboiling on thiamin protein and fat of rice', *J Sci Food Agri*, **25**, 697–701
PLANTALECH L C, CHAPUY M C and GUILLAUMONT M (1990), 'Impaired carboxylation of serum osteocalcin in elderly women: effect of vitamin K_1 treatment,' in *Osteoporosis 1990*, C Christiansen and K Overgaard (eds), Copenhagen, Osteopress Aps, 345
PLATT B S (1958), 'Clinical features of endemic beri-beri', *Fed Proc* **17**(suppl), 8–20

POWERS H J (1999), 'Current knowledge concerning optimum nutritional status of riboflavin, niacin and pyridoxine', *Proc Nutr Soc*, **58**, 435–40

PRICE P A (1988), 'Role of vitamin-K-dependent proteins in bone metabolism', *Ann Rev Nutr*, **8**, 565–83

REICHEL H, KOEFFLER H P and NORMAN A W (1989), 'The role of the vitamin D endocrine system in health and disease', *New Engl J Med*, **320**, 980–91

REID I, GALLAGHER D J and BOSWORTH J (1986), 'Prophylaxis against vitamin D deficiency in the elderly by regular sunlight exposure', *Age and Ageing*, **15**, 35–40

ROSS A C (1996), 'The relationship between immunocompetence and vitamin A status', in *Vitamin A Deficiency: Health, Survival and Vision*, A Sommer and K P West (eds), New York, Oxford, Oxford University Press, 251–73

ROSS A C (1999), 'Vitamin A and retinoids', in *Modern Nutrition in Health and Disease*, 9 ed, M E Shils, et al (eds), Baltimore, Lippincott Williams & Wilkins, 305–27

ROSS A C and HAMMERLING U (1994), 'Retinoids and the immune system', in *The Retinoids: Biology, Chemistry and Medicine*, M B Sporn, A B Roberts and D S Goodman (eds), New York, Raven Press, 521–44

SAKAMOTO N, NISHIIKE T, IGUCHI H and SAKAMOTO K (1999), 'The effect of diet on blood vitamin K status and urinary mineral excretion assessed by food questionnaire', *Nutr Health*, **13**, 1–10

SAUBERLICH H E (1975), 'Vitamin C status: methods and findings', *Ann NY Acad Sci*, **258**, 438–50

SAUBERLICH H E, HODGES R E, WALLACE D L, KOLDER H, CANHAM J E, HOOD J, RAICA N and LOWRY L K (1974), 'Vitamin A metabolism and requirements in the human studied with the use of labeled retinol', *Vitamins and Hormones*, **32**, 251–75

SAUBERLICH H E, HERMAN Y F, STEVENS C O and HERMAN R H (1979), 'Thiamin requirements of the adult human', *Am J Clin Nutr*, **32**, 2237–48

SCHAAFSMA A, MUSKIET F A J, STORM H et al (2000), 'Vitamin D_3 and vitamin K_1 supplementation of Dutch postmenopausal women with normal and low bone mineral densities: effects on serum 25-hydroxyvitamin D and carboxylated osteocalcin', *Eur J Clin Nutr*, **54**, 626

SCHAUMBURG H, KAPLAN J and WINDEBANK A (1983), 'Sensory neuropathy from pyridoxine abuse: a new megavitamin syndrome', *New Engl J Med*, **309**, 445–8

SCOTT J (2000), 'Folate (folic acid) and vitamin B_{12}', in *Human Nutrition and Dietetics*, 10 ed, J S Garrow, W P T James and A Ralph (eds), Churchill Livingstone, London, 271–80

SCOTT J M, WEIR D G and KIRKE P N (1994), 'Prevention of neural tube defects with folic acid: a success but . . .' *Quarterly Journal of Medicine*, **87**, 705–7

SHEARER M J (1995), 'Vitamin K', *Lancet*, **45**, 229–34

SHEARER M J (2000), 'Fat-soluble vitamins: vitamin K (phylloquinone and menaquinone)', in *Human Nutrition and Dietetics*, 10 ed, J S Garrow, W P T James and A Ralph (eds), London, Churchill Livingstone, 236–47

SHERMAN S S, HOLLIS B W and TOBIN J D (1990), 'Vitamin D status and related parameters in a healthy population: the effects of age, sex and season', *J Clin Endocrinol Metabol*, **71**, 405–13

SHIRAKI M, SHIRAKI Y, AOKI C and MIURA M (2000), 'Vitamin K_2 (menatetrenone) effectively prevents fractures and sustains lumbar bone mineral density in osteoporosis', *J Bone Mineral Res*, **15**, 515

SIEGAL B V (1993), 'Vitamin C and the immune response in health and disease', in *Nutrition and immunology series: human nutrition: a comprehensive treatise*, New York, Plenum Press, 167–96

SIES H and STAHL W (1995), 'Vitamins E and C, beta-carotene, and other carotenoids as antioxidants', *Am J Clin Nutr*, **62**, (suppl), 1315S–21S

SINCLAIR H M (1982), 'Thiamin', in *Vitamins in medicine*, B M Barker and D A Bender (eds), London, Heinemann Medical Books, 1–71

SIPE J D (1985), 'Cellular and humoral components of the early inflammatory reaction', in *The Acute Phase Response to Injury and Infection*, A H Gordon and A Koj (eds), New York, Elsevier, 3–21

SMITH J L and HODGES R E (1987), 'Serum levels of vitamin C in relation to dietary and supplemental intake of vitamin C in smokers and non-smokers', *Ann NY Acad Sci*, **498**, 144–52

SMITH R (2000), 'Clinical nutrition and bone disease', in *Human Nutrition and Dietetics*, 10 ed, J S Garrow, W P T James and A Ralph (eds), London, Churchill Livingstone, 641–50

SMITHELLS R W, SHEPPARD S and SCHORAH C J (1976), 'Vitamin deficiencies and neural tube defects', *Arch Dis Childh*, **51**, 944–50

STADTMAN E R (1991), 'Ascorbic acid and oxidative inactivation of proteins', *Am J Clin Nutr*, **54**, 1125S–8S

STEPHENS N G, PARSONS A, SCHOFIELD P M, KELLY F, CHEESEMAN K and MITCHINSON M J (1996), 'Randomised controlled trial of vitamin E in patients with coronary heart disease: Cambridge Heart Antioxidant Study (CHAOS)', *Lancet*, **347**, 781–6

STEVENSON N R (1974), 'Active transport of L-ascorbic acid in the human ileum', *Gastroenterology*, **67**, 952–6

STOCKSTAD E L R (1990), 'Historical perspective on key advances in the biochemistry and physiology of folates', in *Contemporary Issues in Clinical Nutrition: Folic Acid Metabolism in Health and Disease*, 13, M F Picciano, E L R Stokstad and J F Gregory (eds), New York, Wiley-Liss, 1–21

SUDA T, SHINKI T and TAKAHASHI N (1990), 'The role of vitamin D in bone and intestinal cell differentiation', *Ann Rev Nutr*, **10**, 195–211

SUTTIE J W (1995), 'The importance of menaquinones in human nutrition', *Ann Rev Nutr*, **15**, 399

SZULC P, CHAPUY M-C, MEUNIER P J and DELMAS P D (1993), 'Serum undercarboxylated osteocalcin in a marker of the risk of hip fracture in elderly women', *J Clin Invest*, **91**, 1769–74

SZULC P, ARLOT M, CHAPUY M-C, DUBOEUF F, MEUNIER P J and DELMAS P D (1994), 'Serum undercarboxylated osteocalcin correlates with hip bone mineral density in elderly women', *J Bone Mineral Res*, **9**, 1591–5

TAKAHASHI M, NAITOU K, OHISHI T, KUSHIDA K and MIURA M (2001), 'Effect of vitamin K and/or D on uncarboxylated and intact osteocalcin in osteoporotic patients with vertebral or hip fractures', *Clin Endocrinol*, **54**, 219–24

TANG C M, WELLS J C, ROLFE M and CHAM K (1989), 'Outbreak of beri-beri in The Gambia', *Lancet*, **ii**, 206–7

TANG G, DOLNIKOWSKI G G and RUSELL R M (2000), 'Vitamin A equivalence of β-carotene in a woman as determined by stable isotope reference method', *Eur J Nutr*, **39**, 7–11

TANNER J M (1976), 'Population differences in body size, shape and growth rate: a 1976 review', *Arch Dis Child*, **51**, 1–2

TANPHAICHITR V (1999), 'Thiamin', in *Modern Nutrition in Health and Disease*, 9 ed, M E Shils, et al (eds), Baltimore, Lippincott, Williams & Wilkins, 381–9

THURNHAM D I (1994), 'β-Carotene, are we misreading the signals in risk groups? Some analogies with vitamin C', *Proc Nutr Soc*, **53**, 557–69

THURNHAM D I (1997), 'Impact of disease on markers of micronutrient status', *Proceedings of the Nutrition Society*, **56**, 423–31

THURNHAM D I (2000), 'Vitamin C and B vitamins, thiamin, riboflavin and niacin', in *Human Nutrition and Dietetics*, 10 ed, J S Garrow, W P T James and A Ralph (eds), London, Churchill Livingstone, 249–68

THURNHAM D I, MIGASENA P, VUDHIVAI N and SUPAWAN V (1971), 'A longitudinal study on dietary and social influences on riboflavin status in pre-school children in Northeast Thailand', *SE Asian J Trop Med Pub Health*, **2**, 552–63

THURNHAM D I, DAVIES J A, CRUMP B J, SITUNAYAKE R D and DAVIS M (1986), 'The use of different lipids to express serum tocopherol: lipid ratios for the measurement of vitamin E status', *Ann Clin Biochem*, **23**, 514–20

United States Department of Health and Human Services, F A D A (1996), 'Food standards: amendment of the standards of identity for enriched grain products to require the addition of folic acid', *Federal Register*, **61**, 8781–880

VALLANCE B, HUME R and WEYERS E (1978), 'Reassessment of changes in leucocyte and serum ascorbic acid after acute myocardial infarction', *Br Heart J*, **40**, 684–9

VAN HET HOF K H, BROUWER I A, WEST C E, HADDEMAN E, STEEGERS-THEUNISSEN R P M, VAN DUSSELDORP M, WESTSTRATE J A, ESKES T K A B and HAUTVAST J G A J (1999), 'Bioavailability of lutein from vegetables is 5 times higher than that of β-carotene', *Am J Clin Nutr*, **70**, 261–8

VAN LIESHOUT M (2001), *Bioavailability and Bioefficacy of β-carotene Measured using ^{13}C-labeled β-carotene and Retinol: Studies in Indonesian Children*, PhD thesis, Wageningen, The Netherlands, Wageningen University

VAN LIESHOUT M, WEST C E, MUHILAL, PERMAESIH D, WANG Y, XIAOOYING X, VAN BREEMEN R B, CREEMERS A F L, VERHOEVEN M A and LUGTENBURG J (2001), 'Bioefficacy of β-carotene dissolved in oil studied in children in Indonesia', *Am J Clin Nutr*, **73**, 949–58

VAN VLIET T, SCHEURS W H P and VAN DEN BERG H (1995), 'Intestinal β-carotene absorption and cleavage in men: response of β-carotene and retinyl esters in the triglyceride-rich lipoprotein fraction after a single oral dose of β-carotene', *Am J Clin Nutr*, **62**, 110–16

VERMEER C, JIE K-S G and KNAPEN M H J (1995), 'Role of vitamin K in bone metabolism', *Ann Rev Nutr*, **15**, 1–22

VILLAREAL D T, CIVITELLI R, CHINES A and AVIOLI L V (1991), 'Subclinical vitamin D deficiency in postmenopausal women with low vertebral bone mass', *J Clin Endocrin Metabol*, **71**, 405–13

WAGNER K H (1940), 'Die experimentelle avitaminose A beim Menschen (Experimentally low vitamin A status in humans)', *Z Physiol Chem*, **264**, 153–88

WARD M (2001), 'Homocysteine, folate and cardiovascular disease', *Int J Vit Nutr Res*, **71**, 173–8

WARD M, MCNULTY H, MCPARTLIN J, STRAIN J J, WEIR D G and SCOTT J M (1997), 'Plasma homocysteine, a risk factor for cardiovascular disease is lowered by physiological doses of folic acid', *QJ Med*, **90**, 519–24

WATKINS M L, ERICSON J D, THUN M J, MULINARE J and HEATH C W JR (2000), 'Multivitamin use and mortality in a large prospective study', *Am J Epidemiol*, **152**, 149–62

WEBER P (2001), 'Vitamin K and Bone health', *Nutrition*, **17**, 880–7

WEIR D G and SCOTT J M (1995), 'Biochemical basis of neuropathy in cobalamin deficiency', in *Megaloblastic Anaemias, Clinical Haematology*, S N Wickramasinghe (ed), London, Bailliere Tindall, 479–97

WEIR D G and SCOTT J M (1998), 'Cobalamins: physiology, dietary sources and requirements', in *Encyclopaedia of Human Nutrition*, vol 1, M T Sadler, B Caballero and J J Strain (eds), Academic Press, 394–401

WEIR D G and SCOTT J M (1999), 'Vitamin B$_{12}$ "Cobalamin",' in *Modern Nutrition in Health and Disease*, 9 ed, M E Shils et al (eds), Baltimore, Lippincott, Williams & Wilkins; London, Academic Press, 447–58

WHITEHEAD R G (1991), *The new British Dietary Reference Values, Comments*, London, HMSO, 41

WHITEHEAD R G (1992), 'Dietary reference values', *Proc Nutr Soc*, **51**, 29–34

WHITEHEAD A S, GALLAGHER P, MILLS J L, KIRK P N, BURKE H, MOLLOY A M, WEIR D G, SHIELDS D C and SCOTT J M (1995), 'A genetic defect in 5,10 methylenetetrahydrofolate reductase in neural tube defects', *Q J Med*, **88**, 763–6

WICKRAMASINGHE S N (1995), 'Preface to megaloblastic anaemia', in *Clinical Haematology*, vol 8, S N Wickramasinghe (ed), London, Bailliere Tindall, ix
WILLIAMS R R (1961), *'Towards the Conquest of Beriberi'*, Cambridge, Massachusetts, Harvard University Press
WILLIAMS R R, MASON H L and WILDER R M (1943), 'The minimum daily requirement of thiamine in man', *J Nutr*, **25**, 71–97
WILLS L (1931), 'Treatment of "pernicious anaemia of pregnancy" and "tropical anaemia" with special reference to yeast extract as a curative agent', *B M J*, **1**, 1059–64
WRIGHT A J A, SOUTHON S, CHOPRA M et al (2002), 'Comparison of LDL fatty acid and carotenoid concentrations and oxidative resistance of LDL in volunteers from countries with different rates of cardiovascular disease', *Brit J Nutr*, **87**, 21–9
XU D P and WELLS W W (1996), 'Alpha-lipoic acid dependent regeneration of ascorbic acid from dehydroascorbic acid in rat liver mitochondria', *J Bioenergetics Biomembranes*, **28**, 77–85
YANG S, SMITH C and DE LUCA H F (1993), '1 alpha, 25-Dihydroxyvitamin D_3 and 19-nor-1 alpha, 25-dihydroxyvitamin D_2 suppress immunoglobulin production and thymic lymphocyte proliferation in vivo', *Biochim Biophys Acta*, **1158**, 279–86
ZEIGLER R G, MAYNE S T and SWANSON C A (1996), 'Nutrition and lung cancer', *Cancer Causes Controls*, **7**, 157
ZILE M H (2001), 'Function of vitamin A in vertebrate embryonic development', *J Nutr*, **131**, 705–8

4
Minerals

C. Reilly, Oxford Brookes University

4.1 Introduction

Minerals are the inorganic elements, other than carbon, hydrogen, oxygen and nitrogen, which remain behind in the ash when food is incinerated. They are usually divided into two groups – macrominerals and microminerals (or trace elements). The terms are historical in origin and originated at a time when the development of analytical equipment was still in its infancy and 'trace' was used to refer to components whose presence could be detected, but not quantified. Modern analytical equipment that allows determination of elements at levels in the nano- and even picogram range, can show the presence of most of the minerals in almost any food. Some are present in minute amounts, but others are at significant levels.

The minerals are classified as either essential or non-essential, depending on whether or not they are required for human nutrition and have metabolic roles in the body. Non-essential elements are also categorised as either toxic or non-toxic. Table 4.1 lists elements that occur in food and are important in human nutrition. In addition to the essential elements, some others, including arsenic, silicon and boron, have been shown to be required by certain animals and may also play beneficial roles in the human body.

This section will present an overview of the principal essential minerals, covering their chemical characteristics, basic roles in human health, dietary origins (from food and supplements), and their Reference Nutrient Intakes (RNI), including Safe Intakes (SI). This will be followed by consideration of a number of selected minerals that are of particular interest at the present time. Attention will be given particularly to their nutritional significance, including their possible roles as functional ingredients of food. The elements to be discussed in detail are

Table 4.1 Mineral elements in food

Macrominerals (g/kg)	Microminerals (mg/kg)	Toxic minerals (mg/kg)
Calcium (<1–12)	Chromium (<0.02–0.95)	Cadmium (0.001–0.07)
Magnesium (1–4)	Cobalt (0.008–0.32)	Lead (0.01–0.25)
Phosphorus (1–6)	Copper (<0.2–3.3)	Mercury (<0.001–0.18)
Potassium (1–6)	Iodine (0.04–0.66)	
Sodium (1–19)	Iron (<0.2–92)	
Sulphur (<2–6)	Manganese (<0.10–14.0)	
	Molybdenum (0.004–1.29)	
	Selenium (<0.001–0.34)	
	Zinc (0.2–8.6)	

data from Reilly C (2002) *Metal Contamination of Food*, 3rd ed. Blackwell science: Oxford.

calcium, iron, and zinc. Two other elements, iodine and selenium, will also be considered, though in less detail. A final section will provide suggestions for further reading.

4.2 Chemical characteristics

Nearly all the minerals required by the body are elements of low atomic number, from sodium (11) to selenium (34); the exceptions are molybdenum (42) and iodine (53). In living matter, these elements are present in a number of different states: as inorganic compounds, as free ions in body fluids, or combined with organic compounds (Coultate, 1985).

Approximately 99% of the body's calcium and 85% of its phosphorus are in the hard mineral component of bone. The two elements are combined together to form a compound similar to hydroxyapatite, $Ca_{10}(OH)_2(PO_4)_6$. Other inorganic elements, such as fluoride (F^-), magnesium sodium and potassium are also incorporated into the bone mineral to form the partly amorphous and partly crystalline structure of bone.

In contrast to calcium in the skeleton, the element iron occurs almost entirely as part of co-ordination compounds based on the porphyrin nucleus involved in the transport of oxygen. Several of the other trace elements are also mainly present in biological tissues as organic compounds, such as selenium in the metalloenzyme glutathione peroxidase, and molybdenum in superoxide dismutase.

4.3 Impact on health, absorption and recommended intakes

Minerals function mainly in three ways in the body:

1. As structural components, e.g. calcium, phosphate and magnesium in bones and teeth.

2. In organic combinations as physiologically important compounds, e.g. phosphorus in nucelotides, zinc in enzymes such as carbonic anhydrase, iodine in thyroid hormone.
3. In solution in body fluids to maintain pH, help conduct nerve impulses, control muscle contraction, e.g. sodium and potassium in blood and intracellular fluids.

The macrominerals are mainly involved in functions 1 and 3, and the microminerals in function 2.

A normal diet, composed of a mixture of both plant and animal foodstuffs, should supply all the minerals required by the body. When such a diet is not available, or in some other situations, it may be necessary to provide the missing elements in the form of supplements or by fortifying the diet with additional minerals. The minerals ingested in food are absorbed after digestion from the gut into the blood stream, which transports them to the sites where they function or are stored. Not all minerals are absorbed to the same extent. Some, including sodium and potassium, are readily absorbed as ions or as simple compounds. Others, such as calcium, magnesium and phosphorus may be combined as indigestible or insoluble compounds in food and are less easily taken up from the gut. A few others, especially some of the trace elements such as iron, are poorly absorbed.

Uptake of certain minerals from food can be affected by other components of the diet. Thus phytic acid and phytates in cereals can inhibit absorption of iron and zinc. The same effect can be caused by oxalate in certain vegetables. Iodine absorption can be limited by sulphur-containing compounds known as goitrogens, which occur in certain plants, such as some brassicae and cassava. Consumption of these vegetables can acerbate iodine deficiency and increase the likelihood of goitre.

If an essential element is at a low level in the diet, a nutritional deficiency may occur, with specific symptoms. Thus an inadequate intake of iron can cause anaemia when there is insufficient haemoglobin to meet the needs of the body for oxygen transport. A deficiency of iodine can lead to goitre when the body tries to compensate for a low production of the iodine-containing thyroid hormone by increasing the size of the thyroid gland. Inadequate zinc may result in growth failure in children. Usually these conditions are corrected when intake of the missing element is increased by improving the diet or by providing supplements.

An excessive intake of a mineral may also have serious consequences for health. Too much sodium in the diet may be associated with high blood pressure and increased risk of a stroke. A condition known as siderosis, in which an excess of iron is deposited in the body, can result when too much iron is absorbed. Selenosis, a sometimes fatal effect of an excessive intake of selenium is known to occur in parts of China where high levels of the element enter locally grown foods from selenium-rich soil. Less serious effects, such as nausea, can be caused by a high intake of zinc.

Table 4.2 Reference nutrient intakes and safe intakes for minerals

Mineral	male (19–50 years)	female (19–50 years)
Calcium (RNI) mg/day	700	700
Phosphorus (RNI) mg/day	550	550
Magnesium (RNI) mg/day	300	270
Sodium (RNI) mg/day	1600	1600
Potassium (RNI) mg/day	3500	3500
Chloride (RNI) mg/day	2500	2500
Iron (RNI) mg/day	8.7	14.8+
Zinc (RNI) mg/day	9.5	7.0
Copper (RNI) mg/day	1.2	1.2
Selenium (RNI) µg/day	75	60
Iodine (RNI) µg/day	140	140
Manganese (SI) mg/day	above 1.4	above 1.4
Molybdenum (SI) µg/day	50–400	50–400
Chromium (SI) µg/day	above 25	above 25
Fluoride (SI) mg/kg body weight/day	0.5	0.5

+ insufficient for women with high menstrual losses where the most practical way of meeting iron requirements is to take iron supplements.
adapted from Department of Health (1991) *Dietary Reference Values for Food Energy and Nutrients for the United Kingdom*. HMSO: London.

Health authorities in most countries have established recommendation for intake levels of essential minerals which both meet the nutritional requirements of consumers and at the same time prevent excessive intakes. In the UK, Reference Nutrient Intakes (RNI) for 11 minerals have been published by the Department of Health to meet the requirements for the different age groups and sexes in the Community (Department of Health, 1991). The RNI is defined as 'an amount of the nutrient that is enough, or more than enough, for about 97 per cent of people in a group'. In addition Safe Intakes (SI) have been established for another four minerals. The SI is 'a term used to indicate intake or range of intakes of a nutrient for which there is not enough information to estimate RNI . . . it is an amount that is enough for almost everyone but not so large as to cause undesirable effects'. The RNI for minerals for adult men and women are given in Table 4.2.

4.4 Dietary sources, supplementation and fortification

Because our food is almost entirely made up of components that were once parts of living organisms and since there is a broad similarity between the nutritional requirements and cellular biochemistry of most forms of animal and plant life, it is to be expected that our needs for the mineral nutrients will be met by a conventional mixed diet (Coultate, 1985). It is usually only in exceptional situations, where, for example, there is a reliance on locally produced food in an area where

Table 4.3 Good food sources of minerals

Mineral	cereal	vegetable	Food dairy	meat	Fish	other
Ca		*green	*		*	nuts
Mg	*					nuts
Fe	*fortified	*green			*	
Zn	*			*	*	
Cu				*	*	
Se	*			*	*	nuts
I			*		*	iodised salt
Mn	*			*	*	tea
Mo	*					
Cr	*			*	*	Brewer's yeast

the soil is deficient in a particular mineral, or where the diet is deliberately restricted to a limited number of food types, that problems of mineral deficiencies occur.

Some food sources are better than others as sources of minerals. Plant foods are generally poor in iron and zinc, with the exception of certain dark green vegetables such as spinach. Dairy products are generally an excellent source of calcium. Red meat and offal, such as liver, are the best dietary sources of easily absorbed iron. Many of the trace elements are found in relatively high concentrations in fish and other seafoods. Table 4.3 lists some of the best food sources of a number of the essential minerals. As is indicated in the table, there are some unusually good sources of a number of these minerals. Milk, for example, is often an excellent source of iodine because of the presence of residual iodine-containing compounds used to sterilise dairy equipment. Tea is a major source of manganese in the UK diet. An important source of chromium in the diet of some people is canned food which picks up the metal that is one of the ingredients of the alloy used to produce 'tin'cans (Reilly, 2002).

For many people supplements are an important source of minerals. It has been estimated that as many as 40% of the US population consume them, and up to 60% in the UK, either as 'over-the-counter' self-selected products or prescribed by a physician or other health advisor (Balluz et al, 2000).

Mineral supplements are available in a number of chemical forms, either as inorganic compounds, such as ferrous sulphate and calcium carbonate, or as organic preparations such as selenium yeast and zinc gluconate. The products vary in the amounts of the different elements they contain, in their absorbability and in other qualities and while undoubtedly their use can make a definite contribution in some cases to nutritional health, there can also be problems such as over-dosing and interactions with other components of the diet (Huffman et al, 1999).

The addition of minerals and other nutrients to foods to increase their nutritional value is widely practised. In the 1920s iodised salt was introduced in some countries to help combat endemic goitre. Iodised salt, as well as other iodised foods such as bread and monosodium glutamate, are today widely used in parts of the world where iodine deficiency diseases (IDD) are still endemic, such as India, and China, Papua New Guinea, Central Africa and the Andean region of South America.

Legislation was introduced in several countries during World War II which required the addition of iron and calcium, as well as of certain water-soluble vitamins, to bread and flour in order to combat nutritional deficiencies caused by food restrictions. The success of these measures in improving health led to the extension of the legislation into peacetime. Some countries, such as the UK, still require that bread and flour be fortified with calcium and iron (Statutory Instrument, 1984).

Bread and flour are the only foodstuffs required by law to be fortified with minerals in the UK. There is, in addition, legal provision for the voluntary addition by food processors of other minerals to other foodstuffs, with the exception of alcoholic drinks. This has given manufacturers the opportunity to produce a variety of foods enriched with other minerals. Most ready-to-eat (RTE) breakfast cereals are enriched with iron and zinc. Some varieties will also contain added iodine and other minerals. These are normally added at levels which are well below those which might cause toxic effects (Brady, 1996). Fortified RTE cereals have been shown to make a significant contribution towards meeting the nutritional requirements of consumers for iron, as well as for copper, manganese and zinc (Booth et al, 1996). Currently a considerable amount of research is being carried out on methods, such as fortification of a variety of commonly used foods with minerals and other nutrients, as a way of improving nutritional status in countries where deficiency problems regularly occur (Gibson and Ferguson, 1998).

In recent years there has been a growth in the production of foods, which have been deliberately selected or formulated to provide, according to their promotors, specific physiologic, health promoting and even disease-preventing benefits. They have been given a variety of names such as 'designer food', 'nutraceuticals', 'functional foods' and, officially in Japan, 'foods for specific health use' (FOSHU). Several of these products contain minerals such as selenium (Reilly, 1998).

4.5 Calcium

Without an adequate supply of the macromineral calcium in the diet calcification of the skeleton will be adversely affected. During early growth and development the supply of calcium for this purpose is particularly critical and for this reason the amount required by a child is proportionally greater than for an adult (British Nutrition Foundation, 1989).

4.5.1 Calcium absorption

Uptake of calcium from food in the gut is not very efficient. Only about 30% is absorbed, with 70% lost in faeces. Absorption is a complex process, which is under the control of the cholecalciferol (vitamin D)-parathyroid hormone system. Calcium is transported across the intestinal mucosa bound to a special carrier protein. Synthesis of this protein is stimulated by an activated form of cholecalciferol, 1,25-dihydroxycholecalciferol (1,25-DHCC). If vitamin D levels are low, calcium absorption will be restricted and a deficiency will occur.

To be absorbed, calcium must be in the soluble ionic form. Several food components can prevent this happening. These include phytic acid (inositol hexaphosphate) in cereals, and oxalate in certain dark green vegetables, such as spinach, and in rhubarb. Uronic acid in dietary fibre can have a similar effect, as can free fatty acids and certain other dietary factors, including sodium chloride and a high protein intake.

4.5.2 Functions of calcium in the body

Over 99% of body calcium is in the skeleton, where it both provides structural support and serves as a reservoir for maintaining plasma levels. Calcium in plasma plays a number of roles, for example in muscle contraction, neuromuscular function and blood coagulation. To maintain these roles, calcium levels in the plasma must be very stable. If for any reason they are altered, they are immediately restored to normal levels by an increased secretion of parathyroid hormone and the formation of 1,25-DHCC. In children this increase in plasma calcium means that less of the mineral goes into bones, while in adults calcium is withdrawn from the skeleton. In either case there can be significant implications for bone structure.

4.5.3 Osteoporosis

Osteoporosis is a condition which is characterised by loss of bone tissue from the skeleton and deterioration of bone structure with enhanced bone fragility and increased risk of fracture. It is relatively common in the elderly, especially females, but may also occur in the young. In the UK one in three women and one in twelve men over the age of 50 years can expect to have an osteoporotic fracture during the remainder of their lives (Prentice, 2001).

The causes of osteoporosis, in spite of extensive research, remain elusive. The higher rate in women seems to be associated with a number of factors: the lower skeletal mass in women compared to men, a greater rate of calcium loss and a fall in oestrogen production with age. Lifetime history is also important. Higher intakes of calcium, especially in adolescence and early adulthood, ensure greater bone density. In addition, physical exercise can help increase calcium deposition, while high consumption of alcohol, coffee, meat, salt and cola beverages may contribute to decreased bone density (Sakamoto et al, 2001).

Although there is considerable debate about the effectiveness of calcium supplements in preventing osteoporosis, the weight of evidence points towards a role for calcium deficiency in its genesis and for calcium therapy in its prevention and management, at least in postmenopausal women (Heaney, 2001). Increases in bone mineral density (BMD) have been observed following calcium supplementation in young, as well as in elderly subjects. However, although dietary calcium does play a major role in optimisation of bone mineralisation it is by no means the only factor involved (Prentice, 1997).

4.5.4 Recommended intakes of calcium

There is at present no international consensus regarding calcium requirements and levels in the diet necessary to meet optimum requirements. Recommended intakes differ widely between countries, partly because different methods have been used to arrive at the recommendations. While some authorities have focused on meeting nutritional requirements, others have aimed at optimising bone density (Wynne, 1998). There is also the fact that actual intakes of calcium vary widely world-wide, without, in many cases, an apparent effect on bone development. In parts of Africa and Asia intake of dietary calcium is as low as 300–400 mg/day, while in Northern Europe it can be 1500 mg/day or more.

In the UK the Panel for Dietary Reference Values of COMA (the Committee on Medical Aspects of Food Policy) of the Department of Health, while noting the difficulty of assessing the adequacy of the dietary supply of calcium, has established RNIs for calcium for different groups in the population (Department of Health, 1991). Since the panel's experts found that no single approach to the estimation of these values was considered to be satisfactory, these intakes are not considered to represent true basal dietary requirements, but rather to describe the apparent calcium requirements of healthy people in the UK under prevailing dietary circumstances.

The UK RNI for adults aged 19–50 years is 700 mg/day, with an additional 550 mg/day for lactating women. In the US an intake of 1000 mg/day is recommended for the same age group, with no additional allowance for lactation (Institute of Medicine, Food and Nutrition Board, 1998). In contrast, WHO/FAO in 1974 proposed 400–500 mg/day for this group, with additional intakes for pregnant and lactating women.

4.5.5 Dietary sources of calcium

Milk and dairy products are the major sources of calcium in many diets. In countries such as the UK where addition of calcium to flour is required by law, bread and other cereal products also make an important contribution to intake. Sardines and other small fish, which are eaten whole, are also good sources. In countries where dairy products are not used in quantity and where fortification of flour is not required, requirements may be met by green leafy vegetables, roots, nuts and pulses. Where domestic water is 'hard', with a high calcium content, it can make a significant contribution to intake.

4.5.6 High intakes of calcium

The consumption of calcium supplements is widely practised, especially by the elderly as a precaution against the development of osteoporosis. Although there is little evidence that a high intake of calcium resulting from supplement consumption causes adverse health effects, in the US an Upper Intake Level (UL) has been set for the mineral at 2.5 g/day. A Safe Intake (SI) level has not been set in the UK on the grounds, according to the Department of Health, that calcium metabolism is under such close homeostatic control that an excessive accumulation in the blood (hypercalcaemia) or in tissues (calcification) from overconsumption is virtually unknown (Department of Health, 1991).

4.6 Iron

In spite of the fact that iron is the second most abundant metal in the earth's crust, iron insufficiency is probably the most common nutritional deficiency in the world. Even among the inhabitants of well-fed developed countries it continues to be common, especially in women (Looker et al, 1997).

4.6.1 Iron absorption

The uptake of iron is a complex and highly regulated operation. Once the element is absorbed from the intestine into the blood, only small amounts are lost from the body, except when bleeding occurs. There is no physiological mechanism for secretion of iron, so iron homeostasis depends on its absorption. Thus the healthy individual with a good store of iron is able to maintain a balance between the small normal losses and the amounts of the element absorbed from food. Normally only a very small amount of iron, about 1 mg/day, needs to be absorbed. The metal first enters the intestinal mucosal cells where it is bound into ferritin, an iron-storage protein. This is a large molecule from which the iron can be readily mobilised when required. Some of the incoming iron may be transferred directly by a transport protein, transferrin, to bone marrow and other tissues to be used in the synthesis of haemoglobin and myoglobin.

Iron absorption is apparently regulated by the existing iron status of the body. If this is low, the absorption mechanism can be stimulated to increased activity. When iron stores are high, absorption is slowed down. There is evidence that other mineral elements, such as zinc, can compete with iron for the active absorption pathway. Several other dietary factors can affect absorption, including phytate and fibre, which inhibit absorption, and ascorbic acid and protein, which increase uptake. The pH of the gut also has an effect, with food iron mainly in the more readily absorbed ferrous state under acid conditions.

4.6.2 Functions of iron

Iron is an essential nutrient for all living organisms, with the exception of certain bacteria. It has two major roles in human physiology. As a component of haemoglobin, the red pigment of blood and myoglobin in muscle, iron atoms combine reversibly with oxygen to act as its carrier from the lungs to the tissues. In a variety of enzymes, such as the cytochromes, iron atoms, present in the ferrous and ferric states, interchange with gain or loss of an electron, as part of the electron chain responsible for the redox reactions necessary for release of energy in cellular catabolism and the synthesis of large molecules (Brock et al, 1994).

In addition to its major functions in oxygen transport and as a cofactor in many enzymes, iron also plays an important role in the immune system. Although the mechanisms involved are complex, there is good evidence that an abnormal iron nutritional status can lead to impaired immune function, with serious consequences for health (Walter et al, 1997).

4.6.3 Iron deficiency anaemia

Iron deficiency ultimately results in failure of the body to produce new blood cells to replace those that are constantly being destroyed at the end of their normal 120-day life span. Gradually the number of blood cells falls and, with this, the amount of haemoglobin in the blood. The cells become paler in colour and smaller in size. These undersized cells are unable to carry sufficient oxygen to meet the needs of tissues, so energy release is hindered. This is what is known technically as microcytic hypochromic anaemia, or, simply, as iron deficiency anaemia (IDA) (Expert Scientific Working Group, 1985). Because the fall in red blood cells occurs gradually, IDA can exist for a considerable time before it is clearly detected. By then iron stores have suffered a critical fall and the person affected shows symptoms of chronic tiredness, persistent headache, and, in many cases, a rapid heart rate on exertion. There may also be other functional consequences of iron deficiency, including a decreased work capacity, a fall in intellectual performance, and a reduction in immune function (Brock and Mulero, 2000). There is today growing concern at the possibility that iron deficiency in infancy and childhood can have serious consequences, such as morbidity in the newborn, defects in growth and development of infants and impaired educational performance in schoolchildren (Cook, 1999).

4.6.4 Recommended intakes

The UK RNI is 1.7–8.7 mg/day for both males and females from birth to 10 years of age. This rises to 14.8 mg/day for females from 11 to 50 years, when it is reduced to 8.7 for the post-child bearing years. Women with a high menstrual loss are recommended to increase their iron intake by taking a supplement. The RNI for males from 11 to 18 years is set at 11.3 mg/day, with a drop to 8.7 mg/day for later years (Department of Health, 1991).

The UK recommendations are similar to those published in the US (National Research Council, 1989), but lower than those of WHO. They are also less than recommendations in many developing countries. In Indonesia, for instance, an intake of 14–26 mg/day is recommended for women of child-bearing age, with an additional 30 mg/day during pregnancy (Muhilal, 1998). The reason for such differences between recommendations in the UK and in developing countries relates to the composition of the diets normally consumed by their citizens. According to the Food and Agricultural Organization (FAO), a diet typical of most segments of the population in industrialised countries includes generous amounts of meat, poultry, fish and/or foods containing high amounts of ascorbic acid (FAO, 1988). Iron absorption from such diets can be assumed to be 15%. In contrast, the less varied, high cereal diet of Indonesia and countries with a similar diet, may have a lower iron content with an absorption level of 5% or less.

4.6.5 Dietary sources of iron

One of the richest sources of dietary iron is animal offal, especially liver. Other animal products, in particular red meat, are also rich in iron. This iron is organically bound haem iron, which is easily absorbed. Plant foods are generally poor sources of iron and what is present is in the inorganic form. Depending on the total composition of the diet, absorption of iron from vegetables will be as low as 2–5%. In contrast to most other vegetables, dark green species such as spinach are relatively rich in iron. While cereals in general are low in iron, breakfast cereals which are fortified, voluntarily, by manufacturers, and flour to which the addition of iron is required by law, make major contributions to intake in the UK and elsewhere.

4.6.6 High intakes of iron

Iron toxicity can occur as a result of ingestion of large amounts of iron compounds. This is most unlikely to be caused by iron in normal foods, but by accidental intake of a chemical substance. A lethal dose for adults is about 100 g, while in children, among whom most cases of iron poisoning are reported to occur, it is 200–300 mg/kg body weight (Department of Health, 1991). The source of the iron in most childhood poisoning appears to be supplement pills used by their mothers which the children mistake for sweets (Barr and Fraser, 1968).

A high intake of iron can be a serious problem for persons with the hereditary disorder of haemochromatosis. This condition, in which there is a gradual accumulation of iron in tissues and can result in liver failure, occurs in nearly one per cent of Europeans and more frequently in people of African origin. There is evidence that in some cases iron overload is caused by excessive intake of the metal as a result of consumption of foods and beverages prepared in iron cooking pots and containers (Bothwell et al, 1964).

4.7 Zinc

While zinc was known to be an essential nutrient for plants and certain animals from early in the twentieth century, zinc deficiency in humans only began to be recognised in the 1960s, when zinc-responsive dwarfism was detected in children in Egypt (Prasad, 1990). Although there was some uncertainty among researchers about the possibility of more general zinc deficiency among humans because of the element's ubiquity in the environment (it is the 23rd most abundant element in the earth's crust), subsequent clinical studies of children with acrodermatitis enteropathica, a hereditary error of zinc metabolism, and numerous studies of other zinc-related conditions, have confirmed the essential role played by zinc in human metabolism (Brown et al, 2001). Today zinc is known to be a key nutrient of world-wide significance, and has joined iodine and iron among trace elements whose deficiency problems urgently need to be addressed (Ranum, 2001).

4.7.1 Zinc absorption from food

An adult human contains between 1.5 and 2.5 grams of zinc, almost as much as iron and more than 200 times the amount of copper which is the third most abundant trace element in the body. Absorption from the diet, which occurs in the small intestine, is affected by a number of factors. Uptake has been reported to range from less than 10 to more than 90%, with an average of 20–30% (Forbes and Erdman, 1983). Various components of the diet can affect uptake. Competition for absorption occurs between zinc and other elements, especially copper, iron and cadmium. Phytate, fibre, and calcium can limit gastrointestinal uptake, whereas animal protein enhances it. A diet rich in wholemeal bread, for instance, which contains these three antagonists, has been shown to cause deficiency of the element.

Zinc absorption is believed to be related to the presence of endogenous zinc binding ligands. Most of the zinc that is absorbed from the intestine is found intracellularly, primarily in muscle, bone, liver and other organs (Jackson, 1989). Zinc in plasma is mainly loosely bound to albumin and is also transported attached to transferrin. In the liver it is bound to the low molecular weight metal-binding protein, metallothionin.

Most of the body's zinc reserves turn over slowly and are not readily available for metabolism. Only about 10% makes up a readily available pool, which is used to maintain various zinc-dependent metabolic functions. The body's zinc content is regulated by homeostatic mechanisms, mainly through control of absorption of exogenous zinc from the gut and by regulation of excretion of endogenous zinc in pancreatic and other gastrointestinal secretions (King et al, 2000). Since only about 0.2% of the body's total zinc is in plasma, a small change in uptake by or release from muscle or other tissues can have profound effects on levels in plasma (Hambidge et al, 1989). Plasma zinc concentrations can be affected by stress, surgery, physical exercise, infection and several other factors (Brown et al, 2001). Consequently, plasma levels do not give a reliable measure of total body zinc stores under all circumstances.

4.7.2 Functions of zinc in the body

Zinc is an essential component of more than 200 enzymes in the living world, of which as many as 50 play important metabolic roles in animals. It occurs in all six classes of enzymes. In addition, the metal provides structural integrity in many proteins. Zinc ligands help maintain the structure of cell membranes and of some ion channels. 'Zinc finger protein' is involved in processes of transcription factors that link with the double helix of DNA to initiate gene expression (Berg and Shi, 1996). The expression of certain genes is known to be regulated by the quantity of zinc absorbed from the diet. It is also believed that zinc has an intracellular role that includes regulation of cell growth and differentiation.

While some zinc-dependent biological activities are organ-specific, such as the role of the metal in neuronal transmission (Frederickson et al, 2000), many of the wide range of zinc-dependent metabolic processes are required by all cells. This can explain why the consequences of zinc deficiency are so many and so varied and why they are also non-specific. This could also account for the special importance of the metal during prenatal and early growth, and in systems such as the immune system, in which cells have a rapid turnover (Hambidge and Krebs, 2001). Clinical signs seen in persons suffering from marginal zinc deficiency include depressed immunity, impaired taste and smell, night blindness, impaired memory, and decreased spermatogenesis in men (Walsh et al, 1994). Severe zinc deficiency is characterised by severely depressed immune function, frequent infections, bulbous pustular dermatitis, diarrhoea, alopecia and mental disturbances. An inadequate intake of zinc retards growth and can result in stunting, dwarfism, and failure to mature sexually.

4.7.3 Zinc requirements and dietary reference values

Considerable problems have been encountered in trying to establish dietary zinc requirements. This is largely due to the difficulty of assessing zinc status and optimal zinc nutriture in humans. As has already been mentioned, measurement of plasma levels may not give a true measure of the body's available zinc. Other biomarkers of zinc status, such as activity of zinc-dependent enzymes, are not sufficiently specific to be more than of supportive value (Hambidge and Krebs, 1995). The use of estimates of habitual intake in populations without evidence of zinc deficiency can be of some use, but lacks precision and also does not take sufficiently into account the problem of bioavailability in different types of diet. In practice, a factorial approach, which is based on the quantity of absorbed zinc required to match endogenous excretion of the element, has been used to estimate requirements in several countries. Although not ideal, the factorial approach is widely accepted as offering a useful strategy for estimating zinc requirements and has been adopted for this purpose in the UK and the US. Its use, however, has not produced uniform recommendations. Thus, while the UK RNI for adult males and females are 9.0 mg/day, with an additional 2.5 to 6.0 mg/day for lactating women, but with no allowance for pregnancy, the 1989 US recommendation was 15 mg/day for adult males and 12 mg/day for women up to the age of 50 years, with an extra 16–19 mg/day for lactating women, on top of an additional 15 mg/day all through pregnancy.

4.7.4 Zinc levels in foods and dietary intakes

In Western societies upwards of 70% of zinc consumed is provided by animal products, especially meat (Welsh and Marston, 1982). Liver and other organ meats are particularly rich in the element, as are most seafoods. Another good source is oysters which may, in some cases, contain as much as 1000 mg/kg of the metal. Other foods which contain high levels are seeds and nuts, as well as wholegrain cereals. However, these and other plant foods also contain phytate that can decrease bioavailability of the element.

The average zinc intake by UK adults is about 9–12 mg/day, which means that many people are on the borderline for meeting their requirements. The zinc content of a typical adult US mixed diet is between 10 and 15 mg/day and it is estimated that as many as two thirds of the population fail to meet their recommended level of intake. Intakes are especially low in children, adolescent females and women during their reproductive years, and the elderly. Similar discrepancies between actual intakes and recommendations are seen in a number of European countries (Van Dokkum, 1995). In many Asian countries zinc intakes are particularly low because of the absence of appreciable amounts of animal products and the presence of phytate-rich plant foods in the customary diet. There is evidence that zinc deficiency is widespread, especially in children, in several countries, such as Bangladesh (Osendarp et al, 2001). Considerable efforts are currently being made by health authorities in such areas to improve zinc nutriture by provision of zinc supplements as well as by other methods, including fortification (Gibson and Ferguson, 1998).

4.7.5 High intakes of zinc

It is generally assumed that zinc is non-toxic because of the strong homeostatic regulation of absorption and endogenous excretion of the metal. However, large doses can cause gastrointestinal problems and are emetic (Failla, 1999). This has been known to occur when water, which has been stored in galvanised (zinc-plated steel) containers has been consumed. Prolonged exposure to high intakes of zinc is believed to result in copper deficiency and subsequent anaemia. It may also interfere with iron metabolism. Because of evidence that similar effects may be produced by ingestion of high doses of zinc supplements, an intake of more than 15 mg/day in this way is not recommended (Department of Health, 1991).

4.8 Other minerals: iodine and selenium

Three other trace minerals for which there are DRVs in the UK are copper, iodine, and selenium. Copper is considered in detail elsewhere in this volume and will not be discussed further here. In this section, the roles of iodine and selenium will be reviewed briefly.

4.8.1 Iodine

The non-metallic element iodine is an essential nutrient that, apparently, has a single function in the body as a component of the thyroid hormones thyroxine (T4) and triiodotyronine (T3). These hormones are necessary for a range of body processes, the most important of which are the control of metabolic rate, cellular metabolism, growth and neural development. Production of T4 and T3 is controlled by tissue demands which are mediated by the secretions of the pituitary gland and by the supply of iodine in the diet.

Deficiency of iodine can result in a number of diseases, ranging from severe cretinism with mental retardation to barely visible enlargement of the thyroid gland. Goitre is the name given to enlargement of the gland that occurs as the body attempts to compensate for a reduction of its supply of iodine by increasing the size of the gland. The amount of enlargement is related to the degree of iodine deficiency. The condition is widespread throughout the world, with up to a billion people affected (Hetzel and Mano, 1989). It occurs especially in poorer remote areas where the soil is depleted of iodine and the general diet is limited and lacks useful sources of the mineral. Goitre was once endemic in parts of the UK and other European countries, before the introduction of iodised salt and an improvement in the general diet.

Seafood is the major natural source of iodine in the diet. Fish, crustaceans and seaweeds are rich in the element. Milk is another good, though adventitious, source of dietary iodine as a result of the use of iodine-containing chemicals to sterilise dairy equipment. This practice has now ceased in many countries, with the result that dairy products are decreasing in value as a source of the nutrient. Cereals, vegetables and meat are generally poor sources. Iodised salt (sodium chloride) was introduced in many countries in the mid-twentieth century to combat endemic goitre and its use led to a significant improvement in the iodine nutritional status. Today, a reduction in the availability of iodised salt, coupled with an overall decrease in consumption of table and cooking salt, has resulted in a fall in iodine intakes. There is some concern that as a result, goitre may return to countries where it was once endemic (Solcà et al, 1999).

The RNI for iodine in the UK is 140 µg/day for adults, close to the US RDI of 150 µg. These levels are easily achieved by consumption of a normal diet. Higher intakes of more than 1 mg/day may cause toxicity. This can be the result of excessive use of iodine supplements or, in certain cases, even of natural iodine-rich foods (such as certain seaweeds that can contain more than 4 mg/kg of iodine). Paradoxically, high intakes of iodine depress thyroid function and produce goitre in certain individuals. Because some people, especially the elderly, may be sensitive to high iodine intakes, a Safe Limit of not more than 1 mg/day is recommended in the UK.

4.8.2 Selenium

The metalloid selenium, although one of the rarest of the elements, is an essential trace nutrient for humans and all animals, but not for plants. Its essentiality was only recognised in the 1970s when the enzyme glutathione peroxidase was shown to be a selenoprotein (Rotruck et al, 1973). Previously the element had been known only for its toxicity (Reilly, 1996a).

Selenium, in the form of the unique amino acid selenocysteine, is the co-factor in several important functional metalloproteins. At physiological pH, the selenium in the selenocysteine is almost totally ionised and is an extremely efficient redox catalyst. At least 30 selenoproteins have been shown to occur in mammalian cells. Several of these have been fully characterised and their functions determined in human tissues. One group, the glutathione peroxidases, plays a role in intracellular antioxidant systems. Selenium is also an essential cofactor in the iodothyronine deiodinases, which are enzymes involved in thyroid hormone metabolism. Another important selenoenzyme is thioredoxin reductase which helps to control cell growth and division. Several other selenoproteins, including selenoprotein P and selenoprotein W, also occur in human tissues where they appear to have antioxidant and redox roles (Arthur and Beckett, 1994).

Selenium deficiency is associated with several diseases of major economic importance in farm animals. In humans chronic low intake of dietary selenium is responsible for Keshan disease, a sometimes fatal cardiomyopathy which occurs especially in children and young women, as well as for Kashin-Beck disease, a chronic osteoarthropathy, which also affects mainly children. These diseases are found in parts of China and other areas of Central Asia where soil levels of selenium are very low. Several other selenium-responsive conditions occur in humans, including cardiomyopathies and muscular problems in patients on total parenteral nutrition (TPN) if there is inadequate selenium in the fluid. Normal function of the thyroid gland is also dependent on an adequate supply of the element (Arthur et al, 1999). There is evidence that selenium deficiency can cause a wide range of other problems including immunodeficiency (Beck, 1999), increased susceptibility to various forms of cancer and to coronary arterial disease.

Selenium has been added relatively recently to the dietary recommendations in some countries as evidence establishing its important role in human health has become officially accepted. The UK RNI of 60 µg/day for adult females and 75 µg/day for adult males, is higher than the current US Dietary Reference Intake of 55 µg/day for adults (Institute of Medicine, Food and Nutrition Board, 2000). It is believed, however, by some health experts that these intakes are insufficient to meet human needs since they do not take into consideration the element's critically important protective role against oxidative damage.

Selenium is widely distributed, but normally at levels of less than 1 mg/kg, in most foods. The richest sources are organ meat, such as liver (0.05–1.33 mg/kg), muscle meat (0.06–0.42 mg/kg) and fish (0.05–0.54 mg/kg). Though cereals contain only 0.01–0.31 mg/kg, cereal products make a major contribution to intake because of the relatively large amount of such foods consumed in most diets. Another good source of the element is nuts, particularly Brazil nuts which are the richest food source of the element known (Reilly, 1999). Vegetables, fruit and dairy products are poor sources.

Levels of selenium in plant foods, and in animals that feed on them, reflect levels in soils on which they grow. Soil concentrations are subject to considerable regional variations, and consequently levels in different foods can show a wide range. This has important consequences for dietary intakes in some countries. Thus, in the US where much of the food-producing regions have selenium-rich soils, the average intake of the element is 62–216 μg/day. In parts of China, where the soil is severely depleted, intakes are as low as 3–22 μg/day. In the UK, where, as in other European countries, soil levels are relatively low, average selenium intake is about 40 μg/day.

There is concern among some nutritionists about the possible adverse health effects of low selenium intakes and steps have been taken in some countries to protect the population against them. In Finland the law requires that selenium be added to all fertilisers and, as a result, the selenium status of the population has been more than doubled in recent years. In New Zealand the law permits but does not require farmers to use selenium-enriched top dressings on grazing land, to combat selenium deficiency in farm animals. Self-medication with selenium dietary supplements is widely practised by individuals, and is actively promoted by the pharmaceutical industry and the media in many countries (Reilly, 1996b).

Selenium toxicity, or selenosis, has been well documented in farm animals. It has also occurred in humans in some parts of China where very high levels occur in the soil. There have also been reports of selenosis in individuals who consume excessive amounts of selenium supplements. There is some debate about the levels of intake that will cause toxicity. Residents of some high soil areas appear to have no symptoms of selenium toxicity, although they consume as much as 700 μg/day. According to the Environmental Protection Agency in the US, a daily intake of 5 μg/kg body weight (350 μg for a 70 kg adult) is not toxic. In the UK the recommended maximum safe selenium daily intake from all sources for adults in 6 μg/kg body weight or 450 μg for an adult male (Department of Health, 1991).

4.9 Sources of further information and advice

BEARD J L, DAWSON H and PIÑERO DJ (1996), 'Iron metabolism: a comprehensive review', *Nutr Revs*, **54**, 295–317

BOGDEN J D and KLEVAY M (2000), *Clinical Nutrition of Trace Elements*, Totowa NJ, Humana Press

GARROW J S, JAMES W P T and RALPH A (2000), *Human Nutrition and Dietetics* (10th ed), Chapter 10: *Bone Minerals*, 165–76; Chapter 11: *Iron, zinc and other trace elements*, 177–210. London, Churchill-Livingstone

HURRELL R (2001), *Mineral Fortification of Food*, Leatherhead, Leatherhead Food Research Association

NORDIN B E C (1990), 'Calcium', in Truswell AS, *Recommended Nutrient Intakes*, Sydney, Australian Professional Publications, 199–219

4.10 References

ARTHUR J R and BECKETT G J (1994), 'New metabolic roles for selenium', *Proc Nut Soc*, **53**, 615–24
ARTHUR J R, BECKETT G J and MITCHELL J H (1999), 'The interaction between selenium and iodine deficiencies in man and animals', *Nutr Res Rev*, **12**, 55–73
BALLUZ L S, KIESZAK S M, PHILEN R M and MULINARE J (2000), 'Vitamin and mineral supplement use in the United States', *Arch Family Med*, **9**, 258–62
BARR D B G and FRASER D K B (1968), 'Acute iron poisoning in children: role of chelating agents', *Br Med J*, **i**, 737
BECK M A (1999), 'Selenium and host defence towards viruses', *Proc Nutr Soc*, **58**, 707–11
BERG J M and SHI Y (1996), 'The galvanising of biology: a growing appreciation for the roles of zinc', *Science*, **271**, 1081–5
BOOTH C K, REILLY C and FARMAKALIDES E (1996), 'Mineral composition of Australian ready-to-eat breakfast cereals', *J Food Comp Anal*, **9**, 135–47
BOTHWELL T H, SEFTEL H C, JACOBS P, TORRANCE J D and BAUMSLAG N (1964), 'Iron overload in Bantu subjects. Studies on the availability of iron in Bantu beer', *Am J Clin Nutr*, **14**, 47–51
BRADY M C (1996), 'Addition of nutrients: current practice in the UK', *British Food J*, **98**, 12–8
BRITISH NUTRITION FOUNDATION (1989), *Report of Task Force on Calcium*, London, British Nutrition Foundation
BROCK J H and MULERO V (2000), 'Cellular and molecular aspects of iron and immune function', *Proc Nutr Soc*, **59**, 537–40
BROCK J H, HALLIDAY J W, PIPPARD M J and POWELL L W (1994), *Iron Metabolism in Health and Disease*, London, WB Saunders
BROWN K H, WUEHLER S E and PEERSON J M (2001), 'The importance of zinc in human nutrition and estimation of the global prevalence of zinc deficiency', *Food Nutr Bull*, **22**, 113–25
COOK J D (1999), 'Defining optimal body iron', *Proc Nutr Soc*, **58**, 489–95
COULTATE T P (1985), *Food, the Chemistry of its Components*, 2nd ed, Cambridge, Royal Society of Chemistry
DEPARTMENT OF HEALTH (1991), *Dietary Reference Values for Food Energy and Nutrients in the United Kingdom*, London, HMSO
EXPERT SCIENTIFIC WORKING GROUP (1985), 'Summary of a report on assessment of the iron nutritional status of the United States population', *Am J Clin Nutr*, **42**, 1318–30
FAILLA M L (1999), 'Considerations for determining optimal nutrition for copper, zinc, manganese and molybdenum', *Proc Nutr Soc*, **58**, 497–505
FOOD AND AGRICULTURAL ORGANIZATION (1988), *Requirements of Vitamin A, Iron, Folate and B_{12}. Report of a Joint FAO/WHO Consultation*, Rome, FAO
FORBES R M and ERDMAN J W Q (1983), 'Bioavailability of trace mineral elements', *Ann Rev Nutr*, **3**, 213–31
FREDERICKSON C J, SUH S W, SILVA D and THOMPSON R B (2000), 'Importance of zinc in the central nervous system: the zinc-containing neuron', *J Nutr*, **130**, 1471S–83S
GIBSON R S and FERGUSON E L (1998), 'Nutrition interventions to combat zinc deficiencies in developing countries', *Nutr Res Rev*, **11**, 115–31
HAMBIDGE K M and KREBS N F (1995), 'Assessment of zinc status in man', *Indian J Pediatr*, **62**, 169–80
HAMBIDGE M and KREBS N F (2001), 'Zinc metabolism and requirements', *Food Nutr Bull*, **22**, 126–32
HAMBIDGE K M, GOODALL M J, STALL C and PITTS J (1989), 'Postprandial and daily changes in plasma zinc', *J Trace Elem Electrolytes Health Dis*, **5**, 55–7
HEANEY R P (2001), 'Calcium needs of the elderly to reduce fracture risk', *J Am Coll Nutr*, **20**, 192S–7S

HETZEL B S and MANO M T (1989), 'A review of experimental studies of iodine deficiency', *J Nutr*, **119**, 145–51

HUFFMAN S L, BAKER J, SHUMANN J and ZEHNER E R (1999), 'The case for promoting multiple vitamin and mineral supplements for women of reproductive age in developing countries', *Food Nutr Bull*, **20**, 379–94

INSTITUTE OF MEDICINE, FOOD AND NUTRITION BOARD (1998), *Dietary Reference Intakes for Thiamin, Riboflavin, Niacin, Vitamin B-6, Folate, Vitamin B-12, Pantothenic Acid, Biotin, and Choline*, Washington DC, National Academy Press

INSTITUTE OF MEDICINE, FOOD AND NUTRITION BOARD (2000), *Dietary Reference Intakes for Vitamin C, Vitamin E, Selenium, and Carotenoids*, Washington DC, National Academy Press

JACKSON M J (1989), 'Physiology of zinc: general aspects', in *Zinc in Human Biology*, ed. CF Mills, London, Springer Verlag, 1–14

KING J C, SHAMES D M and WOODHOUSE L R (2000), 'Zinc homeostasis in humans', *J Nutr*, **130**, 1360S–6S

LOOKER A C, DALLMAN P R, CARROLL M D, GUNTER E W and JOHNSON C L (1997), 'Prevalence of iron deficiency in the United States', *J Amer Med Assoc*, **227**, 973–6

MACKEY M, HILL B and GUND C K (1994), 'Health claims regulations: impact on food development', in *Nutritional Toxicology*, eds. FN Kotsonis, M Mackey and J Hielle, 251–71, New York, Raven Press

MUHILAL (1998), 'Indonesian Recommended Dietary Allowance', *Nutr Revs*, **56**, S19–S20

NATIONAL RESEARCH COUNCIL (1989), *Recommended Dietary Allowances*, 10th ed, Washington DC, National Academy Press

OSENDARP S J M, VAN RAAIJ J M A, DARMSTADT G L, BAQUI A H, HAUTVAST J G A J and FUCHS G J (2001), 'Zinc supplementation during pregnancy and effects on growth and morbidity in low birthweight infants: a randomised placebo controlled trial', *Lancet*, **357**, 1080–5

PRASAD A S (1990), 'Discovery of human zinc deficiency and marginal deficiency of zinc', in Tomita H, *Trace Elements in Clinical Medicine*, Tokyo, Springer, 3–11

PRENTICE A (1997), 'Is nutrition important in osteoporosis?,' *Proc Nutr Soc*, **56**, 357–67

PRENTICE A (2001), 'The relative contribution of diet and genotype to bone development', *Proc Nutr Soc*, **60**, 45–52

RANUM P (2001), 'Zinc enrichment of cereal staples', *Food Nutr Bull*, **22**, 169–72

REILLY C (1996a), *Selenium in Food and Health*, London, Blackie

REILLY C (1996b), 'Selenium supplementation – the Finnish experiment', *BNF Nutr Bull*, **21**, 167–73

REILLY C (1998), 'Selenium: a new entrant into the functional food arena', *Trends Food Sc Technol*, **9**, 114–8

REILLY C (1999), 'Brazil nuts – a selenium supplement?' *BNF Nutr Bull*, **24**, 177–84

REILLY C (2002), *Metal Contamination of Food*, 3rd ed, Oxford, Blackwell science

ROTRUCK J T, POPE A, GANTHER H E, SWANSON A B, HAFEMAN D and HOEKSTRA W G (1973), 'Selenium: biological role as a component of glutathione peroxidase', *Science*, **179**, 588–90

SAKAMOTO W, NISHIHIRA J, FUJIE K, IIZUKA T, OZAKI M and YUKAWA S (2001), 'Effect of coffee consumption on bone metabolism', *Bone*, **28**, 332–6

SOLCÀ B, JAEGGI-GROISMAN S E, SAGLINI V and GERBER H (1999), 'Iodine supply in different geographical areas of Switzerland: comparison between rural and urban populations in the Berne and the Ticino regions', *Eur J Clin Nutr*, **53**, 745–55

STATUTORY INSTRUMENT (1984), *Statutory Instrument No. 1304. The Bread and Flour Regulations*, London, HMSO

VAN DOKKUM W (1995), 'The intake of selected minerals and trace elements in European countries', *Nutr Res Rev*, **8**, 271–302

WALSH C T, STANSTEAD H H, PRASAD A S, NEWBERNE P M and FRAKER P J (1994), 'Zinc health effects and research priorities for the 1990s, *Environ Health Perspect*, **102**, 5–46

WALTER T, OLIVARES M, PIZARRO F and MUÑOZ C (1997), 'Iron, anaemia and infection', *Nutr Revs*, **55**, 111–24

WELSH S O and MARSTON R M (1982), 'Zinc levels in the US food supply: 1909–1980', *Food Technol*, **36**, 70–6

WYNNE A (1998), 'Breaking new ground: calcium and bone health, *BNF Nutr Bull*, **23**, 167–72

5

Measuring intake of nutrients and their effects: the case of copper

L. B. McAnena and J. M. O'Connor, University of Ulster

5.1 Introduction

In this chapter, copper is considered as a case study for the measurement of the effect of nutrient intake. The importance of the role of copper in biological systems is first explored in a brief review of selected human cuproenzymes. Worldwide estimates of dietary copper requirements, and dietary recommendations, are discussed. Although dietary sources of copper are numerous, many Western diets appear to be barely adequate in copper. While clinical copper deficiency is rare, usually seen only in malnourished children and premature babies or as a consequence of malabsorption, a proposed link between copper deficiency and degenerative diseases makes the question of suboptimal status an important issue. Copper toxicity, acute or chronic, is also rare, but sound limits for total intake and for levels of copper in drinking water are essential nonetheless. The assessment of nutrient intake, in general, is made difficult by the limitations associated with the available methods. Putative or traditional indicators of copper status are also subject to problems and limitations, and rarely fulfil all of the essential criteria for a good index of copper status. Functional copper status is the product of the interactions of copper with a variety of factors. Foods vary in copper content and digestibility, and the mechanisms involved in absorption are affected by a variety of luminal and systemic factors. Distribution of copper around the body occurs in two phases: transport from the intestine to the liver; and subsequent delivery to other tissues. Problems specific to the assessment of copper absorption are discussed. Some recent advances in copper metabolism research are outlined, along with promising new areas for future study.

5.2 The nutritional role of copper

Copper was identified as an essential trace element, first for animals[1] and subsequently for humans[2] when anaemia was successfully treated by supplementing the diet with a source of copper. Since then the full significance of its role in biological systems has continued to unfold as it has been identified in a large number of vital metalloproteins, as an allosteric component and as a cofactor for catalytic activity. These proteins perform numerous important roles in the body, relating to the maintenance of immune function, neural function, bone health, arterial compliance, haemostasis, and protection against oxidative and inflammatory damage. However, the accurate assessment of copper status is problematic. Functional copper status is the product of many interacting dietary and lifestyle factors, and an adequate marker of body copper status has yet to be identified. Accurate measurement of dietary copper intake is difficult because while a number of dietary factors are known to limit copper bioavailability, the precise molecular mechanisms of copper absorption and metabolism are not completely understood.

Shown in Table 5.1 is a selection of the copper-containing enzymes and proteins known to be important in human systems. A number of these enzymes exhibit oxidative/reductive activity and use molecular oxygen as a co-substrate. In these redox reactions, the ability of copper to cycle between cupric and cuprous states is crucial to its role as electron transfer intermediate. Cytochrome-*c*

Table 5.1 Human copper-containing proteins, and their functions

Protein	Function
Cytochrome-*c* oxidase	Cellular energy production
Ferroxidase I (Caeruloplasmin)	Iron oxidation and transport; free radical scavenging; amine and phenol oxidation; acute-phase immune response
Ferroxidase II	Iron oxidation
Hephaestin	Iron metabolism
Copper/zinc superoxide dismutase	Antioxidant defence
Extracellular superoxide dismutase	Antioxidant defence
Monoamine oxidase	Brain chemistry
Dopamine β-hydroxylase	Brain chemistry
Diamine oxidase	Limitation of cell growth, histamine deactivation
Lysyl oxidase	Connective tissue formation
Peptidylglycine α-amidating monooxygenase	Peptide hormone activation
Prion protein PrP	Antioxidant defence and/or copper sequestration and transport
Tyrosinase	Melanin synthesis
Albumin	Metal binding in plasma and interstitial fluids
Chaperone proteins	Intracellular copper delivery to specific target proteins
Chromatin scaffold proteins	Structural integrity of nuclear material
Clotting factors V and VIII	Thrombogenesis
Metallothionein	Metal sequestration
Transcuprein	Copper binding in plasma

oxidase, embedded in the inner mitochondrial membrane, is the terminal link in the electron transport chain. It catalyses the reduction of oxygen to water. One molecule of cytochrome-c oxidase contains three copper atoms and possesses two active sites. At one site two copper atoms receive, from the electron-carrier cytochrome-c, electrons which are then transferred to the second active site, where the third copper atom functions as a reducing agent.[3] Because this is the rate-limiting step in electron transport, cytochrome-c oxidase is considered the single most important enzyme of the mammalian cell.

Ferroxidases I and II are plasma glycoproteins. Ferroxidase I, also known as caeruloplasmin, oxidises Fe (II) to Fe (III) without formation of hydrogen peroxide (H_2O_2) or oxygen radicals. It is primarily this role which gives rise to caeruloplasmin's well-known antioxidant function. It also scavenges H_2O_2, superoxide and hydroxyl radicals, and inhibits lipid peroxidation and DNA degradation stimulated by free iron and copper ions.[4] Caeruloplasmin is also an acute-phase protein: in acute response to inflammatory cues caeruloplasmin concentration rises, binding free circulating iron and limiting the amount available to participate in oxidative reactions. One molecule of caeruloplasmin contains six copper ions, of which three provide active sites for electron transfer processes, while the remaining three together form an oxygen-activating site for the enzyme's catalytic action.[5] Superoxide dismutase (SOD) is another important and well-studied enzyme. In human systems, it exists in several forms, of which two contain copper: the cytosolic copper/zinc variety sometimes termed SOD1, present in most cells; and the extracellular SOD2, found in the plasma and also in certain cell types in the lung, thyroid and uterus.[6] SOD catalyses the dismutation of superoxide radicals to hydrogen peroxide and oxygen.

In several amine oxidases, copper acts as an allosteric component, conferring the structure required for catalytic activity. Monoamine oxidase (MAO) inactivates, by deamination, substrates such as serotonin and catecholamines including adrenalin, noradrenalin and dopamine. Tricyclic antidepressants are MOA inhibitors. Diamine oxidase (DAO) deaminates histamine and polyamines involved in cell proliferation. It is present at low levels in the plasma, but at higher concentrations in the small intestine where histamine stimulates acid secretion, in the kidney where it likely inactivates diamines filtered from the blood, and in the placenta, where it is thought to inactivate foetal amines in maternal blood. Lysyl oxidase deaminates lysine and hydroxylysine, which are present as sidechains of immature collagen and elastin molecules. It thereby enables the formation of crosslinks which lend strength and flexibility to mature connective tissue.

Peptidyl-glycine α-amidating mono-oxygenase (PAM) is found in the plasma and in a number of tissues, including the brain. It produces mature, α-amidated, peptide hormones from their glycine-extended precursors. The enzyme contains two copper atoms per molecule.[7] Dopamine β-hydroxylase (DβM) is a mono-oxygenase similar to PAM in structure and activity. Found in the adrenal gland and the brain, it catalyses the synthesis of the catecholamines adrenalin and noradrenalin from dopamine. Tyrosinase, or catechol oxidase, is the only enzyme involved in the synthesis of melanin from tyrosine. Tyrosinase first hydroxylates the amino acid to dopa, then oxidises it to dopaquinone. Subsequent reactions

Table 5.2 Dietary Reference Values for copper

Dietary Reference Value	Copper (mg/d)	Source
US EAR	0.7	Food and Nutrition Board, 2001
US RDA	0.9	Food and Nutrition Board, 2001
UK RNI	1.2	Department of Health, 1991
WHO AROI	1.2 to 2 or 3	WHO International Programme on Chemical Safety, 1998

leading to melanins occur spontaneously *in vitro*. Regulation of pigment formation is also provided by tyrosinase, as it can remove substrates from this pathway by catalysing alternative reactions for them.[8] Congenital deficiency of tyrosinase results in albinism.

In the nucleus, copper has a structural role as an essential component of chromatin scaffold proteins, which contribute to nuclear stability.[9,10] It does not, however, appear to be required for DNA synthesis in mammalian cells. Although in yeast cells, copper has been identified as a component of gene regulatory mechanisms, if equivalent proteins exist in human cells they remain to be identified.[11]

5.3 Dietary copper requirements

Despite the known essentiality of copper in humans, dietary requirements are still uncertain. World-wide, a number of Dietary Reference Values are recommended for copper intake (see Table 5.2) but the variability between them is indicative of the lack of consensus between advisory bodies. Making dietary recommendations, even of Estimated Average Requirements (EAR), is difficult owing to a lack of adequate data. In the UK, the Department of Health considers the available data on human copper requirements to be insufficient to determine an EAR.[12] In the US, an EAR of adults for copper was derived from a combination of biochemical indicators of copper requirement, as no single indicator was judged as sufficiently sensitive, specific and consistent to be used alone.

A Recommended Daily Allowance (RDA) can be calculated by extrapolating the EAR to account for inter-individual variation in requirements. The US RDA, like the UK Reference Nutrient Intake (RNI) is intended to provide enough copper for about 97% of adults. The World Health Organization has loosely defined an Acceptable Range of Oral Intake (AROI). Its upper limit could not be specifically confirmed because of the limited information available on the level of intake that would provoke adverse heath effects. It is apparent that more data are needed if sound and defensible guidelines are to be derived.

5.4 Sources of copper

In most diets, sources of copper are numerous because copper is widespread in foods. Rich sources include organ meats, nuts, shellfish, seeds, legumes and the germ portion of grains. Other foods including cereals, meats, mushrooms, potatoes, tomatoes, bananas and other dried fruits provide sufficient copper in a normal diet to ensure that overt copper deficiency is rare in human populations. Nonetheless, many Western diets are estimated to supply a level of copper only barely adequate to meet the body's requirements. Published estimates of copper intake vary around 1–2 mg/d, with few diets containing more than 2 mg/d.[13,14,15,16,17]

5.5 Copper deficiency

Clinical copper deficiency is seen mainly in malnourished and recovering children, in premature babies, in patients receiving total parenteral nutrition (TPN) and as a consequence of malabsorption. Copper deficiency also occurs as the result of Menkes syndrome, a rare inherited defect of copper transport. Malnourished children are reported to be at particular risk of copper deficiency. A diet consisting exclusively or predominantly of cow's milk, with its poor bioavailability of copper, increases the likelihood of copper malabsorption. During nutritional recovery, growth rate can be 5–10 times the normal rate, increasing copper requirements beyond the dietary intake.[3] Copper deficiency during this period has been shown to impair growth rate[18] and to be associated with increased incidence of respiratory infection.[19]

Preterm babies are also at particular risk of copper deficiency, for several reasons. Copper stores are acquired late in foetal development, as metallothionein-bound copper accumulates in the foetal hepatocyte nuclei over the last trimester.[11] Although neonates appear not to absorb copper well, particularly from highly-refined carbohydrate-based diets or cow's milk[20], full-term infants have well-developed copper stores which can be mobilised during the first six months' rapid growth, to supplement dietary intake.[21] Full-term infants are therefore independent of dietary intake for the first weeks of life.[22] Premature babies, especially those with very low birth-weight, do not have such a resource. They also have higher growth rate than full-term babies, with accordingly higher copper requirements.[23]

Clinical copper deficiency in adults was unknown until the introduction of TPN, which is now well known to result in elevated urinary copper output and a net depletion of copper status.[20] Although copper is now usually added to TPN infusates, it is often withheld from cholestatic patients since their impaired biliary excretion is expected to result in reduced intestinal losses. The complex interactions between disease states and copper metabolism, however, make individuals' requirements difficult to anticipate, and TPN-related copper deficiency continues to occur.[24,25]

A number of malabsorption syndromes have been reported to result in increased intestinal copper losses leading to deficiency. Such conditions include coeliac disease[26], cystic fibrosis[27], shortened intestine following surgery[28], and chronic or recurrent diarrhoea.[29,30] Menkes disease is an X-linked recessive disorder of copper metabolism in which mutations in the MNK gene impair copper transport from cells. The disease is manifest as copper deficiency, because although copper is absorbed by gut cells, very little is transported to the tissues where it is required for enzyme function. Symptoms usually appear within the first months of life, and can result in death in early childhood.[31] In clinical copper deficiency, the most common defects are: cardiovascular and haematological disorders including iron-resistant anaemia, neutropenia and thrombocytopenia; bone abnormalities including osteoporosis and fractures; and alterations to skin and hair texture and pigmentation.[23] Immunological changes have also been indicated.[19,32] These changes may be accompanied by depressed serum copper and blood cuproenzymes, with caeruloplasmin concentrations observed at 30% of normal.[6]

It has been clearly demonstrated that very many of the changes induced by severe copper deficiency are also risk factors for ischaemic heart disease in humans. Human copper depletion studies have produced impaired glucose clearance,[33] blood pressure changes,[34] electrocardiographic irregularities and significantly increased LDL cholesterol with decreased HDL cholesterol.[21] In copper-deficient animals, cardiovascular disorders observed include lesion and rupture of blood vessels, cardiac enlargement, myocardial degeneration and infarction (MI).[33] It has been argued that copper deficiency is the only nutritional deficit known to affect adversely so many risk factors for ischaemic heart disease.[35] The proposed link between copper deficiency and cardiovascular disease is supported by data gathered from studies of cardiovascular patients. Post-mortem measurement of tissue copper has revealed lower-than-normal copper concentrations in ischaemic hearts, in the liver and heart of individuals with severe atherosclerosis, and in leucocytes of patients with highly occluded coronary arteries.[33]

A variety of mechanisms may contribute to the cardiovascular effects of copper deficiency. There is evidence for alterations in the activity of copper-dependent enzymes, increased oxidative stress and damage to biomolecules, and interference with the maintenance of blood pressure. An interaction of these three mechanisms of damage has been proposed to have even further potential for harm,[36] which need not be limited to cardiovascular defects. The adverse effects elicited by copper deficiency are numerous and as varied as the roles of copper in health. In the light of this, it has been proposed that long-term sub-clinical copper deficiency may contribute to the pathogenesis of a number of degenerative and inflammatory conditions.[37]

5.6 Copper toxicity

Copper toxicity is rare because levels in food and water are generally low and because increased dietary intake results in decreased absorption and increased excretion.[38] Cases of both acute and chronic poisoning have, however, been reported. Acute toxicity has been known to result from accidental or deliberate consumption of copper salts and, more commonly, from contamination of drinks by copper containers.[6] A 1957 report of contamination of cocktails stored for just two hours in a metal cocktail shaker was used in 1988 by US Environmental Protection Agency (EPA) Office of Drinking Water to derive drinking water regulations which are still in place.[39] Acute toxicity results, initially, in symptoms such as abdominal pain, nausea, vomiting and diarrhoea. These gastrointestinal effects are often sufficiently severe and prompt to prevent systemic toxicity which, like chronic copper poisoning, is associated with liver damage. Chronic toxicity has most often been caused by contaminated water supplies, and occasionally by contamination of haemodialysis equipment by copper parts.[40]

The highest intake which has been shown experimentally to produce no adverse effects is defined as the No-Observed-Adverse-Effects-Level (NOAEL). While a NOAEL of 4 mg/l in drinking water has been observed for acute effects,[41] a higher NOAEL of 10 mg supplemental copper per day has been demonstrated to provoke no ill effect upon liver function after 12 weeks.[42] The US Food and Nutrition Board have used the latter value to calculate a theoretical Tolerable Upper Intake Level (UL), defined as the highest level of daily intake considered likely to pose no threat to the health of almost all individuals. The UL is in agreement with the World Health Organization's provisional maximum tolerable daily intake (PTDI), an estimate of the amount that can be ingested daily over a lifetime without appreciable risk to health.

In drinking water, copper levels vary considerably depending on factors including the pH and hardness of the water supply and the length of piping. In some systems, copper salts are added to control the growth of algae.[16] Suggested upper limits for copper in drinking water differ world-wide, and while some are based on health issues, others consider only aesthetic values. The issue is currently under review by several international groups.[39] Table 5.3 shows current permissible levels of copper in drinking water, and recommended limits of total copper intake.

A number of disorders of copper homeostasis can result in toxicity leading to liver cirrhosis at dietary copper levels which are tolerated by the general population. Copper-induced cirrhosis is mainly restricted to children, possibly because

Table 5.3 Recommended limits of copper intake

Reference Value	Copper limit	Source
In drinking water (mg/l)		
UK standard	3.0	Water Supply (Water Quality) Regulations, 1989
WHO standard	2.0	WHO Guidelines for Drinking Water Quality, 1993
EU standard	2.0	EU Directive 98/83 L330, 32–54
US maximum contaminant level	1.3	EPA Drinking Water Regulations, 1988
Total intake (mg/d)		
US UL	10.0	Food and Nutrition Board, 2001
WHO PTDI	10.0 (women) 12.0 (men)	World Health Organization, 1996

of the lower capacity of their biliary excretory mechanisms.[38] Indian Childhood Cirrhosis (ICC) is a fatal condition of copper metabolism which was, at one time, a major cause of infant mortality on the Indian subcontinent. ICC sufferers, usually infants aged between 6 months and 5 years, are often found to have been exposed at an early age to milk contaminated with copper from untinned brass or copper vessels.[43] High copper intake, however, is not thought to be the sole cause of the illness; both environmental and genetic components are thought to contribute.[44] Cases of a similar infantile condition have been reported in Germany and in the Tyrol, Austria.[45,46] Incidence of both ICC and Tyrolean Infantile Cirrhosis has dropped in recent years. One possible explanation is reduced use of brass vessels, while an alternative is the dilution of the responsible gene by increased population mobility and fewer consanguineous marriages.

A rare inherited disorder of copper metabolism leads to Wilson's disease, in which copper cannot be properly transported out of the liver and so accumulates to toxic levels. When the hepatocytes die, copper is released into the plasma and deposited in other tissues including the central nervous system.[47] Treatment of Wilson's disease is aimed at removing copper from the body and preventing its reaccumulation.

5.7 General limitations in assessing nutrient intake

As for any nutrient where deficiency and toxicity are issues, the reliable assessment of intake is paramount. The ultimate aim of defining optimal dietary intakes is hampered by difficulties in determining certain key facts, namely, individual copper intakes and status. Dietary intake can be assessed by a number of methods, involving either the recording of actual consumption (prospective) or the assessment by questionnaires of diet in the recent past (retrospective). At each stage in the application of any method, errors are introduced, producing as a result either a systematic bias or random deviations from the true values. Of the methods in common use, the weighed dietary record is widely accepted to be the most accurate, but it requires a considerable amount of co-operation from human subjects. This disadvantage may give rise to substantial bias, most likely toward underreporting habitual dietary intakes.[48] In clinical practice the most frequently used method of dietary assessment is the diet history, which is highly dependent on accurate recall by the individual. It is possible to verify these reports, to some extent, by independent methods. Under- and over-estimation of an individual's total food intake can be identified by measuring total energy expenditure, either directly, using the doubly-labelled water technique, or indirectly, by calculating basal metabolic rate. Another check is a comparison of the individual's 24-hour urinary nitrogen output with the reported protein intake. The accuracy of these methods is limited either by the involvement of estimates, or by reliance on the assumption that body weight is constant.

One means of assessing nutrient requirements is the metabolic balance study. The aim of a balance study is to compare the intake of a nutrient with the amount

Measuring intake of nutrients and their effects: the case of copper

leaving the body. A constant daily intake of the nutrient in question is provided throughout the study period, and collection of stools and urine are made. Crucial to the success of the investigation is the accuracy of measurement of intake and excretion. For this reason, balance studies demand careful planning and execution, good facilities for food preparation, sample collection and sample storage, and good laboratory services. A major limitation is that balance studies provide little information about nutrient transport or utilisation within the body.[22]

Nutrient intake can also be assessed by the use of experimental diets with different mineral intakes. The use of experimental diets to determine nutrient requirements depends on the selection and measurement of a biochemical endpoint, to serve as a marker of nutrient sufficiency. However, experimental diets must be carefully constituted to minimise the possibility that other dietary components may modify absorption of the nutrient, or even influence directly the chosen marker.[23] A limitation of this method is that it permits the estimation of the basal nutrient requirements, but not the amount needed to maintain bodily nutrient reserves.

Epidemiological studies such as the US Total Diet Study[13] or the North/South Ireland Food Consumption Survey[15] are often carried out with the aim of estimating the fraction of the population at risk from deficiency or excess intake. Attempts are made to assess long-term average intake of populations from data gained using short-term measures of intake. Few studies have reported testing the validity of such an extrapolation, but a recent study which examined values calculated from up to six samples, spaced over a year, found significant temporal variability for individual subjects.[49] In addition, when the reliability of short-term (4-day) samples was estimated by comparing individual values to the aggregate value, results suggested that three short-term samples would be required to achieve a strong correlation ($r = 0.9$) between short- and long-term values. Traditional reliance on short-term measures for estimation of long-term copper status could produce erroneous results.

5.8 Putative copper indicators

Determination of copper status suffers from the lack of sensitive, reliable and easy measures for detecting marginal copper status. Copper levels in the hair, nails or saliva do not appear to reflect copper status.[50] Urinary copper is normally extremely low, and although it can decline in extreme copper deficiency, this is usually seen only after changes are seen in other copper indices.[17] In copper depletion and repletion studies, cuproenzyme activities have appeared relatively insensitive to change.[51]

The traditional and most commonly used putative indicator of copper status is serum or plasma copper. Under normal circumstances, strong homeostatic mechanisms maintain the range between 0.64 and 1.56 µg/ml.[50] Although in severe copper depletion it has been known to fall to very low levels, and to recover upon copper repletion, it does not appear to reflect dietary levels when intake is close to normal.[17] It does not increase after a meal or decrease during short-term fasting and has been shown to correspond poorly with reported dietary intakes.[52] In some studies of copper depletion, serum copper responses have been absent even in the presence of other biochemical or physiological changes.[53]

Serum copper is known to be altered by a number of factors not directly related to copper status. Concentrations are low in infancy and rise to adult levels over the first 4–6 months, or longer following a low birth weight. In adult women, serum copper concentration is generally higher than in men, and is further raised during pregnancy and by oestrogen treatments.[54] There is also a normal diurnal variation with a slight peak in the morning. Plasma copper fluctuates with age, and is raised in a number of other conditions including exercise, rheumatoid arthritis, dilated cardiomyopathy and anticonvulsant chemotherapy. Between 60 and 95% of serum copper is associated with caeruloplasmin, so serum copper levels often mirror those of caeruloplasmin.[11]

Normal levels of serum or plasma caeruloplasmin protein are 180–400 μg/ml.[17] Like serum copper, caeruloplasmin has shown variable responses to marginal depletion. Its concentration and activity fall with severe copper deficiency and return to normal with copper repletion; but because of its role as an acute phase protein, caeruloplasmin concentration in the plasma reflects oxidative status more reliably than copper status. Copper depletion may be masked by caeruloplasmin elevated in response to exercise, infection or inflammation, liver disease, malignancy and MI.[55] Like serum copper, normal caeruloplasmin values also vary with age and gender, and during pregnancy.[23]

Erythrocyte copper/zinc SOD concentration is normally 0.471 ± 0.067 mg/g protein.[50] SOD activity has appeared in some studies to be more sensitive than caeruloplasmin to changes in copper status, while in other studies its activity has fallen with depletion but failed to respond to repletion.[56] Copper/zinc SOD activity has been reported to rise in response to physical exercise.[57] As an antioxidant enzyme, SOD is likely to respond to conditions of oxidative stress. A further complicating factor is that SOD measured in erythrocytes is unlikely to reflect short-term changes in dietary intake owing to the 100-day lifetime of erythrocytes. Leucocyte copper has been found to decline along with other indices of copper status.[51] Platelet copper has been shown to decline with copper depletion and to recover with copper repletion.[56] However, there are not yet sufficient experimental data to confirm the validity of leucocyte or platelet copper as indicators of suboptimal copper status. DAO has been indicated in some studies of copper depletion as a possible marker of copper status.[58] Its measurement is currently difficult because of its extremely low levels in plasma. Furthermore, its use as an indicator may be limited because it is elevated during pregnancy, after heparin treatment and in some conditions of intestinal damage.

A valid functional index must respond sensitively, specifically and predictably to changes in the dietary supply or stores of copper, and must be measurable and accessible for measurement. Validation of a candidate marker would require demonstration of a cause and effect relationship between the marker and copper status and also, ideally, between copper status and health measures.[59]

5.9 Functional copper status

The body's total copper content is the end result of a balance achieved between absorption and biliary excretion. In comparison to other trace elements, relatively little copper is present in the body, usually about 100 mg. The largest tissue pool of copper is in the skeleton, followed by the muscle;[60] however, the major site for storage of exchangeable copper is the liver,[61] which contains 4–6 µg/g wet weight.[60] This is followed by the brain, kidney and heart.

Functional copper status, however, is not dependent only on the absolute copper content of the body. Utilisation of absorbed copper is also modulated by the interactions of copper with a number of other factors, deriving from the general status and requirements of the body. Furthermore, individual organs have the potential to modulate copper status by retaining copper in response to dietary restriction. This capacity is highly organ-specific, being stronger and/or more sensitive in some tissues than in others. Depletion studies in animals have found plasma to possess almost no copper conservation mechanisms, whereas the heart and brain were shown to conserve most of their endogenous copper during periods of restriction.[62] Liver copper conservation mechanisms, while induced only after levels had dropped to around 60% of normal, were thereafter found to operate so strictly that almost no copper was exported into the plasma, and biliary copper excretion was also significantly reduced.

5.10 Mechanisms of copper absorption

Copper absorption in humans has been found to depend on a number of factors, of which the most important is probably dietary copper intake.[6] The efficiency of copper absorption is regulated to maintain body copper status, with levels of uptake rising to 70% during periods of deficiency,[63] and falling to 12% in high-copper diets.[61] This modulation of absorption, which provides a means of adapting to changing dietary intake, appears to develop during childhood, with copper absorption in infants operating at a lower level than in adults.[38] While a low level of copper absorption occurs in the stomach, the main site of absorption is the duodenum. Copper absorption from the gut lumen by enterocytes involves both passive and active carrier-mediated systems, which uptake copper across the brush-border, and transport it across the basolateral membrane into the plasma.

Most of the copper in foods is found as a component of macromolecules. Inorganic mineral salts are present in dietary supplements but otherwise probably do not contribute substantially to dietary copper intake.[64] In the UK only 1–2% of adults report taking supplements containing copper[65] although in the US the figure may be as high as 15%.[17] The sulphate, nitrate, chloride and acetate are easily absorbed, but copper oxide and copper porphyrin are unavailable.[63] Gastric acid can solubilise the carbonate and facilitate the release of copper from macromolecules.[64]

Most of the copper in human diets is supplied by vegetable foods, and vegetarian diets generally provide a higher intake. Plant materials, however, are generally less digestible than animal tissues. A substantial proportion of the copper in whole grains is associated with lectins and glycoproteins. Vegetable tissues frequently require more enzymatic attack to digest the copper-binding matrix than do animal proteins, which are generally more easily solubilised, so that percentage copper absorption may in fact be substantially higher from an animal protein diet than from a plant-protein diet.[66] Even so, the greater copper content of a vegetarian diet is likely to provide more available copper.[67] Dairy products contain relatively little copper, with cow's milk being particularly poor. Absorption is estimated at 24% for human milk and 18% for cow's milk. The quaternary protein structure is thought to exert an effect on the availability of copper in food, as cooked meat has been found to supply more available copper than raw.[64] The efficiency of absorption from food is modified by a variety of luminal factors including copper intake levels, other dietary factors and aspects of the intestinal environment. Dietary components known to modify absorption include protein, amino acids, zinc, manganese, iron, tin, molybdenum, sugars, dietary fibre and ascorbate.[55]

Studies of dietary protein and copper retention in young women have found highest retention with a diet high in protein.[68] However, copper bioavailability in high-protein foods may be decreased by heat treatments which promote condensation reaction, such as the Maillard Reaction, between sugars and amino acids.[69] The formation of products such as lactulosyl-lysine and lysinoalanine depletes the food of free amino acids. This leaves fewer sites available for the formation of organo-metallic complexes, from which copper is highly bioavailable.[70] The bioavailabilities of copper-lysine and copper-methionine complexes, relative to copper sulphate, have been reported as 120% and 96% respectively.[71]

Copper uptake by the intestinal mucosa is strongly influenced by chelation of copper ions by amino acids. Chelation may even be a mandatory requirement for copper absorption.[64] Yet, although dietary amino acids can enhance copper absorption, when present in excess they may result in copper malabsorption, possibly by competing with binding proteins on the enterocyte membrane. The ratio of chelate to metal may determine whether there is a net inhibition or promotion of copper uptake. In one human study, methionine supplementation was found to increase copper absorption.[72] Animal studies have provided less straightforward results. One study of rats found that excess dietary methionine decreased indices of copper status.[73] Jejunal copper uptake has been found to be decreased by high levels of dietary proline or histidine,[74] while excessive cystine and cysteine have been shown to exacerbate the effects of dietary copper deficiency.[75] Cysteine is thought to decrease copper bioavailability by reducing Cu (II) to Cu (I).[71]

The high bioavailability of copper in human milk, compared to cow's milk, may be a consequence of the two foods' protein and amino acid content. Ruminant milk has a higher level of low-molecular-weight ligands, which can inhibit copper absorption. In addition, copper is differently-distributed among the milks' constituents: human milk has a much larger fraction of its copper content bound to whey, as well as to lipids.[64] The antagonistic nature of the copper-zinc relationship has been known for decades. In animals, dietary zinc intake has an inverse relationship with copper absorption.[76] In patients with Wilson's disease, zinc salts are given orally to lower copper status by limiting absorption.[77]

Copper in the gut lumen competes for absorption with zinc, as well as iron and other divalent metal ions. Divalent metals, with their similar electron configurations, can form similar co-ordination complexes.[65] This could reduce absorption by displacing copper from specific transporter molecules on the brush border membrane[78] or by competing for ligands which are necessary for uptake by these receptors.[55] After uptake by enterocytes, intracellular zinc may exert a further antagonistic effect on copper transport. High zinc concentrations are thought to induce the metal-binding protein metallothionein, which has a higher affinity for copper than for zinc. This binding blocks the export of copper, as well as zinc, across the basolateral membrane.[55] Recent studies have elucidated a further aspect of the copper-zinc relationship.[79] Dietary zinc inadequacy was found to be more detrimental to copper status than moderately high zinc intake, suggesting a degree of interdependence. Although at high levels of intake the two metals act antagonistically, adequate zinc levels are beneficial for copper utilisation.

Copper status can also be impaired by high intakes of manganese.[80] Iron and tin, in their divalent forms, have also been shown in animals to compete with copper when present in the diet at high levels.[81] Both metals have been known to contaminate food from cooking vessels. Animal studies have suggested that high iron intake affects copper absorption only when copper status is low or marginal.[65] In the context of a copper-normal diet its influence on copper absorption in adults may be minimal. However, babies fed an iron-enriched formula have been found to absorb less copper than infants on the same, but lower-iron, formula.[82] In rhesus monkeys, which are excellent models of human babies, infants fed a commercially-available iron-enriched formula for 5 months had significantly lower copper status than those fed a lower-iron formula.[83]

In sheep and other ruminants, interactions between copper and molybdenum have frequently been observed. Chronic molybdenum poisoning in livestock (teart disease) can depress tissue and blood copper levels and produce anaemia and bone deformities, generally symptoms of copper deficiency. In humans, high molybdenum intake has been found to increase urinary copper excretion and result in lowered blood copper.[121] The symptoms of excessive molybdenum intake can generally be improved by increasing copper intake.[122] Molybdenum is also known to influence intestinal copper absorption: the unabsorbable molybdenum complex, thiomolybdate, inhibits intestinal copper uptake and has been used as a treatment for Wilson's disease.[85]

Dietary carbohydrate choice can also influence copper status. The interactions of dietary sugars with copper absorption in humans are not yet well understood, but there is evidence to suggest both systemic and luminal influences upon copper absorption. Glucose polymers are thought to enhance copper uptake by increasing mucosal water uptake.[64] Dietary fibres such as phytate may somewhat decrease copper uptake, but it is likely that other divalent ions are more strongly bound. Dephytinisation, a process frequently used by food processors to improve the bioavailability of metals, can therefore indirectly reduce absorption of dietary copper by increasing the availability of free, competing, divalent ions.[64]

In animals, palmitic and stearic acids have been found to reduce the rate of copper uptake from the jejunum.[86] In the literature on humans, there is little data regarding the relationship between dietary lipid intake and copper absorption. One human study of the influence of fatty acids on metal absorption indicated that polyunsaturated fatty acids have no effect on copper uptake.[87] High dietary levels of ascorbate are thought to reduce Cu (II) to Cu (I), thereby lowering its intestinal absorption rate.[88] Conversely, however, utilisation of copper is increased by tissue ascorbate, as it facilitates the release of copper from caeruloplasmin.[22] High intakes of ascorbate have been found to decrease serum caeruloplasmin activity and serum copper.[89] A moderately raised intake (605 mg ascorbate/day) has proved sufficient to lower caeruloplasmin activity by 21% without altering intestinal absorption or other markers of copper status.[90] Other organic acids, including citric acid, have also been shown to form soluble complexes with copper. It is probably for this reason that fruit intake has a positive effect on copper status.[91] The efficiency with which any dietary nutrient is absorbed *and utilised* in the body is described as bioavailability. It is an essential consideration in the nutritional evaluation of foods and diets.[12]

In studies of the bioavailability of some minerals, the degree of utilisation may be inferred by measuring some functional endpoint such as the level of synthesis, or activity, of certain biomolecules. Iron bioavailability, for instance, can be determined by measuring the incorporation of a stable isotope into haemoglobin. For copper, however, no single index of utilisation has yet been identified. As a result, estimates of bioavailability have previously focused on measuring intestinal absorption, or bodily retention, rather than utilisation.[92] Nonetheless, copper utilisation is influenced by a number of endogenous factors not directly related to luminal absorption rates. By exerting nonluminal effects upon copper utilisation, such factors may result in impaired copper status.

The copper-depleting effect of excess dietary histidine in rats is associated with increased urinary excretion of chelated copper.[93] The high level of low-molecular-weight chelates in cow's milk may help to explain the copper deficiency sometimes observed in infants fed on unmodified cow's milk. This may be particularly relevant during periods of anabolic activity, such as recovering from malnutrition.

An association has also been observed between very high intake of fructose or sucrose and a worsening of the effects of copper deficiency in rats,[94,95] but not in pigs.[96] In humans, similar experiments[97] have produced changes including cardiac arrhythmia and reduction of erythrocyte SOD activity with apparently increased copper balance, suggesting that high fructose intake acts systemically to raise body copper requirements. Experimental evidence implicating high fat

5.11 Copper distribution in the body

Copper distribution around the body appears to operate in two phases.[60] In the first phase, copper ions are exported from enterocytes into the circulation. This is controlled by specific copper transporting proteins, including ATP7A, a P-type ATPase localised to the trans-Golgi network. It is also known as the Menkes protein MNK, because hereditary deficiency results in Menkes disease.[99]

Copper ions secreted from the intestinal mucosa are immediately bound to the high-affinity plasma proteins albumin and transcuprein.[60] In physiological conditions, copper is almost always protein-bound, resulting in extremely low plasma concentrations of free ionic copper, perhaps as low as 10^{-18} Molar. Protein-bound copper is transported to the liver and kidney. Of the copper taken up by liver parenchymal cells, approximately 80% is excreted in the bile.[100] Intestinal excretion provides the major mechanism for body copper homeostasis, urinary copper excretion being normally less than 0.1 mg/d. Several pathways involving sequential protein-to-protein transfers are believed to be involved in copper transport across the hepatocyte.[101] Cytoplasmic carrier proteins deliver copper to sites of synthesis of cytoplasmic cuproenzymes such as superoxide dismutase. Carrier proteins also supply copper to specific organelle-bound transporter proteins which control its incorporation into mitochondrial proteins, or entry into the hepatocyte secretory pathway.[60] The trans-Golgi network protein ATP7B is involved both in bile formation and in caeruloplasmin secretion.[99] Congenital deficiency of this enzyme results in Wilson's disease.

The second phase of body copper transport involves its efflux from liver and kidney and delivery to other tissues. It is secreted into the plasma, from liver and kidney cells, bound mainly to caeruloplasmin.[60] From studies using radioisotopes to trace body copper transport, caeruloplasmin appears to be the main copper carrier around the body. Most tissues have been shown to have specific surface receptors for caeruloplasmin-copper, and to take it up from solution,[102] either by endocytosis of the complex or by transfer of the copper to an intracellular receptor. There remains some uncertainty, however, concerning the importance of caeruloplasmin's role in body copper distribution. The protein is not thought to be crucial to copper transport because the genetic defect acaeruloplasminaemia does not severely disrupt copper metabolism. It appears that there is redundancy in the system, with copper also available to tissues from non-caeruloplasmin sources including proteins and other ligands. Current thinking is that tissues absorb copper preferentially from caeruloplasmin, but can utilise other sources if caeruloplasmin is not available.[60]

Hephaestin is a recently discovered membrane-bound glycoprotein. A homologue of caeruloplasmin, it appears to play a role in iron metabolism and has been most highly localised to the small intestinal villi, the site of iron absorption.[103]

5.12 Assessment of copper absorption

Early research into human copper metabolism involved studies of copper intake and excretion, copper balance and tissue concentrations, which permitted the estimation of bodily requirements and dietary recommendations.[104] Studies on laboratory animals, and the use of *in vitro* techniques such as intestinal perfusion and the creation of sacs from everted duodenal segments, have contributed much to our understanding of intestinal mechanisms. The use of balance studies to examine copper metabolism poses certain difficulties. Firstly, the regulation of copper absorption according to dietary intake is a process which may require a period of adaptation. For absorption to reflect bodily requirement accurately, therefore, a balance study must be of considerable duration.[92] Secondly, the estimation of losses is difficult owing to a current scarcity of data concerning copper levels in sweat, integument, hair, nails, menstrual blood and semen. Thirdly, balance studies of children must account for the changing copper requirements associated with growth, about which little information is available.[105]

The introduction of isotopic tracers as an investigative tool has permitted detailed examination of absorption mechanisms, dose effects and interactions with other minerals and food components. Findings in mammals of a saturable, carrier-mediated transport mechanism are compatible with the dose-related reduction in absorption which has been demonstrated in humans. The absorption of stable and radioactive isotopes of copper may be determined after oral administration by monitoring either their disappearance from the gut lumen or their incorporation into biomolecules.[106] Copper has seven radioisotopes, of which only ^{64}Cu and ^{67}Cu have half-lives long enough to be useful in metabolic research – 12.8 h and 58.5 h respectively. These relatively short half-lives limit the use of radioisotopes to short-term studies.

Longer-term studies require the use of stable isotopes which have several additional advantages: because they emit no radiation, they are safe to use in high-risk population groups; and because there is no decay, samples can be stored without loss of signal. Copper has two stable isotopes, ^{63}Cu and ^{65}Cu, which both have high natural abundances – 69.2% and 30.8% respectively. To act as a tracer, an isotope must be 'enriched' to a higher proportion than in nature. The production of enough ^{63}Cu or ^{65}Cu to detect above background levels is costly. The use of such large doses raises further problems. The intravenous administration of non-physiological quantities of the mineral may alter normal metabolism[107] while the labelling of food with ^{65}Cu has been found to change its copper content substantially.[108] In studies of trace minerals, the simultaneous use of multiple stable isotopes offers a means to study the effects of different compounds and different routes of administration. Such studies are necessarily impossible for copper, because with only two stable isotopes, only one can be enriched at a time.

Biological samples obtained in stable isotope studies are analysed by determining isotopic ratios. Available methods are generally slow and expensive, and require access to sophisticated analytical equipment. Neutron Activation

Analysis, Electron Ionisation Mass-Spectrometry and Gas-Chromatography Mass-Spectrometry all offer relatively poor precision, while Thermal Ionisation Mass-Spectrometry is laborious and slow. Inductively Coupled Plasma Mass-Spectrometry, used since the 1980s for trace-element quantification, offers acceptable precision with faster analysis and a lower limit of detection than the other methods.[109] Most radioisotopes can be measured by whole-body counting of gamma-emissions, but this method of detection is not readily applicable to copper, owing to the radioisotopes' short half-life. It has, however, been applied in studies of abnormal copper absorption and retention.[110]

Faecal monitoring, of stable or radioisotopes, is currently the most widely used method for assessing copper absorption. A stool marker may be given simultaneously to test for completeness of faecal collection, and may consist of indigestible beads or a non-absorbable chemical marker. In this method, the relatively rapid re-excretion of absorbed copper necessitates special consideration. Even before the non-absorbed fraction of an oral dose has left the body – a process which has been found to take five to seven days – re-excretion of the absorbed isotope will have begun. To correct for this, the rate of endogenous excretion must be determined. Owing to the large inter-individual variation,[110] it should be measured in each individual. Faecal monitoring of a radioisotope for longer than five days would require more than the maximum safe dose[106] so endogenous excretion must be determined on a separate occasion using an intravenous dose.

One application of tracer data obtained from isotope studies is the development of compartmental models of metabolism. In this technique, modelling software is used to compile extensive data on copper distribution and transport into a model simulating whole-body copper metabolism. This provides a powerful tool to describe and predict copper kinetics and to determine dietary requirements.[111] Kinetic modelling provides a means to correlate experimental data from previous studies. Existing information including tissue concentrations, fractional transfer and turnover rates can be assembled into a system in which known components are viewed in perspective. This can have the effect of highlighting areas requiring further research. It can also be used to improve experimental design by simulating in advance the system of interest.

5.13 Current research and future trends

Research into copper metabolism has benefited from recent advances in several areas, with development of novel techniques and refinement of existing methods for the measurement of copper absorption, utilisation and excretion; and ongoing investigations into the biological roles of copper. A recent development in faecal monitoring techniques has been the validation of a novel method to distinguish the non-absorbed portion of an oral label from the absorbed but re-excreted portion.[112] While, previously, this was achieved by a separate test of endogenous excretion rate, it is now possible to measure true absorption by use of the rare earth metal holmium as a faecal marker. Because its excretion pattern parallels that of copper, it can safely be assumed that all label recovered after complete holmium clearance, is re-excreted copper. While other rare earth metals have been used to check for completeness of faecal collection, their excretion pattern differs from that of copper, precluding their use for estimating true absorption. Owing to the limitations of faecal collection, a plasma indicator of absorption may be preferable. This approach requires that newly-absorbed, albumin- and transcuprein-bound copper be distinguishable from the caeruloplasmin-copper pool. Whereas the movement of injected isotopes between the two compartments is readily traceable, orally-administered isotopes are more slowly transported into plasma, resulting in a problematic temporal overlap of the two copper pools. This issue has recently been addressed in a novel method of separating tracer-bound albumin by dialysis.[113]

Recent research using both stable and radioisotopes has benefited from the development of detectors with ever-lower detection limits and the ability to distinguish different isotopes. An increasing range of software applications for the mathematical modelling of biological systems has also contributed to ongoing developments. One such application is SAAMII, produced in the University of Washington, Seattle. A recent mass spectrometry technique currently being applied to human nutrition studies is Inductively-Coupled Plasma Mass-Spectrometry. With a reported lower limit of detection below 1.4 ng/ml human plasma,[114] it has recently been used to evaluate apparent copper absorption from vegetarian and non-vegetarian diets.[67] Accurate assessment of functional copper status has long been hindered by the current lack of a plasma or tissue parameter suitable for use as an index of copper utilisation. Ongoing investigations attempt to identify such a marker. Although numerous copper-containing biomolecules have been observed to change in response to clinical copper deficiency, none has yet been verified as a valid index of marginal copper status.

PAM, DβM and tyrosine mono-oxygenase have all been indicated in animal studies as potential markers of marginal copper status.[115,116] PAM activity in Menkes patients is reduced, but is modifiable *in vitro* by addition of copper, thereby obtaining a copper stimulation index. This technique could provide an indicator of copper status, but requires validation in human trials. Animal studies have suggested tissue activities of cytochrome-c oxidase and lysyl oxidase as early indicators of copper deficiency.[53,117] Experimental copper depletion in humans has produced decreased cytochrome-c oxidase activity in leucocytes and in platelets, but the latter measure has sometimes failed to respond to copper repletion.[56] In human skin, lysyl oxidase activity has been seen to decline with copper depletion and to respond to copper repletion.[118] Too few data are currently available to determine whether these enzymes may be feasible indices of marginal copper status. In addition, the invasive nature of biopsy makes tissue enzymes assays undesirable for general use.

Measurements of blood copper concentration and cuproenzyme activities have not so far proved to be a sensitive method for the evaluation of nutritional status at the tissue, organ and systemic levels. Tissue sampling is generally not a feasible option for use in the general population. One suggested alternative to biochemical testing is the measurement of some other aspect of biological function which is known to be dependent on copper sufficiency. If the adequacy of response to a stressor is regulated by copper status, then response will be adverse or deleterious when status is suboptimal.[119] Potential parameters for functional testing may, in theory, include any aspect of physiological or psychological function which can be shown to be altered by copper depletion and supplementation. One candidate is blood-pressure response to isometric work.

In young women undertaking a standardised hand-grip exercise, the blood pressure response was exaggerated when dietary copper was restricted to 0.65 mg/d.[34] This was observed in the absence of significant changes in copper balance or plasma copper, but with reduced caeruloplasmin activity. Good correlations were found, for individual subjects, between blood pressure response and caeruloplasmin concentration, demonstrating a relationship between the biochemical and physiological indices of copper status. The application of performance-related indices in parallel with biochemical measurements allows potential novel indicators of copper status to be evaluated.

Recent research into the stimulatory effect of copper deficiency upon hepatic lipid synthesis has examined the mechanisms behind the observed increase in transcription of lipogenic gene expression.[120] Findings suggest that copper deficiency stimulates the expression of the fatty acid synthase gene by increasing the nuclear localization of a mature transcription factor, sterol regulatory element binding protein-1.

There is clearly a need to identify more closely the role of copper in biological systems, both in health and in disease states. According to the WHO, there is a great need for standardised sampling and analytical procedures for the determination of dietary copper and copper in drinking water. There appears, also, to be a case for revision of the existing guidelines for copper in drinking water. Whereas the US EPA has used acute toxicity data to derive its guideline, the WHO has used data on total copper intake and chronic toxicity. A greater degree of consensus on the criteria used would be instrumental in the establishment of sounder, more defensible guidelines.

In Western societies an emerging issue is the identification of the requirements for optimal nutrition. The importance of developing such markers can hardly be overemphasised. With these tools, appropriate studies can be used to establish recommendations for optimal copper intake of individuals and of populations.

5.14 Sources of further information and advice

World Health Organization: http://www.who.int/home-page/
International Programme on Chemical Safety: http://www.inchem.org
European Commission Scientific

Committee on Food: http://www.europa.eu.int/comm/food/index_en.html
UK Food Standards Agency: http://www.food.gov.uk/
The Nutrition Society: http://www.nutsoc.org.uk/
US National Institute of Medicine,
Food and Nutrition Board: http://www.nationalacademies.org/sitemap/
Ministry of Agriculture,
Fisheries and Food:
http://archive.food.gov.uk/dept_health/pdf/evmpdf/erm9919.pdf

5.15 References

1 HART E B, STEENBOCK H, WADDELL J and ELVENHJEM C A (1928), 'Iron Nutrition. VII. Copper is a supplement to iron for hemoglobin building in the rat', *J Biol Chem* **77**, 797–812
2 MILLS E S (1930), 'The treatment of idiopathic (hypochromic) anemia with iron and copper', *Can Med Assoc J* **22**, 175–8
3 UAUY R, OLIVARES M and GONZALEZ M (1998), 'Essentiality of copper in humans', *Am J Clin Nutr* **67**(suppl), 952s–9s
4 JOHNSON M A, FISCHER J G and KAYS S E (1992), 'Is Copper an Antioxidant Nutrient?', *Critical Reviews in Food Science and Nutrition* **32**(1), 1–31
5 ZAITSEVA V N, ZAITSEVA I, PAPIZ M and LINDLEY P F (1999), 'An X-ray crystallographic study of the azide inhibitor and organic substrates to ceruloplasmin, a muli-copper oxidase in the plasma', *Journal of Biological Inorganic Chemistry* **4**(5), 579–87
6 TURNLUND J (1999), 'Copper', in: Shils M, Olson J, Shike M and Ross A (eds) *Modern Nutrition in Health and Disease*. 9 ed. Baltimore: Williams & Wilkins, 241–52
7 PRIGGE S T, KOLKEHAR A S, EIPPER B A, MAINS R E and AMZEL L M (1997), 'Amidation of bioactive peptides: the structure of peptidylglycine alpha-amidating monooxygenase', *Science* **278**(5341), 1300–5
8 MATHEWS C K and VAN HOLDE K E (1990), *Biochemistry*. Redwood City, California: Benjamin/Cumming Publishing Company
9 BRYAN S E, VIZARD D L, BEARY D A, LA BICHE R A and HARDY K L (1981), 'Partitioning of zinc and copper within subnuclear nucleoprotein particles', *Nucleic Acids Res* **9**(21), 5811–23
10 AGARWAL K, SHARMA A and TALUKDER G (1989), 'Effects of copper on mammalian cell components', *Chemico-Biological Interactions* **69**(1), 1–16
11 LINDER M C (2001), 'Copper and genomic stability in mammals', *Mutation Research* **475**, 141–52
12 DEPARTMENT OF HEALTH (1991), *Dietary Reference Value for Food Energy and Nutrients for the UK*. London: Committee on Medical Aspects of Food Safety
13 PENNINGTON J A and YOUNG B E (1991), 'Total diet study nutritional elements, 1982–1989', *J Am Diet Assoc* **91**, 179–83
14 KEHOE C A, TURLEY E, BONHAM M P, O'CONNOR J M, MCKEOWN A, FAUGHNAN M S, COULTER J S, GILMORE W S, HOWARD A N and STRAIN J J (2000), 'Response of putative indices of copper status to copper supplementation in human subjects', *British Journal of Nutrition* **84**(2), 151–6
15 KIELY M (2001), *IUNA North/South Ireland Food Consumption Survey: Food and Nutrient Intakes, Anthropometry, Attitudinal Data and Physical Activity Patterns*. Dublin: Irish Universities Nutrition Alliance

16 MA J and BETTS N M (2000), 'Zinc and copper intakes and their major food sources for older adults in the 1994–96 continuing survey of food intakes by individuals (CSFII)', *Journal of Nutrition* **130**(11), 2838–43
17 FOOD and NUTRITION BOARD (2001), Copper. *Dietary Reference Intakes: Vitamin A, Vitamin K, Arsenic, Boron, Chromium, Copper, Iodine, Iron, Manganese, Molybdenum, Nickel, Silicon, Vanadium and Zinc*. Washington, DC: National Academy Press, 7.1–7.27
18 CASTILLO-DURÁN C and UAUY R (1988), 'Copper deficiency impairs growth of infants recovering from malnutrition', *Am J Clin Nutr* **47**, 710–14
19 CASTILLO-DURÁN C, FISBERG M, VALENZUELA A, EGAÑA J and UAUY R (1983), 'Controlled trial of copper supplementation during the recovery from marasmus', *Am J Clin Nutr* **37**(6), 898–903
20 BESHGETOOR D and HAMBIDGE M (1998), 'Clinical conditions altering copper metabolism in humans', *Am J Clin Nutr* **67**, 107s–21s
21 INTERNATIONAL PROGRAMME ON CHEMICAL SAFETY (1998), *Environmental Health Criteria 200: Copper*. Geneva: World Health Organization
22 THOMAS B (ed.) (1994), *Manual of Dietetic Practice*, 2 ed. Oxford: Blackwell Scientific Publications
23 OLIVARES M and UAUY R (1996), 'Copper as an essential nutrient', *Am J Clin Nutr* **63**(5), 791S–796
24 SPIEGEL J E and WILLENBUCHER R F (1999), 'Rapid development of severe copper deficiency in a patient with Crohn's disease receiving parenteral nutrition', *Journal of Parenteral and Enteral Nutrition* **23**(3), 169–72
25 FUHRMAN M P, HERRMANN V, MASIDONSKI P and EBY C (2000), 'Pancytopenia after removal of copper from total parenteral nutrition', *Journal of parenteral and enteral nutrition* **24**(6), 361–6
26 GOYENS P, BRASSEUR D and CADRANEL S (1985), 'Copper deficiency in infants with active celiac disease', *J Pediatr Gastroenterol Nutr* **4**(4), 677–80
27 PERCIVAL S, BOWSER E and WAGNER M (1995), 'Reduced copper-enzyme activities in blood-cells of children with cystic fibrosis', *Am J Clin Nutr* **62**(3), 633–8
28 SCHLEPER B and STUERENBURG H J (2001), 'Copper deficiency-associated myelopathy in a 46-year-old woman', *J Neurol* **248**, 705–6
29 RODERIGUEZ A, SOTO G, TORRES S, VENEGAS G and CASTILLO-DURÁN C (1985), 'Zinc and copper in hair and plasma of children with chronic diarrhea', *Acta Paediatr Scan* **74**(5), 770–4
30 CASTILLO-DURÁN C, VENEGAS G, VILLALOBOS J C, GATICA L and RODERIGUEZ A (1998), 'Trace mineral balance in acute diarrhea of infants. Association to etiological agents and lactose content of formula', *Nutrition Research* **18**(5), 799–808
31 MERCER J B (2001), 'The molecular basis of copper-transport diseases', *Trends in Molecular Medicine* **7**(2), 64–9
32 HOPKINS R G and FAILLA M K (1997), 'Copper deficiency reduces interleukin-2 (IL-2) production and IL-2 mRNA in human T-lymphocytes', *J Nutr* **127**, 257–62
33 KLEVAY L M (2000), 'Cardiovascular disease from copper deficiency – a history', *The Journal of Nutrition* **130**, 489s–92s
34 LUKASKI H C, KLEVAY L M and MILNE D B (1988), 'Effects of dietary copper on human autonomic cardiovascular function', *European Journal of Applied Physiology and Occupational Physiology* **58**(1–2), 74–80
35 KLEVAY L M (2000), 'Dietary copper and risk of coronary heart disease', *Am J Clin Nutr* **71**(5), 1213–14
36 SAARI J T (2000), 'Copper deficiency and cardiovascular disease: Role of peroxidation, glycation and nitration', *Canadian Journal of Physiology and Pharmacology* **78**(10), 848
37 STRAIN J J (1994), 'Newer aspects of micronutrients in chronic disease: copper', *Proc Nut Soc* **53**, 583–9

38 BREMNER I (1998), 'Manifestations of copper excess', *Am J Clin Nutr* **67**(suppl), 1069s–73s
39 FITZGERALD D J (1998), 'Safety guidelines for copper in water', *Am J Clin Nutr* **76**(suppl), 1098s–102s
40 LYLE W H, PAYTON J E and HUI M (1976), 'Haemodialysis and copper fever', *Lancet* **1**, 1324–5
41 ARAYA M, MCGOLDRICK M C and KLEVAY L M (2001), 'Determination of an acute no-observed-adverse-effect-level (NOAEL) for copper in water', *Regulatory Toxicology and Pharmacology* **34**(2), 137–45
42 PRATT W, OMDAHL J and SORENSON J (1985), 'Lack of effects of copper gluconate supplementation', *Am J Clin Nutr* **42**(4), 681–2
43 O'NEILL N C and TANNER M S (1989), 'Uptake of copper from brass vessel by bovine milk and its relevance to Indian childhood cirrhosis', *J Pediatr Gastroenterol Nutr* **9**(2), 167–72
44 SETHI S, GROVER S and KHODASKAR M B (1993), 'Role of copper in Indian childhood cirrhosis', *Annals of Tropical Paediatrics* **13**(1), 3–5
45 MÜLLER-HÖCKER J, MEYER U, WIEBECKE B, HÜBNER G, EIFE R, KELLNER M and SCHRAMEL P (1988), 'Copper storage disease of the liver and chronic dietary copper intoxication in two further German infants mimicking Indian childhood cirrhosis', *Pathol Res Pract* **183**, 39–45
46 MULLER T, FEICHTINGER H, BERGER H and MULLER W (1996), 'Endemic Tyrolean infantile cirrhosis: An ecogenetic disorder', *Lancet* **347**(9005), 877–80
47 LOUDIANOS G and GITLIN J D (2000), 'Wilson's Disease', *Seminars in Wilson's Disease* **20**(3), 353–64
48 LIVINGSTONE M B E, PRENTICE A M, STRAIN J J, COWARD W A, BLACK A E, BARKER M E, MCKENNA P G and WHITEHEAD R G (1990), 'Accuracy of weighed dietary records in studies of diet and health', *Br Med J* **300**, 708–12
49 PANG Y, MACINTOSH D L and RYAN B P (2001), 'A longitudinal investigation of aggregate oral intake of copper', *J Nutr* **131**(8), 2171–6
50 TURNLUND J R (1988), 'Copper nutriture, bioavailability and the influence of dietary factors', *J Am Diet Assoc* **88**(3), 303–10
51 TURNLUND J, SCOTT K, PEIFFER G, JANG A M, KEYES W R, KEEN C L and SAKANASHI T M (1997), 'Copper status of young men consuming a low-copper diet', *Am J Clin Nutr* **65**(1), 72–8
52 KONIG J S and ELMADFA I (2000), 'Plasma copper concentration as a marker of copper itake from food', *Annals of Nutrition and Metabolism* **44**(3), 129–34
53 MILNE D B (1998), 'Copper intake and assessment of copper status', *Am J Clin Nutr* **67**(suppl), 1041s–5s
54 MILNE D B and JOHNSON P E (1993), 'Assessment of copper status – effect of age and gender on reference ranges in healthy adults', *Clinical Chemistry* **39**(5), 883–7
55 COUSINS R J (1985), 'Absorption, transport and hepatic metabolism of copper and zinc: Special reference to metallothionein and ceruloplasmin', *Physiol Rev* **65**, 238–309
56 MILNE D and NIELSEN F (1996), 'Effects of a diet low in copper on copper-status indicators in postmenopausal women', *Am J Clin Nutr* **63**(3), 358–64
57 LUKASKI H, HOVERSON B, GALLAGHER S and BOLONCHUK W (1990), 'Physical training and copper, iron, and zinc status of swimmers', *Am J Clin Nutr* **51**(6), 1093–9
58 KEHOE C A, FAUGHNAN M S, GILMORE W S, COULTER J S, HOWARD A N and STRAIN J J (2000), 'Plasma diamine oxidase activity is greater in copper-adequate than in copper-marginal or copper-deficient rats', *J Nutr* **130**, 30–3
59 STRAIN J (2000), 'Defining optimal copper status in humans: concepts and problems', in: Roussel (ed.) *Trace Elements in Man and Animals 10*. New York: Plenum Publishers, 923–8

60 LINDER M C, WOOTEN L, CERVEZA P, COTTON S, SCHULZE R and LOMELI N (1998), 'Copper Transport', *Am J Clin Nutr* **67**(suppl), 965s–71s
61 TURNLUND J R (1998), 'Human whole-body copper metabolism', *Am J Clin Nutr* **67**, 960S–4S
62 LEVENSON C (1998), 'Mechanisms of copper conservation in organs', *Am J Clin Nutr* **67**(suppl), 978s–81s
63 GARROW J S, JAMES W P T and RALPH A (eds) (2000), *Human Nutrition and Dietetics*. 10 ed. London, Churchill Livingstone
64 WAPNIR R A (1998), 'Copper absorption and bioavailability', *Am J Clin Nutr* **67**, 1054S–60S
65 BOOBIS S (1999), *Review of Copper*. Expert Group on Vitamins and Minerals, London: Ministry of Agriculture, Fisheries and Food
66 TURNLUND J, SWANSON C and KING J (1983), 'Copper absorption and retention in pregnant women fed diets based on animal and plant protein', *J Nutr* **113**, 2346–52
67 HUNT J R and VAN DER POOL R A (2001), 'Apparent copper absorption from a vegetarian diet', *Am J Clin Nutr* **74**(6), 803–7
68 PRICE N O, BUNCE G E and ENGEL R W (1970), 'Copper, manganese and zinc balance in preadolescent girls', *Am J Clin Nutr* **23**(3), 258–60
69 LANGHENDRIES J P, HURRELL R F, FURNISS D E, HISCHENHUBER C, FINOT P A, BERNARD A, BATTISTI O, BERTRAND J M and SENTERRE J (1992), 'Maillard reaction products and lysinoalanine: urinary excretion and the effects on kidney function of preterm infants fed heat-processed milk formula', *J Pediatr Gastroenterol Nutr* **14**(1), 62–70
70 ANDIEUX C and SACQUET E (1984), 'Effect of Maillard's reaction products on apparent mineral absorption in different parts of the digestive tract. The role of microflora', *Reprod Nutr Dev* **25**, 379–86
71 BAKER D H and CZARNECKI-MAULDEN G L (1987), 'Pharmacologic role of cysteine in ameliorating or exacerbating mineral toxicities', *J Nutr* **117**, 1003–10
72 KIES C, CHUANG J H and FOX H M (1983), 'Copper utilization in humans as affected by amino acid supplements', *FASEB Journal* **3**, A360 (abstr)
73 STRAIN J J and LYNCH S M (1990), 'Excess dietary methionine decreases indexes of copper status in the rat', *Annals of Nutrition and Metabolism* **34**(2), 93–7
74 WAPNIR R A and BALKMAN C (1991), 'Inhibition of copper absorption by zinc – effect of histidine', *Biological Trace Element Research* **29**(3), 193–202
75 WAN Q, YANG B S and KATO N (1996), 'Feeding of excessive cystine and cysteine enhances defects of dietary copper deficiency in rats by differential mechanisms involving altered iron status', *Journal of Nutritional Science and Vitaminology* **42**(3), 185–93
76 FISCHER P W, GIROUX A and L'ABBE M R (1981), 'The effect of dietary zinc on intestinal copper absorption', *Am J Clin Nutr* **34**(9), 1670–5
77 BREWER G, YUZBASIYAN-GURKAN V, LEE D-Y and APPELMAN H (1989), 'Treatment of Wilson's disease with zinc. VI. Initial treatment studies', *J Lab Clin Med* **114**, 633
78 VULPE C D and PACKMAN S (1995), 'Cellular Copper Transport', *Annu Rev Nutr* **15**, 768–73
79 MILNE D B, DAVIS C D and NIELSEN F H (2001), 'Low dietary zinc alters indices of copper function and status in postmenopausal women', *Nutrition* **17**, 701–8
80 JOHNSON M A, SMITH M M and EDMONDS J T (1998), 'Copper, iron, zinc and manganese in dietary supplements, infant formulas, and ready-to-eat breakfast cereals', *Am J Clin Nutr* **67**(suppl), 1035s–40s
81 WAPNIR R, DEVAS G and SOLANS C (1993), 'Inhibition of intestinal copper absorption by divalent cations and low-molecular-weight ligands in the rat', *Biol Trace Elem Res* **36**, 291–305
82 HASCHKE F, ZIEGLER E E, EDWARDS B B and FOMAN S J (1986), 'Effect of iron fortification of infant formula on trace mineral absorption', *J Pediatr Gastroenterol Nutr* **5**, 768–73

83 LONNERDAL B, KELLEHER S L, LIEN E L (2001), 'Extent of thermal processing of infant formula affects copper status in infant rhesus monkeys', *Am J Clin Nutr* **73**(5), 914–19
84 AASETH J and NORSETH T (1986), in: Friberg L, Nordberg G F and Vouk V B (eds) *Handbook on the toxicology of metals*. 2 ed. Amsterdam, London: Elsevier/North-Holland Biomedical Press
85 BREWER G J, DICK R D, YUZBASIYAN-GURKAN V, TANKANOW R, YOUNG A B and KLUIN K J (1991), 'Initial Therapy of patients with Wilson's Disease with tetrathiomolybdate', *Arch Neurol* **48**, 42–7
86 WAPNIR R and SIA M (1996), 'Copper intestinal absorption in the rat: effect of free fatty acids and triglycerides', *Proc Soc Exp Biol Med* **211**, 381–6
87 LUKASKI H C, KLEVAY L M, BOLONCHUK W W, MAHALKO J R, MILNE D B, JOHNSON L K and SANDSTEAD H H (1982), 'Influence of dietary lipids on iron, zinc and copper retention in trained athletes', *Federation Proceedings* **41**(3), 275
88 VAN CAMPEN D R and GROSS E (1968), 'Influence of ascorbic acid on the absorption of copper by rats', *J Nutr* **95**, 617–22
89 FINLEY E B and CERKLEWSKI F L (1983), 'Influence of ascorbic acid supplementation on copper status in young adult men', *Am J Clin Nutr* **37**(4), 553–6
90 JACOB R A, SKALA J H, OMAYE S T and TURNLUND J R (1987), 'Effect of varying ascorbic acid intakes on copper absorption and caeruloplasmin levels in young men', *J Nutr* **117**(12), 2109–15
91 SABLE-AMPLIS R, SICART R and REYNIER B (1987), 'Apparent retention of copper, zinc and iron in hamsters: influence of a fruit-enriched diet', *Nutr Rep Int* **35**, 811–18
92 FAIRWEATHER-TAIT S J (1992), 'Bioavailability of trace elements', *Food Chemistry* **43**, 213–17
93 HARVEY P W, HUNSAKER H A and ALLEN K G D (1981), 'Dietary L-histidine induced hypercholesterolemia and hypocupremia in the rat', *J Nutr* **111**(4), 639–47
94 FIELDS M, FERRETTI R J, SMITH J C, JR and REISER S (1984), 'The interaction of type of dietary carbohydrates with copper deficiency', *Am J Clin Nutr* **39**(2), 289–95
95 REISER S, FERRETTI R J, FIELDS M and SMITH J J (1983), 'Role of dietary fructose in the enhancement of mortality and biochemical changes associated with copper deficiency in rats', *Am J Clin Nutr* **38**, 214–22
96 SCHOENEMANN H M, FAILLA M L and STEELE N C (1990), 'Consequences of severe copper deficiency are independent of dietary carbohydrate in young pigs', *Am J Clin Nutr* **52**, 147–54
97 HOLBROOK J T, SMITH J C, JR and REISER S (1989), 'Dietary fructose or starch: effects on copper, zinc, iron, manganese, calcium, and magnesium balances in humans', *Am J Clin Nutr* **49**(6), 1290–4
98 WAPNIR R and DEVAS G (1995), 'Copper deficiency: interaction with high-fructose and high-fat diets in rats', *Am J Clin Nutr* **61**(1), 105–10
99 HARRIS Z L and GITLIN J D (1996), 'Genetic and molecular basis for copper toxicity', *Am J Clin Nutr* **63**(5), 836S–41S
100 WINGE D R and MEHRA R K (1990), 'Host defenses against copper toxicity', *Int Rev Exp Pathol* **31**, 47–83
101 HARRIS E D (2000), 'Cellular copper transport and metabolism', *Annual Review of Nutrition* **20**, 291–310
102 FLORIS G, MEDDA R, PADIGLIA A and MUSCI G (2000), 'The physiopathological significance of ceruloplasmin – a possible therapeutic approach', *Biochemical Pharmacology* **60**(12), 1735–41
103 EISENSTEIN R S (2000), 'Discovery of the caeruloplasmin homologue hephaestin: New insight into the copper/iron connection', *Nut Rev* **58**(1), 22–6
104 LEVERTON R M and BINKLEY E S (1944), 'The copper metabolism and requirement of young women', *J Nutr* **27**, 480–6

105 OLIVARES M and UAUY R (1996), 'Limits of metabolic tolerance to copper and biological basis for present recommendations and regulations', *Am J Clin Nutr* **63**(5), 846s
106 FAIRWEATHER-TAIT S J, FOX T E, HARVEY L J, TEUCHER B and DAINTY J (2001), 'Methods for analysis of trace-element absorption', in: Lowe N, Jackson M (eds) *Advances in Isotope Methods for the Analysis of Trace Elements in Man*. Boca Raton: CRC Press, 60–80
107 ABRAMS S A and MULLER H (1999), 'Using stable isotopes to assess mineral absorption and utilization by children', *Am J Clin Nutr* **70**, 955–64
108 JOHNSON P E and CANFIELD W K (1989), 'Stable zinc and copper absorption in free-living infants fed breast milk or formula', *Journal of Trace Elements in Experimental Medicine* **2**, 285
109 TURNLUND J (2001), 'Copper status and metabolism studies with metabolic tracers', in: Lowe N, Jackson M, (eds) *Advances in Isotope Methods for the Analysis of Trace Elements in Man*. Boca Raton: CRC Press, 117–27
110 HANSEN M, ISAKSSON M and SANDSTROM B (2001), 'Advances in Radioisotope Methodology', in: Lowe N, Jackson M, (eds) *Advances in Isotope Methods for the Analysis of Trace Elements in Man*. Boca Raton: CRC Press, 23–41
111 BUCKLEY W T (1996), 'Application of compartmental modeling to determination of trace element requirements in humans', *J Nutr* **126**(9s), 2311s–2319s
112 HARVEY L J, MAJSAK-NEWMAN G, DAINTY J R, WHARF S G, REID M D, BEATTIE J H and FAIRWEATHER-TAIT S J (2002), 'Holmium as a faecal marker for copper absorption studies in adults', *Clinical Science* **102**(2), 233–40
113 BEATTIE J H, REID M D, HARVEY L J, DAINTY J R, MAJSAK-NEWMAN G and FAIRWEATHER-TAIT S J (2001), 'Selective extraction of blood plasma exchangeable copper for isotope studies of dietary copper absorption', *Analyst* **126**, 2225–9
114 BUCKLEY W T, VANDERPOOL R A, GODFREY D G and JOHNSON P E (1996), 'Determination, stable isotope enrichment and kinetics of direct-reacting copper in blood plasma', *Journal of Nutritional Biochemistry* **7**, 488–94
115 PROHASKA J R, BAILEY W R and LEAR P M (1995), 'Copper deficiency alters rat peptidyl-glycine α-amidating monooxygenase activity', *J Nutr* **125**(6), 1447–54
116 PROHASKA J R and BROKATE B (2001), 'Dietary copper deficiency alters protein levels of rat dopamine β monooxygenase and tyrosine monooxygenase', *Exp Biol Med* **226**(6), 199–207
117 RUCKER R B, RUCKER B R, MITCHELL A E, CUI C T, CLEGG M, KOSONEN T, URIU-ADAMS J Y, TCHAPARIAN E H, FISHMAN M and KEEN C L (1999), 'Activation of chick tendon lysyl oxidase in response to dietary copper', *J Nutr* **129**, 2143–6
118 WERMAN M J, BHATHENA S J and TURNLUND J R (1997), 'Dietary copper intake influences skin lysyl oxidase in young men', *Nutritional Biochemistry* **8**, 201–4
119 LUKASKI H C, C H and PENLAND J G (1996), 'Functional changes appropriate for determining mineral element requirements', *J Nutr* **126**(9s), 2354s–62s
120 TANG Z, GASPERKOVA D, XU J, BAILLIE R, LEE J H and CLARKE S D (2000), 'Copper deficiency induces hepatic fatty acid synthase gene transcription in rats by increasing the nuclear content of mature sterol regulatory element binding protein-1', *Journal of Nutrition* **130**(12), 2915–21
121 PISCATOR M (1979), 'Copper' In *Handbook on the toxicology of metals* Eds. Friberg L, Nordberg G F and Vouk V B. Elsevier/North-Holland Biomedical Press, Amsterdam 411–20
122 FRIBERG L (1979), 'Molybdenum' In *Handbook on the toxicology of metals*, Eds. Friberg L, Nordberg G F and Vouk V B. Elsevier/North-Holland Biomedical Press, Amsterdam 531–9

6

Consumers and nutrition labelling

L. Insall, Food and Drink Federation, London

6.1 Introduction: the problem of providing nutrition information

Developments in nutrition research and improved scientific understanding of the relationship between diet and health have led to increasing interest in the nutritional aspects of the food supply. This interest is shared by academics, health professionals, government officials, consumers and the food and supplement industries alike, although not always for the same reasons and generally at different levels of knowledge and understanding. Interest in nutrition, in respect of both total diet and individual foods, is second only to concern about food safety and is sometimes confused with the safety aspects of the food supply. Pick up any newspaper or general magazine in the UK and you will almost certainly find several column inches devoted to some aspect of food, either as the latest 'scare' or controversial issue, or as a feature about the most recent fashionable food trend or restaurant or celebrity chef. However, despite extensive media coverage and take-up of food issues and master classes in cookery, knowledge and understanding about food – how to prepare and cook it, and what constitutes a healthy, balanced diet – remain poor, particularly in the younger generations and lower socio-economic groups. The nutritional content of the diet is blamed for a wide range of health problems such as obesity, cardiovascular disease and certain cancers, i.e. long-term chronic diseases as opposed to the type of short-term acute illnesses that are usually associated with food safety problems.

Improving the overall diet in the UK with a view to reducing the incidence and severity of certain diet-related chronic diseases has been a major plank in UK government health strategy for several years and now involves several key departments: Education and Employment (DfEE), Health (DH), and the Food

Standards Agency (FSA); the last-named has taken over responsibility for this area from the (now defunct) Ministry of Agriculture, Fisheries and Food (MAFF) since April 2000.

Nutrition information is, therefore, an aspect of a very broad debate, often highly politicised, about the nutritional quality of the modern food supply, and specifically about the contribution to the modern diet, and therefore to the health of the population, made by pre-packed 'convenience' foods which, together with 'fast food' restaurants and take-aways, make a substantial contribution to the total dietary intake of a significant proportion of the UK population. In terms of issues, the provision of nutrition information ranks very high in the diet and health debate. The UK has possibly been more absorbed by this subject than have most other European Member States, a reflection, perhaps, of the cultural attitude towards food as fuel and the growing obsession with fitness and body form in a population inclining towards obesity. Where food has traditionally been enjoyed as one of life's great pleasures, notably France, the most important factor is what the product tastes like, not the 'vital statistics' of its content. These cultural differences across Europe have had a significant bearing on the regulatory controls governing food labelling, including nutrition information, and are in part responsible for what is generally regarded as a somewhat 'user unfriendly' approach to nutrition labelling. This will be discussed in greater detail later in the chapter, but firstly the current application of nutrition labelling will be considered.

The provision of nutrition information, as with the provision of any other form of information, is an enabling mechanism intended to assist the purchaser to make a reasoned choice about the product he or she is considering buying. The degree of interest in this particular segment of the mass of information printed on a food label is a matter which will be discussed in greater detail in section 6.4, but two essential points should be borne in mind:

- The provision of nutrition information on a label is voluntary, *unless a claim is made*.
- Approximately 80% of pre-packed foods manufactured in the UK carry nutrition labelling; this is far higher than in most other EU Member States.

The strict and detailed regulatory requirements which govern the presentation of nutrition information are set out below, and it will be clear from a brief glance that the legislation was not drafted with consumer understanding in mind. This is not necessarily a criticism of the lawyers – laws are, after all, drafted and interpreted by lawyers, not by the general public. So whilst the formulaic nature of the required presentation may appear unnecessarily prescriptive, there is good reason for this. The intention of the current legislation was to encourage the provision of nutrition information in a prescribed format which would allow consumers to compare the nutritional content of various products. The effectiveness of this policy is another issue which will be discussed in greater detail in a later section, but it is not arbitrary and reflects the complexity of negotiating legislation on a contentious issue to cover a large trading block made up of a dozen European Member States, risen to 15 at the time of writing. These states have diverse geographic and cultural backgrounds, and there are therefore differences in local food supply and eating patterns. If criticism is due, it should perhaps be aimed at those authorities whose job it is to explain the existence and meaning of legislation in lay terms, but this too can be a complex communication issue and many attempts have been made to bridge the gap between legislator and consumer, and in the case of nutrition information are still on-going. This aspect will be developed later.

6.2 Current EU nutrition information

Legislation on nutrition labelling was developed as a means of providing consumers with information about the nutrient content of the foods they were choosing in a standardised format recognisable across the European Community, thereby also promoting the freedom of movement of goods in the Single Market.

An essential part of the philosophy behind the Nutrition Labelling Directive, the principal EU legislative instrument in this area,[1] was the growing recognition of the link between diet and health and the need to encourage consumers to make an informed choice about the foods they consume. It was considered that knowledge of the basic principles of nutrition and the provision of nutrition labelling would contribute significantly in this and act as a tool in the nutrition education of the public. To this end, it was deemed that the information provided should be simple and easily understood, with a standardised format that would allow comparison of one product with another. This means that the dual principles underlying EU legislation on nutrition labelling are consumer information and education and the removal of technical barriers to trade.

As usual in the development of harmonised legislation, one of the driving forces was the divergence in national legislation that risked causing reciprocal barriers to trade after completion of the Single Market on 31 December 1992. In the UK there was no specific legislation on nutrition information, but the Food Advisory Committee (FAC) had issued guidelines on nutrition labelling, which had been widely adopted by the industry. The FAC was abolished in December 2001 because its functions have now been taken over by the Board of the Food Standards Agency, but its advice at the time in question carried considerable weight. The Ministry of Agriculture, Fisheries and Food (MAFF) indicated its intention to introduce national legislation on the compulsory indication of fat content. This spurred the European Commission into pushing its own proposals forward, on the basis that the UK's freedom to legislate in this area was constrained by its Community obligations under the Food Labelling Directive, 79/112/EEC (updated and consolidated in 2000 as Directive 2000/13/EC).

Work on European harmonisation began in 1988, when the Commission put forward two linked proposals, one on compulsory nutrition labelling and the other

---

[1] *Official Journal of the European Communities*, No. L 276/40-44, 6.10.90

setting out what that labelling should be. The Directive eventually adopted in 1990, Directive 90/496/EEC on nutrition labelling for foodstuffs, did not require compulsory labelling, except where a claim is made, and focused more on the nature and format of the labelling, about which it goes into great detail.

Interestingly, for a piece of legislation for which one of the primary aims is the provision of information regarded as being of benefit to the consumer, it is a highly technical Directive, unlikely to be understood by anyone without some knowledge of food science or food legislation, and ideally both. To understand and use it requires detailed analysis. The following are its main provisions.

6.2.1 Provisions of the current legislation: format

The provision of nutrition labelling is voluntary, unless a nutrition claim is made, e.g. 'reduced fat', 'high fibre', 'low sodium'. If nutrition information is given, it must be in one of two formats:

either • Group 1 information: energy, protein, carbohydrate and fat (in that order).
or • Group 2 information: energy, protein, carbohydrate, sugars, fat, saturates, fibre and sodium (in that order).

These formats are commonly referred to as 'The Big 4' and 'The Big 4 plus Little 4'. Quantities must be given per 100 g or 100 ml of the food or drink, or per 100 g/100 ml *and* per serving. The Directive requires that the information be given in one place, in tabular format, with the numbers aligned if space permits.

Declarations may also be made in respect of vitamins and minerals, provided they are listed in the Annex of the Directive and are present in 'significant amounts', currently defined as 15% of the Recommended Daily Amount (RDA), supplied per 100 g or 100 ml of the food, or per package if the package contains only a single portion. The vitamins and minerals currently listed and their RDAs are:

Vitamin A (µg)	800	Vitamin B_{12} (µg)	1
Vitamin D (µg)	5	Biotin (mg)	0.15
Vitamin E (mg)	10	Pantothenic acid (mg)	6
Vitamin C (mg)	60	Calcium (mg)	800
Thiamin (mg)	1.4	Phosphorus (mg)	800
Riboflavin (mg)	1.6	Iron (mg)	14
Niacin (mg)	18	Magnesium (mg)	300
Vitamin B_6 (mg)	2	Zinc (mg)	15
Folacin (µg)	200	Iodine (µg)	150

A declaration may also be given in respect of one or more of the following:

* starch
* polyols
* mono-unsaturates
* polyunsaturates
* cholesterol

but if a declaration is made in respect of polyunsaturates, mono-unsaturates or cholesterol, the amount of saturates must also be given.

6.2.2 Calculation of energy value

For the purpose of calculating the energy value for these nutrients, the Directive specifies the values on which they are to be calculated by means of the following conversion factors:

- carbohydrate (except polyols)   4 kcal/g   –   17 kJ/g
- polyols   2.4 kcal/g   –   10 kJ/g
- protein   4 kcal/g   –   17 kJ/g
- fat   9 kcal/g   –   37 kJ/g
- alcohol (ethanol)   7 kcal/g   –   29 kJ/g
- organic acid   3 kcal/g   –   13 kJ/g

6.2.3 Definitions

The Directive, like most pieces of legislation, must specify to what it refers so that all the nutrients are defined scientifically. So, for example, the Directive states that:

> 'protein' means the protein content calculated by using the formula:
> protein = total Kjeldahl nitrogen × 6.25

and

> 'saturates' means fatty acids without a double bond

This exemplifies the earlier comment that it is a Directive written for the food scientist rather than for the average consumer.

The Directive also defines 'average value'. This is necessary because the composition of foods is subject to natural variation due, for example, to variations in cultivar, weather, growing location, conditions and practices (crops) and in breed, seasonality, rearing conditions and practices (animal-derived materials). The Directive therefore states that: 'average value' means the value which best represents the amount of the nutrient which a given food contains, and reflects allowances for seasonal variability, patterns of consumption and other factors which may cause the actual value to vary.'

6.2.4 Declared values

These are the average values of the nutrients, as defined above, based on:

1. The manufacturer's analysis of the food.
2. A calculation from the known or actual average values of the ingredients used.
3. A calculation from generally established and accepted data.

The amounts declared must be for the food as sold. However, where appropriate they may relate to the foodstuff after preparation, provided that sufficiently detailed instructions for preparation are given and the information relates to the food as prepared for consumption.

The Directive provides for the use of the Standing Committee procedure in the event of discrepancies being found between the declared values and those established during the course of official analysis. The Standing Committee is convened from experts from all Member States who will adjudicate on the matter(s) placed before them. In the UK, the term 'typical' is preferred to 'average' and is more generally used as a more representative indication of value than the average.

6.2.5 Nutrition claims

As stated earlier, the provision of nutrition information is voluntary unless a claim is made. So, for example, if a claim is made that a product is 'low in fat', at least Group 1 information must be given. Very often the full Group 2 information is given, but this would only be compulsory if the claim were for one of the 'Little 4' nutrients, i.e. 'saturated fat' rather than 'fat'.

The Directive defines as a nutrition claim:

> 'any representation and any advertising message which states, suggests or implies that a foodstuff has particular nutrition properties due to the energy (calorific value) it
> – provides,
> – provides at a reduced or increased rate or
> – does not provide
> and/or due to the nutrients it
> – contains,
> – contains in reduced or increased proportions or
> – does not contain.'

Only generic advertising is excluded from this, so if a producer decided to launch a campaign to persuade people to eat more fresh green vegetables and claimed that green vegetables are low in fat, he would not have to include the nutrition information alongside his images of leafy greens.

6.2.6 Timescale

The Directive came into force in September 1990 and required that trade in products complying with the Directive be permitted by 1 April 1992 and that products not complying with the Directive be prohibited with effect from 1 October 1993. The Directive also required that, eight years from its notification, the Commission would submit to the European Parliament and the Council a report on the application of the Directive and any appropriate proposals for amendment. This review, due in autumn 1998, has not yet taken place at the time of writing and will be discussed further in sections 6.5 and 6.6.

6.2.7 Implementation

Most legislation is only as good as its implementation and enforcement and the application of these procedures has been variable in the case of the Nutrition Labelling Directive. Some Member States were tardy in including it in their national legislation and some, the UK being a prime example, did it so clumsily that it would have been a deterrent to use had the Directive itself not already been familiar to most UK food and drink manufacturers and its provisions already widely used on a voluntary basis. Reports from elsewhere in Europe suggest that national implementing rules, which invariably entail a degree of interpretation, have indeed been a deterring factor and have acted as a disincentive in providing nutrition information voluntarily. The UK's record of some 80% of manufactured food and drink products voluntarily carrying nutrition information remains a matter of surprise, admiration and consternation in other Member States.

UK implementation of the Nutrition Labelling Directive is via the *Food Labelling Regulations 1996* (as amended). These are complex Regulations covering all the essentials of food labelling from batch marking to medicinal claims. Implementation of the Nutrition Labelling Directive, which took place in 1994, carried with it the usual burden of complexity that comes with turning the positive approach of EU legislation (you are not allowed to do it unless the Directive says so) into the negative style of UK Regulations (you can do what you like unless the Regulations state that 'No person shall . . .'). The transposition of Article 4.1 of Directive 90/496/EEC, which states simply that 'Where nutrition labelling is provided, the information to be given shall consist of either group 1 or group 2 in the following order:

Group 1
(a)　energy value;
(b)　the amounts of protein, carbohydrate and fat.

Group 2
(a)　energy value;
(b)　the amounts of protein, carbohydrate, sugars, fat, saturates, fibre and sodium.'

became in Schedule 6A Part I of The Food Labelling (Amendment) Regulations 1994 a half page single table listing both Group 1 and Group 2 nutrients, plus all the additional nutrients allowed to be mentioned, such as polyols under carbohydrates and polyunsaturates under fats, with a complex set of cross references to Part II of the Schedule and subsequent paragraphs of Part I to explain the two separate groups and how they should be set out. It is no wonder that MAFF needed to issue explanatory guidance notes to accompany the amendment to the Regulations.[2]

---

[2] MAFF *Guidance Notes on Nutrition Labelling*, issued 18 March 1994

6.2.8 General requirements

It is important that nutrition information is correct. Not only is it a legal requirement that any labelling information must be accurate and not misleading, but periodically consumer organisations run checks on the values given for the various nutrients and publicise embarrassing inaccuracies. The manufacturer also has an obligation to ensure that the label is understandable in the market(s) in which the product is sold. However, this requirement has not yet been extended to ensure that the consumer understands the nutrition information *per se*, only the language in which it is provided. Regrettably, it cannot be assumed that consumers throughout the EU understand the nutrition information if given in the language of the country of manufacture even though it is set out in a recognised format and order of nutrients. On the other hand, consumers may well express interest in the nutritional attributes of the product, whether or not nutrition information is provided. Many manufacturers and retailers produce leaflets to help explain nutrition labelling and how it can help them to choose a balanced diet, or refer their customers to some of the organisations and resources referred to in section 6.7.

6.3 Consumer expectations and understanding of nutrition labelling

Of the many factors governing food choice, of which price is likely to be quite high on most people's lists, nutrition information may not figure strongly for many. But the enormous number and variety of food products available on the market today including imports of exotic foods and ingredients from all over the world, resulting from the increasing interest in ethnic dishes generated by long-haul travel and TV cooks, not to mention new ranges of products inspired by these developments, means that the consumer needs ever greater knowledge and information to allow him or her to choose from this vast range. At point of purchase it is the food label that provides the information that will enable the consumer to make the choice between products. If diet and health are important to the consumer, the provision of nutrition information on the pack may be a deciding factor between purchasing the product and leaving it on the shelf or a more careful study of the nutrition panel later in the home may influence a repeat purchase.

A further influence on the provision (or not) of nutrition information may be the intermediate customer, namely the retailer, rather than the end consumer. The major UK supermarket chains exert an enormous influence on the highly competitive retail market for food and therefore on food production. All major retailers stock a wide range of 'own label' products, manufactured to their own specification by a variety of food manufacturers. The specification will cover not only the composition of the product but also the details of the food label. This will almost certainly include 'full' nutrition labelling, i.e. the 'Big 4' and 'Little 4' nutrients (see section 6.2.1) and possibly additional, supplementary voluntary information, which is discussed in detail in sections 6.5 and 6.6. Most retailers and many food brands now carry a range of 'healthy' products, in which the composition is strictly formulated to meet specified nutrition criteria such as reduced fat content, lower sodium content, lower calorie, high fibre or any combination of these. They will invariably carry 'full' nutrition information, but consumers interested in a healthier diet may find some of the research work taken out of their shopping expeditions if such ranges of products meet their needs, tastes and pockets. Consumers may also exert their purchasing power by choosing not to buy a product which does not provide nutrition information. In the UK, it has become a general accusation of consumer groups against those manufacturers who choose, for whatever reason, not to provide nutrition information, that they have got something to hide, i.e. it is a 'bad' food containing high levels of sugar, fat or salt.

It is a long-held view of many nutritionists and dieticians that nutrition labelling alone cannot educate the consumer to select a healthy balanced diet, but that it should provide the cornerstone of any nutrition education policy. Research has shown that relatively few consumers actually read the nutrition information provided, and even fewer of them understand it. Nevertheless, consumer organisations have continuously requested greater clarity and use of nutrition information, at least Group 2 nutrition labelling, and on a mandatory basis. In this context, research conducted by the UK Consumers' Association in 1995 revealed some interesting results. A survey conducted in March/April 1995 questioned consumers on a number of issues about food purchases. The research was both qualitative and quantitative; the qualitative research consisted of four discussion groups held with women responsible for choosing and buying food. The quantitative research involved personal interviews with a representative sample of 1454 people in Great Britain aged over 15 years who were responsible for choosing food and doing any of the food shopping.

Respondents were asked which of the following were important to them when shopping for food:

	Most important Base 1454	Important at all (more than 1 answer) Base 1454
Price/value for money	34%	87%
Quality	21%	77%
Nutrition/how healthy it is	16%	61%
Family's/personal preference	12%	53%
How quick/easy to prepare	5%	33%
How fattening it is	4%	33%
Brand name/label	3%	28%
Special diet for medical reasons	3%	10%
Ethical/religious considerations	1%	3%

The following statements make interesting reading both for nutritionists and marketing departments:

Agreement with statements about information given on food labels:

	Agree (Base 1454)	Neither	Disagree
I believe all of the health messages and claims that appear on products nowadays	33%	17%	48%
I never believe the nutrition claims on food packaging and always check the label for more information	47%	24%	27%
I find it difficult to work out from the nutrition information panel on food products what is good for me and what is not	49%	18%	32%
Nutrition information panels should be laid out in the same way for all food products	90%	7%	3%
Claims are a quick and easy way of seeing how healthy a food product is	54%	17%	25%
Health messages and nutrition claims should all be regulated	84%	10%	3%
It is important that nutrition information is shown on all food products	88%	8%	3%

6.4 The use of nutrition panels

The majority of UK food manufacturers and retailers provide nutrition information on most of their products, at least the 'Big 4', and in many cases the 'Big 4 plus Little 4' (see 'format' under Section 6.2.1 above). However, for as long as a voluntary regime continues, the decision as to whether or not to provide nutrition information is largely a commercial one. The arguments for change will be discussed in detail later in this chapter, but taking points 3, 6 and 8 from the Consumers' Association's research into the factors which are important to consumers when shopping for food as relevant to nutrition, diet and health, 23% of respondents consider this the most important aspect when shopping for foods, and a much higher number of some importance, even though nutrition and health ranked third after price/value for money and quality. Of those asked, 86% recognised a nutrition information panel, although of these only 42% took notice of it, with 33% stating that it was what they took most notice of.

Clearly, nutrition panels are very familiar and the circumstances in which nutrition information panels are used are of note: 36% when buying food not bought very often or never bought before; 34% when comparing two different makes or types of the same product; 26% when checking the nutrition claims made on the front of the pack; 15% never use this information; 15% every time food is bought that has this information on it; 14% have never seen this information.

If we focus on the preferences expressed by those who participated in the survey for presentation of the nutrition panel and the aspects and terms of the current format they found difficult to understand: the easiest to use were those that were clear and easy to read e.g. large print/good for poor eyesight (50%); good layout (general) e.g. simple, clear, neat, in order (in a column) (22%); easy to understand (9%); (other points were: use of highlighting or bold print; distinction between medium and high; showing value per 100g; familiar/used to it/seen most often.) The most difficult to use were those with poor layout e.g. crammed together, jumbled, a muddle, words run together, cluttered (41%); difficult to read/indistinct/small print (34%); not tabulated nor itemised, not in columns (9%); hard to pick out a particular piece of information (4%).

Terms on a nutrition information panel that were found confusing:

% RDA	80%
kJ	53%
kcals	41% calories (2%)
sodium	14%
saturates	11%
per 100 grams	8%
per serving	7%

Leaving aside the 88% desire for nutrition information on all food products against the 42% who actually take any notice of it, the provision of nutrition information is evidently the expectation and the norm. The next hurdle is making it helpful and meaningful to consumers.[3]

Alongside the results of the UK Consumers' Association's research, it is also pertinent to consider the Nutrition Labelling Study Report prepared for the UK Ministry of Agriculture, Fisheries and Foods (MAFF) by Research Services Ltd and published in April 1995.[4] The purpose of this study was to conduct a quantitative survey on consumers' awareness of nutrition labelling on food products, with the main objective of the research being to find out the extent to which consumers use and understand this type of information. This was particularly timely in terms of baseline information as the new Regulations on nutrition labelling i.e. implementation of the Nutrition Labelling Directive, came into force in March 1995. The study looked at the level of use of nutrition labelling; any problems in its presentation; and dietary habits, including changes in dietary patterns and what consumers thought they should be eating more or less of. The areas examined were:

- The level of usage of nutrition labelling, including level of awareness; who uses nutrition labelling; the nutrients respondents were aware of/looked for

---

[3] Reference: *Consumers' Association Nutrition Labelling Research, Brief Summary of Quantitative Survey, 1995* (Tables reproduced by kind permission of the Consumers' Association)
[4] Study Report, Research Services Limited (RSL), *MAFF J1366*, April 1995

on the label; use of 100 g or per serving information and which was most useful; and how the labelling was used, i.e. to compare different foods or to assess the nutritional profile of individual foods and whether this was in the context of an individual meal or the whole diet.
- Any problems with the way in which the nutrition information was presented, including whether or not the nutrients shown were understood, e.g. energy, sodium, protein and the relationship between carbohydrate and sugar, fat and saturates; whether the units and other terms were understood, i.e. kilojoules, kilocalories, calories, grams, percent RDA; could consumers understand the relationship between per 100 g and per portion information? Were consumers able to compare nutrient levels in different products on a 100 g and per portion basis? And were consumers able to make judgements about products across the range of nutrients, i.e. products that may be high in fat but differ in their content of saturates?
- The type of diet followed at the moment, including special dietary requirements; changes in diet over the last few years; what people think they should be eating more or less of.

A nationally representative sample of 1000 interviews was used, following an initial qualitative phase for which actual knowledge was tested in a hall test situation. Those interviewed had to be personally responsible for shopping for food for the household or play a significant part in choosing what food was to be bought for themselves or their household. Further tests were incorporated to distinguish between those who were 'nutritionally aware' and those who were less well informed.

Most respondents were aware of nutrition labelling when asked about the information which could be found on foods, 62% mentioning nutrients whilst only 45% mentioned ingredients. The sample was more likely to look for nutrition labelling than look for the ingredients. Nutrition labelling was found to be the primary source of information about the content of foods. Around half the sample claimed to take this information into account when buying or using foods. People who were health conscious were more likely to take nutrition labelling into account than any other subgroup.

Within the nutrition panel, the information of most interest was fat levels (68%). About half those who looked at labels looked for energy levels, whilst sugar, protein and fibre were of less interest.

Overall, 'per serving' information was preferred to 'per 100 g' information. (65% of those who looked at labels preferred per serving information against 21% who preferred per 100 g information). However, the perceived usefulness of the 'per 100 g' information increased among respondents who could understand labels and had a high knowledge of nutrition.

Respondents were most likely to use nutrition information to compare two brands of the same product (49% of those who looked at labels claimed this). They were less likely to use it to compare two different products (only 15% claimed this). They were slightly more likely to use the information to assess products in terms of their whole diet rather than see how products fitted in with the rest of the meal.

The sample was equally divided between those who considered nutrition information useful and those who did not. However, certain subgroups believed it to be more helpful than others did. A large majority (68%) of those who were health conscious considered the information useful. The researchers stated 'if it is the aim of nutrition labelling to be helpful to those who *want to use it*, it would make sense to see this group as the 'target group', therefore a result of over two-thirds finding nutrition information useful seems encouraging'. Some 53% of females compared to 44% of males claimed nutrition information to be quite useful or very useful. Younger age groups were more likely to find the information useful (62% of those aged 16 to 34, 51% of those aged 35 to 44, 48% of those aged 45 to 64 and 33% of those aged over 65), as were those from higher social grades (60% of ABs, 53% of C1s, 48% of C2s, 43% of DEs). Other subgroups which found the information more useful were those with children in the household (57%); those whose education finished at the age of 19 or over (65%); those who were working (55%); those who were in the household with someone who had a special diet (60%) and those with high nutritional knowledge (61%).

Suggestions for improvement, apart from 'make it easier to understand' were generally in terms of making the print larger and giving more explanation of what the names and numbers meant.

With regard to understanding of the nutrients, fat was the most widely recognised nutrient and the one that respondents considered they knew most about (89% claimed to know something about it). The vast majority stated that individuals should cut down on fat. When comparing two products, over half the respondents cited a lower level of fat as a healthier difference. By comparison, saturates, polyunsaturates and monounsaturates were less well recognised or understood. A proportion of the sample was aware of the need to cut down on saturates and increase polyunsaturates intake. However, compared with the number of respondents looking at fat levels on labels, very few claimed to look for saturate levels. When comparing two products, a very small number cited a lower level of saturates being a healthier difference. The researchers concluded 'it appears that there is a need for people to be made more aware of the implications of high saturate intake'.

Carbohydrate was very widely recognised, but around 25% of the sample claimed not to be sure what it was. Some 27% of respondents claimed carbohydrate intake should be increased whilst 17% believed intake should be reduced. When comparing two products, opinion was divided as to whether carbohydrate should be looked for in higher or lower levels. Fat, sugars, protein, fibre and energy were all more likely to be looked for on a nutrition label than carbohydrate. Sugar and starch were at least as well recognised as carbohydrate, sugar being understood and looked for more than carbohydrate. The vast majority of the sample believed sugar levels should be reduced. However, respondents were also far more likely to believe that starch intake should be reduced. The researchers concluded 'there is a need to educate people on the healthiness of this nutrient'.

Protein was widely recognised, but as with carbohydrate, about a quarter of the sample were not sure what it was. The majority of respondents agreed that intake of protein was beneficial and, when comparing two products, about half of them cited a higher level of protein as a healthier difference.

Fibre was better recognised and understood than either protein or carbohydrate were. Some 84% of the sample claimed to know something about fibre. Over two-thirds of the sample believed fibre intake should be increased, and around half of the sample cited a higher level of fibre to be a healthier difference when comparing two products.

Energy was perceived by respondents as 'calories'. Most respondents (67%) claimed to know something about energy although, again, about a quarter of the sample were not sure what it was. After fat, it was the item of most interest on the nutrition label.

The term 'sodium' was much less well understood than 'salt'. Some 62% of respondents felt salt intake should be reduced, compared with 22% believing that sodium should be reduced. Sodium levels were rarely inspected by those who looked at nutrition labels. A majority of the sample mentioned that a lower level of sodium was beneficial when there was a substantial difference in sodium levels between two products. Only 15% of the sample gave the same answers when comparing salt and sodium levels between two products, suggesting that relatively few respondents were able to equate sodium levels with salt levels.

'Calories' was a term recognised by almost all the sample, and most respondents correctly defined it as a measure of energy. By comparison, the terms 'kilocalories' and 'kilojoules' were less well recognised and understood. Grams were recognised and correctly defined as a measure of weight by the vast majority of respondents. Few claimed to be aware of the term 'percentage RDA', only about one in ten being able to correctly define this term.

As far as visualising what amount of food constitutes 100 g, the sample's performance was generally quite poor, though this was dependent upon the foodstuff in question. Where respondents were given three different amounts of the food to choose from, 28% of the sample gave the correct answer for fish fingers, 30% gave the correct answer for digestive biscuits and 16% gave the correct answer for raisins.

When asked to read figures from a nutrition label, or to make comparisons of nutrient levels between two labels, almost a third of respondents were unable to answer each time. When no calculation was required, the majority of the sample could read 'per 100 g' or 'per packet' information from a label. The declaration 'of which saturates' or 'of which sugars' was understood as well as any other part of the label. Calorific information confused some respondents, bringing the proportion of those who could read this particular statement of information down to around 50%. If a simple calculation was required, less than half of the sample was able to obtain the correct answer. This also applied when comparing nutrient levels between two labels. Most people did not have the ability to make the necessary calculations in their head to convert 'per 100 g' information into information for the whole packet, either when comparing two products or when assessing one product.

The researchers wanted to test how well respondents could assess the product's healthiness taking into account *all* as opposed to *individual* nutrients. In comparisons between two products, respondents were good at recognising the healthier product when the healthier differences between the products were to do with the most well known nutrients, for example lower in fat, higher in fibre, higher in protein. Respondents were less likely to recognise the healthier product when the healthier differences between the products involved nutrients which were less well known, for example, lower in saturates, lower in sodium.

Few respondents claimed to be in a household with someone who had special dietary requirements, the most common being a slimming diet which was mentioned by one in ten respondents. However, most individuals claimed to have changed their diet over the last few years, and the most commonly given reason was to 'be healthier'. The foods people were most likely to believe they should be eating less of were fatty foods and sweet things. In terms of what the sample felt they should be eating more of, the most likely responses were fruit and vegetables. The researchers concluded 'most respondents claimed to be concerned about the healthiness of foods although less than half claimed to always choose a healthier food. A strong feeling for enjoying the foods they were eating emerged.' Geographically, respondents in Wales and southern England performed better than those in the Midlands and the north of England. Respondents from Scotland and Northern Ireland were relatively less well informed.

The results of this research galvanised the food industry, both retail and manufacturing, into seeking ways of providing nutrition information in a manner which would be more helpful to consumers.

Further research commissioned and conducted in the UK by the Institute of Grocery Distribution (IGD) in 1996 showed that of those consumers who use the nutrition information on the label, most focus on energy, and to a lesser extent fat, and this finding is slightly at odds with the RSL Report. The research also indicated that many consumers have little knowledge of how much energy, in terms of kilocalories or kilojoules, they need per day and little idea of what guideline targets are with respect to fat. As indicated in the previously listed research results, few understood the meaning of the term 'saturates', especially in the given format where it is indicated under fats as 'of which . . .', and the concept of kilojoules was not understood at all. Most respondents said that 'per serving' information was generally found to be more helpful than 'per 100 g/100 ml', although the latter was useful when making comparisons between products at point of sale.

As a result of this research, proposals were drawn up for highlighting calories and fat on the nutrition label, and the UK Ministry of Agriculture, Fisheries and Foods (MAFF) and Department of Health (DH) were consulted about Guideline Daily Amounts of calories and fat and values were agreed for both men and women. Various formats were tested on consumers and, as a result, a scheme for supplementary voluntary nutrition labelling was launched in February 1998.[5] The details of this scheme are set out in the next section.

---

[5] *Voluntary Nutrition Labelling Guidelines to Benefit the Consumer – Supplementary to legislative nutrition labelling requirements*, Institute of Grocery Distribution, 1998

6.5 Improved nutrition labelling

Since the advent of the European Nutrition Labelling Directive and an agreed regulatory basis for the provision of nutrition information, there has been little scope for divergence from the statutory format, except via additional off-label information to assist consumers to understand and use the information on the pack by providing leaflets, customer helplines and other sources of assistance. However, this does not necessarily help at point of purchase.

Feedback from consumers informs businesses about what their customers want and expect and the results of the UK consumer research outlined in section 6.4 above came as no great surprise to the food industry. Some major UK retailers had already begun to highlight information about specific nutrients below the standard nutrition panel in response to dietary advice in the (then UK Government's) health strategy 'Health of the Nation' White Paper[6] recommendations to reduce consumption of fat, and especially saturated fat, and to reduce levels of obesity.

In pursuit of UK Government strategy in respect of nutrition goals, a Nutrition Task Force (NTF) was established to consider a range of aspects which might assist in improving consumers' eating habits including, unsurprisingly, the use of nutrition information. A group of experts commissioned the consumer research project, described above, which concluded that current nutrition information was not helpful to many consumers.

The industry began to look at the possibilities, within the constraints of the existing legislation, for providing additional voluntary nutrition labelling as a tool to help consumers choose a healthy diet. The initiative was formalised in May 1995 under the auspices of the Institute of Grocery Distribution (IGD), a research organisation which draws its membership from every stage of the food supply chain and has links with a number of consumer organisations.

The existing scientific, consumer and company research was reviewed, including that described in section 6.4, and new research commissioned to identify a labelling format for food products which would provide consumers with information to enable them to gain an improved understanding of the amount of fat and energy they consume in their daily diets. The objective was that the labelling format should provide relevant information and the nutrition information be expressed in a format useful to consumers: it should help them to understand and manage the type and balance of nutrients (fat and energy) they were consuming in their diet. The information should be clear and simple to understand, for which reason the study focused on three nutrients in order not to confuse consumers with overly complex or detailed information. The choice of nutrients, fat, saturates and calories resulted from the identification that such a focus would be a significant step forward in providing supplementary nutrition labelling, and that simpler supplementary nutrition labels would assist more consumers in selecting healthy diets.

---

[6] *The Health of the Nation – a strategy for health*, HMSO, 1992

A two-step research programme was conducted. Step one consisted of qualitative research (five focus groups) which explored consumer attitudes towards nutrition labelling and provided guidance for the design of the larger quantitative research. Step 2, the quantitative research, covered 2300 adult consumers in a nationally representative study to assess the performance of a number of nutrition labelling formats. The research was designed to assess consumers' ability to use the label, i.e. their performance, rather than their preference for different labelling formats.

The main findings of the research were as follows:

- Current levels of nutrition understanding are low.
- Current nutrition information is too complicated, frustrating and often illegible.
- Fat and calories were the most monitored nutrients, followed by protein and sugar with fibre and sodium stimulating little concern.
- Many people only monitor the nutritional quality of their food if they are dieting or ill.
- The terms carbohydrate, saturates and sodium were not understood.
- Kilojoules are perceived as irrelevant to adult consumers.
- Consumers' ability to assess accurately the calorie content in foods was quite good. However, their ability to assess accurately the fat content in foods was poor. Products were rated as high or low in fat with very few intermediate assessments.
- Nutrition information is read whilst in the supermarket.
- There was genuine support for guideline daily amounts. Consumers felt that this was new information which helped them to place nutrition information in context, making the whole label more valuable and useful.
- Consumers preferred the use of whole numbers to decimal places and could not understand the relevance of having the information expressed to a tenth of a gram.
- 'Per serving' information was preferred over 'per 100 g', although the 'per 100 g' information was used when comparing the nutrient content of similar products at the point of purchase.

The IGD's guidance on Voluntary Nutrition Labelling was formulated after thorough analysis and discussion of the research results. The concept of Guideline Daily Amounts (GDAs) was central to the labelling formats tested and the underlying purpose of the supplementary voluntary nutrition information, i.e. to assist consumers choice of a healthier diet in line with 'Health of the Nation' recommendations. A number of companies were already promoting daily 'amounts' for fat and calories in company literature, and it clearly made sense to work to a common standard to avoid confusing consumers. The GDAs recommended by the IGD were agreed following discussion with MAFF and the DH. They are based on the predicted daily consumption of an average consumer eating a diet conforming to Committee on Medical Aspects of Food Policy (COMA) recommendations. They are not intended as targets to aim for, but guidance to

Consumers and nutrition labelling 159

assist consumers in their understanding of their daily consumption of calories, fat and saturates. The recommended Guideline Daily Amounts are:

	Women	Men
Calories	2000	2500
Fat	70 g	95 g
Saturates	20 g	30 g

It was recognised that consumer understanding of saturates is low, but the GDA was provided for those companies which choose to offer this information.

There are four other recommendations. The first of these concerns additional on-pack information. In line with the research results which indicated that consumers were most interested in fat and calorie content, and on a per serving basis, the IGD recommends that this information be illustrated independently of the nutrition panel in a separate box, as shown in Tables 6.1 and 6.2. Where this is not possible because of the pack size or layout, it is suggested that this information be highlighted in colour within the nutrition panel. The 'per serving' measures must be stated and be appropriate to consumers, who show a preference for household units, e.g. per teaspoon, per half pack, per biscuit, per slice.

The next recommendation is that the column order in the nutrition information panel should be changed so that 'per serving' information comes before the 'per 100 g' information.

The IGD also recommended that a consumer education programme is required to improve consumer understanding about saturates and their role in the diet. Companies are recommended to use Group 2 nutrition information thereby ensuring that saturates appear on the label.

Table 6.1 Nutrition information: typical values

Nutrition information	
Typical values	per 100 ml
Energy	280 kj
	67 kcal
Protein	3.2 g
Carbohydrates	4.8 g
of which sugars	4.8 g
Fat	3.9 g
of which saturates	2.6 g
fibre	0.0 g
sodium	0.1 g

Table 6.2 Nutrition information: per serving

Per serving (a cup)	
67 calories	3.9 g fat

The final issue is that of legibility. The IGD referred to its June 1994 publication *Packaging Legibility – Recommendations for Improvements* as guidance to assist consumers to read the information provided. The scheme has been widely adopted on UK supermarket 'own label' products. Uptake on branded foods has been less enthusiastic, for two reasons. Firstly, the recommended supplementary format is, strictly speaking, illegal. This was recognised by the IGD, and was stated in the published Guidelines:

> MAFF point out that, in the strictest interpretation of the current legislation, this information would likely fall within the definition of 'nutrition information' in Article 1(4)(a). Under Article 4, which sets out the order in which information should be given and the eighth Whereas clause, which prohibits any other form of nutrition labelling than that specified in the Directive, the presentation of fat and Calories as recommended by the IGD Nutrition Group would be prohibited. However, LACOTS [Local Authorities Co-ordinating body on Food and Trading Standards] supports nutrition labelling which assists consumers to make informed dietary choices and takes the view that the IGD recommendations go some way to achieving this aim and therefore welcomes the IGD recommendations. Whilst noting the current legal constraints local authorities will carefully consider pragmatic approaches which will benefit consumers. In the longer term LACOTS strongly supports changes to existing legislation to enable alternative forms of information to be given.

Secondly, most major food producers operate in a European environment and package and market accordingly. The supplementary information, especially the Guideline Daily Amounts, would not necessarily be appropriate to consumers elsewhere in Europe, and would almost certainly fall foul of local enforcement authorities. Many UK manufacturers have therefore opted not to display the supplementary information on the pack, but to include it in their company leaflets and promotional literature.

The IGD is committed to reviewing the effectiveness of the supplementary voluntary labelling, and to considering other nutrients. Sodium/salt has been uppermost in recent discussions.

The establishment of the Food Standards Agency (FSA) with its statutory responsibilities to the consumer sparked a major review of food-labelling requirements from the perspective of consumer needs. An eighteen point Action Plan was agreed by the FSA's Board in September 2000. Its broad themes are the 'progressive development of a more transparent labelling regime based on consumers' priorities and a common set of EU rules, promotion of good labelling practice and the improvement of consumer education and advice'. Points 4 and 7 of the Action Plan are:

- To press for EU rules requiring nutrition labelling on all foods.
- To commission consumer research to define the ideal content and format for nutrition labelling.

Results of the qualitative research into possible new formats were published in March 2002. The formats used in the research took into account the existing statutory formats described in section 6.2 and the IGD voluntary labelling supplementary format. The study, based on group and individual in-depth interviews, compared eight different specimen labels to see which layouts were easiest to read and understand.

It is interesting to compare the results of this research with the 1995 survey. The main findings were that consumers check the calorie and fat content first, are more likely to check nutritional values 'per serving' than 'per 100 g', and cannot do sums.

In summary, the research found:

- People generally check calories first.
- Fat content was widely checked and the most commonly avoided nutrient.
- Salt was preferred to sodium as a clearer labelling term.
- People understood that 'trace' meant a small amount, and felt that replacing it with '0' would be inaccurate and misleading.
- Putting nutritional values as a percentage of Guideline Daily Amounts (GDAs) confuses people.

The research found that consumers would value some reordering of important nutrients such as salt in food labels, and putting some in bold or in a separate text box, but this could risk downgrading the perceived value of others, particularly sugars. The FSA also pointed out that, although salt is regularly listed on labels and is useful for people with conditions such as high blood pressure who need to reduce their salt intake, sodium occurs in ingredients other than salt, e.g. sodium bicarbonate that is added to bakery products.

Again the research found that consumers do not always check labels, particularly for items they buy regularly. Also, of the eight specimen labels shown to consumers, the one which grouped together fat, saturates and salt (linked to coronary heart disease) was considered sensible. So, little has changed since 1995.

The FSA states that the report will help inform its submission to any future discussions about nutrition labelling in Brussels. It will be interesting to see how our European neighbours respond from a regulatory viewpoint. Most importantly, will the proposed changes actually help consumers make healthier choices within a total diet context and encourage those who do not currently use nutrition information to do so, or help those who would like to use it but do not understand it? One thing for certain is that change is unlikely to be rapid.

6.6 Future trends

The application of the Nutrition Labelling Directive and its usefulness to consumers has remained under constant review since it entered into force. The anticipated arrival of the formal deadline of October 1998 for the European Commission to provide its report and any proposals for amendment provided an additional focus, as did the Commission's 1997 Green Paper on The General Principles of Food Law in the European Union. The review of the Directive is at the time of writing more than three years overdue and it is high time to consider proposals for change.

In May 2001 the European Commission published a discussion paper on Nutrition Claims and Functional Claims (SANCO/1341/2001). Whilst this was not a review of the nutrition labelling Directive as such, clearly any such discussion cannot ignore the issue of general nutrition labelling and it would seem sensible to consider the entire package. The FSA response to the discussion paper, following extensive consultation with stakeholders, was that the scope of any proposal should embrace all nutrition and health claims, but also that harmonised rules on nutrient claims would help to improve the quality of information available to help consumers choose a healthy diet. It also urged the Commission to initiate the Community-wide debate on the mandatory use of 'full' nutrition labelling (Group 2) as the Agency view is that consumers will not be able to make fully informed choices between the foods available to them until all foods carry it.

In the light of experience and research into consumer use and understanding of nutrition information, the UK response to the need for change can be summed up in a single word: simplification. Most pre-packed food and drink products sold in the UK already carry at least Group 1 information, and many provide Group 2. Nutrition labelling could, if appropriate supporting education programmes were put in place, help consumers to construct a healthy balanced diet from the wide variety of products available to them.

A concept enshrined in the Directive is that nutrition information should be simple and easily understood. Highlighting specific information believed to be of most use to consumers, as recommended by the IGD, and removing any unnecessary clutter would therefore appear to be a step in the right direction.

The debate on whether nutrition labelling should be on a voluntary or mandatory basis has been going on since before the Directive was adopted. Many consumer groups call for nutrition information to be mandatory on all pre-packed foods and drinks. However, it should be remembered that no information comes without a price or a trade-off. Consider the amount of compulsory labelling on any food product: the name of the food; the supplier; a full list of ingredients; a use-by or 'best before' date; storage instructions; cooking or usage instructions to name but a few. Information overload can be off-putting. Possibly more focus should be placed on the general change in eating patterns and the tendency to consume more of our food outside the home, in restaurants and other catering establishments? At present the Directive concerns nutrition labelling of 'foodstuffs to be delivered as such to the ultimate consumer'. It also applies to foodstuffs supplied to restaurants, hospitals, canteens and other similar mass caterers, but how often do we see nutrition declarations on a menu or on any food sold loose over the counter?

In any future trends, perhaps there is a need to reconsider the primary purpose of nutrition information and whether or not current practice is actually achieving it. Consumer information and consumer education are not necessarily the same thing. The primary purpose of the food label is to inform the consumer, not to educate, but the information, as indicated in section 6.4, is of little or no use without some pre-existing knowledge. Responsibility for providing this background knowledge has always been shared between Government, consumer and health organisations, the media and the trade, but the goal appears not to have been reached. It would appear that the lead needs to come from Government, in the UK specifically from the Food Standards Agency, that has responsibility for food labelling and consumer information, and that, unlike its predecessors, seems to be gaining the trust of consumers. If the provision of nutrition information is to assist consumers to choose a more healthy, balanced diet, they must first know what that diet should consist of, then how to use nutrition information to help achieve it. Consistency and simplicity in the messages would be a good start, followed by consistency and simplicity on the label. The growing use of electronic information, including in store, offers opportunities not previously dreamt of. If such a medium can provide each individual consumer with every iota of information he or she wishes to know about any product, why try to cram more and more on the label? Perhaps future policy should gravitate towards providing only the more essential information on the label, and giving interested consumers quick and easy access to any other nutrition information they may wish to know via another medium. The debate on diet and health will continue indefinitely. Arguments over the provision of nutrition information will probably do likewise.

6.7 Sources of further information and advice

British Dietetic Association, 7th Floor, Elizabeth House, 22 Suffolk Street, Queensway, Birmingham B1 1LS Telephone +44 (0)121 616 4900

British Nutrition Foundation, High Holborn House, 52–54 High Holborn, London SW1V 6RQ Telephone +44 (0)171 404 6504

Camden and Chorleywood Food RA, Chipping Campden, GL55 6LD Telephone 0386 840319

Food and Drink Federation, 6 Catherine Street, London WC2B 5JJ Telephone +44 (0)171 836 2460

Food Standards Agency, Aviation House, 125 Kingsway, London WC2B 6NH Telephone +44 (0)20 7276 8000

Institute of Grocery Distribution, Grange Lane, Letchmore Heath, Watford, Herts WD2 8DQ Telephone +44 (0)1923 857141

Leatherhead Food RA, Randalls Road, Leatherhead, KT22 7RY Telephone +44 (0)0372 376761

6.8 References

Consumers' Association Nutrition Labelling Research, *Brief Summary of Quantitative Survey*, London 1995

Council Directive of 24 September 1990 on nutrition labelling for foodstuffs (90/496/EEC), *Official Journal of the European Communities* No. L276/40-44, 6 October 1990

Department of Health, *Guidelines on Educational Materials concerned with Nutrition*, London, HMSO, 1996

Department of Health, *The Health of the Nation: a strategy for health*, London, HMSO, 1992

Dietary Reference Values for Food Energy and Nutrients for the United Kingdom, Report of the Panel on Dietary Reference Values of the Committee on Medical Aspects of Food Policy, London, HMSO, 1991

The Food Labelling Regulations 1996, Statutory Instrument 1996 No. 1499, London, HMSO

Food Standards Agency (FSA), *Nutritional Labelling Qualitative Research*, Final Report, November, 2001

Hunt, M.A., *Nutrition Labelling: European Perspectives*, The Encyclopaedia of Human Nutrition, ed Michèle J Sadler et al, London, Academic Press, 1998

MAFF Foodsense Leaflet *Use Your Label: Making Sense of Nutrition Information*, London, MAFF, 1991

MAFF Guidance Notes on Nutrition Labelling, London, MAFF, 1994

McCance and Widdowson's *The Composition of Foods*, 5 ed, Cambridge, The Royal Society of Chemistry and London, MAFF, 1991

Nutrition Labelling Study Report, Research Services Limited (RSL), MAFF J1366, April 1995

Voluntary Nutrition Labelling Guidelines to Benefit the Consumer: Supplementary to legislative nutrition labelling requirements, Institute of Grocery Distribution, Watford, Herts, 1GD, 1998

7

New approaches to providing nutritional information

J. A. Monro, New Zealand Institute for Crop & Food Research

7.1 Introduction

Both food processors and consumers have a basic need for valid and relevant nutritional information; on the one hand to guide production and marketing of genuinely functional products, and on the other to allow selection of products according to efficacy. Data on product efficacy that are relevant, in the sense of being easily communicated, understood and appropriately applied are, however, often unavailable. There is little to guide evidence-based food choice to meet such widespread health challenges as control of blood glucose levels, and maintenance of large bowel function, two examples that will be considered in detail in this chapter.

New approaches to nutritional information must, therefore, focus not only on data that validly represent physiological changes linked to health, but also on transforming the data to show meaningfully the relative efficacy with which products can bring about change. This chapter focuses on new approaches to nutritional information that attempt to link food choice to health end-points through effective communication.

7.2 Why food processors need new types of nutritional information

Food processing has been shown to have large effects on a range of nutritional properties.[1] Changes in macronutrients, such as starch and protein,[2,3] and the destruction of vitamins during food processing,[4] have been well documented, and are updated in this book. Most studies have been constrained by experimental design to a few foods and conditions, and apart from effects on nutrient levels measured in standard food analyses, nutritional information that reflects the effects of processing does not generally reach consumers in a form in which it can be widely used to choose foods. Similarly, food processors often do not have available means to apply, either accurately or practically, relevant nutritional criteria to select prototype products during development. Below are listed several reasons for the need for new nutritional information.

7.2.1 Showing effects of food properties on nutritional qualities

Much of the impact of processing on nutritional quality comes about through changes in physicochemical properties of food polymers, such as dietary fibre,[5] that cannot be represented by food composition values. Changes in structure associated with such processes as starch hydration and gelatinisation,[6] milling,[7] and extrusion,[8] can have an large impact on the rate and extent of digestion, and consequently on a range of physiological markers linked to disease end-points. For example, the impact of cereals on blood glucose and insulin responses is increased markedly as particle size is reduced by milling,[7] or as starch is gelatinised.[6,9]

7.2.2 Tracking changes in nutritional quality

Information from rapid, valid, but relevant tests is needed to guide processing to healthy products. Because of the expense, time, ethics, compliance and other issues involved in clinical trials, human subjects are not usually suitable for monitoring effects of processing until potential products have been identified.

Food processing for improved nutrition may require pragmatic choice of different tests at different stages in product development, to maintain momentum in product development. Active ingredients and formulations may be identified with screening tests, using indirect predictors of health effects, such as ingredient properties. Responses in animal models may guide food processing further, and most promising products then taken into clinical trials, in which effects on biomarkers with established links to health end-points are measured,[10,11] before a claim of efficacy is made. Increasing rigour in nutritional evaluation of functional properties during the course of product development is illustrated in Table 7.1.

As a general principle, the properties of foods that affect physiology should be measured under conditions as close as is reasonable to those in which the food property acts *in vivo*. Developing a soluble fibre-enriched product to lower blood cholesterol is an example. Ingredients of high soluble fibre content could be identified using soluble fibre analysis under simulated gastrointestinal conditions.[12] As hypocholesterolaemic effects of soluble dietary fibres result from increased intestinal viscosity,[13] fibre viscosity should be measured, followed by *in vitro* digestion of products containing selections of viscous fibre sources, with measurement of digesta viscosity. Promising products could be subjected to animal trials to establish that predicted gut viscosity and blood lipid changes occur

Table 7.1 Types of nutritional tests that may be used in food processing at different stages of product development

Level of evidence	Use in food processing	Comments
Ingredient properties	Identifying ingredients with desired properties.	May change in processing. Affected by food matrix and gut milieu. Cheap and quick.
Food composition	Defining nutrient retention. Meeting labeling requirements.	Ignores physiochemical properties, bioavailability, and bioactivity, but relatively cheap.
In vitro digestion	Predicting responses to gut conditions.	May give an indication of effects of digestion on food properties, but not take other important food-host interactions into account.
Animal models	Predicting effects in the whole body context.	May be physiologically different to humans. Require validation. Compliance good.
Human studies[95]	Usually limited application until nearing final product.	Costly, slow, ethically difficult, study population variable, compliance may be poor. Intermediate endpoints required.
Epidemiology	Identifies possible health-relevant food factors.	Associations identified, but not cause-effect relationship (uncertain). Ecologically valid. Not suitable for product testing.
Case-control	Identifying possible food factors in health by association.	Less controlled than experimental methods leaving room for doubt about cause-effect.
Experimental	Provides basis for a health claim.	Most rigorous, but findings apply to the experimental conditions – may lack external validity.

in vivo. Final selections could then be clinically evaluated, to establish firmly their potential as functional foods for humans.

7.2.3 Avoiding unjustified extrapolation between products

The complexity of processing effects on food matrices makes nutritional properties susceptible to processing conditions, and extrapolation of function between different products uncertain.[14] Nonetheless, it is a common cost-cutting measure for marketers to use a functional effect of a bioactive in one product, to promote other foods containing the bioactive, but with a different processing history. To reduce unjustified extrapolation, information is required from tests that are practical and inexpensive enough to use for detecting nutritional effects of different processing conditions in large numbers of samples.

7.2.4 Helping consumers choose foods for health

Food properties can be used to select foods for health only if supported by useable efficacy data.[15] Information from tests of the nutritional and functional properties of foods needs to be easily used by both processors and consumers, to discriminate between products. Without scientific but communicable efficacy data, food processors cannot develop or ethically promote foods, and consumers cannot choose foods for real health effects.

7.2.5 Gaining consumer confidence

Consumer confidence in a product or company requires that claimed benefits are delivered. Distrust is associated with perceptions of deliberate distortion of information, and having been proven wrong in the past.[16] Therefore, the more that the benefits of a food product are exaggerated and overextrapolated, while scrutiny by food regulators and nutritionists continues, the greater the likelihood of generating mistrust. Investment in tests to demonstrate real differences in efficacy of products is, therefore, a prudent strategy.

7.3 Limitations of food composition data in food processing

A number of related reasons why simple direct relationships between constituent levels in foods and effects on health cannot be assumed are outlined below.

7.3.1 People eating foods are complex systems consuming complex systems

Food composition data are obtained from standardised analyses of discrete nutrients, whereas the nutritional effects of food components are modulated by multiple interactions within the food matrix,[17] within the gut,[18] and within the body after absorption.[19] Effects of nutrients in foods are, therefore, seldom the same when consumed in a food, as they would be if consumed as a pure nutrient. Yet, food composition is often used as a measure of 'nutritional quality', and nutrient information panels have been the consumers' main guide to healthy food selection. The ability to make informed food choices for health has therefore been quite restricted.

7.3.2 Analytical data may not reflect bioactivity[20]

Bioactivity is determined by response of the body to food. Several metabolic steps may converge to contribute more to a response than might be expected from amounts of a single active component in a food. For instance, vitamin A activity may be obtained not only from vitamin A as retinal, but also from a range of provitamin A carotenoid precursors.[21] Therefore, analytical methods must measure not only vitamin A in a food, but also carotenoids with the potential for conversion to active vitamin A, as vitamin A equivalents. Similarly, blood lipid is a biomarker that depends on more than dietary lipids as lipid type and carbohydrate intake, for instance, may also affect blood lipids.[22]

7.3.3 Availability or extraction in analytical systems may not equate with bioavailability[23]

Analyses are usually designed to measure all of a component of interest in a food, rather than the bioavailable fraction. Most samples are finely ground to facilitate complete extraction with an effective solvent.[24] As a result, food components may be much more soluble during food analysis than during digestion in the gut. Soluble dietary fibre is a good example; as prescribed in the American Association of Analytical Chemists method for soluble fibre analysis,[25] food samples must be finely ground and extracted in hot buffer at 100 °C, whereas in the gut extraction is normally at 36.4 °C, from a mixture of particles. Soluble fibre extraction in gut conditions may therefore be much less than in fibre analysis.[26]

7.3.4 Physiological effects of food constituents depend on prior physiological state

The effects of food constituents are emergent consequences of the interaction between food and body, and subject to the existing physiological state. A viscous polysaccharide may, for instance, lower blood cholesterol in subjects with hypercholesterolaemia, with much less effect in normals.[27] Similarly, the impact of a food carbohydrate on blood glucose levels is affected by the capacity of the body's cells to absorb glucose, which may be affected by insulin release, by sensitivity to insulin, and by the state of muscle glycogen reserves as a result of exercise.[28]

The body may modulate uptake and utilisation of a nutrient in response to nutrient status; iron uptake is increased in states of iron deficiency,[29] and vitamin C is excreted when uptake exceeds requirements.[30]

7.3.5 A single analytical value may represent a group of compounds differing in nutritional properties

Physiological effects often depend on physicochemical properties that vary within a food constituent class that is represented by a single analytical value. Total dietary fibre as a single value in a food table is a family of compounds of diverse form, physicochemical properties, and physiological effects.[31] Dietary fibres exist as insoluble faecal bulking materials, such as wheat bran, that have little impact on blood cholesterol,[32] or as viscous, fermentable, cholesterol-lowering polysaccharides, such as guar gum,[33] that have relatively little impact on faecal bulk.[34]

7.3.6 Food matrix properties may strongly modulate nutritional effects[35]

Food processing may give products of the same composition, with markedly different physiological effects, because of differences in structure and physicochemical properties. For instance, digestion in a porous starch-protein matrix in the form of bread takes place much more rapidly than in a solid, non-porous matrix of similar composition, in the form of pasta or whole kernels, which consequently have less impact on blood glucose levels.[36,37]

7.4 Foundations for practical nutritional information

Several characteristics of nutritional information for evidence-based food choices for health, are summarized below and will be illustrated with reference to data sets for managing blood glucose (Table 7.2) and large bowel function respectively (Table 7.3). In a nutshell, health end-points need to be selected, markers

Table 7.2 Developing nutritional data sets related to health end-points associated with elevated blood glucose

Consideration	Relevance to blood glucose
End-points	Disorders from glycation and glycaemia, including vascular disease of retina, kidneys, nerves. Heart disease. Polyuria.
Intermediate end-point or marker of effect	Postprandial glycaemic response: blood glucose elevation underlies many long term complications of diabetes mellitus, involving hyperinsulinaemia and glycation.
Currently used indices	Sugars and available carbohydrate: not dependable indicators of blood glucose response, which depends on digestion rate of available carbohydrates and on their monosaccharide composition. Glycaemic index (GI): A percentage based on glycaemic response to food carbohydrate compared with response to glucose. Use restricted to equicarbohydrate comparisons and does not respond to food intake. Not useful for accurate blood glucose control.
Relevant index	Relative glycaemic potency (RGP):[58] A percentage based on comparison of food with glucose. RGP ranks whole foods by their glycaemic impact on an equal weight basis, but does not respond to food intake. Suitable for food comparisons on an equal weight basis.
Practical units	Glycaemic glucose equivalents (GGE):[44] Derived from RGP. A measure of glycaemic impact based on foods. Responsive to food quantity. Useful for communicating efficacy. Can be applied to food items of any weight.
Validation	Clinical measurements have shown that GGE intake predicts glycaemic response to foods of different GI, carbohydrate content, and intake at carbohydrate doses consumed in most meals.[61]

identified that can be causally linked to the end-points, valid indicator variables that predict changes in markers identified for practical tests, and measurements communicated so they can be easily understood.

7.4.1 End-points that are important to well-being

A number of health and disease end-points, affecting a large proportion of the population, need to be addressed in developing healthy foods. Some, such as cardiovascular disease, colorectal cancer, osteoporosis, and constipation are associated with a combination of ageing and unhealthy dietary patterns. Others, such as obesity, are largely the result of food processors and marketers successfully providing foods that appeal to the basic human preferences for sweetness and fats, in all age groups. It would be best to design foods with a number of end-points in mind, and evaluate them with a battery of tests to demonstrate nutritional balance. Producing foods for specific functions or using foods as medicines risks unbalanced nutrient intake.

7.4.2 Biomarkers that are relevant[38]

To be health-relevant and useable, food information needs to relate to practically measurable but valid markers linked to health end-points,[10,38] such as blood cholesterol in relation to cardiovascular disease,[39] or alterations in faecal components

Table 7.3 Developing nutritional data sets related to health end-points associated with insufficient faecal bulk

Consideration	Relevance to faecal bulk
End-points	Various large bowel disorders including constipation, diverticulosis, colorectal cancer.
Intermediate end-point or biomarker	Faecal mass, representing distal colonic bulk.
Currently used index	Dietary fibre: does not reliably predict faecal bulk because bulking effects depend on fermentability, water holding capacity and bacterial growth.
Relevant index	Faecal bulking index (FBI):[34] The impact of a whole food on faecal bulk as a percentage of the effect of an equal weight of wheat bran. Usable for measuring efficacy on an equal weight basis.
Practical units	Wheat bran equivalents (WBE_{fb}):[42] Expressed as a content in foods. May be used to communicate relative efficacy. Applicable to food items of any weight.
Validation	Faecal bulking response measured as mass of rat faecal pellets after hydration closely reflects response in humans.[85]

in relation to colon cancer,[40] and to be obtained with standardised procedures that can be applied to a wide enough range of foods for comparisons to be made.

Biomarkers are required because human death, disease and sub-optimal health are not permissible dependent variables, and many are the result of cumulative changes over long periods. Instead, intermediate biomarker 'end-points', markers of exposure to a food component, and food properties that research has already established as causal in disease and health must be used to assess health effects of food processing. Intermediate end-points must be either causal factors or correlated with changes that lead to end-points. For instance, hyperlipidaemia is an intermediate biomarker that is causally related to a true end-point – atherosclerosis.[39] However, as many factors are involved, evidence for the benefit of a product would be more convincing if several relevant biomarkers were measured. At present most biomarkers require clinical or laboratory measurement and are not widely used to monitor nutritional changes in the course of product development. A good deal of further work is required to develop tests that are useful to industry.

7.4.3 Validity that is balanced with practicality

Validation is a crucial step in selecting variables that indicate effects of foods and food processes on biochemical precursors of health end-points. Because most foods are complex systems, ideal experimental trials in which one food factor is varied while all other variables are kept constant are not often possible, and there is a need to balance practical requirements of food processing with degree of nutritional validation. Given that final products should be comprehensively evaluated, progress in food processing will often best be maintained by being prepared to sacrifice some degree of validity for expediency by appropriate choice of tests, as discussed in section 7.2.3 and illustrated in Table 7.1.

7.4.4 Nutrition information that is up-to-date

Nutrition science is constantly advancing, and as hard data throws new light on the relationship between a food property or component and a health end-point, indices of food effects on health are likely to change. For instance, heart disease is now considered to be influenced less by intake of fat than by intake of specific fatty acids such as saturated and *trans*-fatty acids.[41] Such changes are not a sign that nutrition science cannot be relied on but that continuing research leads to clarification.

A food company that had not kept abreast of nutritional knowledge recently formulated a new 'diabetic muesli bar', replacing all sucrose sources with dextrins, in the belief that 'sugar' replacement would improve blood glucose control. However, such wisdom was obsolete, because sucrose, being half fructose, induces a much lower blood glucose response than dextrins, which are rapidly digested glucose polymers. The new 'diabetic' bar had a greater glycaemic impact than the unmodified version.

7.4.5 Relevant indices that are based on factors that confer relevance on food data

The relevance of food information is determined by validity, sufficiency, practicality, and communicability. Is an index a true reflection of a change in a biomarker or end-point, is it sufficient on its own to predict a change in the end-point, is it a variable that can be measured easily, and expressed in terms that users understand well enough to use in food choice?

7.4.6 Food data that is easily understood

Food data is not relevant if it cannot accurately link consumer behaviour to health end-points, in other words, if it cannot guide food choice for health. To do so it should be easily used. The relative efficacy of foods may, for instance, be expressed in terms of equivalents to a familiar reference that exhibits a specified effect to a known degree, as in wheat bran equivalents and faecal bulking.[42] Glycaemic index (GI), on the other hand, is an example of a number that is supposed to represent the glycaemic potency of a food.[43] However, unlike intake of a nutrient, GI does not change with the composition, serving size, or intake of food, so it makes little sense to consumers, and cannot be used accurately to modify eating patterns that affect blood glucose.[44]

7.5 Limitations of food composition data: the case of carbohydrates

The above framework for building practical, evidence-based data sets linked to health end-points is illustrated below by reference to two physiological effects of food carbohydrates: postprandial glycaemia (post-meal elevation of blood glucose), and faecal bulking. Postprandial glycaemia is determined largely by carbohydrate digestibility,[45] and faecal bulk largely by non-digestible, non-fermentable polysaccharides.[46]

7.5.1 Limitations of carbohydrate composition data

Standard food analyses do not account for the large effects of the structure of carbohydrate molecules and foods in the carbohydrate nutrition. Monosaccharide composition and order, glycosidic bonds, degree of polymerisation, chain configurations, non-covalent interactions between chains, and crosslinks that carbohydrates readily form may all greatly affect physicochemical properties,[6,47] and the physiological effects that depend on such properties. Furthermore, food structure, such as particle size, may considerably modulate the ability of food carbohydrates to express their potential properties,[35] by limiting solubility, extraction, and access of digestive enzymes. Beyond effects on extraction, interactions between carbohydrates and other food components in the intestine are multiple and complex.[18] The amounts of carbohydrate fractions in foods are therefore not usually reliable guides to their physiological effectiveness.[33,48]

174 The nutrition handbook for food processors

Postprandial glycaemia and distal colonic bulk are both physiological markers that are strongly influenced by the effects of food properties on carbohydrate availability, but which cannot be reliably predicted from food composition data. New nutritional information is required for control of postprandial glycaemia (Table 7.2) and distal colonic bulk (Table 7.3), taking into account end-points, biomarkers of exposure, current indices, relevant indices, their validation, and communication discussed above.

7.6 Relative glycaemic potency and glycaemic-glucose equivalents

Control of postprandial glycaemia – the blood glucose response to food intake – is an increasingly important health issue. Diabetes mellitus, marked by an inability to control blood glucose levels, is increasing rapidly in many developed countries, in which an over-supply of high energy and highly digestible carbohydrate foods is coupled with predisposing factors, including physical inactivity, obesity, and inheritance.[28] Many consumers need to be able to manage postprandial glycaemia by selecting foods and food combinations according to glycaemic impact, but food labels at present give them little assistance.

7.6.1 End-point

Health consequences of hyperglycaemia are multiple and most evident in the diabetes mellitus syndrome.[28,49,50] Persistently raised blood glucose causes protein glycation throughout the body, leading to cumulative, diffuse damage, emerging as pathology in a number of organ systems. Basal membrane damage is commonly an underlying factor in changes to micro-vessels involving the eyes, kidneys and nerves.[51] Intense insulin production in response to diabetic hyperglycaemia, or to repeated acute glucose loading from large intakes of highly digestible carbohydrate, is thought to contribute to the progression of glucose intolerance, through β-cell toxicity, leading to loss of the capacity of the pancreas to produce insulin.[52] Hyperinsulinaemia as a response to elevated blood glucose favours elevated blood lipids, obesity and hypertension, all risk factors in heart disease.[49,50,51]

Post-prandial glycaemia may also lead to a number of acute and sometimes serious disorders, as the body attempts to counter the osmotic effects of high blood sugar levels. The excretion of sugar by the kidneys leads to water loss, excessive thirst, and in extreme cases, to fatal electrolyte imbalances.[53]

7.6.2 Markers

As blood glucose response is causal in glycation, insulin response, osmotic effects and other aspects of diabetic pathology, it is a highly relevant marker of the influence of foods and carbohydrates on progression towards disease end-points related to diabetes. Indeed, persistent elevation of blood glucose is clinically a defining feature of diabetes mellitus.

7.6.3 Current indices

Glycaemic carbohydrate components most commonly seen on food labels are 'carbohydrate', 'available carbohydrate', 'complex carbohydrate' (starch), and 'sugars'. One of the main reasons for distinguishing between sugars and complex carbohydrates is the once-held belief that sugars have a more acute impact on blood glucose levels than starch. However, some starches are so rapidly digested that they induce a blood glucose response similar to that of pure glucose. For instance, starch in rice bubbles has a glycaemic index (GI) of 97 (gives 97% of the response to an equicarbohydrate dose of glucose) and baked potato a GI of 85, whereas starch in noodles has a GI of 46.[54] The relative amounts of sugar versus complex carbohydrate in a food is not, therefore, a reliable guide to its impact on blood glucose.

Sugar type is another reason that 'sugar' content does not indicate glycaemic effect. Sucrose ('cane sugar') for instance has a GI of 61 because it is a disaccharide containing a fructose (GI = 23) and a glucose (GI = 100) unit.[55] While dietary sugars include sucrose, lactose, fructose, glucose, and other mono- and disaccharides, 'blood sugar' is blood glucose.

GI is now being used to classify and promote foods by glycaemic impact. The GI of a food is the incremental effect of carbohydrate in a food on blood glucose, as a percentage of the effect of an equal weight of glucose. It is usually based on the glycaemic effect of enough food to provide a 50 g dose of carbohydrate, compared with the effect of 50 g glucose, or its carbohydrate equivalent in white bread, as the reference.

$$\text{GI} = \frac{\text{Blood glucose increment due to } 50\,g \text{ } carbohydrate \text{ } in \text{ } a \text{ } food}{\text{Blood glucose increment due to 50 g glucose}} \times 100 \quad [7.1]$$

The glycaemic index was devised to take account of the relative differences in the impact of food carbohydrates on blood glucose resulting from the types of carbohydrate and their rates of digestion.[43]

Two intrinsic characteristics of GI make it difficult to use alone in accurate blood glucose management. Firstly, because GI is based on an equicarbohydrate comparison it should be used to compare foods only at equal carbohydrate doses whereas most foods differ enormously in available carbohydrate content. It is often incorrectly stated that GI ranks foods according to their impact on blood glucose,[56] but it ranks carbohydrates in food, not foods, and ranks foods only if they contain equal amounts of carbohydrate. Secondly, as a percentage, GI does not change with food quantity, so cannot be used to predict relative glycaemic responses to servings or intakes of food. It is an example of an impractical index.

Table 7.4 Foods within food groupings ranked by glycaemic index (GI), with corresponding values for glycaemic glucose equivalents (GGE) per common standard measure (CSM), and GGE per 100 g (RGP).[44] Rankings by GI did not similarly rank either RGP or GGE/CSM, showing that GI does not rank foods by glycaemic impact

Food grouping	Nature of CSM	CSM wt(g)	%CHO	GI	Glycaemic impact	
					RGP	GGE/CSM
Bakery products						
Doughnut ring	doughnut	42	44	76	33	14
Bagels, plain	bagel	74	47	72	33.8	25
Bread, roll, white, soft	roll	51	49	70	34.3	17.5
Bread, white, sliced	med slice	26	43	70	30.1	7.8
Bread, wholemeal	med slice	28	37	69	25.5	7.1
Croissants	small	57	39	67	26.1	14.9
Crispbread, rye	biscuit	6	64	65	41.6	2.5
Biscuit, digestive	biscuit	14	63	58	37	5
Cake, sponge	slice	89	60	46	28	25
Bread, multigrain 'heavy'	med slice	28	37	52	19.2	5.4
Breakfast cereals						
Puffed rice	cup	14	78	89	69	10
Corn flakes, Kelloggs	serving	30	85	84	71.4	21.4
Wheat, puffed	cup	14	64	74	47.4	6.6
Wheat biscuit, 'Weet-Bix'	biscuit	15	62	70	43.4	6.5
Porridge, prepd. (milk & w)	cup	260	10.5	61	6.4	16.7
Muesli, non toasted	cup	107	57	56	32	31.9
Muesli, toasted, sweet	cup	110	53	43	22.8	25.1

7.6.4 Relevant indices

To overcome the limitations of GI, a food-based 'GI', termed Relative Glycaemic Potency (RGP), was calculated, and defined as the theoretical response to 50 g of a *food* as a percentage of the response to 50 g glucose:[57,58]

$$\text{RGP} = \frac{\text{Blood glucose increment due to } 50\,g\,food}{\text{Blood glucose increment due to 50 g glucose}} \times 100 \quad [7.2]$$

RGP is simply GI adjusted for the carbohydrate content of a food (%CHO), and it allows a comparison of foods, rather than food carbohydrates, on an equal weight basis. Adjustment for the carbohydrate content of a food results in a completely different ranking of foods than is obtained with GI, as shown in Table 7.4.

7.6.5 Practical units

Because they are based on whole foods, RGP values can easily be expressed as practical units that are related to food intakes. RGP is a percentage of the effect of glucose, so the RGP of a food can be regarded as the amount of glucose that would be equivalent to 100 g of the food in its glycaemic impact. In other words, an RGP 30 can be expressed as 30 glycaemic glucose equivalents (GGE) per 100 g food:

$$RGP = (\% \ CHO/100) \cdot GI \quad [7.3]$$

$$= GGE/100\,g \ food \quad [7.4]$$

The number of GGEs donated by a food item or meal may be termed its relative glycemic impact (RGI):

$$RGI = GGE \ intake \ at \ a \ time \quad [7.5]$$

$$= Food \ weight \cdot GGE/g \ of \ food \quad [7.6]$$

$$= \sum (no. \ CSMs \ food \cdot CSM \ weight \cdot (\%CHO \cdot GI)/10\,000) \quad [7.7]$$

Glycaemic impact (RGI), as GGE intake, then becomes a function, not of GI alone, but of GI, carbohydrate content, and serving size or food intake, so it takes into account all of the factors determining the RGI of a food, and gives freedom from the equicarbohydrate limitation of GI. The term 'glycaemic loading' is similar to RGI, but has been used in epidemiology to express cumulative or chronic exposure to glycaemia in response to foods over periods of months,[59] whereas RGI refers to acute impact. The inaccuracy of food classifications for glycaemic control based on GI alone, when foods differ in carbohydrate content and serving size, is shown in Fig. 7.1.

Expressing glycaemic potency as a content of GGEs enables it to be treated like a nutrient, so that RGI and nutrient intake can be presented simultaneously, allowing complete nutritional management, and use in computer-based diet management systems.[44] GGEs should also enable the combined effect of foods in meals to be gauged, because the GGE contents of different foods may, in theory, be added to give the glycaemic impact of the meal.

Table 7.5 The glycaemic index (GI) of foods does not indicate relative glycaemic impact (glycaemic glucose equivalents per common standard measure; GGE/CSM). GI is not a useful guide to food choice for blood glucose control unless carbohydrate intakes are equal

Common standard measure of food	Weight (g)	GI	GGE/CSM
1 apricot	54	57	3
1 banana	128	58	18
2 scoops ice-cream	50	61	6.5
1 blueberry muffin	80	59	24
1 can Fanta™	375	68	35
2 slices pineapple	125	66	6.6
1 glass orange juice	256	46	9.9
1 slice banana cake	80	47	22
1 slice dark rye bread	70	86	19
1 apple muffin	80	44	19
1 cup broad beans	160	79	14.2
1 cup spaghetti	180	41	23

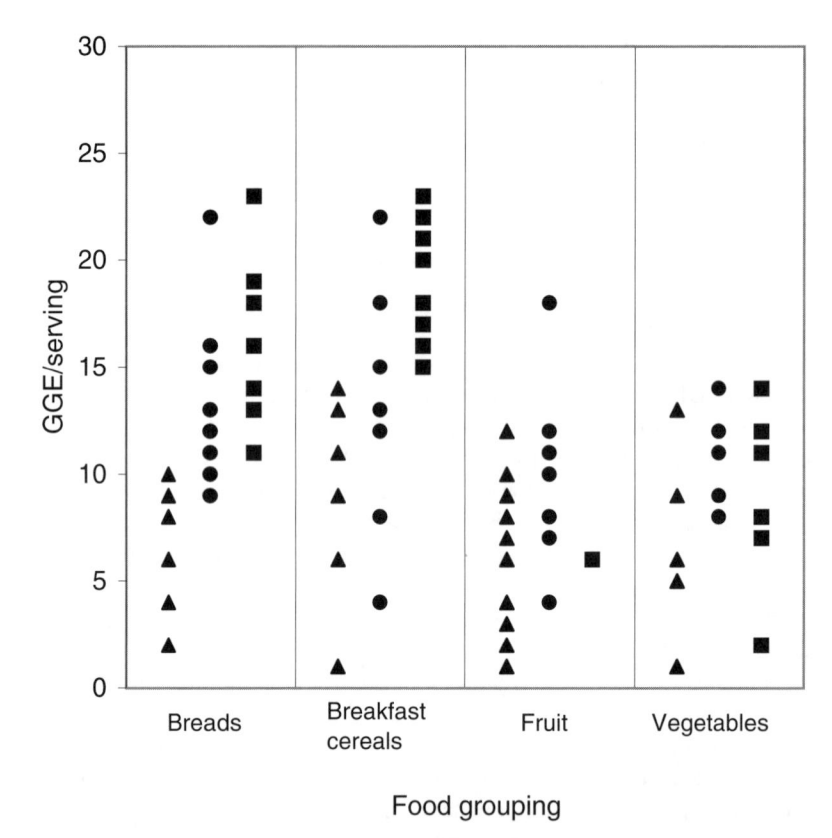

Fig. 7.1 Glycaemic impact as glycaemic glucose equivalents (GGE) per serving of foods classified as low (<55; ▲), medium (55–70; ●) and high (>70; ■) glycaemic index (GI), in each of the food groupings breads, breakfast cereals, fruit and vegetables. GI has not usefully classified foods in each food grouping by glycaemic impact, as GGE contents in the different GI classes overlap.

GGE has potentially great practical advantages over GI in dietary management of glycaemia and in food labelling. Responsiveness of GGE intake to food intake could greatly improve the precision with which glycaemia could be managed by diet, insulin and medication. GGE values on food labels would allow the relative glycaemic impact of any food item or quantity to be directly specified, as the examples in Table 7.5 show.

Because atherosclerosis is a common long-term complication of diabetes mellitus, food products for diabetes should also contain a low proportion of saturated fat. Less than 7% of energy from saturated fat is the recommended guideline of the American Heart Association.[60]

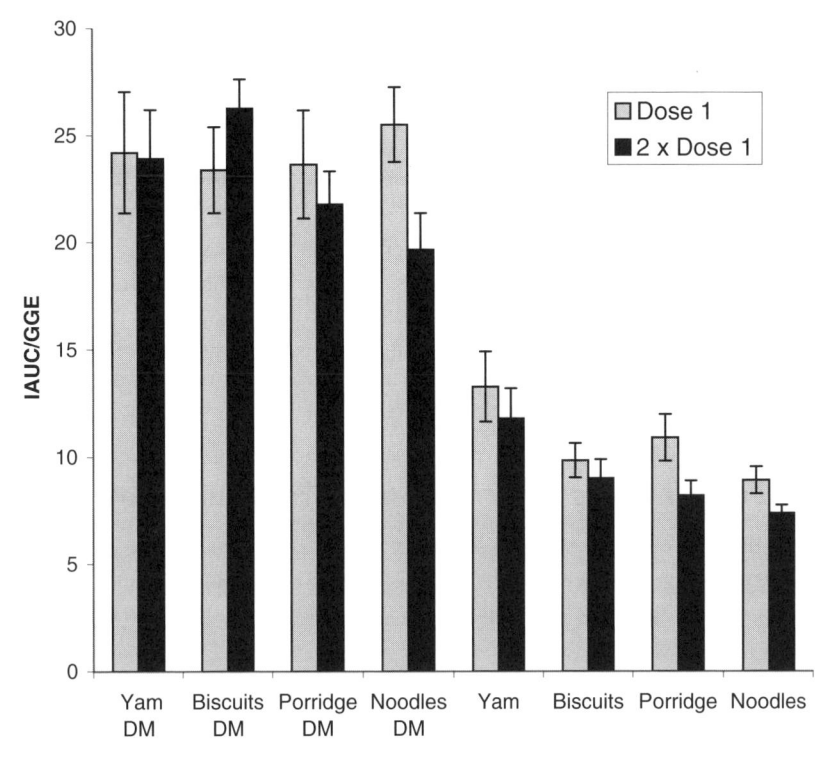

Fig. 7.2 Glycaemic responses (IAUC; mmol·min/L) per glycaemic glucose equivalent (GGE) for foods of differing glycaemic index (GI), carbohydrate (CHO) content, and intake, consumed at a single and a double GGE dose, by subjects with (DM) and without Type 2 diabetes. Yams, (GI, 35; CHO, 8.84%; intakes: 10 GGE, 323.2 g; 20 GGE, 646.4 g), biscuits (GI, 49.5; CHO, 72.9%; intakes: 10 GGE, 27.7 g; 20 GGE, 55.4 g), porridge (GI, 67.5; CHO, 13.1%; intakes: 10 GGE, 132.4 g; 20 GGE, 246.8 g), noodles (GI, 48; CHO, 16%; intakes: 24 GGE, 323.2 g; 48 GGE, 646.4 g). Results show that GGE content is a robust measure of glycaemic impact.

7.6.6 Validity of GGE intake in predicting glycaemic response

GGE is a new concept, and only one study to date has directly tested the predictive validity of GGE intake *per se*.[61] But GGEs are a combination of GI and carbohydrate dose so studies of joint effects of GI and carbohydrate dose on blood glucose are a test of GGE, and have shown that both amount of carbohydrate and its glycaemic potency (GI) in a food determine glycaemic response.[62,63] We fed subjects several foods, each at two GGE doses, one double the other. After adjusting for individual glycaemic responsiveness, glycaemic responses per unit GGE intake were similar across food types and doses to over 100 g carbohydrate intake. Figure 7.2 shows the increment in blood glucose response per GGE for several foods of differing GI, carbohydrate content and intake; it confirms that GGEs are a robust predictor of glycaemic impact.

7.6.7 Product screening for GGE content

GGE content is calculated from GI which is a clinical measurement of relative blood glucose responses that may not be feasible to use in a food processing context. However, several tests of *in vitro* digestibility that correlate well with glycaemic responses in humans are now available and are suitable for screening starchy foods to gauge their relative glycaemic potencies.[64,65,66] Glucose release after 20 min of starch digestion appears to predict glycaemic response well.[66] More slowly digested starch has less impact on blood glucose, because the slower rate of glucose loading into the blood does not exceed the rate of cellular glucose uptake enough to produce an acute glycaemic response.

The most accurate measurement of GGE content requires measurement of blood glucose responses to foods in humans, but, because of costs and time, *in vitro* digestion is a more practical option for the product development stages.

7.7 Faecal bulking index and wheat bran equivalents

Faecal bulking capacity is an important property of foods because bulk in the large bowel has a crucial role in large bowel function and health (Table 7.6). The direct relationship between faecal bulk and 'regularity' is of concern to a large

Table 7.6 Putative links between properties and effects of bulk in the large intestine

Property/effect	Consequent effect
Bulkiness	Bulk transfer.
Bulk transfer	Toxin removal, colonic exposure reduced, decreased transit time. Replenishment of substrates for fermentation – decreased colon cancer risk.
Decreased transit time	Less protein putrefaction to harmful nitrogenous products – decreased colon cancer risk. Less time for dehydration and stool hardening.
Increased water load	Diluted colon contents, stool softening, pressure distribution – decreased risk of diverticulosis and haemorrhoids.
Replenishment	Provides substrates for bacterial growth. Butyrate produced by fermentaion protects against colorectal cancer. Short chain fatty acid production decreases pH and solubility of carcinogenic bile acids.
Binding	Reduced toxin/carcinogen activity.
Pressure distribution	Reduces risk of diverticulosis and haemorrhoids by reducing localised pressure points.
Distension	Stimulates defaecation, preventing stagnation.
Defecation	Comfort and continued flow, sense of well-being.

proportion of the population, who assume that dietary fibre is the food component responsible,[67] a point well used by food marketers. Countless foods and supplements are promoted as containing dietary fibre, implying that they will promote regularity, but with no supporting efficacy data other than dietary fibre content.

Dietary fibre values can, in fact, be a poor guide to faecal bulking.[34,68] Faecal bulk is a result of multiple interactions between the food, the host, and the gut ecosystem – food composition, digestion, endogenous secretions, fermentation, bacterial biomass, water-holding capacity, and particle structure will all play a role.[69] Materials that do not analyse as dietary fibre contribute to faecal bulk,[46] and the combined loss of polysaccharide and its water-holding capacity can be only partly compensated for by bacterial growth.[70] Pectin, for example, is a much less effective faecal bulker than psyllium gum,[34] because it is readily fermented, whereas psyllium is fermentation-resistant and remains highly hydrated in the colon. Both pectin and psyllium are non-starch polysaccharides, and therefore dietary fibre, but dietary fibre analysis gives no indication of the important differences in their physiological actions.

7.7.1 End-points

Normal large bowel function and health are general end-points which, it is almost universally agreed, depend on a supply of bulk to the distal colon.[69,71] More specific effects of bulk in the colon were summarised in Table 7.6. Colonic bulk has been related to a number of health end-points in a number of ways. It is a direct stimulus to defecation, dilutes various toxins and distributes intracolonic pressure, reducing the risk of diverticulosis.[69,72] The defecation that it induces allows movement of fermenting material into the distal colon, where it produces butyrate, thought to protect against colorectal cancer.[73] Replenishment of carbohydrates in the distal colon may also reduce formation of carcinogenic nitrogenous compounds, formed when proteins are used as a carbon source in fermentation after exhaustion of carbohydrate substrates.[74]

Simple constipation resulting from an inadequate supply of moist bulk to the distal colon is one of the most widespread consequences of Western eating patterns.[75] If only to prevent constipation, faecal bulking efficacy deserves attention.

7.7.2 Markers

Distal colonic bulk is a highly relevant marker of large bowel health because of the number of direct and indirect effects that it has (Table 7.6), and because it is a major factor in laxation.

7.7.3 Current indices

Dietary fibre has traditionally been relied on to indicate the potential of a food to promote regularity of bowel function. Indeed, fibre analysis for human foods originated from the physiological concept of dietary fibre as roughage – plant cell wall material not digested by human enzymes in the gut, and responsible for stool bulk.[76] The plant cell wall still remains central to most definitions of dietary fibre and corresponding methods of analysis,[77] although, the definition is being extended to include added non-digestible polysaccharides and oligosaccharides that have beneficial effects.[78,79] But 'beneficial effects' specified as part of the definition of dietary fibre include blood cholesterol-lowering and blood glucose-lowering effects, and are not confined to those associated with faecal bulking, so the definition has become too broad to be useful. In fact, dietary fibre analysis has never been congruent with the original physiological concept of dietary fibre as faecal bulking 'roughage', because it measures materials resistant to digestion by foregut proteases and amylases, while faecal bulk depends also on resistance to hind gut fermentation. Food components that are both resistant to digestion and to fermentation are not discretely analysed in fibre analysis.

There is an overall statistical relationship between dietary fibre intake and faecal bulk,[80] but because of the large amount of variability in foods of low fibre content, fibre cannot be used as a guide to choosing any individual food for bulk, as the results in Fig. 7.3 show. Each food needs to be individually tested before it can be chosen for its faecal bulking efficacy.

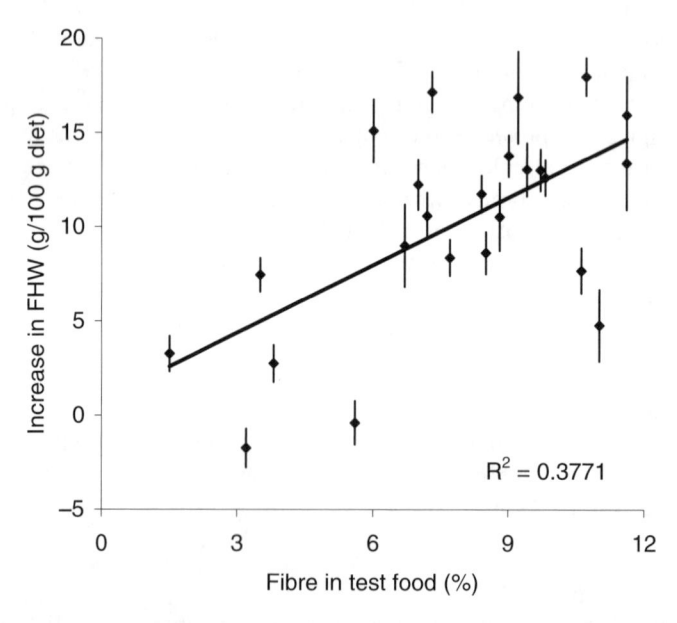

Fig. 7.3 Increase in hydrated faecal weight (FHW) induced by breakfast cereals fed to rats at 50% of the diet. The results show that dietary fibre content is not a reliable predictor of faecal bulking in most breakfast cereals.

7.7.4 Relevant indices

The faecal bulking index (FBI) has been developed as an index of the distal colonic bulking efficacy of a food.[34] FBI is defined as the increment in hydrated faecal mass induced by a food as a percentage of the increase due to a wheat bran reference.

$$\text{FBI} = \frac{\text{Increase in weight of rehydrated faeces per g of test food}}{\text{Increase in weight of rehydrated faeces per g of reference food}} \times 100$$

[7.8]

FBI allows foods to be ranked by relative bulking efficacy, on an equal weight basis. Ranking by FBI of a representative sample of Australasian breakfast cereals is shown in Fig. 7.4.

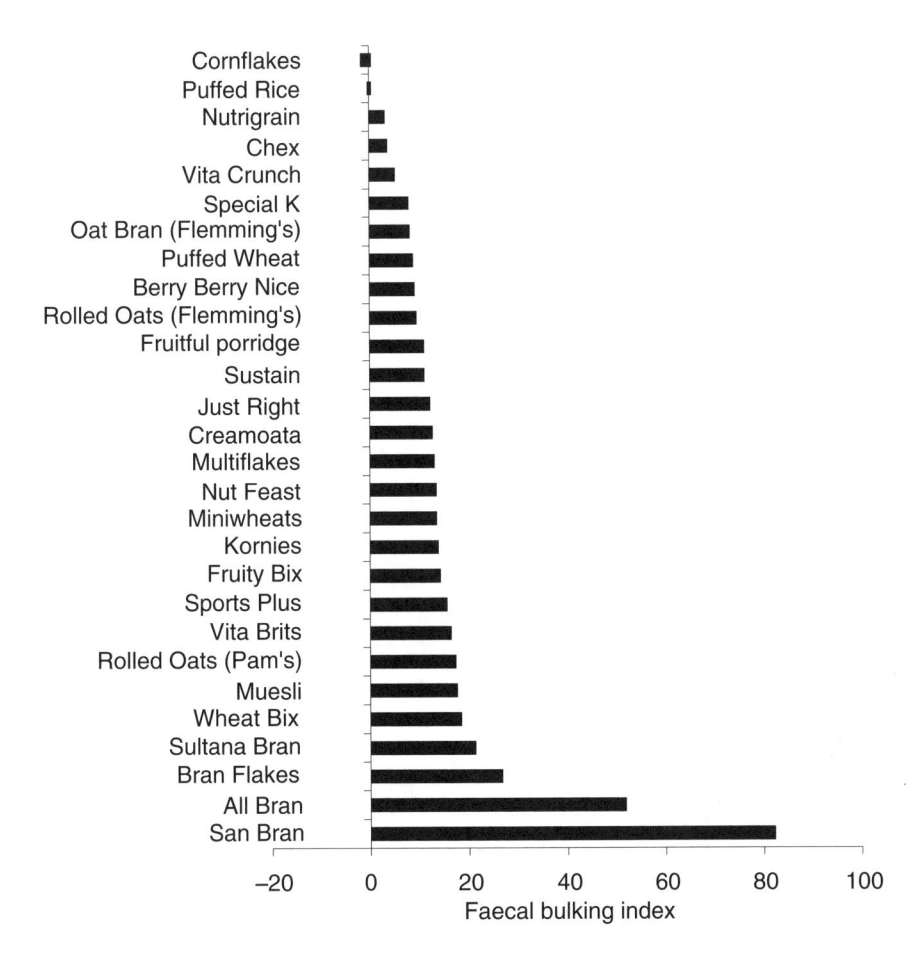

Fig. 7.4 Faecal bulking indices (FBI) of a representative selection of Australasian breakfast cereals. FBI gives the increment in faecal bulk indiced by a food relative to that induced by an equal weight of wheat bran.

To measure FBI, rats are fed a nutritionally complete baseline diet containing 5% mixed dietary fibre and 50% sucrose, and the increase in hydrated faecal bulk when a proportion of the sucrose is replaced by a test food is compared with the increment induced by an equal weight of wheat bran reference. In the case of the breakfast cereals, all of the sucrose was replaced by cereal.

7.7.5 Valid measurement

A crude estimate of faecal bulking would be resistance to fermentation by colonic bacteria *in vitro*.[81] But, because of the complex of host and food factors determining faecal bulk, it is best measured *in vivo*, and ideally in humans. However, for the purposes of product screening in food processing, an animal model giving a valid representation of human responses would be expedient, to avoid the difficulties of human research. The laboratory rat gives a reasonable prediction of the relative effects of foods on faecal bulk,[34,82] because, like humans, it is monogastric, and food residues from the small intestine undergo extensive mixed bacterial fermentation in the hind gut, where extent of digestion will be limited more by substrate characteristics than by the availability of microbes. As in humans, dominant factors determining faecal dry matter are the mass of material resistant to mixed bacterial fermentation, bacterial mass, and endogenous secretions.[81]

Transit time in the rat is shorter than in man,[83] the rat concentrates faecal dry matter as pellets, and is a caecal rather than a colonic fermenter. Its validity as a model is improved by using large rats (>250 g), preadapting them to mixed dietary fibre, and making sure that test foods are fed at realistic levels to avoid overloading the gut or exceeding normal fermentation capacity. The problem of faecal dehydration is overcome if the rat faecal pellets are allowed to imbibe water passively to their full water-holding capacity, when their water content rises to that of fresh human stools, and the increase in faecal bulk per gram of wheat bran fibre is almost identical to that measured in humans.[84]

The FBI assay gives a relatively quick *in vivo* measure of relative faecal bulking efficacy. However, as material entering the colon depends on diet composition, not on one component of it, absolute effects may be influenced by other foods in the diet.

7.7.6 Practical units

FBI is a percentage based on comparison of equal weights of foods, so, like GI, it is not a function of food quantity. This problem is addressed by expressing faecal bulking efficacy in terms of content of equivalents to a familiar faecal bulking reference material, so that choice of food type (content), and quantity, can be a guide in choosing foods.[42]

To be consumer-friendly such a reference should be:

- Widely available.
- Familiar/identifiable – well known to consumers.

- Understood – known for its effectiveness.
- Relevant – occurring widely in the normal diet.
- Constant – not varying in the relevant properties.
- Effective – exhibiting the property of interest to at least a moderately high degree.

Hard red wheat bran is a relevant reference for faecal bulking: it is widely available, familiar, well known for its bulking effects, widely consumed, and although it may vary between batches, it is available as an American Association of Analytical Chemists reference material for dietary fibre analysis.

With wheat bran as the reference ($FBI_{wheat\ bran} = 100$), faecal bulking efficacy may be expressed as the weight of wheat bran that would contribute the same faecal bulk as the given quantity of food, that is, as the content of wheat bran equivalents for faecal bulk (WBE_{fb}) in the food.

WBE_{fb} in a weight w_A of Food A, with an FBI value of FBI_A is:

$$WBE_{fb} = w_A \cdot (FBI_A/100) \text{ (g)} \qquad [7.9]$$

The faecal bulking efficacies of some of the breakfast cereals in Fig. 7.4, expressed as WBE_{fb} per serving, are shown in Table 7.7.

WBE_{fb} content allows direct comparison of different amounts of different products and can therefore be useful to both food processors and consumers. WBE_{fb} allows the potential contributions to faecal bulk by food in a meal or diet to be monitored, in theory, by adding the WBE_{fb} contributions of each food. Then, based on a desired daily WBE_{fb} intake, any shortfall can be determined by difference, and remedied with an appropriate food or bulking supplement.

Individual WBE_{fb} requirements will vary greatly, but once established, cumulative intake of WBE_{fb} per day could be used to ensure that dietary goals are met. An average adult daily reference value for faecal bulking (DRV_{fb}) of 67.6 WBE_{fb} per day has been calculated,[84] from associations between faecal weight and protection against large bowel disease measured in epidemiological studies.[80,85]

7.7.7 Application of FBI assay to product screening

An evaluation of the faecal bulking efficacy of Australasian breakfast cereals is an example of how the FBI assay might be used in product screening.[82] The results are shown in Fig. 7.5. Faecal bulking efficacies, as wheat bran equivalents per serving, were classified according to associated nutrient claims for dietary fibre. The results show that most breakfast cereals provided less than the average bulk per serving required to provide the DRV_{fb} on current intakes of dietary fibre sources (10 servings per day; 6.7 WBE_{fb} per serving required), or on recommended intakes (16 servings per day; 4.2 WBE_{fb} per serving required).

It was concluded that nutrient claims for dietary fibre in most breakfast cereals probably exaggerated their faecal bulking efficacy, although the findings would be best confirmed in human trials with some selections of the cereals.

Table 7.7 Relative faecal bulking efficacy of breakfast cereals as faecal bulking indices (FBI), and as wheat bran equivalents for faecal bulk (WBE_{fb}) per serving

	FBI (= WBE_{fb}/100 g)	Serving size (g)	WBE_{fb}/serving (g)
All Bran	51.3	45	23.1
Berry Berry Nice	8.6	30	2.6
Bran flakes	26.2	30	7.9
Chex	3.3	30	1.0
Cornflakes	−1.7	30	−0.5
Creamoata	12.2	30	3.7
Fruitful porridge	10.5	40	4.2
Fruity Bix	13.8	40	5.5
Just right	11.7	45	5.3
Kornies	13.4	30	4.0
Miniwheats	13.0	30	3.9
Muesli	17.2	50	8.6
Multiflakes	12.6	45	5.7
Nut Feast	13.0	45	5.9
Nutrigrain	2.7	30	0.8
Oat Bran	7.7	30	2.3
Puffed rice	−0.4	30	−0.1
Puffed wheat	8.4	30	2.5
Rolled Oats (Fleming's)	9.0	30	2.7
Rolled Oats (Pam's)	16.9	30	5.1
San Bran	81.7	45	36.8
Special K	7.5	30	2.2
Sports plus	15.1	50	7.6
Sultana bran	20.8	45	9.4
Sustain	10.6	45	4.7
Vita Brits	15.9	30	4.8
Vita crunch	4.8	60	2.9
Wheat biscuits	18.0	30	5.4
Wheat bran (reference)	100.0	67.5	67.5

7.8 Conclusion and future trends

The discussion in this chapter has focused on the need for new tests of the nutritional functionality of foods, and on making information from such tests relevant in the sense of helping consumer choice for wellbeing. Without such data, neither food processors nor consumers will be able to make the choices required for the development of healthier food products on the one hand, and healthier diets on the other. The primary justification for objective nutrition research is that it improves health, and if food choice is part of that, nutritional information needs to facilitate healthy food choice to be truly relevant.

It has been estimated that the market for functional foods in the USA will be worth US$ 34 billion in 2010,[86] and that 'do it yourself' health, based on supplements and functional/fortified foods is at present a US$ 42 billion oppor-

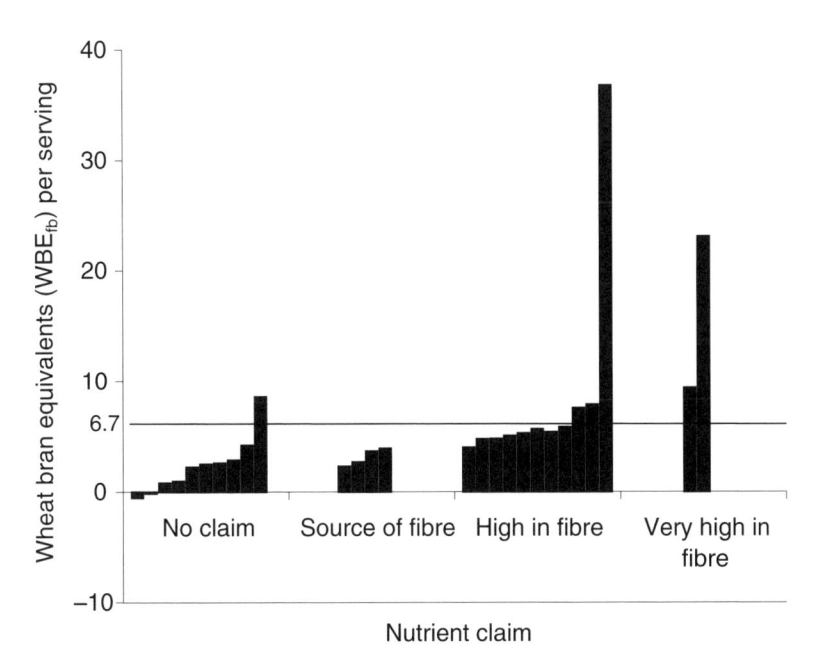

Fig. 7.5 Faecal bulking efficacy as wheat bran equivalents (WBE$_{fb}$) per serving of breakfast cereals classified by the nutrient claims for dietary fibre in Australasia (no claim, <1.5 g fibre/serving; source of fibre, 1.5–3 g fibre/serving; high in fibre, 3–6 g fibre/serving; very high in fibre, >6 g dietary fibre/serving), relative to the mean WBE$_{fb}$ contribution per serving (6.7) required to satisfy average adult requirements in a diet containing 10 servings per day of dietary fibre sources.

tunity.[87] But there have also been signs that consumer support for some functional foods is faltering. Given the flood of functional foods onto the market, coupled with inadequate information for discriminatng between products, confusion and mistrust generated by extravagant claims, and apparently conflicting statements from nutritionists, some resistance in consumers who do not know what to believe or what to choose, is understandable.

For the future, then, several needs must be met:

1. New information on the health–relevant food properties of specific foods from new tests of nutritional efficacy.
2. More comprehensive data sets to supplement food composition tables with data that better reflects health effects of foods.
3. Forms of data that are meaningful, for use in healthier food selection at point of sale.
4. Education to help give meaning to nutritional information for healthier food choices.

The need for new tests and biomarkers to assess nutritional functionality is well recognised,[88] and detailed attention has been given to characteristics required of tests for them to be valid predictors of food effects on health end-points.[38] Such discussions will give impetus to further work required to identify valid biomarkers and other measures for predicting effects of food components and properties on health.

The properties of individual processed foods have been the focus of this chapter, but at a higher level of complexity, interactions between foods in meals, and the place of foods in dietary patterns will be important determinants of health. Even when the efficacy of a food has been well established, its role in the diet, and the ways that other foods may modulate its effectiveness will need to be clarified.

Many of the properties of foods that are beneficial to health are characteristic of unprocessed or 'whole' foods, and there is a movement to exploit the benefits of natural structure, as seen in the recent promotion of whole grains.[89,90] The same tests that are used to monitor nutritional effects of food processing in formulated products will be valuable in identifying processes that preserve the intrinsic value of natural foods.

7.9 Sources of further information and advice

The need for new approaches to providing nutritional information has arisen from the recent interest in functional foods. Recent reviews focusing on tests of food function and biomarkers include entire issues of the *British Journal of Nutrition*,[91,92] and the *American Journal of Clinical Nutrition*,[93] and a book devoted to the subject.[94]

7.10 References

1 HENRY C J K and HEPPELL N J (1998), *Nutritional aspects of food processing and ingredients*, London, Aspen
2 ELIASSON A C and GUDMUNDSSON M (1996), 'Starch: physicochemical and functional aspects', in Eliasson, A C (ed), *Carbohydrates in Food*, New York, Marcel Dekker, 431–503
3 FRIEDMAN M (1992), 'Dietary impact of food processing', *Ann Rev Nutr* **12**, 119–37
4 WAHLQVIST M (1997), 'Vitamins and vitamin-like compounds', in Wahlqvist M L (ed), *Food and Nutrition*, NSW Australia, Allen & Unwin, 222–48
5 POUTANEN K (2001), 'Effect of processing on the properties of dietary fibre', in McLeary B V and Prosky L (eds), *Advanced dietary fibre technology*, Oxford, Blackwell Science, 277–82
6 BJÖRK I (1996), 'Starch: Nutritional aspects', in Eliasson A C (ed), *Carbohydrates in Food*, New York, Marcel Dekker, 505–53
7 HEATON K W, MARCUS S N, EMMETT P M and BOLTON C H (1988), 'Particle size of wheat, maize, and oat test meals: effects on plasma glucose and insulin responses and on the rate of starch digestion *in vitro*', *Am J Clin Nutr* **47**, 675–82
8 CAMIRE M E, CAMIRE A and KRUMHAR K (1990), 'Chemical and nutritional changes in foods during extrusion', *Crit Rev Food Sci Nutr* **29**, 35–57
9 GRANFELDT Y, HAGANDER B and BJÖRK I (1995), 'Metabolic responses to starch in oat

and wheat products. On the importance of food structure, incomplete gelatinisation or presence of viscous dietary fibre', *Eur J Clin Nutr* **49**, 189–99

10 MILNER J A (1999), 'Biomarkers for evaluating benefits of functional foods' *Nutr Today* **34**, 146–9

11 WEBER P (2001), 'Role of biomarkers in nutritional science and industry – a comment' *Br J Nutr* **86**, S93–S95

12 MONRO J A (1993), 'A nutritionally valid procedure for measuring soluble dietary fibre', *Food Chem* **47**, 187–93

13 LAIRON D (2001), 'Dietary fibres and dietary lipids', in McLeary B V and Prosky L (eds), *Advanced dietary fibre technology*, Oxford, Blackwell Science, 177–85

14 PARIZA M W (1999), 'Functional foods: technology, functionality, and health benefits', *Nutr Today* **34**, 150–1

15 MONRO J (2000), 'Evidence-based food choice: the need for new measures of food effects', *Trends Food Sci Tech*, **11**, 136–44

16 FREWER L J, HOWARD C, HEDDERLY D and SHEPHERD R (1996), 'What determines trust in information about food-related risks? Underlying psychological constructs', *Risk Anal* **16**, 473–86

17 PHILLIPS R D and FINLEY J W (1989), '*Protein quality and the effects of processing*', New York and Basel, Marcel Dekker

18 MONRO J A, LEE J and SINCLAIR B R (1992), 'Bile acid activity in the presence of dietary fibres, casein, calcium, phospholipid, fatty acid and cholesterol: factorial experiments *in vitro*'. *Food Chem* **44**, 325–9

19 CREWS H, ALINK G, ANDERSON R, BRAESCO V, HOLST B, MAIANI G, SCOTTER M, SOLFRIZZO M, VAN DEN BERG R, VERHAGEN H and WILLIAMSON G (2001), 'A critical assessment of some biomarker approaches linked with dietary intake', *Br J Nutr* **86**, S5–S35

20 GRUSAK M A, DELLAPENNA D and WELCH R M (1999), 'Physiologic processes affecting the content and distribution of phytonutrients in plants' *Nutr Rev* **57**, S27–S33

21 OLSON J A (1996), 'Vitamin A', in Ziegler E E and Filer L J (eds), *Present Knowledge in Nutrition, 7 ed.*, Washington, ILSI Press, 109–19

22 BAUM C L and BROWN M (2000), 'Low-fat, high-carbohydrate diets and atherogenic risk', *Nutr Rev*, **58**(5), 148–51

23 GIBSON R S (1990), *Principles of Nutritional Assessment*, Oxford, UK, Oxford University Press

24 LICHON M (1996), 'Sample preparation', in Nollet L (ed), *Handbook of Food Analysis*, New York, Marcel Dekker, 1–19

25 PROSKY L, ASP N-G, SCHWEIZER T F, DEVRIES J W and FURDA I (1992), 'Determination of soluble dietary fibre in food products: collaborative study', *J AOAC Int*, **77**, 690–4

26 MONRO J A (1991), 'Dietary fibre pectic substances: source of discrepancy between methods of fibre analysis', *J Food Comp Anal* **4**, 88–99

27 KAHLON T S (2001), 'Cholesterol-lowering properties of cereal fibres and fractions', in McLeary B V and Prosky L (eds), *Advanced dietary fibre technology*, Oxford, Blackwell Science, 206–20

28 HORTON E S and NAPOLI R (1996), 'Diabetes mellitus', in Ziegler E E and Filer L J (eds), *Present Knowledge in Nutrition, 7 ed.*, Washington DC, ILSI Press, 445–55

29 YIP R and DALLMAN P R (1996), 'Iron', in Ziegler E E and Filer L J (eds), *Present Knowledge in Nutrition, 7 ed.*, Washington DC, ILSI Press, 277–92

30 LEVINE M, RUMSEY S, WANG Y, PARK J, KWON O, XU W and AMANO N (1996), 'Vitamin C', in Ziegler E E and Filer L J (eds), *Present Knowledge in Nutrition, 7 ed.*, Washington DC, ILSI Press, 146–59

31 MORRIS ER (1992), 'Physico-chemical properties of food polysaccharides', in Schweizer T F and Edwards C A (eds), *Dietary Fibre – A Component of Food: Nutritional Function in Health and Disease*, London, UK, Springer-Verlag, 41–56

32 JENKINS D J A, SPADAFORA P J, JENKINS A L and RAINEY-MACDONALD C G (1993), 'Fiber

in the treatment of hyperlipidaemia', in Spiller G A (ed), *CRC Handbook of Dietary Fiber in Human Nutrition 2 ed.*, Boca Raton, CRC Press, 419–38
33 EDWARDS C A and PARRET A M (1996), 'Plant cell wall polysaccharides, gums, and hydrocolloids: Nutritional aspects', in Eliasson A-C (ed), *Carbohydrates in Food*, New York, Marcel Dekker, 319–45
34 MONRO J A (2000), 'Faecal bulking index: a physiological basis for dietary management of bulk in the distal colon', *Asia Pac J Clin Nutr*, **9**, 74–81
35 ELLIS P R, RAYMENT P and QI W (1996), 'A physico-chemical perspective of plant polysaccharides in relation to glucose absorption, insulin secretion and the entero-insular axis', *Proc Nut Soc*, **55**, 881–98
36 GRANFELDT Y, BJÖRK I and HAGANDER B (1991), 'On the importance of processing conditions, product thickness and egg addition for the glycaemic and hormonal responses to pasta: a comparison with bread made from 'pasta ingredients', *Eur J Clin Nutr* **45**, 489–99
37 GRANFELDT Y, ELIASSON A-C and BJÖRK I (2000), 'An examination of the possibility of lowering the glycaemic index of oat and barley flakes by minimal processing', *J Nutr* **130**, 2207–14
38 ILSI EUROPE (1999), 'Scientific concepts of functional foods in Europe consensus document', *Br J Nutr* **81**, S1–S27
39 LICHTENSTEIN A H (1996), 'Atherosclerosis', in Ziegler E E and Filer L J (eds), *Present Knowledge in Nutrition, 7 ed.*, Washington DC, ILSI Press, 430–7
40 BRANCA F, HANLEY A B, POOL-ZOBEL B and VERHAGEN H (2001), 'Biomarkers in disease and health', *Br J Nutr* **85**, S55–S92
41 KRITCHEVSKY D (2000), 'Overview: dietary fat and atherosclerosis', *Asia Pac J Clin Nutr* **9**, 141–5
42 MONRO J A (2001), 'Wheat bran equivalents based on faecal bulking indices for dietary management of faecal bulk', *Asia Pac J Clin Nutr* **10**, 242–8
43 JENKINS D J, WOLEVER T M S, TAYLOR R H, BARKER H, FIELDEN H, BALDWIN J M, BOWLING A C, NEWMAN H C, JENKINS A L and GOFF D V (1981), 'Glycaemic index of foods: a physiological basis for carbohydrate exchange', *Amer J Clin Nutr*, **34**, 362–6
44 MONRO J A and WILLIAMS M (2000), 'Concurrent management of postprandial glycaemia and nutrient intake using glycaemic glucose equivalents, food composition, and computer-assisted meal design', *Asia Pac J Clin Nut* **9**, 67–73
45 JENKINS D J A, GHAFARI H, WOLEVER T M S, TAYLOR R H, BARKER H M, FIELDER H, JENKINS A L and BOWLING A C (1982), 'Relationship between the rate of digestion of foods and post-prandial glycaemia', *Diabetologia* **22**, 450–5
46 CHEN H-L, HAACK V S, JANECKY C W, VOLLENDORF N W and MARLETT J A (1998), 'Mechanisms by which wheat bran and oat bran increase stool weight in humans', *Amer J Clin Nutr* **68**, 711–19
47 WHISTLER R L and BEMILLER J N (1997), *Carbohydrate Chemistry for Food Scientists*, Minnesota, USA, Eagen Press,
48 ASTRUP A and RABEN A (1996), 'Mono- and disaccharides: nutritional aspects', in Eliasson, A-C (ed), *Carbohydrates in Food*, New York, Marcel Dekker, 159–89
49 DE FRONZO R A and FERRANNINI E (1991), 'Insulin resistance: a multifaceted syndrome responsible for NIDDM, obesity, hypertension, dyslipidemia, and atherosclerotic cardiovascular disease, *Diabet Care*, **14**, 173–94
50 LIU S (1998), 'Insulin resistance, hyperglycaemia and risk of major chronic diseases – a dietary perspective', *Proc Nutr Soc Aust* **22**, 140–50
51 SZEPESI B (1996),'Carbohydrates', in Ziegler E E and Filer L J (eds), *Present Knowledge in Nutrition, 7 ed.*, Washington DC, ILSI Press, 33–43
52 ATKINSON M and MACLAUREN N (1994), 'The pathogenesis of insulin dependent diabetes mellitus', *New Eng J Med*, **xx: 331**, 1428–38

53 GUYTON A C (1991), *Textbook of Medical Physiology*, Philadelphia, PA, W B Saunders
54 FOSTER-POWELL K and BRAND-MILLER J (1995), 'International tables of glycaemic index', *Amer J Clin Nut* **62**, 871S–893S
55 WOLEVER M S and BRAND MILLER J (1995), 'Sugars and blood glucose control', *Amer J Clin Nutr*, **62**, 212S–227S
56 BRAND MILLER J, FOSTER-POWELL K, COLAGIURI S and LEEDS A (1996), *The G.I. Factor*, Rydalmere, Australia: Hodder Headline Australia Pty
57 MONRO J A (1997), 'Glycaemic index and available carbohydrates in exchanges of New Zealand foods', *Proc Nutr Soc NZ* **22**, 241–8
58 MONRO J A (1999), 'Available carbohydrate data and glycaemic index combined in new data sets for managing glycaemia and diabetes', *J Food Comp Anal* **12**, 71–82
59 LIU S, WILLETT W C, STAMPFER M J, HU F B, FRANZ M, SAMPSON L, HENNEKENS C H and MANSON J E (2000), 'A prospective study of dietary glycemic load, carbohydrate intake, and risk of coronary heart disease in US women', *Amer J Clin Nutr* **71**, 1455–61
60 LAUBER R P and SHEARD N F (2001), 'The American Heart Association dietary guidelines for 2000; a summary report', *Nutr Rev* **59**, 298–306
61 LIU P W W, PERRY T and MONRO J A (2001), 'Validation of glycaemic glucose equivalents in the dietary management of diabetes mellitus', Proc NZ Dietetic Assoc Ann Conf, Christchurch, 5–7 Sept. *J NZ Dietetic Assoc* (in press)
62 WOLEVER T M S and BOLOGNESI C (1996), 'Source and amount of carbohydrate affect postprandial glucose and insulin in normal subjects', *J Nutr* **126**, 2798–806
63 COLAGIURI S, BRAND J C, MILLER J C, SWAN V, COLAGIURI M and PETOCZ P (1997), 'Glycaemic equivalents: exchanges based on both the glycaemic index and carbohydrate content', *Proc Nutr Soc Aust* **21**, 137
64 GIACCO R, BRIGHENTI F, PARILLO M, CAPUANO M, CIARDULLO A V, RIVIECCIO A, RIVELLESE A A and RICCARDI G (2001), 'Characteristics of some wheat-based foods of the Italian diet in relation to their influence on postprandial glucose metabolism in patients with type 2 diabetes', *Br J Nutr* **85**, 33–40
65 GÕNI I, GARCIA-ALONSO A and SAURA-CALIXTO F (1997), 'A starch hydrolysis procedure to estimate glycaemic index', *Nutr Res* **17**, 427–37
66 ENGLYST K N, ENGLYST H N, HUDSON G H, COLE T J and CUMMINGS J H (1999), 'Rapidly available glucose in foods: an *in vitro* measurement that reflects the glycaemic response', *Am J Clin Nutr* **69**, 449–54
67 ONIANG'O R K (1998), 'Fibre: implications for the consumer', *Nut Res* **18**, 661–9
68 CUMMINGS J H (1993), 'The effect of dietary fibre on faecal weight and composition', in Spiller G A (ed), *CRC Handbook of Dietary Fibre in Human Nutrition*, Boca Raton, CRC Press, 263–349
69 EASTWOOD M (1993), 'Diet, fibre and colorectal disease: a critical appraisal', in Philips S F, Pemberton J H, and Shorter R G (eds), *The Large Intestine: Physiology, Pathophysiology, and Disease*, New York, Raven Press, 209–22
70 HA M-A, JARVIS M C and MANN J I (2000), 'A definition of dietary fibre', *Eur J Clin Nutr* **54**, 861–4
71 GALLAHER D D and SCHNEEMAN B O (1996), 'Dietary fiber', in Ziegler E E and Filer L J (eds), *Present Knowledge in Nutrition, 7 ed.*, Washington DC, ILSI Press, 87–97
72 SCHNEEMAN B O (1998), 'Dietary fibre and gastrointestinal function' *Nutr Res* **18**, 625–32
73 YOUNG G P, CHAI F and ZALEWSKI P (1999), 'Polysaccharide fermentation, butyrate and apoptosis in the colonic epithelium', *Asia Pac J Clin Nutr* **8**, S27–S31
74 BIRKETT A, MUIR J, PHILLIPS J, JONES G and O'DEA K (1996), 'Resistant starch lowers fecal concentrations of ammonia and phenols in humans', *Amer J Clin Nutr* **63**, 766–72
75 TOPPING D and BIRD A R (1999), 'Foods, nutrients and digestive health', *Aust J Nutr Dietet* **56**, S22–S34
76 TROWELL H C (1974), 'Definition of dietary fibre', *Lancet* **I** 503

77 MONRO J A (1996), 'Dietary fibre' in Nollet L M L (ed), *Handbook of Food Analysis*, New York, Marcel Dekker, 1051–88
78 PROSKY L (2001), 'What is dietary fibre? A new look at the definition', in McLeary B V and Prosky L (eds), *Advanced dietary fibre technology*, Oxford, Blackwell Science, 63–76
79 Panel on the Definition of Dietary Fibre, Standing Committee on the Scientific Evaluation of Dietary Reference Intakes, Food and Nutrition Board, Institute of Medicine (2001), 'Proposed definition of dietary fiber', *Nutr Today*, **36**, 190
80 CUMMINGS J H, BINGHAM S A, HEATON K W and EASTWOOD M A (1992), 'Fecal weight, colon cancer risk, and dietary intake of nonstarch polysaccharides (dietary fibre)', *Gastroenterol* **103**, 1783–9
81 EDWARDS C A, ADIOTOMRE J and EASTWOOD M A (1992), 'Dietary fibre: the use of *in vitro* and rat models to predict action on stool output in man', *J Sci Food Agric* **59**, 257–60
82 MONRO J A (2002), 'The faecal bulking efficacy of Australasian breakfast cereals', *Asia Pac J Clin Nutr* (in press)
83 MCBURNEY M I and VANSOEST P J (1991), 'Structure-function relationships: lessons from other species', in Phillips S F, Pemberton J H, Shorter R G (eds), *The large intestine: physiology, pathophysiology, and disease*, New York, Raven Press, 37–49
84 MONRO J A (2002), 'Dietary fibre content and nutrient claims relative to the faecal bulking efficacy of breakfast cereals', *Asia Pac J Clin Nutr* (in press)
85 BIRKETT A M, JONES G P, DE SILVA A M, YOUNG G P and MUIR J G (1997), 'Dietary intake and faecal excretion of carbohydrate by Australians: importance of achieving stool weights greater than 150g to improve faecal markers relevant to colon cancer risk', *Eur J Clin Nutr* **51**, 625–32
86 REA P (2001), 'Functional foods report 2001', *Nutr Bus J*, Jan
87 SLOAN A E (2001), '"Do-it-yourself" health' *Funct Foods* **3**(16), 10–11
88 WEBER P (2001), 'Role of biomarkers in nutritional science and industry – a comment', *Br J Nutr* **86**, S93–S95
89 JACOBS D, PEREIRA M, SLAVIN J and MARQUART L (2000), 'Defining the impact of whole grain intake on chronic disease', *Cereal Fd World* **45**, 51–3
90 RICHARDSON D P (2000), 'The grain, the wholegrain and nothing but the grain: the science behind wholegrain and the reduced risk of heart disease and cancer', *Nutr Bull* **25**, 353–60
91 BELLISLE F, DIPLOCK A T, HORNSTRA G, KOLETZKO B, ROBERFROID M, SALMINEN S and SARIS W H M (eds) (1998), 'Functional food science in Europe', *Br J Nutr* **80** Supplement S1–S193
92 CREWS H M, HANLEY A B, VERHAGEN H and WILD C (eds) (2001), 'Biomarkers of exposure and effect in relation to life and human risk assessment', *Br J Nutr* **86** Supplement S1–S127
93 HARPER A E (ed.) (2000), 'Physiologically active food components: Their role in optimising health and ageing' *Amer J Clin Nutr* **71**, 1653S–1743S
94 GIBSON G R and WILLIAMS C M (eds.) (2001), '*Functional foods: concept to product*' Cambridge, UK, Woodhead
95 WAHLQVIST M, HSU-HAGE B H-H and LUKITO W (1999), 'Clinical trials in nutrition' *Asia Pac J Clin Nutr* **8**, 231–41

Part 2

Processing and nutritional quality

8

The nutritional enhancement of plant foods

D. Lindsay, CEBAS-CSIC, Spain

8.1 Introduction

The question of why it is necessary to improve the nutritional value of plant foods is one that at first hand might seem difficult to justify. What evidence is there that this is a problem? In the developed world there are no overt signs of malnutrition even amongst strict vegans. The reasons for this are that many processed plant foods are fortified with essential nutrients. Fortification is utilised to replace nutrients lost in the heat processing of foods and through oxidation. Few vegetarians are dependent on a single plant source to provide their basic nutritional needs. In addition, vegetarians frequently consume vitamins as supplements and the growth in this industry has been rapid. The fact that people are resorting to the consumption of vitamins as supplements is a reflection of their belief that more of a good thing will result in an improvement in their health. This is a very dubious argument. Nonetheless, it is important to recognise that the recommended intakes of nutrients, that have been determined by expert groups of nutritionists, are based on the evidence that a specific intake level for a nutrient is required to ensure healthy growth and development. They do not reflect the growing body of evidence that suggests different, and often higher, intakes of these same nutrients are required to optimise health and lead to an active life through the prevention of chronic degenerative diseases associated with ageing.[1,2,3] The critical issue is to determine what intakes are required to optimise health rather than to compromise it.

8.2 The nutritional importance of plants

Plants are the staple food for the vast majority of the world's population. It is known that many staple plant foods are deficient in essential nutrients and, consequently, malnutrition is widespread. It has been estimated that over 100 million children worldwide are vitamin A deficient and improving the vitamin A content of their food could prevent as many as two million deaths annually in young children.[4] This is apart from the deficiencies in iodine intake, resulting in goitre, and in iron-deficient anaemia which are estimated to affect millions in the developing world. There is also an important need to improve the amino acid content of legume proteins that are deficient in essential sulphur amino acids. Nutritional deficiencies can lead to a reduction in immune responsiveness, rather than a specific attributable disorder, making it difficult to establish clearly how many people are suffering from malnutrition.[5]

In the developed world all public health authorities are urging consumers to consume more plant-based foods as part of a healthy diet. There is a significant body of evidence to suggest that the traditional Mediterranean diet, rich in plant foods, reduces the risk of many age-related diseases. Epidemiological studies show a strong and consistent inverse relationship between fruit and vegetable intake and the risk of cardiovascular diseases and some cancers.[2] An explosion of interest in trying to define what are the factors in fruit and vegetables which might be responsible for these observations has not yet led to a clear set of explanations although many theories abound.

Plants contain 17 mineral nutrients, 13 vitamins and numerous phytochemicals that have been shown to have potentially beneficial effects on health especially against the initiation or progression of degenerative diseases. Almost all human nutrients can be obtained from plant foods, the exceptions are vitamins B_{12} and D. However, the adequacy of a plant diet in delivering a health benefit from a specific component will depend on the amount ingested and its bioavailability. Many beneficial plant compounds that are associated with the plant cell wall are not easily bioavailable. Any way in which overall levels can be increased will help overcome this difficulty.

8.3 Strategies for nutritional enhancement

There is no single approach to the improvement of the nutritional quality of plant foods since this is affected by a wide variety of factors. Amongst these are:

- The application of traditional breeding methods to select for varieties with an increased level of the bioactive compound.
- A reduction in the content of antinutritional factors.
- The use of genetic manipulation to introduce new traits in plants.
- Improvements in handling, storage and food processing technologies.

Each of these approaches has a role to play but genetic manipulation provides a mechanism for the improvement of nutritional quality that overcomes the problem of the absence of a specific biochemical pathway in a staple crop.

8.3.1 Application of 'traditional' breeding methods

Plant varieties have not been selected to date on the basis of nutritional qualities but there are wide natural variations that can be found in the gene pool of crop plants. Examples of where significant variations in the nutrient content of genotypes have been documented include a:

- 2-fold variation in calcium concentration in beans.[6]
- 4-fold variation in β-carotene concentrations in broccoli.[7]
- 4-fold variation in folates in beetroot.[8]
- 2–3-fold variation in iron and zinc levels in maize.[9]

In the case of the pro-vitamin A carotenoids, plants provide highly variable amounts depending on their colour. Varieties of sweet potato may contain levels varying from 0.13 mg to 11.3 mg g^{-1} dry weight β-carotene.[10] Similar variations in levels can be found in carrots and cassava. In the case of the tomato, genes have been identified that are associated with high and low lycopene content. Incorporation of genes that increase lycopene content and/or elimination of genes that decrease the lycopene content can be achieved by pedigree selection and backcross programmes. Such techniques have produced hybrids with a three- or four-fold increase in content of lycopene in tomato fruits.[11]

8.3.2 Reduction in antinutritional factors

The interest in reducing antinutritional factors in plants has been predominantly focused around improving the nutritional value of feedstuffs. Phytates are present in many plant seeds and limit phosphorus uptake as well as other elements. The potential for introducing a phytase gene into feedstuffs has been explored.[12] However, there are other strategies that seem to be of greater overall value in human nutrition. Thioredoxin is thought to be an activator of the germination process in seeds.[13] It is able to activate proteins to degradation by proteolysis and results in improved digestibility.[14] It also has the potential advantage of being able to reduce allergenicity, presumably because of its capacity to break disulphide bonds by the action of the reduced thiol groups in the molecule and ensure the tertiary structure of the protein is accessible to degradation by proteases.[14] The insertion of the wheat thioredoxin gene into barley has produced a transgenic plant where thioredoxin accounts for 7% of the total protein content in the barley and is a good source of sulphur amino acids.[15]

8.3.3 The application of genetic manipulation

Genetic engineering is being applied to enhance levels of functional compounds in food crops. Indeed, for some purposes it will be the only approach feasible especially where there are widespread deficiency diseases and the population is dependent on staple crops which are not sources of the nutrient required. There are many examples where the technology has been applied with success although there are no products which have yet reached the marketing stage where nutritional benefits have been the main focus.

Potential strategies for the enhancement of specific metabolites could target on:

1. Over-expression of enzymes that control the final steps in the biosynthesis of a metabolite.
2. Over-expression of rate-limiting enzymes.
3. Silencing of genes whose expression causes the metabolite to be degraded.
4. Increased expression of genes that are not subject to metabolic feedback control.
5. Increasing the number of plastids in a plant.
6. Increasing metabolic flux into the pathway of interest.
7. Expression in storage organs using site-specific promoters.

The strategy that has had the greatest success at present is the first one, especially in conjunction with the last strategy. In practice, if a substantial increase in the concentration of a metabolite is required, the use of specific promoters directing the synthesis to a particular organelle normally used for storage purposes, or where the plant normally synthesises the metabolite, is essential. Failure to use these approaches could cause toxicity in the plant by interfering with the production or function of other essential metabolites. However, this strategy presupposes the metabolite of interest is the final one in a particular pathway.

Few strategies have yet been applied where multiple gene insertions are necessary to produce the metabolite, although these are progressing rapidly, and none where plastid numbers have been increased. However, the accumulation of sequence data of both chromosomal DNA and expressed sequence tags of plants and other species is providing rapid advances in knowledge of the genetic make-up and functions of several plants, and it is expected that these other possibilities will soon be feasible.

8.4 The priorities for nutritional enhancement

8.4.1 For the developed world

Although it is known that the distribution and processing of food can lead to a significant loss in nutritional quality, there are few instances where present evidence suggests there is a need to change current practices. There is very little evidence for nutritional deficiencies. In those cases where public health authorities have thought there is a potential problem, food supplementation with nutrients is a commonly adopted policy. The use of nutritional supplements is widespread. Whilst the focus of current interest is on the need to consider nutrients and other phytochemicals as protective against the development of disease in later life, the levels of intake that may be necessary to optimise protection are far from resolved at the present time.

The only plant-derived food product on the market where nutritional health benefits are claimed (as opposed to implied) is the enrichment of margarines with plant sterol and stanol esters for the reduction in plasma cholesterol levels (Fig.

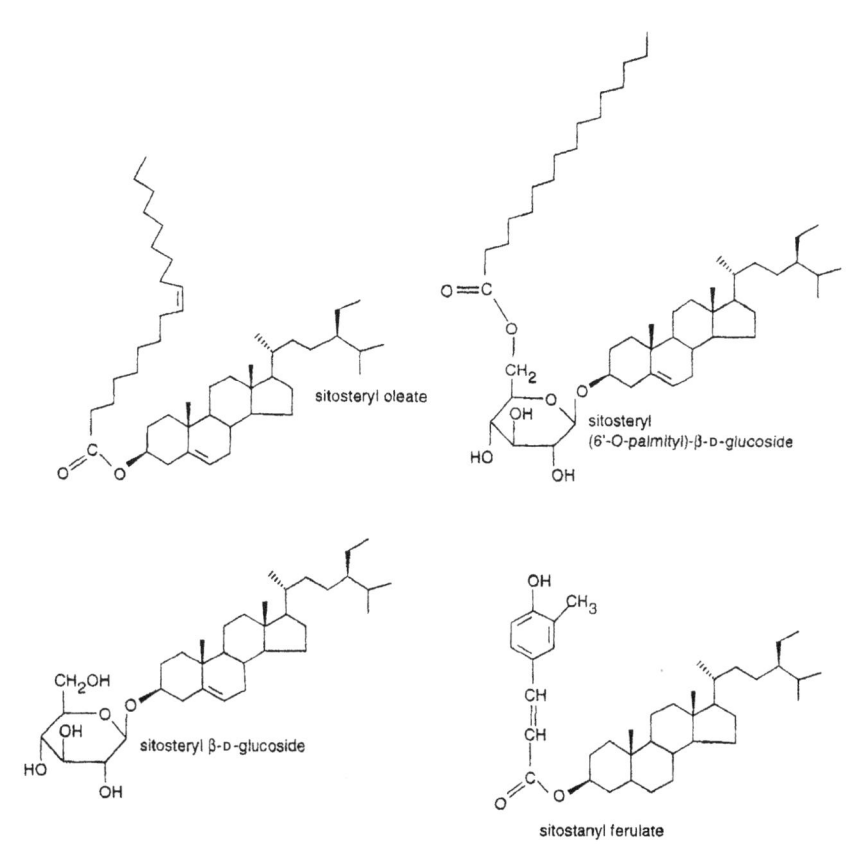

Fig. 8.1 Structure of plant sterol and stanol esters.

8.1) These products do not require the development of specifically bred plants since it is possible to extract stanols and sterols from existing plants (albeit in the case of the stanols from the bark of a tree) for use in their manufacture.

Experiments with plant stanol esters were shown to lower serum cholesterol consistently by about 10–15% and LDL-cholesterol by about 20% in patients with high serum cholesterol levels as well as in normal individuals.[16, 17] Similar effects have been seen with plant sterol esters but at least 1 g/day of plant sterols need to be consumed.[18] Consequently, they require extraction and addition to foods.

Plant sterols can be in the free form or predominantly esterified with long chain fatty acids or with phenolic acids as in rice-bran oil (ferulate) and shea butter (cinnamates). Sterol esters are better absorbed than the free sterols and most sterol esters are hydrolysed to the free sterols in the intestine.

As campesterol esters are better absorbed than sitosterol esters, serum levels of campesterol could rise to those levels that are found in the very few people who suffer toxic symptoms from phytosterolemia. Thus there may be a benefit in increasing the sitosterol to campesterol ratio in plants.

The ideal situation would be for sufficient sterols to be present in our diets to ensure that plasma cholesterol levels are kept reasonably low without the need to buy a specific functional food, and that they would be in a fat-soluble form for effective uptake. The evidence favours, in increasing order of preference, the use of:

1. Plant sterol esters with low campesterol contents.
2. Sterol esters from tall oil (derived from pine wood) which have a higher stanol content than edible oils.
3. Plant stanol esters.

A vegetable oil rich in plant stanols, especially in sitostanol esterified with polyunsaturated fatty acids, would also have the benefit of being less susceptible to oxidation at frying temperatures than the sterols. The potential health benefits of this class of bioactive compounds are unlikely to be met by the use of classical plant breeding methods but genetic engineering could make these targets feasible.

8.4.2 For the developing world

The world-wide deficiency of vitamin A is being tackled both through conventional plant breeding and by genetic manipulation. However, the use of conventional plant breeding to deliver adequate intakes is dependent on the availability of carotenoid-rich staple foods. Often these are available for very restricted times of the year in some societies. In those countries where rice is a dietary staple the problem is particularly severe and the deficiency is likely to be corrected only by the introduction of rice that has been genetically manipulated to produce β-carotene. However, yellow rice is produced and this may give rise to problems of acceptability to consumers used to white rice.

Manipulation of the carotenoid pathway in rice
The nature of the challenges faced in manipulating plant secondary metabolites is well illustrated through the attempts that have been made to produce carotenoids in rice plants. A simplified version of the pathways leading to the synthesis of the carotenoids principally found in food plants is shown in Figure 8.2.

Immature rice endosperm is capable of synthesising the early pathway intermediate geranylgeranyl diphosphate (GP). Four plant genes corresponding to the enzymes phytoene synthase (psy) (1), phytoene desaturase (2), zeta carotene desaturase (3) and lycopene cyclase (crt) (4) are required. Enzyme (1) was obtained from the daffodil (*narcissus pseudonarcissus*), (2) from a bacterium *Erwinia uredovora* – which is capable of achieving steps (2) and (3) from the single enzyme, and (4) from the daffodil.

The genes need to be expressed in a tissue-specific manner through the insertion of specific promoters. This has been achieved in rice through the use of the daffodil psy gene.[19] In rice the daffodil psy cDNA insertion is under the control

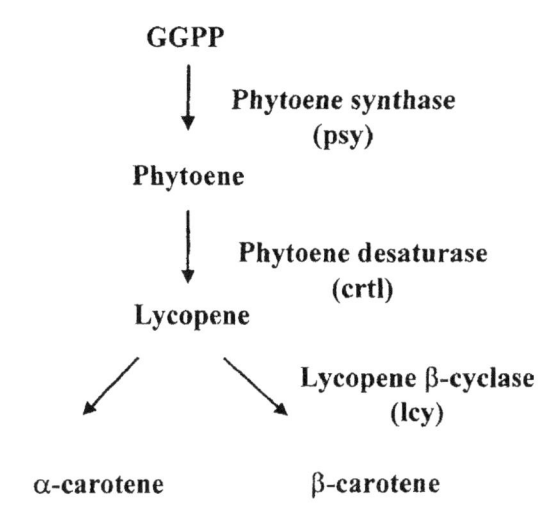

```
        GGPP
          │    Phytoene synthase
          ▼         (psy)
        Phytoene
          │    Phytoene desaturase
          ▼         (crtl)
        Lycopene
         ╱   ╲    Lycopene β-cyclase
        ╱     ╲         (lcy)
   α-carotene   β-carotene
```

Fig. 8.2 The carotenoid biosynthetic pathway (simplified).

of an endosperm-specific promoter. The choice of promoter will very much affect the timing and tissue-specific expression of a gene.

Surprisingly, seeds that expressed psy and crt did not accumulate lycopene. Instead they contained β-carotene and other xanthophylls. Thus it would seem that the enzymes required to make these metabolites are either normally expressed in rice endosperm or are induced if lycopene is formed. The maximum level of carotenoids in the endosperm of plants that were heterozygous for the transgenes was $1.6\,mg\,kg^{-1}$ which is likely to help to meet the nutritional needs of people consuming rice as a staple. Interestingly, good progress is being made in adding a gene coding for ferritin – the iron storage protein found in mammals and plants – to rice.[20] It is likely that this would, in addition, help improve the iron deficiency also seen in these communities if it is shown to be bioavailable.

The controversy over the use of advanced technologies for producing sustainable food in the developing world has been addressed by the developers of modified rice. They have in effect waived all intellectual property rights for exploitation of the technologies in the developing world and are actively involved in assisting the International Rice Research Institute to breed stable and agronomically successful lines for use in vitamin A-deficient areas.

8.5 Relationship of structure to nutritional quality (bioavailability)

The overall content of a given nutrient in a food is not always a useful indicator of its nutritional value because not all of the nutrient present is absorbed. Nutritionists must concern themselves with understanding the proportion of an available nutrient that is digested, absorbed, and ultimately utilised. In the case of nutrients or phytochemicals, whose beneficial effects are directed towards inhibiting degenerative diseases, it is important to know whether or not the nutrient is reaching the particular target organ and in a form which is active. Otherwise the claims for the health benefits of that chemical would not be justified, especially as it is difficult to demonstrate benefits from long-term human studies.

Diet plays an important role in the uptake of specific nutrients and phytochemicals. Those that are lipophilic are absorbed much more readily from a lipid-rich diet. Frying tomatoes in oil dramatically improves the uptake of lycopene compared with the consumption of fresh tomatoes.[21] Raw carrots, which have high levels of pro-vitamin A carotenoids, are poorer sources of β-carotene than gently cooked carrot.[22] The bioavailability of certain trace elements is increased on cooking or processing; for example, the bioavailability of iron is increased in canned spinach.[23]

The chemical form of the phytochemical present in food is very important in determining uptake through the gastro-intestinal tract. Quercitin-β-glucoside is more easily absorbed than the aglycone quercitin. Isorhamnetin-β-glucoside, which is chemically similar to quercitin, differing only by a single methoxyl group, is more readily absorbed. Flavonoid rutinosides (rhamnosyl 1–6 glucosides) are less easily absorbed.[24] Thus whilst some phenols might be better antioxidants than others when tested in *in vitro* systems, this is of little significance in terms of health relevance. What matters is whether the compounds are easily absorbed, are not quickly degraded in tissues, and are able to reach the target sites. Flavonoids that are not absorbed undergo extensive degradation by gut microorganisms, and may play only a limited role in preventing oxidative damage in the colon.

8.6 Nutritional enhancement versus food fortification

The importance of enhancing the levels of a natural protective constituent in plant foods is well illustrated in the case of the folates. There is a good chance that folate status even in affluent countries is not optimal.[25,26] The most important sources of folates in the diet are liver, products derived from yeast, eggs, green vegetables, legumes and certain fruits. Plant foods (vegetables, fruits and potatoes) are by far the single largest contributor to the overall folate intake of adults.[27,28,29] Some 40% of the total folate intake is from fruit and vegetable consumption in these countries even when the average consumption is not very high.

Folates have the effect of reducing the levels of plasma homocysteine which is a sensitive biomarker of folate status. A variety of studies have suggested that increased plasma homocysteine levels are a risk factor for cardiovascular disease and stroke.[30] Human studies have shown that if individuals consume a supplement of 100 g/day of folic acid their plasma homocysteine is reduced to a level of about 7.0 μM/l. Increasing the intake of folic acid beyond that level has no further effect. However, the bulk of the population have homocysteine levels in excess of 7.0 μM/l.

Folic acid is not the natural form of folate that is found in plants where natural folate consists of ten different polyglutamate complexes. Folic acid is, however, the form of folate that is used in the fortification of food as it is more stable. It is also found to be more bioavailable. Natural folates show only 50% or less of the bioavailability of folic acid.[31, 32]

There is good evidence that to achieve the ideal level of plasma homocysteine dietary levels of folate (as opposed to folic acid) would have to increase from the current average of 200 μg/day to 600 μg/day.[33] This increased intake is also likely to have an important impact on the reduction of Neural Tube Defects (NTDs). Women with a low folate status (about 150 μg/l red cell folate) have a 0.7% risk of NTDs in their offspring, whereas supplementation with folic acid at doses of between 100 and 200 g/day resulted in red blood cell folate levels that have been associated with an optimal reduction in NTD incidence. Since average intakes of natural folates are about 100 μg/day from the diet it would require at least 500 mg of natural folate to be consumed (preferably 600 mg/day) to ensure that the incidence of NTD in the population was kept to a minimum.

The fact that supplemental folic acid can achieve these same effects whilst being more stable and bioavailable would imply that there was little purpose in supplementing natural levels of folate. This ignores the intrinsic difference between the cellular metabolism of synthetic pro-vitamin folic acid compared to the natural folates. The mucosa converts all of the natural forms of folate into 5-methylenetetrahydrofolate monoglutamate. This reaction also occurs when folic acid is consumed but the difference is that for folic acid the process can be saturated at around 300 μg. Intakes in excess of this cause un-metabolised folic acid to enter the circulation.[34] The control of how much natural folate is taken up and retained by cells is regulated by the enzyme methionine synthase which acts on 5-methyltetrahydrofolate to conjugate it into a polyglutamate which is then retained in the cell. Folic acid does not pass through the methionine synthase pathway and can be conjugated directly, retained and metabolised.

If folic acid is present in excess of the mucosal capacity to metabolise it can bring about DNA biosynthesis in vitamin B_{12}-deficient cells in cases of pernicious anaemia via the DNA cycle. This causes a haematological response with the risk that the anaemic state is masked and the associated neuropathy is not avoided. Natural folates on the other hand will be poorly metabolised by vitamin B_{12}-deficient cells enabling the anaemia to be detected at an earlier stage. Another concern that has been raised against increasing population levels of folate is that the increased capacity to cause DNA biosynthesis could promote tumour growth. This would be expected to be more of a problem with folic acid than natural folates because of folic acid's less controlled uptake into cells.

8.7 Constraints on innovation

The potential to exploit fully GM technologies is severely limited by constraints on the use of the technology itself, as well as in satisfying the legislation that exists on the pre-market approval of foods that have been produced by the technology, or are in some way novel. These constraints are so severe in Europe that in very few cases will any producer see a return on their investment if nutritional improvement is their goal. This market is also affected by the widespread addition of specific nutrients as additives to certain processed foods. Enhancement of any component considered to be beneficial is likely to be of market value only if positive claims can be made. Whenever possible 'conventional' plant breeding will be used.

8.7.1 Genetic manipulation

There has been a *de facto* European Union moratorium on the approval of GMO products since October 1998. Eighteen products have already been approved under the general EU Directive (90/220/CEE) whilst 14 are pending approval. Five Member States have temporarily banned already approved GM products, which is permitted under the Directive. Two new EU labelling regulations have been drafted but have not been implemented because of a lack of testing methodologies, certifying labels and inspection procedures. The ultimate intention is to ensure that products can be labelled GM free to enable consumers to make an informed choice. It has been argued that products labelled as containing products derived from GM will convey negative messages to consumers. This is likely to be so in the absence of benefits that are clearly seen by consumers. This will occur if plants are used as factories for the production of vaccines and pharmaceutical products. However, it is unclear at present where these benefits will lie in the nutritional field other than for the developing world.

The lack of public confidence in the European food safety system is already causing harm to markets in the US and in developing nations where the technology is already embraced. This is likely to lead to major problems in international trade unless it is resolved.

8.7.2 Safety

No scientific development in food can ignore the very strict regulatory controls that exist before any new or 'novel' product or process can be applied in its production. Food plants produced by 'conventional' plant breeding techniques in general are not subject to any regulatory controls. In some countries voluntary codes of practice have been developed within the plant breeding sector when it was discovered that varieties of potatoes with good agronomic characteristics were found to contain high levels of toxic glycoalkaloids.[35]

At the present time, genetically-modified (GM) foods are regulated applying the concept of 'substantial equivalence'.[36] This concept is applied as the basis from which to determine the extent of the requirements for food safety assessment. If a genetically modified food can be characterised as substantially equivalent, it can be assumed to pose no new health risks over its conventional counterpart and can be marketed without the need to undertake extensive toxicological and nutritional studies to determine its safety-in-use.

The principle of substantial equivalence was adopted into the EU Regulation on Novel Foods and Novel Food Ingredients.[37] The Regulation excludes from its controls foods and food ingredients obtained through traditional propagating or breeding practices and which have a history of safe use. GM plants are considered as 'novel' under the terms of the Regulation. However, the detailed safety evaluation provisions of the Regulation do not apply to foods produced by genetic manipulation 'if on the basis of the scientific evidence available they are substantially equivalent to existing foods with regard to their composition, nutritional value, metabolism, intended use, and the level of undesirable substances present'. The Regulation regards food as 'novel' if the characteristics of the food differ from the conventional food regarding the accepted limits of natural variation of such characteristics. It is clear that most nutritionally enhanced plants would be caught under the definition of a 'novel' food.

The principle of substantial equivalence is vague and difficult to define in many cases. Consequently the whole issue of regulation of GM foods is under intensive debate. Meanwhile the EU has applied a *de facto* moratorium on GM plant introductions. The US attitude to regulation has so far been to regard safety as an issue that relates to the characteristic of the food and not to the process(es) that lead to it. Novel food products, of which products produced by GM are included in the definition, are not subject to any specific approval on safety ground if the constituents of the food are the same, or substantially similar, to substances currently found in other foods.

It is clear that it is never going to be possible to argue that a GM plant is safe any more than it is possible to argue that a plant produced by conventional plant breeding is safe. The very concept can be addressed only in the context of a history of safe use as a human food. Clearly, the overwhelming evidence supports the view that health benefits arise as a consequence of the regular consumption of a variety of fruits and vegetables, few if any of which have any close compositional relationship to the wild types from which they were bred. Similarly their production, storage and distribution has depended on the use of a wide range of chemical fertilisers and pesticides. These chemicals are extensively tested for safety before approval is given for their marketing and use but this has not removed the widely held view amongst consumers that 'organic products' are better for your health. There is no evidence to support this view and any adverse health effects that there might be as a consequence of the use of pesticides appear to be outweighed by the beneficial effects from the consumption of fruit and vegetables. What determines 'safety' is the overall effect of consumption over a period, not the effects of a specific chemical that might be present.

The issue of 'safety' in the context of the ability to market foods which are 'novel' is emotionally charged and without a solid scientific base. Consequently it is unlikely that any industry would want to take on these issues unless they had a product with a potentially large market.

8.8 Future trends

It is clear that the developing world will adopt whatever approach is technically feasible for them to meet the food and nutritional needs of their populations. Genetically modified crops will be used if there are clear benefits. In terms of resistance to disease and adaptation to harsh environments the technology has clear potential. Improvements in nutritional quality can be added to the list of benefits.

In Europe and other developed countries the impetus for improving the nutritional value of foods will occur only if there are clear health benefits in doing so. As there is growing evidence that nutritional needs will vary according to age and genetic susceptibility, it will be hard to convey a consistent message since intakes that benefit one sector of society might not benefit another. The priority is to demonstrate clearly what are the functional effects of nutrients, or beneficial phytochemicals, at the physiological level. The information is generally rudimentary. In those cases where the function is clearer the relationships between dose and effect are not known. When it comes to marketing foods that have been genetically manipulated the benefits will have to be very great indeed if current consumer resistance to their use is to be overcome.

8.9 Further information

Sources of further information about the potential for nutritional enhancement can be found in reviews by Willis, Lencki and Marangoni (1998),[38] Grusak and DellaPenna (1999),[39] Dixon et al., (1996),[40] Yamauchi and Minamikawa (1998).[41] An overview of the subject is contained in Lindsay, D. G. (2000) 'Maximising the functional benefits of plant foods', in: *Functional Foods*. Chapter 8, edited by Williams, C. M. and Gibson, G. R., Woodhead Publishing Ltd. Cambridge, England. pp. 183–208. ISBN 1 85573 503 2.

A account of the issues to be addressed in tackling the nutritional enhancement of plants (including increasing levels of bioactive secondary metabolites) can be found in published reviews commissioned under the EU's concerted action project 'The Nutritional Enhancement of Plant Foods in European Trade (NEODIET)', 2000, *J Sci Food & Agric*. **80**(7): 793–1137. Some of the issues raised in relation to the use of plant biotechnology in food and feed production are discussed in papers contained in a special edition of *Science* (Plant Biotechnology: Food & Feed, 1999, *Science* 285: 367–389).

8.10 References

1 BURING J E and SMITH C V (1997), Antioxidant vitamins and cardiovascular disease *Nutrn Rev*, **55**(1), S53–S58

2 STEINMETZ K A and POTTER J D (1996), Vegetables, fruit and cancer prevention: A review. *J Am Diet Assoc*, **96**, 1027–39
3 AIFR WORLD CANCER RESEARCH FUND (1997), *Food, Nutrition and the Prevention of Cancer – A Global Perspective*, Washington, DC
4 WORLD HEALTH ORGANISATION (1995), Global prevalence of vitamin A deficiencies' Micronutrient deficiency information systems, Working Paper No 2, Geneva, WHO
5 CALDER P C and JACKSON A A (2000), Undernutrition, infection and immune function, *Nutrn Res Rev*, **13**, 3–29
6 QUINTANA J M, HARRISON H C, NIENHUIS J, PALTA J P and GRUSAK M A (1996), Variation in calcium concentration among sixty S1 families and four cultivars of snap bean (*Phaseolus vulgaris* L.), *J. Amer Soc Hort Sci* **121**, 789–93
7 SCHONHOF I and KRUMBEIN A (1996), Gehalt an wertgebenden Inhaltstoffen verschiedener Brokkolitypen (*Brassica oleracea* var *italica* Plenck). *Gartenbauwissenschaft*, **61**, 281–88
8 WANG M and GOLDMAN I L (1996), Phenotypic variation in free folic acid content among F1 hybrids and open-pollenated cultivars of red beets, *J Am Soc Hortic Sci*, **121**, 1040–42
9 IFPRI (1999), International Food Policy Research Institute, *Agricultural strategies for micronutrients.* Http.//www.cgair.org/ifpri/themes/grp06.htm
10 SOLOMONS N W and BULUX J (1997), Identification of local carotene-rich foods to combat vitamin A malnutrition, *Eur J Clin Nutrn* **51**(Suppl.), S39–S45
11 AMITOM (1999) *Role and control of antioxidants in the tomato processing industry*. EU FAIR Project (FAIR CT97–3233). httpl/:www.tomate.org/Antioxidantnetwork.html
12 PEN J, VERWOERD T C, VAN PARIDON P A, BEUDEKER R F, VAN DEN ELZEN P J M, GEERSE K, VAN DER KILS J D, VERSTEEG H A J, VAN OOYEN A J J and HOEKEMA A (1993). Phytase-containing transgenic seeds as a novel feed additive for improved phosphorus utilisation, *Biotechnology*, **11**, 811–14
13 LOZANO R M, WONG J H, YEE B C, PETERS A, KOBREHEL K and BUCHANAN B B (1996) New evidence for a role for thioredoxin h in seedling development and germination, *Planta*, **200**(1), 100–106
14 BUCHANAN B B, ADAMIDI C, LOZANO R M, YEE B C, MOMMA M, KOBREHEL K, ERMEL R and FRICK O L (1997), Thioredoxin-linked mitigation of wheat allergies, *Proc Natln Acad Sci* USA **94**, 5372–77
15 BUCHANAN B B. Unpublished data
16 GYLLING H, RADHAKRISHNAN R and MIETTINEN T A (1997), Reduction of serum cholesterol in postmenopausal women with previous myocardial infarction and cholesterol malabsorption induced by dietary sitostanol ester margarine: women and dietary sitostanol, *Circulation*, **96**, 4226–31
17 GYLLING H and MIETTINEN T A (1999), Phytosterols, analytical and nutritional aspects, In, *Functional foods – a new challenge for the food chemist*. Eds Lasztity R, Pfannhauser V, Simon-Sarkadi L and Tômôskôzi S, Publishing Company of TUB, Budapest. *Proceedings of the Euro Food Chem X*. Vol. 1, 109
18 HENDRICKS H F J, WESTRATE J A, VAN VLIET T and MEIJER G W (1999), Spreads enriched with three different levels of vegetable oil sterols and the degree of cholesterol lowering in normocholesterolemic subjects, *Eur J Clin Nutrn*, **53**, 319–27
19 BURKHARDT P K, BEYER P, WUNN J, KLOTI A, ARMSTRONG G A, SCHLEDZ M, VONLINTIG J and POTRYKUS I (1997), Transgenic rice (*Oryza sativa*) endosperm expressing daffodil (*Narcissus pseudonarcissus*) phytoene synthase accumulates phytoene a key intermediate in pro-vitamin A synthesis, *Plant J*, **11**, 1071–78
20 SHINTANI D and DELLAPENNA D (1998), 'Elevating the vitamin E content of plants through metabolic engineering' *Science*, **282**, 2098–2100
21 GÄRTNER C, STAHL W and SIES H (1997), Increased lycopene bioavailability from tomato paste as compared to fresh tomatoes, *Am J Clin Nutrn*, **66**, 116–122
22 ROCK C L, LOVALVO J L, EMENHISER C, RUFFIN M T, FLATT S W and SCHWARTZ S J (1998),

Bioavailability of beta-carotene is lower in raw than in processed carrots and spinach in women, *J Nutr*, **128**(5), 913–16
23 LEE K and CLYDESDALE F M (1981), Effect of thermal processing on endogenous and added iron in canned spinach, *J Food Sci*, **46**, 1064–67
24 AZIZ A A, EDWARDS C A, LEAN M E J and CROZIER A (1998), Absorbtion and excretion of conjugated flavonols, including quercitin-4'-O-β-glucoside and isorhamnetin-4'-O-β-glucoside by human volunteers after the consumption of onions, *Free Rad Res*, **29**, 257–69
25 WARD M, MCNULTY H, MCPARTLIN J, STRAIN J J, WEIR D G and SCOTT J M (1997), Plasma homocysteine, a risk factor for cardiovascular disease can be effectively reduced by physiological amounts of folic acid, *Quart J Med*, **90**, 519–524
26 SELHUB J, JACQUES P, WILSON P W F, RUSH D and ROSENBERG I H (1993), Vitamin status and intake as primary determinants of homocysteinemia in an elderly population, *J.A.M.A.*, **270**, 2693–2698
27 BAUSCH-GOLDBOHM R A, HULSHOF, K F A M, BRANTS H A M, VAN DEN BERG H and BOUMAN M (1995), TNO Report V95.84 Zeist, The Netherlands, TNO Nutrition and Food Research Institute
28 GREGORY J, FORSTER K, TYLER H and WISEMAN, M (1990), *The dietary and nutritional survey of British adults*, Office of population and surveys, London, HMSO
29 LEE P and CUNNINGHAM K (1990), *Irish Nutrition Survey*. Dublin: The Irish Nutrition and Dietetic Institute
30 BOUSHEY C J, BERESFORD S A A, OMENN G S and MOTULSKY A G (1995), A quantitative assessment of plasma homocysteine as a risk factor for vascular disease: probable benefits of increasing folic acid intake, *J.A.M.A.*, **274**, 1049–57
31 GREGORY J F (1995), The bioavailability of folate, In: *Folate in Health and Disease*. Ed. Bailey L B, New York, Marcel Dekker, pp. 195–235
32 CUSKELLY G J, MCNULTY H and SCOTT J M (1996), Effect of increasing dietary folate on red-cell folate: implication for prevention of neural tube defects, *Lancet*, **347**, 657–59
33 SCOTT J, REBEILLE F and FLETCHER J (2000), Folic acid and folates: the feasibility for nutritional enhancement in plant foods, *J Sci Fd Agric*, **80**, 795–824
34 KELLY P, MCPARTLIN J, GOGGINS M, WEIR D G and SCOTT J M (1997), Unmetabolized folic acid in serum: acute studies in subjects consuming fortified food and supplements, *Amer J Clin Nutrn*, **65**, 1790–95
35 HELLENAS K-E, BRANZELL C, JOHNSSON H and SLANINA P (1995), High levels of glycoalkaloids in Swedish potato variety Magnum-Bonum, *J Sci Fd Agric*, **68**, 249–55
36 OECD. *Safety evaluation of foods derived by modern biotechnology*. OECD, Paris, 1993
37 EU (1997), Regulation No 258/97 of the European Parliament and the Council concerning novel foods and novel food ingredients, *Off J European Communities*, **43**, 1–7
38 WILLIS W M, LENCKI R W and MARANGONI A G (1998), Lipid modification strategies in the production of nutritionally functional fats and oils, *Crit Rev in Food Sci & Nutrn*, **38**, 639–74
39 GRUSAK M A and DELLAPENNA D (1999), Improving the nutrient composition of plants to enhance human nutrition and health, *Annu Rev Plant Physiol.*, *Plant Mol Biol*, **50**, 133–161
40 DIXON R A, LAMB C J, MASOUD S, SEWALT V J H and PAIVA N L (1996), Metabolic engineering: prospects for crop improvement through the genetic manipulation of phenylpropanoid biosynthesis and defense responses a review, *Gene*, **179**, 61–71
41 YAMAUCHI D and MINAMIKAWA T (1998), Improvement of the nutritional quality of legume seed storage proteins by molecular breeding, *J Plant Res*, **111**, 1–6

9

Enhancing the nutritional value of meat

J. D. Higgs, Food To Fit; and B. Mulvihill

9.1 Introduction

The most common dietary problems in developed countries are due mainly to over nutrition. The incidence of overweight, obesity and adult onset-diabetes is increasing steadily. Cancer is now the most common cause of death in many developed countries. The most common cancers are breast, lung, bowel and prostate, which are virtually absent in some developing countries. However, even in our affluent society, we also see signs of nutritional inadequacies. For instance, in the UK nearly half of females aged between 11 and 14 are not getting enough iron in their diet, while more than a third are not getting enough zinc (Gregory et al, 2000). We are living in a society where both signs of over- and under-nutrition occur side by side. To correct for these nutritional paradoxes we as consumers have to get the balance of nutrients, energy and physical activity right. The objective of this chapter is to highlight the nutritional role that meat can play in modern society.

The National Food Survey for 1999 (Ministry of Agriculture Fisheries and Food, 1999) included a special analysis on meat and meat products consumption in the UK. It stated that 'meat, meat products... are important contributors to the intakes of many nutrients in the British diet'. Data from this survey showed that meat and meat products supply: energy 15%, protein 30%, fat 22% (SFA 22%, MUFA 27%, PUFA 15%), vitamin D 19%, B_2 14%, B_6 21%, B_{12} 22%, vitamin A equivalents 20%, niacin 37%, zinc 30%, iron 14%.

Meat has been a major part of the human diet for at least 2 million years. Human genetic make-up and physical features have been adapted over 4.5 million years for a diet containing meat. An example of this adaptation is our present teeth and jaw structure, that has developed to become efficient at chewing and swallowing meat. Meat is a highly nutritious and versatile food. The primary importance of meat as a food lies in the fact that when digested its protein is broken down releasing amino acids, which are assimilated and ultimately used for the repair and growth of cells. Meat is a nutrient dense food, providing valuable amounts of many essential micronutrients. Meat supplies fatty acids, vitamins, minerals, energy and water and is involved in the synthesis of protein, fat and membranes in the body.

Traditionally meat was considered a highly nutritious food, highly valued and associated with good health and prosperity. As such, western societies gradually increased consumption with increasing affluence. The healthy image of red meat gradually became eroded during the 1980s, when research on the role of lipids in heart disease focused attention on the fat contributed from meat. The British Government's Committee on Medical Aspects of Food and Nutrition (COMA) report on coronary heart disease (CHD) in 1984 identified meat as a major source of saturated fat, contributing a quarter of UK intakes (Committee on Medical Aspects of Food Policy, 1984). Although the multifactorial nature of CHD risk is now widely acknowledged (British Nutrition Foundation,1996; COMA, 1994), the health image of red meat remains tarnished due to this negative association. More recently, we have seen the publication of two reports on diet and cancer (World Cancer Research Fund, 1997; COMA, 1998). These reports associated red meat consumption with increased incidence of certain cancers, in particular, colorectal cancer (CRC), despite the existence of conflicting evidence. Both of these reports issued guidelines on the limits of red meat one should consume, to reduce the risk of developing CRC, which negatively influenced the image of red meat.

The 1990s also saw major publicity on non-nutritional issues including animal health concerns such as bovine spongiform encephalopathy (BSE) and more recently the return of foot and mouth disease (FMD) to Britain. The last 25 years have been the most turbulent regarding issues surrounding meat consumption with much of the publicity being negative thus downplaying meat's nutritional value.

9.2 Meat consumption trends

The negative nutritional image that surrounds red meat is in some way responsible for the decrease in expenditure. In 1999, 25.8% of expenditure on home food in Great Britain was spent on meat and meat products (Ministry of Agriculture Fisheries and Food, 1999). This is a significant drop compared with 32.1% in 1979. During this time period there have been major changes in the type of meat that people are buying in the UK. Expenditures on beef, lamb, pork, bacon and ham each fell, whilst expenditure shares on poultry and on other meats have risen. The major growth area in processed meats and meat products has been frozen convenience meat products, meat based ready meals and other meat products such as Chinese and Italian meals containing meat (Ministry of Agriculture

Fisheries and Food, 1999). There are many factors responsible for these changes, the tarnished image of red meat being one such. Other influencing factors include changes in lifestyle trends which saw the drive for convenience foods, and the resultant responsiveness of the industry to this has greatly influenced the changing meat-buying habits of consumers.

9.3 Cancer

Meat consumption has been implicated in many cancers, as being either protective or causative, depending on the type of cancer. Meat consumption has been shown to protect against cancers of the stomach (Hirayama, 1990; Tuyns et al, 1992; Azevedo et al, 1999), liver and the oesophagus (Zeigler et al, 1981; Tuyns et al, 1987; Nakachi et al, 1988). These are three of the top five cancers globally. On the other hand, meat consumption has been implicated as a cause of colorectal (colon and rectal), breast and prostate cancer, with the main emphasis being on CRC. CRC is the fourth most common cancer in the world, but in Europe and other Western countries it is second in terms of incidence and mortality (after lung cancer in men and breast cancer in women) with 190 000 new cases per year in Europe (Black et al, 1997; Bingham, 1996). There is strong evidence from epidemiological studies showing that diet plays an important role in most large bowel cancers, implying that it is a potentially preventable disease (Higginson, 1966; COMA, 1998). The precise dietary components that influence CRC risk have not been fully elucidated. However, epidemiological studies suggest that high intakes of fat, meat and alcohol increase risk, whereas vegetables, cereals and non-starch polysaccharides, found in fruit and many other foods, decrease the risk (Bingham, 1996). For many of these dietary factors the evidence is equivocal. In the case of meat, the evidence is conflicting, early cross-sectional comparisons attributed much of the world-wide variation in CRC incidence to fat and animal protein consumption (Armstrong and Doll, 1975). In contrast, subsequent case-control and cohort studies are much less consistent (Hill, 1999a).

Meat consumption and CRC became a high profile issue during 1997 and 1998 with the global launch of the World Cancer Research Fund report (WCRF, 1997), timed to coincide with the publication of the British COMA report, both on diet and cancer. The WCRF report was particularly negative towards red meat, which fuelled the launch publicity. This stimulated several critical appraisals of the report, all challenging the conclusions regarding meat (Hill, 1999b). The scientific evidence is not sufficiently robust to recommend a maximum of 80 g/day red meat as pronounced by the WCRF and the initial announcement by COMA for a similar recommendation was subsequently revised. Most of the data showing an association between meat consumption and CRC are American, whereas several studies conducted outside the US (many in Europe) have shown no such relationship (Hill, 1999a). On final publication, COMA (1998) reassured UK consumers that average consumption levels (90 g/day of cooked red meat) were acceptable. COMA suggests that high consumers, less than 15% of the UK population, eating above 140 g/day might benefit from a reduction. Equally importantly, this report acknowledged that meat and meat products remain a valuable source of a number of nutrients including iron and that for many a moderate intake makes an important contribution to micronutrient status. The potential effect on iron status of further reductions to red meat intakes was subsequently investigated, as recommended within the COMA report. Given that a 50% reduction in intake would result in a third of women having low iron intakes (below 8 mg/d), the appropriateness of public health messages concerning meat consumption should be carefully considered prior to reaching the media (Gibson and Ashwell, 2001).

Various components of meat (protein, iron, and heterocyclic amines) have been suspected of contributing to the development of CRC. Dietary protein is broken down in the body to amino acids, which are further degraded to ammonia, which may have cancer-initiating effects. The human colon is also rich in amides and amines that are substrates for bacterial nitrosation by nitric oxide (NO) to N-nitroso compounds that are found in human faeces. There is no conclusive evidence that protein derived compounds can increase cancer risk in humans. It is hypothesised, but not yet established, that the intake of iron from meat and other iron-rich foods may increase the risk of cancer via the production of free radicals in the body. Heterocyclic amines are formed by the Maillard reactions that involve amino acids, sugars and creatine during cooking. They are usually produced on the surface of meat during cooking at very high temperatures, such as in frying, grilling or barbecuing but they are minimal when meat is steamed, microwaved or marinated. The heterocyclic amines are known mutagens *in vitro* and carcinogens in rodents. The most abundant heterocyclic amine produced in meat is phenylimadazo pyridine (PhIP), which is a relatively weak carcinogen compared to other heterocyclic amines such as IQ and MeIQ. The role of heterocyclic amines in causing CRC is not fully elucidated in humans.

Truswell summarised the evidence in 2000 and showed that 20 out of 30 case-control studies and 10 out of 14 prospective studies showed no relationship between meat intake and CRC with some of the results of the remaining studies being confused and one prospective study showing an inverse correlation between meat consumption and CRC risk (Hill, 2000). If meat consumption were associated with increased risk for cancer, one would expect mortality from cancer to be much lower among vegetarians. In a recent meta-analysis of five cohort studies, results have shown no significant differences in mortality from cancer in general, and more specifically mortality in stomach, breast, lung, prostate and colorectal cancer between vegetarians and omnivores (Key et al, 1998, 1999). If red meat consumption were associated with increased risk for CRC, one would expect a decrease in the incidence of CRC to occur over time as a result of decreasing meat consumption trends. During the past 30 years, red meat consumption in the UK has decreased by approximately 25%, while during the same time the incidence of CRC has increased by about 50% (Hill, 1999b). Similarly, if meat consumption were associated with increased risk for CRC, one would

Enhancing the nutritional value of meat 213

expect the rates of CRC to be higher in countries with high meat consumption and lower in countries with low meat consumption. People in the Mediterranean countries eat more red meat than do, for instance, the inhabitants of the UK, yet these countries have lower CRC rates (Hill, 2000). Such paradoxical findings are further evidence that, at current levels, meat consumption is not a risk factor for CRC incidence.

Epidemiological associations between dietary components, specific foods or food groups and chronic disease, such as cancer, can identify risk factors, but are generally insufficient to establish cause and effect relationships. Findings from epidemiological studies must be combined with other types of evidence (e.g. animal experiments, human clinical trials) before a persuasive causal relationship can be established. CRC is multi-factorial; it is confounded by diet, smoking, alcohol, physical activity, obesity, aspirin use, age and family history. There are known protective and causative factors. It is well-known that daily consumption of vegetables and meat reduces the risk of cancer at many sites, whereas daily meat consumption with less frequent vegetable consumption increases risk (Hirayama, 1986; Kohlmeier et al, 1995; Cox and Whichelow, 1997). Evidence suggests that it is the reduced intakes of the protective factors such as vegetables and cereals that are the main determinants of CRC risk with meat being coincidentally related.

There is a need to assess the role of meat when consumed in normal quantities, by normal cooking methods, and within the context of a mixed, balanced, diet. The method of cooking meat and the degree of browning are of particular importance to this whole issue. A major effort by International Meat Industry partners has attempted to raise awareness of the complexities of meat preparation and cooking habits and how these differ between countries. Dietary assessment techniques adopted by nutrition scientists currently do not take full account of the diverse differences between meat products world-wide and the consequent influences these may have on the body. For example, it is well recognised that meat is often cooked more evenly through the muscle within Europe, whereas it tends to be 'blackened' on the outside whilst remaining rare on the inside in North America. This may be one reason for the greater negative findings in American studies of the role of meat in CRC, compared with European studies. This hitherto unexplored facet of meat consumption may have far-reaching implications for interpretation of epidemiological data and ultimately for public health recommendations. Certain marinades applied to meat before cooking will reduce the quantity of potential carcinogenic materials present. The application of knowledge in this area to the production of processed meat products with all the nutritional benefits and none of the potentially harmful components would be progressive indeed.

In summary, it is important not only to examine the relationship between meat consumption and CRC alone, but also to look at meat preparation and cooking differences in conjunction with protective factors, such as vegetables and cereals. At a meat and diet workshop, it was stated:

It is time that the meat CRC story was laid to rest, so that we can get back to recommending that young women of childbearing age eat meat as a ready source of available iron. (Hill, 2000)

Nevertheless, it is sensible to consider that there must be an optimal range for meat intakes in order to ensure a balanced diet is achieved whilst optimal weight is maintained. From this practical perspective COMA's (1998) suggested intake range of 90–140g cooked meat per day is sensible as a public health message. The overemphasis on reducing meat, however, rather than encouraging greater accompanying plant food intake has served only to confuse the public (Hill, 1999*b*). Evidence suggests that the risk of cancer will be reduced to a greater extent by increasing intakes of fruit and vegetables than by lowering meat intakes. Once again, the move towards pre-prepared meal solutions provides opportunity for manufacturers to develop recipes with a healthy balance of meat and vegetable ingredients such that the nutritional profile of the dish is optimised.

9.4 Concerns about fat

Regular consumption of red meat is associated epidemiologically with increased risk of coronary heart disease, due to its fat composition. Conversely, a growing bank of evidence is showing that a healthy diet that includes lean red meat can produce positive blood lipid changes (Watts et al, 1988; Scott et al, 1990; Davidson et al, 1999; Beauchesne-Rondeau et al, 1999). Blood cholesterol levels are increased by inclusion of beef fat, not lean beef in an otherwise low-fat diet. Equal amounts of lean beef, chicken, and fish added to low fat, low saturated fat diets, similarly reduce plasma cholesterol and LDL-cholesterol levels in hypercholesterolaemic and normocholesterolaemic men and women.

Meat is a source of arachidonic acid (20:4n-6), both in the lean and visible fat components (Duo et al, 1998). Assumptions that the 20:4n-6 content of meat was responsible for increasing thrombotic tendencies in Western societies are too simplistic. The presence of large amounts of linoleic acid (18:2n-6) in current diets results in plasma increases of linoleic and arachidonic acids only. However, in the absence of linoleic acid, the long chain n-6 and n-3 PUFAs present in lean meat can influence the plasma pool, increasing plasma eicosatrienoic acid (20:3n-6), 20:4n-6, and eicosapentanoic acid (20:5n-3), and probably reducing thrombotic tendencies. It is the imbalance of n-6: n-3 PUFAs in the diet, brought about by excessive 18:2n-6, that causes high tissue 20:4n-6 levels, so encouraging metabolism to eicosanoids (Sinclair et al, 1994; Mann et al, 1997).

Meat contributes between a third and a half of the UK daily cholesterol intake (Chizzolini et al, 1999; British Nutrition Foundation, 1999). Meat's cholesterol content is, for consumers, another negative influence on meat's health image, although it is now accepted that dietary intake of cholesterol has little bearing on plasma cholesterol. A review of the cholesterol content of meat indicates surprisingly that levels of cholesterol are generally not higher in fatty meat or meat products. The cholesterol content of a meat is related to the number of muscle fibres so tends to be higher the more red the muscle.

9.5 Reductions in the fat content of red meat

Twenty years ago red meat and meat products were identified as major contributors to fat intake in the UK. Most of the visible (subcutaneous) fat in the meat was consumed. In the early 1980s the red meat industry began to shift production systems to favour less fat, reflecting more energy-efficient animal husbandry. For many years now there has been emphasis on reducing the fat content of our diets and this continued consumer demand for less fat further prompted the meat industry to consider ways of reducing the fat content of meat. The fat content of the carcase has been reduced in Britain by over 30% for pork, making British pork virtually the leanest in the world, 15% for beef and 10% for lamb, with further reductions anticipated for beef and lamb over the next 5–10 years. The fat content of fully trimmed lamb, beef and pork is now 8%, 5% and 4% respectively (Chan et al, 1995).

These achievements are due to three factors: selective breeding and feeding practices designed to increase the carcase lean to fat ratio; official carcase classification systems designed to favour leaner production; and modern butchery techniques (seaming out whole muscles, and trimming away all intermuscular fat). It is easier to appreciate the process and extent of fat reduction by looking at the changes over time for a single cut of meat such as a pork chop (Fig. 9.1). The reduction in fat for pig meat is well illustrated by the trend downwards in P_2 fat depth between the 1970s and the 1990s (P_2 is fat depth at the position of the last rib) (Fig. 9.2). Since 1992 it has remained stable at around 11 mm.

Although updated compositional figures for British meat were published from 1986 onwards (Royal Society of Chemistry, 1986; 1993; 1996; Meat and Livestock Commission and Royal Society of Chemistry, 1990), it is only since updated supplements to the McCance and Widdowson tables were published in 1995 (Chan et al, 1995 and 1996), that the achievement of the meat industry in reducing the fat content of meat has been more widely acknowledged (Department Of Health, 1994b; Scottish Office, 1996; Higgs, 2000).

A fat audit for the UK, commissioned by the Government's Ministry of Agriculture, Fisheries and Food to trace all fat in the human food chain provides a more accurate picture than National Food Survey (NFS) (Ministry of Agriculture, Fisheries and Food, 1981–99) data for identifying principal sources of fat in the diet, between 1982 and 1992 (Ulbricht, 1995). It illustrates that whereas the fat contributed by red meat decreased by nearly a third, that from fats and oils as a group increased by a third to contribute nearly half of our fat intakes (Fig. 9.3). This striking picture is lost in NFS data since vegetable fats (in particular) are consumed within a broad range of end products – from chips (so here they are hidden within the vegetables section) to meat products (so here they artificially inflate the apparent fat contributed by meat).

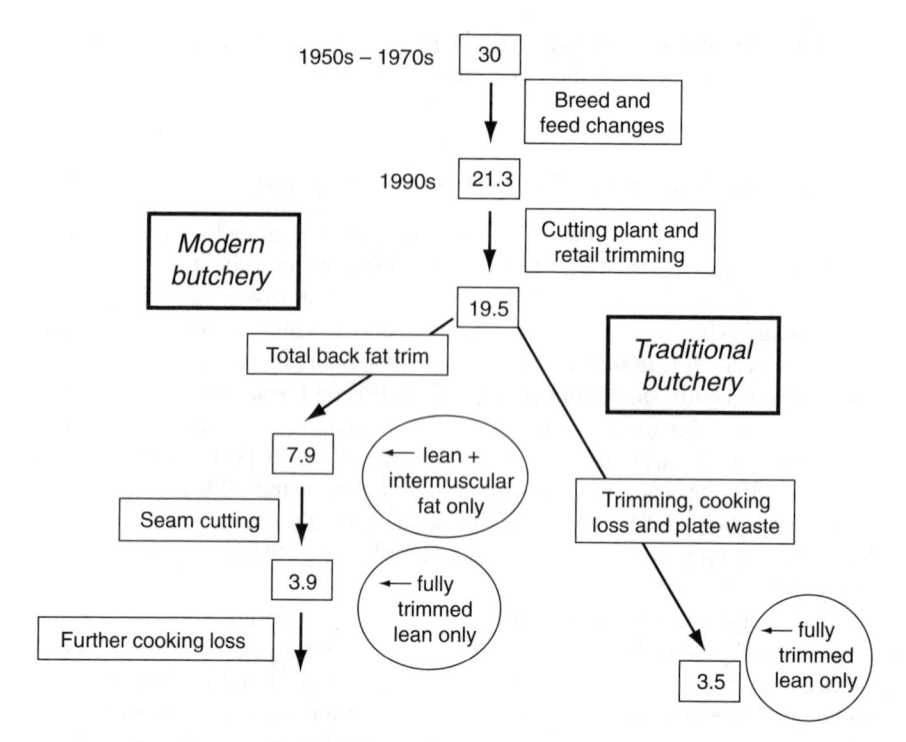

216   The nutrition handbook for food processors

Fig. 9.1 Change in fat content of pork loin for 100 g of raw edible tissue. (Adapted from Higgs JD and Pratt J, 1998) (McCance and Widdowson, 1940, 1960, 1978; Royal Society of Chemistry, 1995; MLC/RSC report to MAFF, 1990)

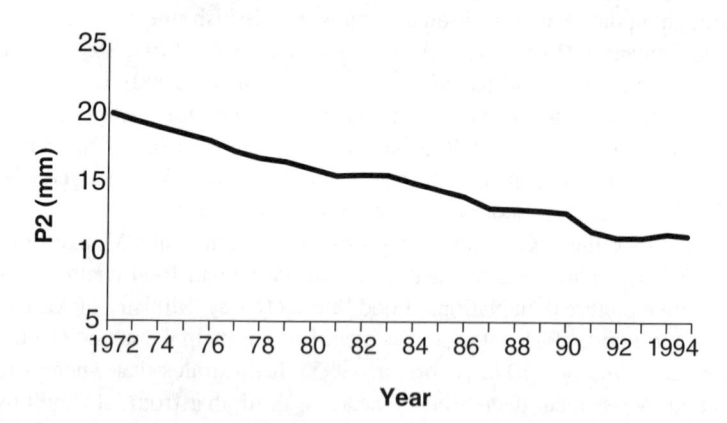

Fig. 9.2 Average P₂ fat depth of British slaughter pigs 1972–1995.

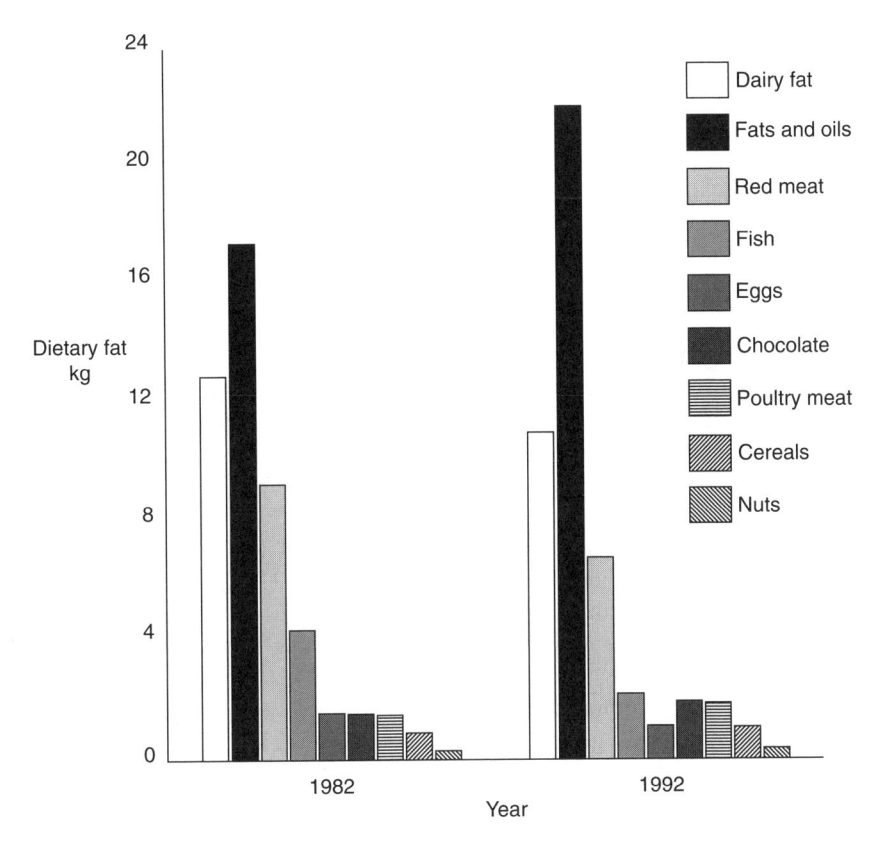

Fig. 9.3 Total fat available for consumption (UK) from different food sources. (Ulbricht TLV, 1995)

The fat content of meat products can vary considerably, dependent on the proportion of lean and fat present and the amount of added non-meat fat (Higgs and Pratt, 1998). Traditional types such as sausages, pastry-covered pies and salami are high in fat (up to 50%) but modern products include ready meals and prepared meats that can be low in fat (5%). The trend downwards in fat for red meat is reflected in the reduced fat content of a number of meat products, such as hams and sausages. Some reduced-fat meat products are now available although the potential for product development in this area has not been fully exploited.

9.6 Fatty acids in meat

The fatty acid composition of food, including meat, has become increasingly important in recent years because of concerns with the effects they have on human health. Fatty acids play a role in many conditions such as CHD, cancer, obesity, diabetes and arthritis. These roles can be protective, causative or relatively neutral, depending on the disease, the fatty acid, and the opposing effects of other dietary components. Current dietary advice emphasises balancing the intake of the different fatty acids. The Department of Health (COMA, 1994) has recommended a reduction in the intake of saturated fat and an increase in the intake of unsaturated fat. Within the unsaturated fatty acids it is recommended to increase the omega-3 (n-3) PUFAs relative to the omega-6 (n-6) PUFAs.

9.6.1 Saturated fatty acids

Probably the main misconception about meat fat is that it is assumed to be totally saturated. Meat contains a mixture of fatty acids both saturated and unsaturated and the amount of saturated fat in meat has been reduced in recent years. At the present time, less than half the fat in pork and beef and 51% of the fat in lamb is saturated. The saturated fat contributed to the diet from red meat and meat products has gradually fallen from 24% in 1979 to 19.6% in 1999. Carcase meats now provide 6.7% of total saturated fat intake (Ministry Of Agriculture Fisheries And Food, 1981). In reality, even this figure is an overestimate, since there is a disproportionate wastage in terms of trimming, cooking losses and plate waste (Leeds et al, 1997).

The predominant saturated fatty acids in meat are stearic acid (C18:0) and palmitic acid (C16:0). In general terms, saturated fats are known as the 'bad' fats as they tend to raise blood cholesterol and cause atherosclerosis. However, not all saturated fats are equal in their effects on blood cholesterol. For instance, stearic acid does not appear to raise blood cholesterol (Bonanome and Grundy, 1988) or other thrombotic risk factors (Kelly et al, 1999, 2001). Stearic acid is a prominent saturated fat in meat, for example; it accounts for approximately one third of the saturated fat in beef. Similarly, palmitic acid, another major saturated fat in meat does not consistently raise blood lipids. On the other hand, myristic acid (C14:0) is the most atherogenic fatty acid, having four times the cholesterol raising potential of palmitic acid (Ulbricht, 1995). Myristic acid is found only in minor quantities in meat.

9.6.2 Monounsaturated fatty acids

Meat contains a mixture of unsaturated fatty acids, polyunsaturated fatty acids and monounsaturated fatty acids (MUFAs). MUFAs are the dominant unsaturated fatty acid in meat and they account for approximately 40% of the total fat in meat. It is a neglected fact that meat and meat products are the main contributors to MUFAs in the British diet, supplying 27% of total MUFA intake (Ministry Of Agriculture Fisheries And Food, 1999). MUFAs are considered to be neutral with respect to blood cholesterol levels. The principal MUFA in meat is oleic acid (*cis* C18:1n-9), which is also found in olive oil and is associated with the healthy Mediterranean diet.

9.6.3 Polyunsaturated fatty acids

The PUFAs have a structural role because they are found in the membrane phospholipids and they are also involved in eicosanoid synthesis. There are two types of polyunsaturated fatty acids, the omega-3 (n-3) and the omega-6 (n-6). Meat and meat products supply 17% n-6 and 19% n-3 PUFA intake (Gregory et al, 1990). Linoleic acid (C18:2 n-6) and α-linolenic acid (C18:3n-3) are essential fatty acids as we cannot synthesise them ourselves, so we are dependent on diet to provide them. In the body these are further elongated and desaturated to longer chain derivatives, arachidonic acid (C20:4n-6), docosapentaenoic acid (C22:5n-6), eicosapentaenoic acid (C20:5n-3) and docosahexaenoic acid (C22:6n-3). These are found in useful quantities in meat. Over the past 30 years there has been a major shift in the intakes of the different fatty acids and the saturated fats have been replaced by the unsaturated fats. The increase in the unsaturated fatty acids was mainly due to an increase in n-6 fatty acids as a consequence of replacing vegetable oils for animal fat.

Today, the usual Western diet contains 10–20 times more n-6 than n-3. For instance, in Britain, the n-6 PUFA intake is now responsible for 87.5% of total PUFA intake, the remainder being the n-3 PUFAs. However, evidence now indicates that it is the n-3 PUFAs which are cardioprotective, in particular, the very long chain n-3 PUFAs, eicosapentaenoic acid (C20:5n-3) and docosahexaenoic acid (C22:6n-3). The GISSI trial showed that 1 g of eicosapentaenoic acid (C20:5n-3) and docosahexaenoic acid (C22:6n-3) daily reduced coronary heart disease deaths by 20% (GISSI, 1999). The exact mechanism for this effect is not clear but they may reduce blood cholesterol. Other beneficial effects of the very long chain n-3 PUFAs include anti-inflammatory and anti-tumourigenic properties. Docosahexaenoic acid (C22:6n-3) also plays a role in neuronal development, cognitive function and visual acuity. It appears that newborn babies have a reduced ability to make the longer chain derivatives and docosahexaenoic acid (C22:6n-3) is an essential fatty acid for the newborn. Meat and fish are the only significant sources of preformed very long chain n-3 PUFAs in the diet. The chief sources of n-3 PUFAs are oily fish and fish oils, however, only one third of the UK population consume oily fish weekly. It is unsurprising, then that in the UK, meat and meat products supply more n-3 PUFAs (19%) than do fish and fish dishes (14%) (Gregory et al, 1990). In a report on n-3 fatty acids the British Nutrition Foundation summarised this fact with the following statement: 'red meat is likely to rival fish as a source of n-3 PUFAs in many people's diet' (BNF, 1999).

Animals can convert α–linolenic acid to 20- and 22-carbon n-3 PUFAs but plants cannot, hence, there are no long chain PUFAs in vegan diets. Diets, which exclude meat and fish, such as vegetarian diets, are practically devoid of very long chain n-3 PUFAs. Vegans rely solely on the endogenous synthesis of very long chain n-3 PUFA from α–linolenic acid. This fact is verified by studies that have shown that vegetarians have lower n-3 PUFA intake than their omnivore counterparts. This imbalance may have nutritional consequences for vegans and vegetarians. For instance, results from a recent observation study showed that the n-3:n-6 ratio in plasma phospholipids was significantly lower among ovo lactovegetarians and vegans compared with meat eaters and this may be responsible for an increased platelet aggregation tendency among vegetarians, which is a risk factor for cardiovascular disease (Li et al, 1999).

Meat is already a valuable source of n-3 PUFAs among omnivores, thus any further increase in the n-3 PUFA content of meat will make useful contributions to their overall intakes. Nowadays, researchers are looking at ways to enhance the n-3 PUFA content of meat. Feeding trials of cattle, pigs and sheep have shown dietary modification to be successful in raising n-3 PUFA content of their meats. The n-3 PUFA content of meat can be enhanced by increasing the amount of n-3 PUFAs in the diet of the animal. For instance, grass is rich in α-linolenic acid (C18:3n-3) and grass-fed meat has a higher n-3 fatty acid content than has grain-fed meat (Enser et al, 1998). Similarly, experiments have shown that including fish oil, marine algae, oils and oilseeds, such as linseed, which are rich sources of n-3 PUFAs, in the animals' diet can enhance favourably the n-3 content of the resultant meat. Enhancing the n-3 PUFA content of meat is much easier to achieve in monogastrics, such as pigs and poultry, than in ruminants. In the rumen, the dietary unsaturated fatty acids are susceptible to biohydrogenation. Biohydrogenation is a process that occurs in the rumen where the dietary unsaturated fatty acids are hydrogenated by ruminant microorganisms to more saturated end products. Evidence indicates that some unsaturated fatty acids appear to be more resistant to biohydrogenation than others. Examples include the very long chain n-3 PUFAs. However, more research is required to clarify this issue. Researchers are looking at ways to overcome biohydrogenation in ruminants by protecting the n-3 PUFA. Altering the fatty acid composition of meat can have negative impacts on the meat quality, its shelf-life, colour and flavour. Therefore animal scientists, food technologists and nutritionists are looking at ways to improve the nutritional quality of meat by enhancing its n-3 PUFA content without causing any adverse sensory qualities or negatively affecting its shelf-life.

The Department of Health (1994b) has issued guidelines regarding the recommended intake of saturated and polyunsaturated fats. The current recommendation for the polyunsaturated:saturated ratio (P:S ratio) is about 0.4. Pork has a higher P:S ratio whereas the P:S ratios of lamb and beef are lower (Table 9.1), as a consequence of biohydrogenation. The Department of Health (1994b) has also issued an index regarding the ratio of n-6:n-3 PUFAs. The recommended value for this ratio (n-6:n-3) is less than 4. The n-6:n-3 ratios of trimmed beef, lamb and pork are approximately 2.2, 1.3 and 7.5, respectively (Table 9.1). Therefore, both beef and lamb have acceptable n-6:n-3 ratios whereas that for pork needs to be reduced to reach acceptable values. The high n-6:n-3 ratio in pork is due to significant amounts of linoleic acid (C18:2 n-6) present in its adipose tissue (Enser et al, 1996). In summary, researchers are focusing on ways of enhancing the n-3 PUFA content of meat and meat products. However, when increasing the n-3 fatty acid composition of ruminant meats such as beef and lamb, they are focusing on ways to increase the P:S ratio whilst retaining the positive n-6:n-3 ratio. On the other hand, for monogastric meat, such as pork,

Table 9.1 Fatty acid ratios related to healthy nutrition

Source of meat	Sample	P:S	n-6:n-3
Beef	Muscle	0.11	2.11
Beef	Adipose tissue	0.05	2.30
Beef	Steak	0.07	2.22
Lamb	Muscle	0.15	1.32
Lamb	Adipose tissue	0.09	1.37
Lamb	Chop	0.09	1.28
Pork	Muscle	0.58	7.22
Pork	Adipose tissue	0.61	7.64
Pork	Chop	0.61	7.57

Values for steaks and chops calculated for whole cut as purchased. Adapted from Enser et al (1996) 'Fatty acid content and composition of English beef, lamb and pork at retail.' *Meat Science* **42**(4): 443–56.

the n-3 PUFA content should be increased, whilst maintaining its positive P:S ratio. Many of the results to date are promising; for instance, beef and lamb liver from animals raised on grass are particularly good sources of n-3 PUFAs with the n-6:n-3 being 0.46 (Enser et al, 1998). Such data highlights the potential for carcase meat with improved fatty acid composition as a highly acceptable and effective vehicle for providing optimal fatty acid intake for the consumer.

9.6.4 Conjugated Linoleic Acid (CLA)

Another emerging dietary benefit for meat, in particular ruminant meat, is the existence within it of conjugated linoleic acid (CLA). CLA is a fatty acid that occurs naturally in ruminant meats such as beef and lamb. The acronym CLA is a collective term used to describe a mixture of positional (7,9-; 8,10-; 9,11-; 10,12- or 11,13-) and geometrical (*c,c*-; *c,t*-; *t,t*- or *t,c*-) isomers of linoleic acid (9*c*,12*c*-18:2). CLA has the same chain length as linoleic acid (18C), but in CLA the double bonds are conjugated. Conjugated double bonds are separated by only one single carbon bond. The *c*9-*t*11-18:2 isomer (rumenic acid) is the predominant isomer of CLA (Kramer et al, 1998). This isomer has been shown to account for at least 60% of total CLA in beef (Shantha et al, 1994; O'Shea et al, 1998). Factors influencing the CLA content of meat include the breed, age and diet of the animal (O'Shea et al, 1998; Mulvihill, 2001). As well as having a high n-3 PUFA content, grass-fed meat also has higher CLA content (Shantha et al, 1994). Since, CLA is formed predominately in the rumen, the CLA content of ruminant meat, beef and lamb, is much higher than non-ruminant meat such as pork, chicken and game (Chin et al, 1992). The best natural dietary sources of CLA are ruminant products such as beef and lamb (Ma et al, 1999). Meat and meat products supply approximately a quarter of dietary CLA in Germany (Fritsche and Steinhart, 1998).

CLA appears to have a variety of potential health benefits. It has been shown to have tumour reducing (Belury, 1995; Ip and Scimeca, 1997; Ip et al, 1991, 1994, 1999) and atherosclerotic reducing properties (Lee et al, 1994; Nicolosi et al, 1997; Gavino et al, 2000). CLA may also reduce adiposity (Park et al, 1997; West et al, 1998) and delay the onset of diabetes (Houseknecht et al, 1998). The different isomers of CLA appear to be responsible for its differing biological effects. For instance, the c-9,t-11 isomer may play an anti-carcinogenic role, while the t-10,c-12 isomer appears to play a role in reducing adiposity. So far, most of the research work demonstrating the health benefits of CLA has been conducted in experimental animals or cell culture models. The jury is still out for its effect on human health. The American Dietetic Association has endorsed beef and lamb as functional foods because of the anti-tumourigenic properties of the CLA they contain (ADA, 1999). We are just beginning to understand fully the effect(s) that CLA has on human health and the role that meat plays in its dietary provision. In a review, Mulvihill (2001) raised a number of questions that need to be answered to improve our knowledge about CLA in meat. They include: how is CLA formed in the rumen? can this be regulated? what CLA isomers are in meat? and can meat consumption influence CLA levels in the human body?

9.6.5 *Trans*-fatty acids

Trans-fatty acids raise LDL cholesterol and decrease HDL cholesterol. It is recommended by the Department of Health (1991) that *trans*-fatty acids contribute less than 2% of total energy. Ruminant meats are a source of *trans*-fatty acids, contributing around 18% of total intakes. These are formed during biohydrogenation in the rumen. In the British diet the main source of *trans*-fatty acids are cereals and cereal products and fat spreads which use partially hydrogenated vegetable and fish oils in their products. Other significant sources include ruminant meat and milk (Gregory et al, 1990). It appears from the analysis of 14 European countries that the fat content of meat does not correlate with the percentage of *trans*-fatty acid content (Hulshof et al, 1999). *Trans*-fats have been highlighted as contributing to atherogenesis, although the hydrogenated fats from vegetable sources used in bakery goods and other processed foods appear to be more of a concern than the natural *tran*-fats found in ruminant meats and milk fat (British Nutrition Foundation, 1995). After assessing the intake of *trans*-fatty acids in 14 European countries (TRANSFAIR study), the conclusion was that the current intake of TFA in most Western European countries including the United Kingdom does not appear to be a reason for major concern (Hulshof et al, 1999; van de Vijver et al, 2000). In fact, the TRANSFAIR study showed that intakes of *trans*-fatty acids did not influence LDL and HDL cholesterol and a weak inverse association was found in total serum cholesterol (van de Vijver et al, 2000). In the USA, where there is a much greater reliance on processed foods, the consequent higher intakes (6% dietary energy) of non- ruminant *trans*-fatty acids are causing some concern.

9.6.6 Cholesterol

Much research has looked at the effect that individual fatty acids have on blood cholesterol rather than the mixture that we digest. It is now obvious that we should be looking at the effect that diet as a whole has on blood cholesterol. In the United States, the National Cholesterol Education Program (NCEP) recommends dietary guidelines for people with hypercholesterolaemia (raised blood cholesterol). The NCEP dietary guidelines are a first-line therapy for the management of high blood cholesterol. A recent study compared the differing effects of lean red meat (beef, veal and pork) and lean white meat (poultry and fish) in the NCEP diet on blood cholesterol of people with hypercholesterolaemia (Davidson et al, 1999). This study showed that the inclusion of approximately 170g lean red meat per day, five to seven times per week in the NCEP diet was as effective as lean white meat in reducing both total and LDL cholesterol while simultaneously raising HDL cholesterol. Thus the inclusion of lean red meat in such a diet had a positive impact on blood cholesterol levels. The authors also indicated that the study participants who consumed the lean red meat were more likely to follow their dietary regimen as they had a wider food choice than those on the white meat diet. This study not only highlights the nutritional value of red meat in such a diet but also the practical value, as no diet can possibly work unless it is adhered to!

An earlier study conducted in the United Kingdom showed similar results, where mildly hypercholesterolaemic men ate 180g of lean meat every day, a quantity we would consider high today. This diet was low fat, low saturated fat and high in PUFA and it proved to be effective in lowering total and LDL cholesterol (Watts et al, 1988). In Canada, a study was conducted comparing the effects of lipid lowering diets containing lean beef, poultry (without skin) and lean fish on plasma cholesterol levels in men with raised blood cholesterol. The results indicated that when compared to the usual diet, the lean beef and poultry diets significantly reduced both total cholesterol and LDL ('bad') cholesterol in men with raised blood cholesterol. Whereas in the fish containing diet, only total cholesterol levels fell significantly when compared to the usual diet (Beauchesne-Rondeau et al, 1999). There is now a wealth of studies showing similar results (Scott et al, 1990; Mann et al, 1997; Davidson et al, 1999), which are not that surprising, as lean red meat is low in fat, low in SFA and contains a mixture of beneficial unsaturated fatty acids, such as linoleic acid, n-3 PUFAs, MUFAs and CLA.

9.7 Protein

Protein is the basic building material for making cells and its adequate intake can be of particular benefit for growing young people or in adults where muscle tissue is being rebuilt, such as athletes or those recuperating after surgery. Meat is a good source of protein and it contains all the essential amino acids. In the United Kingdom, meat and meat products supply 30% of dietary protein intakes (Ministry Of Agriculture Fisheries And Food, 1999). Emphasis on a prudent diet for health that recommended just 11E% (National Advisory Committee on Nutrition Education, 1983) from protein has led us to underplay the potential role of high protein foods in the diet. Recent interest in the use of high protein diets (25E%) for weight reduction have utilised the higher satiating properties of protein, important for dietary compliance, and achieved significantly more weight loss over a 6 months dietary intervention compared to lower (12E%) protein. These results were achieved without adverse effects on renal function (Skov et al, 1999a, 1999b).

Meat protein has a higher biological value than has plant protein because some of the amino acids are limiting in plant protein. For example, lysine is the limiting amino acid in wheat, tryptophan is the limiting amino acid in maize and sulphur-containing amino acids are limiting in soyabean. It is necessary for vegans and vegetarians to eat a wide variety of vegetable protein foods to provide the necessary amounts of each amino acid. Meat is a rich source of taurine. Taurine is considered to be an essential amino acid for newborns, as they seem to have a limited ability to synthesise it. Taurine concentrations in the breast milk of vegans were shown to be considerably lower than in omnivores (Rana and Sanders, 1986). The significance of this finding is unknown.

9.8 The functionality of meat

Typical Western omnivorous diets over the last 40 years have been relatively high in protein and fat with insufficient dietary fibre, fruit and vegetables. Meat intake is by definition the key difference between vegetarian and omnivorous diets, thus comparative studies have tended to exaggerate the health benefits of a vegetarian diet so reinforcing a negative health image for meat. It has long been recognized (Burr, 1988) that although vegetarianism seems to confer some protection against heart disease, it is not clear if this is due to abstinence from meat or high consumption of vegetables. Meat intake has provided a marker for a generally 'unhealthy' diet in the past (American Dietetic Association, 1993; COMA, 1991; Sanders and Reddy, 1994; Thorogood, 1994). Furthermore, vegetarians have tended to be more health conscious, they traditionally smoke less, consume less alcohol, tea, and coffee, and tend to exercise more, thus their good health could be attributed to any or a combination of these habits. CHD and cancer are multifactorial; diet is one factor playing a role in these conditions, but *diet alone* is a very broad term, because within diet there are protective and causative factors. Comparing current omnivorous and vegetarian diets shows that the meat content of the former is not responsible for its higher fat content. Australian research has shown that when the meat component was removed from an omnivore diet, the remaining part of the diet was still significantly higher in total fat, saturated fat and cholesterol than was a vegetarian diet (Li et al, 1999). This suggests that the overall diet rather than the meat is responsible for these diet characteristics.

The significance of meat to nutrient intake depends on the importance given

Enhancing the nutritional value of meat 225

to meat in an individual's, or in a society's diet and culture. With a limited range of foods available in primitive societies throughout history, meat provided a concentrated source of a wide range of nutrients (Davidson and Passmore, 1969; Sanders, 1999). Considering the diet of modern man, where meat is excluded within traditional vegetarian cultures, the nutrients it provides can be supplied from a combination of other foods and this appears at least adequate, provided the diet is not too restrictive and dependent on nutritionally inferior staples such as maize or cassava (Sanders, 1999). With the range and abundance of foods available to developed societies today, the nutritional significance of any one food is reduced.

Traditionally, the vegetarian was likely to consume a wider range of foods than the meat eater. Consequently, vegetarians in Europe and North America historically had similar energy intakes to meat eaters and greater intakes of vitamins B_1, C, E, folic acid, β-carotene, potassium and fibre (Sanders, 1999). Today, vegetarianism cannot be assumed to provide a favourable fatty acid intake. Comparative studies of vegetarian and omnivorous children surveyed from 9 to 17 years old found that saturated fat intakes were no lower in the vegetarian children (Nathan et al, 1994; Nathan et al, 1997; Burgess et al, 2001). There was no significant difference between energy intakes and the percentage energy from fat, or saturated fat intakes between vegetarian and omnivore adolescents in northwest England (Burgess et al, 2001). Vegetarian women have lower zinc intakes and status than their omnivore counterparts (Ball and Ackland, 2000). A recent study in Australia showed vegetarians had a lower intake of beneficial very long chain n-3 PUFAs (Li et al, 1999). A study comparing meat eaters with vegetarians has shown that levels of plasma homocysteine, an independent risk factor for heart disease, among vegetarians were significantly higher than their omnivore counterparts, and this was correlated with a lower intake of vitamin B_{12} among the vegetarians (Mann et al, 1999; Krajcovicova-Kudlackova et al, 2000; Mann 2001b). Vegans have significantly lower intakes of protein, vitamin D, calcium, and selenium but no difference in energy and iron intakes from those of omnivores and the vegans have significantly lower vitamin B_{12} blood concentration (Larsson and Johansson, 2001).

Modern eating habits contribute to erosion of the traditional vegetarian diet in developed countries because there is now a greater dependence on vegetarian convenience foods, coinciding with increased availability and choice. Whilst vegetarian convenience foods may appear attractive in terms of health as well as for ease and speed of preparation, they are not necessarily of superior nutritional value compared with meat-containing equivalents. There is wide variation in the fat content of vegetarian products, ranging from 2% to 58%, with nearly a third supplying more than 50% of their energy from fat (Reid and Hackett, 2001).

Excluding meat whilst paying little attention to selecting appropriate alternative food combinations, to ensure adequate nutrients are supplied, is cause for concern, especially in children and adolescents. Today's busy lifestyles give rise to more erratic dietary practices making it easier to obtain all nutrients required for health by including meat as a component of the diet. The time spent planning and preparing meals is minimal and an increasing proportion of our daily food intake is consumed outside the home as snacks and quick meals. NFS data suggest that in 1998 28% of total expenditure on food and drink was outside the home (MAFF, 1999). Data on the dietary intakes and nutritional status of young people aged between 4 and 18 years in Britain show that energy intakes of young people are now approximately 20% below estimated average requirements (EAR) for age. Growth patterns suggest such intakes are adequate and merely reflect the corresponding lower activity levels of youngsters today, which in itself is a concern. Reduced energy intakes must increase the emphasis on a more nutrient dense diet, particularly in growing children. The survey has recorded intakes of iron, zinc and copper below the RNI particularly in older girls (Gregory et al, 2000). It is possible that the recorded lower meat intakes are partly responsible for this. The decision to become vegetarian should be accompanied by adequate nutritional information and education. Despite popular opinion, vegetarianism *per se* does not guarantee a nutritionally adequate diet. Conversely, using meat as a significant protein source in the diet provides a concentrated nutrient supplement, thus ensuring the diet is nutritionally adequate (Department Of Health, 1994a; Millward, 1999). The potential for producing nutritionally superior, convenience products, that include meat as a functional ingredient, is enormous and deserves more thorough exploitation.

9.9 Meat, Palaeolithic diets and health

Humans are omnivores. Evidence such as dentition, gut structure and ecosystem, enzymic range and adaptability and our dependence on both plant and animal sources for our essential nutrients all support this issue. We begin life as omnivores, because as babies *in utero*, all the nutrients we receive are of animal origin. During the Ice Age, plants could not grow and so humans had to depend on meat as their main source of nutrition. There is much historical evidence and data from carbon isotopes, gut morphology, brain size, cranio-dental features, tools, weapons and rock art depiction of hunting all tracing the evolution of humans as omnivores (Mann, 2001a). There is considerable weight to the argument that our brains evolved because we could eat a variety of foods including meat.

As we begin the new Millennium, some experts are looking at the diet of Palaeolithic (stone-age) man in a search for ways to reduce the incidences of 'modern' diseases such as obesity, cancer and coronary heart disease. Research from hunter-gatherer societies has indicated that these people were relatively free of many of the chronic and degenerative diseases that plague us today; this is in part attributable to the different dietary practices. Investigation of the dietary habits of modern hunter-gatherer societies, as an approximation of Palaeolithic practices, has shown a high reliance on animal foods compared with plant foods for basic energy requirements (Cordain et al, 2000). It has been estimated that the hunter-gatherers obtained approximately 45–65% of their total energy intake from meat, which was either hunted or fished (Cordain et al, 2000). It is only with the relatively recent rise in agriculture that humans have begun to consume high levels of carbohydrates. This is now recognised as a major contributor to 'Western lifestyle' diseases. We have changed from a diet high in meat to a diet where grains and refined foods dominate. The hunter-gatherer diet was high in protein (19–35% E) and low in carbohydrate (22–40% E) whereas today, the opposite prevails – lower in protein (15% E) and much higher in carbohydrates (55% E) (Cordain et al, 2000). The fatty acid profiles of such diets may have differed with higher levels of unsaturated fatty acids in wild animals, compared to domesticated farm animals.

Studies have shown that Australian Aborigines have shown significant health improvements, including a reduction in blood cholesterol levels, after returning to their natural diets, where there is a high reliance on animal foods (O'Dea, 1991). Research of macronutrient proportions in the diet of hunter-gatherer populations shows a clear relationship between high protein content and the evolution of insulin resistance, which offered a survival and reproductive advantage (Brand-Miller and Colagiuri, 1994). However, the advent of agriculture saw the rise of a diet higher in carbohydrate; this has meant that people were unprepared for the high glycaemic load which in turn is responsible for the current incidence of non-insulin dependent diabetes mellitus (Brand-Miller and Colagiuri, 1994). However, we must also remember that humans are not carnivores and thus we cannot exist on protein intakes above 35% energy for extended periods of time. 'A clear role for lean red meat in a healthy balanced diet becomes evident as the diet history of our species is uncovered' (Mann, 2001a).

9.10 Meat and satiety

The prevalence of obesity has increased dramatically in recent years (National Audit Office, 2001). Satiety influences the frequency of meals and snacks, whereas satiation influences the size of meals and snacks. Macronutrients have differing effects on satiety; protein is more satiating than carbohydrates that are more satiating than fat (Hill and Blundell, 1986; Barkeling et al, 1990; Stubbs, 1995). The exact mechanism by which protein exerts its satiating effect is not elucidated, but it may involve changes in the levels and patterns of metabolites and hormones (e.g. amino acids, glucose and insulin), cholecystokinin and amino acid precursors of the neurotransmitters serotonin, noreadenaline and dopamine. A meat-containing meal was shown to have more sustained satiety than a vegetarian meal (Barkeling et al, 1990). Other studies have shown that different meats have different satiating powers (Uhe et al, 1992). These differences may be related to differences in amino acid profiles or digestibilities. More research on the effects that different meats have on satiety will prove invaluable in assessing whether or not meat can, in the future, be promoted as a food that can negatively curb the growing levels of obesity.

9.11 Meat and micronutrients

9.11.1 Iron in meat

Iron deficiency (Schrimshaw, 1991) and iron deficiency anaemia (Walker, 1998) remain the most common nutritional disorders in the world today. Iron deficiency is the only widespread nutrient deficiency occurring in both developed and developing countries. Iron deficiency affects between 20 and 50% of the world's population (Beard and Stoltzfus, 2001). There are many causes of iron deficiency, including hook worm infestation, low iron intakes, low bioavailability of dietary iron and increased demand due to physiological requirements. The most common result of iron deficiency is anaemia. Some of the liabilities associated with iron deficiency and anaemia are defective psychomotor development in infants, impaired education performance in schoolchildren, adverse perinatal outcome in pregnancy and diminished work capacity (Cook, 1999). All of the iron in our body comes from our diet, and meat is a rich dietary source. Concern about iron deficiency is one nutritional reason for recommending eating at least some meat (WHO, 1990; COMA, 1998).

Food iron can be classified as haem iron or non-haem iron. Haem iron is derived from haemoglobin and myoglobin and its chief food source is meat, whereas non-haem iron is derived mainly from cereals, fruits and vegetables. Meat is distinctive as it contains both types of iron, haem (50–60%) and non-haem. Our bodies readily absorb haem iron (20–30%) as it is not affected by other dietary factors. Meat positively influences the bioavailability of non-haem iron. Bioavailability of iron refers to the proportion of ingested iron that is absorbed and utilised by the body (O'Dell, 1989). Only two dietary factors enhance non-haem iron bioavailability, they are vitamin C (Hallberg et al, 1989) and meat (Cook and Monsen, 1976; Taylor et al, 1986; Hazell et al, 1978; Kapsokefalou and Miller, 1991, 1993, 1995; Mulvihill and Morrissey, 1998a, 1998b; Mulvihill et al, 1998). Absorption of non-haem iron from meat is typically 15–25%, compared with 1–7% from plant sources (Fairweather-Tait, 1989). The presence of meat in a meal enhances the bioavailability of non-haem iron contained in the other foods present such as cereals, fruits and vegetables.

The enhancing effect of meat on non-haem iron bioavailability is commonly referred to as the 'meat factor'. The exact mechanism by which the 'meat factor' works still remains unknown despite the fact that numerous efforts have concentrated on this topic. Research indicates that the mechanism of the 'meat factor' may not be due solely to a single factor but due to a number of contributing factors which work together promoting non-haem iron bioavailability. These factors include the release of cysteine-rich small molecular weight peptides during the proteolysis of meat; the ability of these peptides to reduce ferric iron to the more soluble ferrous iron; the chelation of soluble non-haem iron by these peptides; and the ability of meat to promote gastric acid secretion and gastrin release better than other food components do (Mulvihill, 1996).

Glutathione is a tripeptide containing cysteine, and this is considered to play a role in the 'meat factor'. However, reduced glutathione represents only 3% of total cysteine in meat and this is considered too low to have such a profound positive influence on non-haem iron bioavailability (Taylor et al, 1986). Elucidation of the mechanism(s) of the 'meat factor' is extremely important in the search for more effective ways to improve iron nutrition. Isolation of the 'meat factor' will allow the potential to produce stable non-haem iron absorption enhancers which can be added to other foods, thus improving iron bioavailability.

Meat and meat products provide 14% of iron intake (MAFF, 1999); within this, carcase meat and meat products supply 12.5% of total iron intakes. This figure grossly underestimates the value of meat for influencing iron status. Meat has an important influence on iron bioavailability and thus iron status due to its enhancing properties and overall greater absorption capacity.

Low iron intakes and status are common among certain subgroups of the population – toddlers (Gregory et al, 1995; Edmond et al, 1996), adolescents (Nelson et al, 1993; Nelson, 1996), pregnant women (Allen, 1997) and the elderly (Finch et al, 1998). Data from the National Diet and Nutrition Survey of children shows that 20% have low iron stores and 8% have iron deficiency anaemia (Gregory et al, 1995). Iron deficiency anaemia among toddlers is often associated with late weaning practices. A Spanish study showed that children who first ate meat before eight months of age showed a better iron status than those who were introduced to meat later than eight months (Requejo et al, 1999). Another study showed that low iron stores in one- and two-year old children is related to a low meat iron intake (Mira et al, 1996). The COMA report on Weaning and the Weaning Diet recommends that foods containing haem iron should be incorporated into the diets of infants by 6–8 months of age. Soft-cooked puréed meat can be introduced. This goes against the modern trend to delay introduction, the basis for which appears to be non-scientific.

Adolescents have high demands for iron to allow for muscle development, increased blood volume and the onset of menstruation in females, that makes them vulnerable to iron deficiency. Half the female population living in the UK aged between 15 and 18 years have iron intakes below the recommended level. This is reflected by the fact that 27% of that age group have low iron stores (Gregory et al, 2000). The prevalence of low iron stores among adolescent girls in the UK has been cited to be as high as 43% (Nelson et al, 1993). During pregnancy, more lactovegetarians (26%) reported suffering from iron deficiency than omnivores (11%) (Drake et al, 1999). Lyle et al (1992) has demonstrated that meat supplements were more effective than iron tablets in maintaining iron status during exercise in previously sedentary young women. Among the elderly, both low iron intakes and low iron status has been shown to increase with age (Finch et al, 1998).

Serum ferritin, the body's iron store, is strongly correlated with haem iron (Reddy and Sanders, 1990). Bioavailability of iron plays an important role in determining iron status. Studies have shown that despite the fact that vegetarians have either a similar or a higher iron intake than their omnivore counterparts, their iron status is lower (Nathan et al, 1996; Ball and Bartlett, 1999; Wilson and Ball, 1999). Vegetarians should consume iron-rich foods to compensate for the low bioavailability of non-haem iron from the foods they eat.

The importance of meat in iron nutrition cannot be over-emphasised. The effects of meat and meat products on iron nutrition are three-fold. Firstly, they are a rich source of iron. Secondly, they contain haem iron, which is readily absorbed. Thirdly, they promote the absorption of non-haem in the diet.

9.11.2 Zinc in meat

All meats, but in particular beef, are excellent sources of dietary zinc. It takes 41 oz milk, 15 oz tuna or $6\frac{1}{2}$ eggs to equal the amount of zinc in an average 4 oz portion of beef (Hammock, 1987). On average, meat and meat products account for a third of total zinc intakes (MAFF, 1999). Zinc absorption is suppressed by inhibitors such as oxalate and phytate which are found in plant foods (Johnson and Walker, 1992; Zheng et al, 1993; Hunt et al, 1995). On the contrary, meat facilitates the absorption of zinc – 20–40% of zinc is absorbed from meat. For instance, one study showed that female omnivores who had a significantly lower zinc intake than their vegetarian counterparts had a higher zinc status (Ball and Ackland, 2000); such data highlights the role that meat plays in providing an assured source of dietary zinc. Because of the low bioavailability of zinc from plant foods, vegetarians should strive to meet or exceed their RDA for zinc to ensure adequate zinc intakes.

Zinc is necessary for growth, healing, the immune system, reproduction (Aggett and Comerford, 1995) and cognitive development (Sandstead, 2000). Low zinc intakes are becoming more prevalent, especially among adolescents. An NDNS survey showed that a tenth of 7–10 year old girls and a third of 11–14 year old girls have intakes of zinc below the recommended level (Gregory et al, 2000). Long-term, low zinc intakes leads to zinc deficiencies that may become a public health problem in the future (Sandstead, 1995). Iron and zinc deficiencies can often occur simultaneously, in particular among adolescents (Sandstead, 2000). Adolescents often avoid eating meat, in some incidences meat is providing up to just 25% of total zinc intakes compared to 40% of adult intakes (Gregory et al, 1995; Mills and Tyler, 1992; Gregory et al, 2000). Thus including meat in the diet of adolescents can aid in averting both iron and zinc deficiencies in concert, as these minerals in meat are in easily absorbable forms. Similarly, concern over low zinc status among infants prompted the DoH, in its COMA weaning report, to recommend increasing meat portion sizes for infants at the weaning stage (Department of Health, 1994a).

9.11.3 Selenium in meat

Selenium acts as an antioxidant and is considered to protect against coronary heart disease and certain cancers, such as prostate. Meat contains about 10 mg selenium per 100 g, which is approximately 25% of our daily requirement. Beef and pork contain more selenium than does lamb, which may be due to the age of the animal as selenium may collect in the meat over time. Bioavailability of selenium from plant foods was thought to be greater than that from animal foods, but recent data demonstrate that meat, raw and cooked, provides a highly bioavailable source (Shi and Spallholz, 1994).

9.11.4 Other minerals in meat

Meat also contains phosphorus; a typical serving provides roughly 20–25% of an adult's requirement. Phosphorus has important biochemical functions in carbohydrates, fat and protein metabolism. Meat also provides useful amounts of copper, magnesium, potassium, iodine and chloride.

9.11.5 B vitamins in meat

Meat is a significant and an important source of many B vitamins. The B vitamins in meat are thiamin (vitamin B_1), riboflavin (vitamin B_2), niacin, pantothenic acid, vitamin B_6 and vitamin B_{12}. B vitamins are water-soluble, hence lean meat contains more of these vitamins than does fattier meat. Some losses of B vitamins occur during cooking; the amount lost depends upon the duration and the temperature of the cooking method.

Thiamin and riboflavin are found in useful amounts in meats. Pork and its products including bacon and ham are one of the richest sources of thiamin. Pork contains approximately 5–10 times as much thiamin as do either beef or lamb. Thiamin aids the supply of energy to the body by working as part of a coenzyme that converts fat and carbohydrates into fuel. It also helps to promote a normal appetite and contributes to normal nervous system function. Typical servings of pork provide all the daily requirement of thiamin. Offal meats are good sources of riboflavin, for example, a single portion (100 g) of kidney or liver provides more than the daily requirement. Riboflavin, like thiamin, aids in supplying energy and also promotes healthy skin, eyes and vision.

Meat is the richest source of niacin. Half the niacin provided by meat is derived from tryptophan, which is more readily absorbed by the body than that bound to glucose in plant sources. Niacin helps to supply energy to the body as it plays a role in converting carbohydrates and fats into fuel. Meat and meat products supply more than a third of total niacin intakes in Britain (MAFF, 1999).

Liver and kidney are rich sources of pantothenic acid. Although most of this vitamin is leached into the drip loss associated with frozen meat, this is unlikely to be of any nutritional consequence as pantothenic acid is universal in all living matter.

A 100 g portion of veal liver provides half our daily vitamin B_6 needs and other meats provide around a third. Vitamin B_6 is a necessary cofactor for more than 100 different cellular enzyme reactions including those related to amino acid metabolism and inter-conversion. Vitamin B_{12} is exclusively of animal origin as it is a product of bacterial fermentation that occurs in the intestine of ruminant animals such as cattle, sheep and goats. Vitamin B_{12} is required to produce red blood cells and acts as a cofactor for many enzyme reactions. Deficiency of vitamin B_{12} causes megaloblastic anaemia, neuropathy and gastrointestinal symptoms. Groups at risk of vitamin B_{12} deficiency include vegans and strict vegetarians, because vitamin B_{12} is exclusively of animal origin, and the elderly, because their ability to absorb this vitamin from the diet diminishes with age (Allen and Casterline, 1994; Swain, 1995; Baik and Russell, 1999; Drake et al, 1999a). In the past some vitamin B_{12} was provided from the soil of poorly cleaned foods. This may in part explain the apparent absence of deficiency in some vegan groups. Today, with the emphasis on good food hygiene practices, this source can no longer protect against deficiency in vulnerable individuals. Vegans are recommended to take vitamin B_{12} supplements since the quantity consumed from foods fortified with the vitamin is too low (Jones, 1995; Draper, 1991; Sanders and Reddy, 1994). The RNI for vitamin B_{12} among the elderly is 1.5 µg/day (Department of Health, 1991). A 100 g portion of lean trimmed beef contains 2 µg vitamin B_{12}, thus supplying all their daily needs for this vitamin. In Britain, meat and meat products supply more than a fifth of both vitamin B_6 and B_{12} intakes (MAFF, 1999). The need for vitamin B_{12} has been a part of the rationale for recommending the consumption of animal foods among all age groups (WHO, 1990).

Raised homocysteine, an amino acid metabolite, is an independent risk factor for cardiovascular disease. It is estimated that 67% of the cases of hyperhomocysteinemia are attributable to inadequate plasma concentrations of one or more of the B vitamins namely folate, vitamin B_6 and vitamin B_{12}. Some enzymes that reduce homocysteine levels require vitamins B_6 and B_{12} as cofactors. Vitamin B_6 is a cofactor for two enzyme reactions which catabolise homocysteine to cysteine via a transulphuration pathway, they are cystathionine β-synthase and cystathionase. Meanwhile, vitamin B_{12} is a cofactor for the remethylation enzyme, methionine synthase, which converts homocysteine to methionine. Research has shown that low levels of both vitamins B_6 and B_{12} independently correlates with raised homocysteine. For instance, ovo-lactovegetarians or vegans who had significantly lower serum vitamin B_{12} levels than meat eaters had significantly higher levels of plasma homocysteine (Mann et al, 1999; Krajcovicova-Kudlackova et al, 2000; Mann, 2001*b*). Similarly, low doses of vitamin B_6 can effectively lower fasting plasma homocysteine levels (McKinley et al, 2001). The role of meat in regulating homocysteine is intriguing and needs to be addressed further.

9.11.6 Meat and vitamin D

In the body vitamin D acts as a hormone, essential for the absorption of dietary calcium. Thus, vitamin D is essential for skeletal development and severe deficiency is associated with defective mineralisation of the bone resulting in rickets in children or its adult equivalent, osteomalacia (Fraser, 1995; Dunnigan and Henderson, 1997; De Luca and Zierold, 1998; Department of Health, 1998b). More subtle degrees of insufficiency lead to increased bone loss and osteoporotic fractures. Other functions of vitamin D include its role in the immune system, as well as possible protection against tuberculosis, muscle weakness, diabetes, certain cancers and coronary heart disease (Department of Health, 1998b).

It is well established that sunlight exposure on the skin is the main source of vitamin D. However, there are certain subgroups in the population who are more at risk of vitamin D deficiency, and these depend on diet in addition to sunlight in obtaining adequate vitamin D. Such subgroups include infants, toddlers, pregnant and lactating women, elderly and those who have low sunlight exposure, such as certain ethnic minorities and the housebound (Department of Health, 1998a). The prevalence of vitamin D inadequacies among these groups is widespread. For instance, 27% of 2 year old Asian children living in England have low vitamin D status (Lawson and Thomas, 1999), and 99% of elderly people living in institutions are not receiving enough dietary vitamin D (Finch et al, 1998). Vitamin D deficiency among the elderly will become much more apparent and a greater public health problem when we consider that we are living in an increasingly ageing population.

Liver aside, meat and meat products were considered poor sources of vitamin D. However, new analytical data for the composition of meat indicates that this is not true (Chan et al, 1995). Meat and meat products contain significant amounts of 25-hydroxycholecalciferol, assumed to have a biological activity five times that of cholecalciferol. In fact, the meat group is now recognised as the richest natural dietary source of vitamin D, supplying approximately 21% (Gibson and Ashwell, 1997). Vitamin D is present in both the lean and the fat of meat although its exact function in the animal is not yet known. Since interest in the role of meat in supplying vitamin D is a relatively new subject matter, there are certain areas that need to be researched such as the effect of cooking meat on vitamin D levels, the bioavailability of vitamin D from meat and the influence of seasonal variation on the vitamin D content of meat and meat products.

Low intakes of meat and meat products emerged as an independent risk factor for Asian rickets and absent intakes of meat and meat products emerged as an independent risk factor for Asian osteomalacia (Dunnigan and Henderson, 1997). It has been hypothesised by this research group that there may be a 'magic factor' in meat which is protective against rickets and osteomalacia. In Glasgow, at the beginning of the century, the incidence of rickets was high, whereas, between 1987 and 1991, only one case of rickets was reported. This may be explained by the fact that today infants are weaned onto an omnivorous diet from four months of age and this meat inclusion is offering protection against rickets (Dunnigan and Henderson, 1997). Obviously, much more research is required to improve our knowledge on this subject matter. It is also of interest to note that signs of both iron and vitamin D deficiency can occur simultaneously among toddlers (Lawson and Thomas, 1999). For instance, during the winter, half of the toddlers had both low vitamin D and low iron levels (Lawson and Thomas, 1999). Such evidence highlights the potential protective role that meat inclusion can play in a toddler's diet. It is important for toddlers and children to eat foods rich in both iron and vitamin D such as meat and meat products as well as playing out of doors to get sunlight.

9.12 Future trends

As we begin the twenty-first century, we look to the future to predict the likely nutritional problems we will need to tackle. The four major nutritional problems today are heart disease, hypertension, obesity and diabetes. These are likely to remain significant public health problems in the future. The demographic structure of the population is changing. Throughout Europe, both birth and death dates are falling, people are living longer and it is estimated that by the year 2030 more than half the population living in the UK will be over 50 years of age. With this knowledge we shall try to ascertain the likely future nutritional role of meat.

This chapter clearly outlines ways to reduce the fat content of meat and manipulate its fatty acid composition. The meat that is on sale today has never been leaner. Fortunately, most of the valuable nutrients of meat are located in the lean component, so reducing the visible fat of meat has little bearing on its micronutrient status. Researchers are focusing on ways of further improving the fatty acid composition of meat, using the knowledge that grass feeding results in high levels of both n-3 PUFAs and CLA content. Both n-3 PUFAs and CLA may have many possible benefits for human health, and in particular may offer protection against predicted future health problems (Cordain et al, 2002). N-3 PUFAs, in particular those that have very long chains, are cardioprotective and have anti-inflammatory and anti-tumourigenic properties. CLA can prevent formation and slow the growth for tumour development (Ip et al, 1994), reduce atherosclerosis development (Lee et al, 1994) and can help normalise blood glucose levels, which may be shown to prevent adult-onset diabetes (Houseknecht et al, 1998). Studies in human subjects are needed before we realise fully the benefits of CLA on human health. The fat and fatty acid story for meat so far is positive and only research and time will tell whether this story will be further improved.

The prevalence of overweight and obesity is increasing steadily in many developed countries. In the UK, over a quarter of the population are either overweight or obese. Obesity is a risk factor for many conditions. During a 10-year follow-up study, the incidence of colon cancer, diabetes, heart disease, hypertension, stroke (men only) and gallstones increased in line with the degree of overweight among adults (Field et al, 2001). Thus, reducing the incidence of overweight and obesity is a major public health priority. A positive energy balance is the cause of practically all cases of overweight and obesity. Factors regulating food intake are hunger, appetite, satiation and satiety.

Meat-containing meals have higher satiety values than vegetable containing meals (Barkeling et al, 1990). Research needs to be undertaken to determine whether meat can play a role in curtailing obesity, as a result of its high satiety value. Media hype about CLA has concentrated on its ability to reduce body fat and increase lean body mass. Studies have noted that CLA induces a relative decrease in body fat and an increase in lean muscle (Park et al, 1997; West et al, 1998). Trials are currently taking place to confirm whether or not these benefits occur in humans. Lean meat is already low in fat, but other attributes such as its high satiety value and the CLA it contains may be used in the future to market meat as a food that can help to reduce overweight and obesity. Furthermore, the capacity of meat to encourage greater vegetable and salad consumption, due to the way it is eaten, should not be overlooked in this regard.

An increase in the incidence of hip fractures is an inevitable consequence of people living longer. Research has shown that an increase in meat protein consumption among elderly women correlates with a decrease in the risk of hip fracture (French et al, 1997). Decreasing the risk of hip fracture is a public health priority. Vegetarian women tended to have lower spinal bone mineral density than non-vegetarians (Barr et al, 1998). Dunnigan and Henderson (1997) suggested that there may be a 'magic factor' in meat protecting against rickets and osteomalacia. To suggest that meat plays a role in bone health is relatively new and exciting and warrants further investigation.

Another emerging benefit for meat is that it supplies selenium. Up to the middle part of the last century the main source of selenium in the diet was from wheat-containing products. Wheat, which was imported mainly from the United States, was high in selenium. Nowadays, there is a much greater reliance on European wheat, which is much lower in selenium. This has resulted in the fact that our intake of selenium has decreased steadily during the past fifty years, but the proportion of selenium we get from meat has increased. Recent studies have found that selenium may reduce the risk of heart disease and certain types of cancer such as prostate and enhance the body's ability to fight infections.

Meat does provide a wide range of valuable nutrients, for example, one study has shown that young women consuming a high meat diet have greater intakes of thiamine, niacin, zinc and iron than those consuming a low meat diet (Ortega et al, 1998). In a review on optimal iron intakes, iron contained in animal foods is far better assimilated than that from vegetarian foods (Cook, 1999). Meat is one of the richest natural sources of glutathione, an important reducing agent providing a major cellular defence against a variety of toxicological and pathological processes. Moderate levels of glutathione are found in fruit and vegetables and low levels are present in dairy and cereal products. Glutathione inhibits formation of mutagens in model systems (Trompeta and O'Brien, 1998). It also maintains ascorbate in a reduced and functional form. Glutathione importance in the defence against chronic disease provides positive potential for meat and merits further research (Bronzetti, 1994; Trompeta and O'Brien, 1998).

There has never before been such a wide variety and choice of food on sale in western societies and in the recent past we have seen the development of functional foods. A functional food can be loosely described as a food that provides a health benefit beyond its basic nutritional content. In the United States beef and lamb are now described as functional foods (ADA, 1999), because of the CLA they contain. At a Meat Marketing/Communication Workshop, Dr Lynne Cobiac (CSIRO) (Cobiac, 2000) described some nutritive and non-nutritive meat components that may have potential health-promoting properties. They are summarised as follows:

- *Lipoic acid* has antioxidant properties and has been shown to be beneficial in diabetics and in the prevention of cataract development in animal models and cell lines. Organ meats contain higher quantities of lipoic acid than muscle meats.
- *Carnosine* is a dipeptide composed of alanine and histidine. Carnosine is found in meats and its antioxidant properties may confer some protection against oxidative stress. It's an anti-inflammatory agent and has anti-tumourigenic properties in rats and it also plays a role in cellular homeostasis.
- *Biogenic amines* are naturally formed from bacterial decarboxylation of amino acids or natural decarboxylase activity. They have been linked with improving gut health and cognitive performance.
- *Nucleotides* are added to enteral feeds to enhance the general immune function. Organ meats are good sources of nucleotides.
- *Glutathione* is a tripeptide containing the sulphur amino acid cysteine. Glutathione may be the 'meat factor' which enhances non-haem iron absorption.
- *Choline* is now termed a nutrient. In the United States, it is an essential nutrient and the estimated adequate intake is 550 mg/day for men and 425 mg/day for women. Choline is a precursor of the neurotransmitter acetylcholine, it is necessary for central nervous system development, folate/homocysteine metabolism, it plays a role in the immune system, fat metabolism and improves athletic performance. Beef and in particular liver is one of the richest sources of choline.
- *Carnitine* is composed of lysine and methionine. Seventy-five percent of carnitine comes from the diet, mainly from red meat, lamb being a particularly good source. Carnitine carries the long chain fatty acids to the mitochondria for oxidation to give energy and thus can be used to improve athletic performance. It also has antioxidant capabilities and it may be critical for normal brain development by providing acetyl groups to synthesise acetylcholine, a neurotransmitter.

This range of meat components may have the ability to fight against certain cancers, CHD, anaemia and cataracts, enhance immunity and cognition, improve gut and bone health, regulate body weight and may be used in sports nutrition. However, a lot of the evidence indicating beneficial effects of these components comes from animal or cell culture models. Research will have to be conducted in humans to demonstrate their effect on human health. But even glancing at the amount of 'potential' components present in meat does indicate a positive and competitive future for meat.

However, when looking to the future we must also try and visualise what changes are likely to occur that may influence meat consumption. Traditionally, food purchase was predominantly influenced by price and sustenance. Current and future food choice depends on these values but they lie alongside other factors such as health, food safety, convenience and welfare concerns. Changes in our social patterns, such as moving away from the formal family meat-eating patterns to a 'grazing' or 'snacking' habit, will become much more apparent. Increasing loss of culinary skills is already evident and is likely to rise. The market will demand more convenience and processed meat products in place of traditional cuts of meats. Eating outside the home will place a greater emphasis on the catering sector as food providers. Availability of 'exotic' meats will escalate. Demand for organic meat is expected to rise. Competition from other foods will intensify. The emergence of more functional foods is likely to occur. These are some of the factors that will sculpt the future demand for meat and meat products. Meat must adapt to the changing environment. However, the emphasis between food choice and health was never as great and is likely to become even more important. In the past meat responded to consumer demands by decreasing its fat content. Meat is a versatile food. However, it is time that we banish the misinformation that surrounds the nutritional value of meat. Meat is a relatively low fat nutrient dense food.

> Meat and meat products are an integral part of the UK diet and for those who choose to consume meat, it makes a valuable contribution to nutritional intakes.
> (BNF, 1999).

9.13 Conclusion

There has been considerable emotive and public health debate over the last two decades on the relative importance of meat in the diet of modern humans. Early dismissive arguments have more recently been revisited and challenged as a result of the continual progress and review of nutritional science. The early focus on fat as the predominant cause of western style diseases of affluence led, naïvely, to meat being blamed for diet related problems. More recently, the focus on the diets of our ancestors has effectively reversed this thinking and lean red meat has been rediscovered as a mainstay of human diet evolution. The serious health concerns resulting from the epidemic rise in CHD, obesity, diabetes and cancers require more carefully guided public health advice, based on a holistic approach to diet and lifestyle.

Lean meat can be seen as the ultimate natural functional food. Eaten in moderate quantities as part of a meal along with sufficient plant foods, it provides a valuable, arguably essential nutrient-dense supplement to the diet with beneficial effects for health, both in the short and long term. As a key ingredient of modern processed pre-prepared meals, meat, when added as a quality ingredient, can enhance the nutritional benefits of the food product and make a significant, positive contribution to our health. It would be naïve to ignore this potential.

9.14 References

AGGETT P J and COMERFORD J G (1995), 'Zinc and Human Health', *Nutrition Reviews*, **53**, S16–S22

ALLEN L (1997), 'Pregnancy and iron deficiency: unresolved issues', *Nutrition Reviews*, **55**(4), 91–101

ALLEN L H and CASTERLINE J (1994), 'Vitamin B_{12} deficiency in elderly individuals: diagnosis and requirements', *American Journal of Clinical Nutrition*, **60**, 12–14

AMERICAN DIETETIC ASSOCIATION (1993), 'Position of the American Dietetic Association: vegetarian diets', *Journal of The American Dietetic Association*, 1317–19

AMERICAN DIETETIC ASSOCIATION REPORT (1999), 'Position of the American Dietetic Association: functional foods', *Journal of The American Dietetic Association*, **99**, 1278–85

ARMSTRONG B and DOLL R (1975), 'Environmental factors and the incidence and mortality from cancer in different countries with special reference to dietary practices', *International Journal of Cancer*, **15**, 617–31

AZEVEDO L F, SALGUEIRO L F, CLARO R, TEIXEIRA-PINTO A and COSTA-PEREIRA A (1999), 'Diet and gastric cancer in Portugal – a multivariate model', *European Journal of Cancer Prevention*, **8**, 41–8

BAIK H W and RUSSELL R M (1999), 'Vitamin B_{12} deficiency in the elderly', *Annual Reviews of Nutrition*, **19**, 357–77

BALL M and ACKLAND M (2000), 'Zinc intake and status in Australian vegetarians', *British Journal of Nutrition*, **83**, 27–33

BALL M and BARTLETT M (1999), 'Dietary intake and iron status of Australian vegetarian women', *American Journal of Clinical Nutrition*, **70**, 353–8

BARKELING B, ROSSNER S and BJORVELL H (1990), 'Effects of a high protein meal (meat) and a high carbohydrate meal (vegetarian) on satiety measured by automated computerized monitoring of subsequent food intake, motivation to eat and food preferences', *International Journal of Obesity*, **14**, 743–51

BARR S I, PRIOR J C, JANELLE K C and LENTLE B C (1998), 'Spinal bone mineral density in premenopausal vegetarian and nonvegetarian women: cross-sectional and prospective comparisons', *Journal of the American Dietetic Association*, **98**(7), 760–5

BEARD J and STOLTZFUS R (2001), 'Foreward – iron deficiency anaemia: reexamining the nature and magnitude of the public health problem', *Journal of Nutrition*, **131**, 563S

BEAUCHESNE-RONDEAU E, GASCON A, BERGERON J and JACQUES H (1999), 'Lean beef in lipid lowering diet: effects on plasma cholesterol and lipoprotein B in hypercholesterolaemic men', *Canadian Journal of Dietetic Practice and Research*, **60**, June Supplement

BELURY M A (1995), 'Conjugated dienoic linoleate: a polyunsaturated fatty acid with unique chemoprotective properties', *Nutrition Reviews*, **53**, 83–9

BINGHAM S A (1996), 'Epidemiology and mechanisms relating to risk of colorectal cancer', *Nutrition Research Reviews*, **9**, 197–239

BLACK et al (1997), 'Cancer incidence and mortality in the European Union. Cancer registry data and cancer incidence for 1990', *European Journal of Cancer*, **33**, 1075–107

BONANOME A and GRUNDY S M (1988), 'Effect of dietary stearic acid on plasma cholesterol and lipoprotein levels', *New England Journal of Medicine*, **318**, 1244–8

BRAND-MILLER J and COLAGIURI S (1994), 'The carnivore connection: dietary carbohydrate in the evolution of NIDDM', *Diabetologia*, **37**, 1280–6

BRITISH NUTRITION FOUNDATION (1996), *Diet and heart disease: a round table of facts*, 2ed, M Ashwell (ed), BNF, London

BRITISH NUTRITION FOUNDATION (1999), *Meat in the Diet,* Briefing Paper, BNF, London

BRITISH NUTRITION FOUNDATION'S TASK FORCE (1995), *Trans fatty Acids – the Report of the BNF Task Force*, BNF. London

BRONZETTI G (1994), 'Antimutagens In Food', *Trends in Food Science and Technology*, 5 December, 390–5

BURGESS L, HACKETT A F, MAXWELL S and ROUNCEFIELD M (2001), 'The nutrient intakes of vegetarian and omnivorous adolescents in North-West England', *Proceedings of the Nutrition Society*, **60**(4), 69A

BURR M L (1988), 'Heart Disease In British Vegetarians', *American Journal of Clinical Nutrition*, **48**, 30–2

CHAN W, BROWN J, LEE S M and BUSS D H (1995), 'Meat, poultry and game', *Supplement to McCance and Widdowson's 'The Composition of Foods'*, Cambridge Royal Society of Chemistry and London, Ministry of Agriculture, Fisheries and Food, HMSO London

CHAN W, BROWN J, CHURCH S M and BUSS D H (1996), 'Meat Products and Dishes' *Supplement to McCance and Widdowson's 'The Composition Of Foods'*, Cambridge Royal Society Of Chemistry and London, Ministry Of Agriculture Fisheries And Foods HMSO London

CHIN S F, LIU W, STORKSON J M, HA Y L and PARIZA M W (1992), 'Dietary sources of conjugated dienoic isomers of linoleic acid, a newly recognized class of anticarcinogens', *Journal of Food Composition and Analysis*, **5**, 185–97

CHIZZOLINI R, ZANARDI E, DORIGONI V and GHIDINI S (1999), 'Calorific value and cholesterol content of normal and low fat meat and meat products', *Trends in Food Science and Technology*, **10**, 119–28

COBIAC L (2000), 'Could red meat be a functional food of the future?' MARKETING/COMMUNICATION WORKSHOP, July 6–7, 2000, Organised by the International Meat Secretariat and hosted by The Meat and Livestock Commission

COMMITTEE ON MEDICAL ASPECTS OF FOOD POLICY (1984), *Diet and Cardiovascular Disease: Report on Health and Social Subjects*, No. 28, Department of Health and Social Security, HMSO London

COMMITTEE ON MEDICAL ASPECTS OF FOOD POLICY (1991), 'Dietary Reference Values for Food, Energy and Nutrients for the United Kingdom', *Report of the Panel on Dietary Reference Values*, No. 41, HMSO London

COMMITTEE ON MEDICAL ASPECTS OF FOOD POLICY (1994), 'Nutritional Aspects of Cardiovascular Disease', *Report of the working group on diet and cancer*, No. 46, HMSO London

COMMITTEE ON MEDICAL ASPECTS OF FOOD POLICY (1998), 'Nutritional Aspects of the Development of Cancer', *Report of the working group on diet and cancer of the Committee on Medical Aspects of Food and Nutrition Policy*, No 48, HMSO London

COOK J D (1999), 'Defining optimal body iron', *Proceedings of the Nutrition Society*, **58**, 489–95

COOK J D and MONSEN E R (1976), 'Food iron absorption in human subjects III. Comparison of the effect of animal proteins on non-haem iron absorption', *American Journal of Clinical Nutrition*, **29**, 859–67

CORDAIN L, WATKINS B A, FLORANT G L, KELHER M, ROGERS L and LI Y (2002), 'Fatty acid analysis of wild ruminant tissues: evolutionary implications for reducing diet-related chronic disease', *European Journal of Clinical Nutrition*, **56**(3)

CORDAIN L, BRAND-MILLER J, EATON S B, MANN N J, HOLT S H and SPETH J D (2000), 'Plant-animal subsistence ratios and macronutrient energy estimations in worldwide hunter-gatherer diets', *American Journal of Clinical Nutrition*, **71**, 682–92

COX B D and WHICHELOW M J (1997), 'Frequent consumption of red meat is not a risk factor for cancer', *British Medical Journal*, **315**, 1018

DAVIDSON M H, HUNNINGHAKE D, MAKI K C, KWITEROVICH P O and KAFONEK S (1999), 'Comparison of the effects of lean red meat vs lean white meat on serum lipid levels among free-living persons with hypercholesterolaemia', *Archives of Internal Medicine* **159**, 1331–8

DAVIDSON S and PASSMORE R (1969), 'Human nutrition and dietetics', London, Churchill Livingstone

DE LUCA H F and ZIEROLD C (1998), 'Mechanisms and functions of vitamin D', *Nutrition Reviews*, **56**(2), S4–S10

DEPARTMENT OF HEALTH (1991), *Dietary Reference Values for Food Energy and Nutrients for the United Kingdom*, Report on Health and social subjects 41, London, HMSO

DEPARTMENT OF HEALTH (1994a), *Weaning and the Weaning Diet*, Report On Health And Social Subjects 45, London, HMSO

DEPARTMENT OF HEALTH (1994b), *Eat Well! an Action Plan from the Nutrition Task Force to Achieve the Health of The Nation Targets on Diet and Nutrition*, HMSO, London

DEPARTMENT OF HEALTH (1998a), *Nutrition and Bone Health*, Report On Health And Social Subjects 49, The Stationery Office, London

DEPARTMENT OF HEALTH (1998b), *Nutrition and Bone Health: with Particular Reference to Calcium and Vitamin D*. Committee on the Medical Aspects of Food and Nutrition Policy. Working Group on the Nutritional Status of the Population Subgroup on Bone Health. The Stationery Office, London

DEPARTMENT OF HEALTH (1998c), *Nutritional Aspects of the Development of Cancer*, Report On Health And Social Subjects 48, The Stationery Office, London

DRAKE R, REDDY S and DAVIES G J (1999a), 'Dietary and supplement intake of vegetarians during pregnancy', *American Journal of Clinical Nutrition*, **70**(suppl), 627S

DRAKE R, REDDY S and DAVIES G J (1999b), 'Health of vegetarians during pregnancy and pregnancy outcome', *American Journal of Clinical Nutrition*, **70**(suppl), 628S

DRAPER A (1991), 'The energy and nutrient intakes of different types of vegetarians: a case for supplements', *British Journal of Nutrition*, **69**, 3–19

DUNNIGAN M G and HENDERSON J B (1997), 'An epidemiological model of privational rickets and osteomalacia', *Proceedings of the Nutrition Society*, **56**, 939–56

DUO LI, NG A, MANN N J and SINCLAIR A J (1998), 'Contribution of meat fat to dietary arachidonic acid', *Lipids*, **33**(4), 437–40

EDMOND A M, HAWKINS N, PENNICK C, GOLDING J and the ALSPAC CHILDREN IN FOCUS TEAM (1996), 'Haemoglobin and ferritin concentrations in infants at 8 months of age', *Archives of Disease in Childhood*, **74**, 36–9

ENSER M, HALLETT K, HEWITT B, FURSEY G A J and WOOD J D (1996), 'Fatty acid content and composition of English beef, lamb and pork at retail', *Meat Science*, **42**(4), 443–56

ENSER M, HALLETT K G, HEWITT B, FURSEY G A J, WOOD J D and HARRINGTON G (1998), 'Fatty acid content and composition of UK beef and lamb muscle in relation to production system and implications for human nutrition', *Meat Science*, **49**, 329–41

FAIRWEATHER-TAIT S J (1989), 'Iron in foods and its availability', *Acta Paediatrica Scand*, Suppl. **361**, 12–20

FIELD A E, COAKLEY E H, MUST A, SPADANO J L, LAIRD N, DIETZ W H, RIMM E and COLDITZ G A (2001), 'Impact of overweight on the risk of developing common chronic diseases during a 10-year period', *Archives of Internal Medicine*, **161**(13), 1581–6

FINCH S, DOYLE W, LOWE C, BATES C J, PRENTICE A, SMITHERS G and CLARKE P C (1998), 'National diet and nutrition survey: people aged 60 years and over', London HMSO

FRASER D R (1995), 'Vitamin D', *Lancet*, **345**, 104–7

FRENCH S A, FOLSOM A R, JEFFERY R W, ZHENG W, MINK P J and BAXTER J E (1997), 'Weight variability and incident disease in older women: the Iowa Women's Health Study', *International Journal of Obesity Related Metabolic Disorders*, **21**(3), 217–23

FRITSCHE J and STEINHART H (1998), 'Amounts of conjugated linoleic acid (CLA) in German foods and evaluation of daily intake', *Z Lebensm Unters Forsch A*, **206**, 77–82

GAVINO V C, GAVINO G, LEBLANC M and TUCHWEBER B (2000), 'An isomeric mixture of conjugated linoleic acids but not pure *cis*-9, *trans*-11-octadecadienoic acid affects body weight gain and plasma lipids in hamsters', *Journal of Nutrition*, **130**, 27–9

GIBSON S and ASHWELL M (2001), 'Implications for reduced red and processed meat consumption for iron intakes among British women', *Proceedings of the Nutrition Society*, **60**(4), 60A

GIBSON S A and ASHWELL M (1997), 'New Vitamin D values for meat and their implication for vitamin D intake in British adults', *Proceedings of the Nutrition Society*, **56**, 116A

GISSI-PREVENZIONE INVESTIGATORS (1999), 'Dietary supplementation with n-3 PUFAs and vitamin E after myocardial infarction: results of the GISSI-Prevenzione trial', *Lancet*, **354**, 447–55

GREGORY J, FOSTER K, TYLER H and WISEMAN M (1990), *The Dietary and Nutritional Survey of British Adults*, London HMSO

GREGORY J, LOWE S, BATES C J, PRENTICE A, JACKSON L V, SMITHERS G, WENLOCK R and FARRON M (2000), *National Diet and Nutrition Survey: Young People aged 4 to 18 years*, London, The Stationery Office

GREGORY J R, CLARKE P C, COLLINS D L, DAVIES P S W and HUGHES J M (1995), *National Diet and Nutrition Survey; Children aged 1½ To 4½ years*, London HMSO

HALLBERG L, BRUNE M and ROSSANDER L (1989), 'Iron absorption in man: ascorbic acid and dose dependent inhibition by phytate', *American Journal of Clinical Nutrition*, **49**, 140–4

HAMMOCK D A (1987), 'The red meat in our diet – good or bad?' in: *Nutrition 87/88*, C C Cook Fuller (ed.) Sushkin Publishing group, Guildford, Conn, 16–18

HAZELL T, LEDWARD D A and NEALE R J (1978), 'Iron availability from meat', *British Journal of Nutrition*, **39**, 631–8

HIGGINSON J (1966), 'Etiological factors in gastrointestinal cancer in man', *Journal – National Cancer Institute*, **37**, 527–45

HIGGS J D (2000), 'An overview of the compositional changes in red meat over the last 20 years and how these have been achieved', *Food Science and Technology Today*, **14**(1), 22–6

HIGGS J D and PRATT J (1998), 'Meat poultry and meat products: Nutritional Value', Volume 2, 1272–82, in *The Encyclopaedia Of Human Nutrition*, M J Sadler, J J Strain and B Cabalerro (eds), Academic Press Limited, London

HILL A J and BLUNDELL J E (1986), 'Macronutrients and satiety: the effects of a high protein or high carbohydrates meal on subjective motivation to eat and food preferences', *Nutrition and Behavior*, **3**, 133–4

HILL M J (1999a), 'Meat and colorectal cancer', *Proceedings of the Nutrition Society*, **58**, 261–4

HILL M J (1999b), 'Meat and colorectal cancer: a European perspective', *European Journal of Cancer Prevention*, **8**, 183–5

HILL M J (2000), 'Meeting Report: meat and nutrition', Hamburg: 17–18 October 2000, *European Journal of Cancer Prevention*, **9**, 465–70

HIRAYAMA T (1986), 'A large scale cohort study on cancer risks by diet – with special reference to the risk reducing effects of green-yellow vegetable consumption' in T Hayashi et al (eds), *Diet Nutrition and Cancer*, Tokyo, Japan Sci Soc Press and Utrecht, VNU SCI Press 41–53

HIRAYAMA T (1990), *Lifestyle and Mortality: a Large scale Census based Study in Japan*, Basle, Karger

HOUSEKNECHT K L, VANDEN HEUVEL J P, MOYA-CAMARENA S Y, PORTOCARRERO C P, PECK L W, NICKEL K P and BELURY M A (1998), 'Dietary conjugated linoleic acid normalises impaired glucose tolerance in the Zucker diabetic fatty *fa/fa* rat', *Biochemical and Biophysical Research Communications*, **244**, 678–82

HULSHOF K F, VAN ERP-BAART M A, ANTTOLAINEN M, BECKER W, CHURCH S M, COUET C, HERMANN-KUNZ E, KESTELOOT H, LETH T, MARTINS I, MOREIRAS O, MOSCHANDREAS J, PIZZOFERRATO L, RIMESTAD A H, THORGEIRSDOTTIR H, VAN AMELSVOORT J M, ARO A, KAFATOS A G, LANZMANN-PETITHORY D and VAN POPPEL G (1999), 'Intake of fatty acids in western Europe with emphasis on *trans* fatty acids: the TRANSFAIR Study', *European Journal of Clinical Nutrition*, **53**(2), 143–57

HUNT J R, GALLAGHER S K, JOHNSON L K and LYKKEN G I (1995), 'High- versus low-meat diets: effects on zinc absorption, iron status, and calcium, copper, iron, magnesium, manganese, nitrogen, phosphorus, and zinc balance in postmenopausal women', *American Journal of Clinical Nutrition*, **62**, 621–32

IP C and SCIMECA J A (1997), 'Conjugated linoleic acid and linoleic acid are distinctive modulators of mammary carconogenesis', *Nutrition and Cancer*, **27**(2), 131–5

IP C, CHIN S F, SCIMECA J A and PARIZA M W (1991), 'Mammary cancer prevention by conjugated dienoic derivative of linoleic acid', *Cancer Research*, **51**, 6118–24

IP C, SINGH M, THOMPSON H J and SCIMECA J A (1994), 'Conjugated linoleic acid suppresses mammary carcinogenesis and proliferative activity of the mammary gland in the rat', *Cancer Research*, **54**, 1212–15

IP M M, MASSO-WELCH P A, SHOEMAKER S F, SHEA-EATON W K and IP C (1999), 'Conjugated linoleic acid inhibits proliferation and induces apoptosis of normal rat mammary epithelial cells in primary culture', *Experimental Cell Research*, **250**, 22–34

JOHNSON J M and WALKER P M (1992), 'Zinc and iron utilization in young women consuming a beef-based diet', *Journal of the American Dietetic Association*, **12**, 1474–8

JONES D P (1995), 'Glutathione distribution in natural products', *Methods in Enzymology*, **252**, 3–13

KAPSOKEFALOU M and MILLER D D (1991), 'Effects of meat and selected food components on the valence of non-haem iron during *in vitro* digestion', *Journal of Food Science*, **56**, 352–8

KAPSOKEFALOU M and MILLER D D (1993), 'Lean beef and beef fat interact to enhance non-haem iron absorption in rats', *Journal of Nutrition*, **123**, 1429–34

KAPSOKEFALOU M and MILLER D D (1995), 'Iron speciation in intestinal contents of rats fed meals composed of meat and non-meat sources of protein and fat', *Food Chemistry*, **52**, 47–56

KELLY F D, MANN N J, TURNER A H and SINCLAIR A J (1999), 'Stearic acid-rich diets do not increase thrombotic risk factors in healthy males', *Lipids*, **34**, S199

KELLY F D, SINCLAIR A J, MANN N J, TURNER A H, ABEDIN L and LI D (2001), 'A stearic acid-rich diet improves thrombogenic and atherogenic risk factor profiles in healthy males', *European Journal of Clinical Nutrition*, **55**, 88–96

KEY T J, FRASER G E, DAVEY G K, THOROGOOD M, APPLEBY P N, BERAL V, REEVES G, BURR M L, CHANG-CLAUDE J, FRENTZEL-BEYNE R, KUZMA J W, MANN J and MCPHERSON K (1998), 'Mortality in vegetarians and non-vegetarians: a collaborative analysis of 8300 deaths among 76 000 men and women in five prospective studies', *Public Health Nutrition*, **1**(1), 33–41

KEY T J, FRASER G E, THOROGOOD M, APPLEBY P N, BERAL V, REEVES G, BURR M L, CHANG-CLAUDE J, FRENTZEL-BEYME R, KUZMA J W, MANN J and MCPHERSON K (1999), 'Mortality in vegetarians and non-vegetarians: detailed findings from a collaborative analysis of 5 prospective studies', *American Journal of Clinical Nutrition*, **70**(suppl), 516S–524S

KEY T J, DAVEY G K and APPLEBY P N (1999), 'Health benefits of a vegetarian diet' in *Meat or Wheat for the Next Millennium? Proceedings of the Nutrition Society*, **58**(2), 271–5

KOHLMEIER L, SIMMANSEN N and MOTTINS K (1995), 'Dietary modifiers of carcinogenesis', *Environmental Health Perspectives*, **103** Supplement 8, 180–4

KRAJCOVICOVA-KUDLACKOVA M, BLAZICEK P, KOPCOVA J, BEDEROVA A and BABINSKA K (2000), 'Homocysteine levels in vegetarians versus omnivores', *Annual Nutrition Metabolism*, **44**, 135–8

KRAMER J K G, PARODI P W, JENSEN R G, MOSSOBA M M, YURAWECZ M P and ADLOF R O (1998), 'Rumenic acid: a proposed common name for the major conjugated linoleic acid isomer found in natural products', *Lipids*, **33**, 835

LARSSON C L and JOHANSSON G (2001), 'Dietary intake and nutritional status of young vegans and omnivores in Sweden', *Proceedings of the Nutrition Society*, **60**(4), 69A

LAWSON M and THOMAS M (1999), 'Vitamin D concentrations in Asian children aged 2 years living in England: population survey', *British Medical Journal*, **318**, 28–9

LEE K N, KRITCHEVSKY D and PARIZA M W (1994), 'Conjugated linoleic acid and atherosclerosis in rabbits', *Atherosclerosis*, **108**, 19–25

LEEDS A R, RANDLE A and MATTHEWS K R (1997), 'A study into the practice of trimming fat from meat at the table, and the development of new study methods', *Journal of Human Nutrition and Dietetics*, **10**, 245–51

LI D, SINCLAIR A, MANN N, TURNER A, BALL M, KELLY F, ABEDIN L and WILSON A (1999), 'The association of diet and thrombotic risk factors in healthy male vegetarians and meat-eaters', *European Journal of Clinical Nutrition*, **53**, 612–19

LYLE R M, WEAVER C M, SEDLOCK D A, RAJARAM S, MARTIN B and MELBY C L (1992), 'Iron status in exercising women: the effect of oral iron therapy vs increased consumption of muscle foods', *American Journal of Clinical Nutrition*, **56**(6), 1049–55

MA D W L, WIERZBICKI A A, FIELD C J and CLANDININ M T (1999), 'Conjugated linoleic acid in Canadian dairy and beef products', *Journal of Agricultural and Food Chemistry*, **47**(5), 1956–60

MANN N J (2001a), 'The evidence for high meat intake during the evolution of hominids', *Proceedings of the Nutrition Society*, **60**, 61A

MANN N J (2001b), 'Effect of vitamin B_{12} status on homocysteine levels in healthy male subjects', *Proceedings of the Nutrition Society*, **60**, 58A

MANN N J, SINCLAIR A J, PILLE M, JOHNSON L, WARRICK G, REDER E and LORENZ R (1997), 'The effect of short term diets rich in fish, red meat or white meat on thromboxane and prostacyclin synthesis in humans', *Lipids*, **32**(6), 635–43

MANN N J, LI D, SINCLAIR A J, DUDMAN N P, GUO X W, ELSWORTH G R, WILSON A K and KELLY F D (1999), 'The effect of diet on plasma homocysteine concentrations in healthy male subjects', *European Journal of Clinical Nutrition*, **53**(11), 895–9

MCKINLEY M C, MCNULTY H, MCPARTLIN J, STRAIN J J, PENTIEVA K, WARD M, WEIR D G and SCOTT J M (2001), 'Low dose vitamin B_6 effectively lowers fasting plasma homocysteine in healthy elderly persons who are folate and riboflavin replete', *American Journal of Clinical Nutrition*, **73**, 759–64

MEAT AND LIVESTOCK COMMISSION and ROYAL SOCIETY OF CHEMISTRY (1990), *The Chemical Composition Of Pig Meat*. Report to the Ministry Of Agriculture, Fisheries and Food on the Trial to Determine the Chemical Composition of Fresh and Cured Pork from British Pigs of Different Breed Types, Sexes and Origins. Milton Keynes, Meat And Livestock Commission

MILLS A and TYLER H (1992), *Food and Nutrient Intakes of British Infants aged 6–12 months*, Ministry of Agriculture Fisheries and Food, HMSO, London

MILLWARD D J (1999), 'Meat or Wheat for the next millennium?', *Proceedings of the Nutrition Society*, **58**(2), 209–10

MINISTRY OF AGRICULTURE FISHERIES and FOOD (1981), *Household Food Consumption And Expenditure: 1979* National Food Survey Committee, London, HMSO

MINISTRY OF AGRICULTURE FISHERIES and FOOD (1999), *National Food Survey 1999*, London, The Stationery Office

MINISTRY OF AGRICULTURE FISHERIES AND FOOD, FOOD SAFETY DIRECTORATE (1992, 1993, 1995, 1998) *National Food Survey – Household Consumption for 1991, 1992, 1994, 1997*, London, MAFF

MIRA M, ALPERSTEIN G, KARR M, RANMUTHUGALA G, CAUSER J, NIEC A and LILBURNE A M (1996), 'Haem iron intake in 12–36 month old children depleted in iron: case-control study', *British Medical Journal*, **312**, 881–3

MULVIHILL B (1996), *The Effect of Meat Systems on the Bioavailability of Non-haem Iron*, PhD Thesis, University College Cork, Republic of Ireland

MULVIHILL B (2001), 'Ruminant meat as a source of conjugated linoleic acid (CLA)', *Nutrition Bulletin*, **26**(4), 295–300

MULVIHILL B and MORRISSEY P A (1998a), 'Influence of the sulphydryl content of animal proteins on *in vitro* bioavailability of non-haem iron', *Food Chemistry*, **61**(1–2), 1–7

MULVIHILL B and MORRISSEY P A (1998b), 'An investigation of factors influencing the bioavailability of non-haem iron from meat systems', *Irish Journal of Agricultural and Food Research*, **37**(2), 219–26

MULVIHILL B, KIRWAN F M, MORRISSEY P A and FLYNN A (1998), 'Effect of myofibrillar proteins on the *in vitro* bioavailability of non-haem iron', *International Journal of Food Science and Technology*, **49**, 187–92

NAKACHI K, IMAI K, HOSHIYAMA Y and SASABA T (1988), 'The joint effects of two factors in the aetiology of oesphageal cancer in Japan', *Journal of Epidemiology and Community Health*, **42**, 755–61

NATHAN I, HACKETT I F and KIRBY S (1994), 'Vegetarianism and health: is a vegetarian diet adequate for the growing child?', *Food Science and Technology Today*, **8**(1), 13–15

NATHAN I, HACKETT A F and KIRBY S (1996), 'The dietary intake of a group of vegetarian children aged 7–11 years compared with matched omnivores', *British Journal of Nutrition*, **75**(4), 533–44

NATHAN I, HACKETT I F and KIRBY S P (1997), 'A longitudinal study of the growth of matched pairs of vegetarian and omnivorous children aged 7–11 years in the north-west of England', *European Journal of Clinical Nutrition*, **51**, 20–5

NATIONAL ADVISORY COMMITTEE ON NUTRITION EDUCATION (1983), *Proposals For Nutritional Guidelines for Health Education in Britain*, London, Health Education Council

NATIONAL AUDIT OFFICE REPORT (2001), '*Tackling Obesity in England*', London, The Stationery Office

NELSON M (1996), 'Anaemia in adolescent girls: effects on cognitive function and activity', *Proceedings of the Nutrition Society*, **55**, 359–67

NELSON M, WHITE J and RHODES C (1993), 'Haemoglobin, ferritin, and iron intakes in British children aged 12–14 years: a preliminary investigation', *British Journal of Nutrition*, **70**, 147–55

NICOLOSI R J, ROGERS E J, KRITCHEVSKY D, SCIMECA J A and HITH P J (1997), 'Dietary conjugated linoleic acid reduces plasma lipoproteins and early aortic atherosclerosis in hypercholesterolemic hamsters', *Artery*, **22**(5), 266–77

O'DEA K (1991), Traditional diet and food preferences of Australian aboriginal hunter-gatherers', *Philosophical Transactions of the Royal Society of London, B Biological Sciences*, **334**, 233–41

O'DELL B L (1989), 'Bioavailability of trace elements', *Nutrition Reviews*, **42**, 301–8

ORTEGA R, LOPEZ-SOBALER A, REQUEJO A, QUINTAS M, GASPAR M, ANDRES P and NAVIA B (1998), 'The influence of meat consumption on dietary data, iron status and serum lipid parameters in young women', *International Journal for Vitamin and Nutrition Research* **68**, 255–62

O'SHEA M, LAWLESS F, STANTON C and DEVERY R (1998), 'Conjugated linoleic acid in bovine milk fat: a food-based approach to cancer chemoprevention', *Trends in Food Science and Technology*, **9**, 192–6

PARK Y, ALBRIGHT K J, LIU W, STORKSON J M, COOK M E and PARIZA M W (1997), 'Effect of conjugated linoleic acid on body composition in mice', *Lipids*, **32**, 853–8

RANA S K and SANDERS T A B (1986), 'Taurine concentrations in the diet, plasma, urine and breast milk of vegans compared with omnivores', *British Journal of Nutrition*, **56**, 17–27

REDDY S and SANDERS T A B (1990), 'Haemotological studies on pre-menstrual Indian and caucasian omnivores', *British Journal of Nutrition*, **64**, 331–8

REID R L and HACKETT A F (2001), 'A database of vegetarian convenience foods', *Proceedings of the Nutrition Society*, **60**(4), 4A

REQUEJO A M, NAVIA B, ORTEGA R M, LOPEZ-SOBALER A M, QUINTAS E, GASPAR M J and OSORIO O (1999), 'The age at which meat is first included in the diet affects the incidence of iron deficiency and ferropenic anaemia in a group of pre-school children from Madrid', *International Journal for Vitamin and Nutrition Research*, **69**(2), 127–31

ROYAL SOCIETY OF CHEMISTRY (1986), 'Nitrogen factors for pork', *Analyst*, **111**(8), 969–73

ROYAL SOCIETY OF CHEMISTRY (1993), 'Nitrogen factors for beef; a reassessment', *Analyst*, **118**(9), 1217–26

ROYAL SOCIETY OF CHEMISTRY (1996), 'Nitrogen factors for sheep meat', *Analyst*, **121**(7), 889–96

SANDERS T A B (1999), 'The nutritional adequacy of plant based diets' in 'Meat or wheat for the next millennium?' *Proceedings of The Nutrition Society*, **58**(2), 265–9

SANDERS T A B and REDDY S (1994), 'Vegetarian diets and children', *American Journal of Clinical Nutrition*, Supplement 59 **120**(4), 1176S–81S

SANDSTEAD H H (1995), 'Is zinc deficiency a public health problem?' *Nutrition*, **11**, 87–92

SANDSTEAD H H (2000), 'Causes of iron and zinc deficiencies and their effects on brain', *Journal of Nutrition*, **130**(2S Suppl), 347S–9S

SCOTT L E, KIMBALL K T, WITTELS E H, DUNN J K, BRAUCHI D J, POWNALL H J, HERD J A, SAVELL J W and PAPADOPOULOUS L S (1990), 'The effect of lean beef, chicken and fish on lipoprotein profile', in *63rd Scientific Sessions of the American Heart Association*, Nov 12–15, Dallas, Texas

SCOTTISH OFFICE DEPARTMENT OF HEALTH (1996), 'Eating for health – a diet action plan for Scotland', Edinburgh, HMSO

SCHRIMSHAW N S (1991), 'Iron deficiency', *Scientific American*, October, 24–30

SHANTHA N C, CRUM A D and DECKER E A (1994), 'Evaluation of conjugated linoleic acid concentrations in cooked beef', *Journal of Agricultural and Food Chemistry*, **42**, 1757–60

SHI B and SPALLHOLZ J E (1994), 'Selenium peroxidase is highly available as assessed by liver glutathione peroxidase activity and tissue selenium', *British Journal of Nutrition*, **72**(6), 873–81

SINCLAIR A J, JOHNSON L, O'DEA K and HOLMAN T (1994), 'Diets rich in lean beef increase the arachidonic acid and long chain n-3 PUFA levels in plasma phospholipids', *Lipids*, **29**(5), 337–43

SKOV A R, TOUBRO S, RONN B, HOLM L and ASTRUP A (1999a) 'Randomisd trial on protein vs carbohydrate in *ad Libitum* fat reduced diet for the treatment of obesity', *International Journal of Obesity*, **23**, 528–36

SKOV A R, TOUBRO S, BULOW J, KRABBE K, PARVING H-H and ASTRUP A (1999b) 'Changes in renal function during weight loss induced by high vs low-protein diets in overweight subjects', *International Journal of Obesity*, **23**, 1170–7

STUBBS R J (1995), 'Macronutrient effects on appetite', *International Journal of Obesity*, **19**, S11–19

SWAIN R (1995), 'An update on vitamin B_{12} metabolism and deficiency states', *The Journal of Family Practice*, **41**(6), 595–600

TAYLOR P G, MARTINEZ-TORRES C, ROMANO E L and LAYRISSE M (1986), 'The effect of cysteine-containing peptides released during meat digestion on iron absorption in humans', *American Journal of Clinical Nutrition*, **43**, 68–71

THOROGOOD M, MANN J, APPLEBY P and MCPHERSON K (1994), 'Risk of death from cancer and ischaemic heart disease in meat and non-meat eaters', *British Medical Journal*, **308**, 1667–71

TROMPETA V and O'BRIEN J (1998), 'Inhibition of mutagen formation by organosulphur compounds', *Journal of Agricultural and Food Chemistry*, **46**, 4318–23

TUYNS A J, RIBOLI E, DOORNBOS G and PEGUINOT G (1987), 'Diet and esophageal cancer in Calvados (France)', *Nutrition and Cancer*, **9**, 81–92

TUYNS A J et al (1992), 'Diet and gastric cancer. A case-control study in Belgium', *International Journal of Cancer*, Apr 22, **51**(1), 1–6

UHE A M, COLLIER G R and O'DEA K (1992), 'A comparison of the effects of beef, chicken and fish protein on satiety and amino acid profiles', *Journal of Nutrition*, **122**, 467–72

ULBRICHT T L V (1995), *Fat in the Food Chain*, A Report to The Ministry of Agriculture Fisheries and Food, April 1995, London, MAFF

ULBRICHT T L V and SOUTHGATE D A T (1991), 'Coronary heart disease: seven dietary factors', *Lancet*, **338**, 985–92

VAN DE VIJVER L P L, KARDINAAL A F M, COUET C, ARO A, KAFATOS A, STEINGRIMSDOITTIR L, AMORIM CRUZ J A, MOREIRAS O, BECKER W, VAN AMELSVOORT J M M, VIDAL-JESSEL S, SALMINEN I, MOSCHANDREAS J, SIGFUSSON N, MARTINS I, CARBAJAL, A, YTTERFORS A and VAN POPPEL G (2000), 'Association between *trans* fatty acid intake and cardiovascular risk factors in Europe: the TRANSFAIR study', *European Journal of Clinical Nutrition*, **54**, 126–35

WALKER A R P (1998), 'The remedying of iron deficiency: what priority should it have?' *British Journal of Nutrition*, **79**, 227–35

WATTS G, AHMED W, QUINEY J, HOULSTON R, JACKSON P, ILES C and LEWIS B (1988) 'Effective lipid lowering diets including lean meat', *British Medical Journal (Clin Res Ed)*, **296**(6617), 235–7

WEST D B, DELANY J P, CAMET P M, BLOHM F, TRUETT A A and SCIMECA J (1998), 'Effect of conjugated linoleic acid on body fat and energy metabolism in the mouse', *American Journal of Physiology*, **44**, R667–72

WHO (1990), *Diet, Nutrition and the prevention of chronic diseases*, Report of a WHO Study Group, WHO Technical Series 797, World Health Organisation, Geneva, Switzerland

WILSON A and BALL M (1999), 'Nutrient intake and iron status of Australian male vegetarians', *European Journal of Clinical Nutrition*, **53**, 189–94

WORLD CANCER RESEARCH FUND (1997), 'Food nutrition and the prevention of cancer: a global perspective', Washington DC, American Institute Of Cancer Research

ZEIGLER R G, MORRIS L E, BLOT W J, POTTERN L M, HOOVER R and FRAUMENI J F J (1981), 'Esophageal cancer among black men in Washington DC. II Role of nutrition', *Journal – National Cancer Institute*, **67**, 1199–206

ZHENG J J, MASON J B, ROSENBERG I H and WOOD R J (1993), 'Measurement of zinc bioavailability from beef and a ready-to-eat high-fiber breakfast cereal in humans: application of a whole-gut lavage technique', *American Journal of Clinical Nutrition*, **58**, 902–7

10

The stability of vitamins during food processing

P. Berry Ottaway, Berry Ottaway and Associates Ltd

10.1 Introduction

Vitamins, by their definition, are essential to health and have to be obtained from the diet on a regular basis because, with the exception of vitamin D, they cannot be produced by the body. In terms of medicine and nutrition, our knowledge of vitamins is relatively recent. Although James Lind discovered an association between limejuice and scurvy in 1753, it was over 170 years later that vitamin C was eventually isolated. The understanding of vitamin B_{12} goes back only to the 1950s and new roles for folates were still being discovered in the late 1990s. Man's supply of vitamins is obtained from a varied diet of vegetables, cereals, fruits and meats and the quantities of vitamins that are present in the dietary sources can be affected significantly by the processing and storage of the food.

10.2 The vitamins

Vitamins are a heterogeneous group of substances and are vital nutrients that must be obtained from the diet. Although a number of these were termed vitamins between the 1930s and 1950s, nutritional science now recognises only 13 substances, or groups of substances, as being true vitamins. The 13 substances are divided into two categories, the fat-soluble vitamins of which there are four (vitamins A, D, E and K) and the water-soluble vitamins of which there are nine (vitamins C, B_1, B_2, B_6, B_{12}, niacin, pantothenic acid and biotin). They are listed in Table 10.1. Even within the two sub-categories, the vitamins have almost no common attributes in terms of chemistry, function or daily requirements. In terms of requirements some, such as vitamins C, E and niacin, are needed in tens of

Table 10.1 Vitamins and some commonly used synonyms

Vitamin	Synonyms
Fat-soluble	
vitamin A	retinol
vitamin D_2	ergocalciferol
vitamin D_3	cholecalciferol
vitamin E	alpha, beta and gamma tocopherols and alpha tocotrienol
vitamin K_1	phylloquinone, phytomenadione
vitamin K_2	farnoquinone, menaquinone
vitamin K_3	menadione
Water-soluble	
vitamin B_1	thiamin
vitamin B_2	riboflavin
vitamin B_6	pyridoxal, pyridoxine, pyridoxamine
vitamin B_{12}	cobalamins, cyanocobalamin, hydroxocobalamin
niacin	nicotinic acid (vitamin PP)
niacinamide	nicotinamide (vitamin PP)
pantothenic acid	—
folic acid	folacin (vitamin M)
biotin	vitamin H
vitamin C	ascorbic acid

milligrams a day whilst others, such as vitamins D and B_{12}, are only needed in single microgram amounts. It can be seen from these examples that there is no relationship between the form of delivery (i.e. fat or water soluble) and the daily requirements. The heterogeneity also applies to the chemical structure and the functions of the vitamins. Chemically, there are no similarities between the substances. Some are single substances such as biotin, whilst others, such as vitamin E, are groups of compounds all exhibiting vitamin activity.

10.3 Factors affecting vitamin stability

One of the very few attributes that the vitamins have in common is that none is completely stable in foods. The stability of the individual vitamins varies from the relatively stable, such as in the case of niacin, to the relatively unstable, such as vitamin B_{12}. The factors that affect stability vary from vitamin to vitamin and the principal ones are summarised in Table 10.2. The most important of these factors are heat, moisture, oxygen, pH and light.

The deterioration of vitamins can take place naturally during the storage of vegetables and fruits and losses can occur during the processing and preparation

The stability of vitamins during food processing   249

Table 10.2 Factors affecting the stability of vitamins

Factor
• Temperature
• Moisture
• Oxygen
• Light
• pH
• Presence of metallic ions (e.g. copper, iron)
• Oxidising and reducing agents
• Presence of other vitamins
• Other components of food (e.g. sulphur dioxide)
• Combinations of the above

of foods and their ingredients, particularly those subjected to heat treatment. The factors that affect the degradation of vitamins are the same whether the vitamins are naturally occurring in the food or are added to the food from synthetic sources. However, the form in which a synthetic source is used (e.g. a salt or ester) may enhance its stability. For example, the vitamin E (tocopherol) esters are more stable than the tocopherol form itself.

With the increased use of nutritional labelling of food products, vitamin levels in foods have become the subject of label claims that can be easily checked by the enforcement authorities. This poses a number of problems for the food technologist. When more than one vitamin is the subject of a quantitative label claim for a food, it is very unlikely that the vitamins will deteriorate at the same rate. If the amounts of these vitamins are included in nutritional labelling, the shelf life of the food is determined by the life of the most unstable component.

In order to comply with the legal requirements of maintaining the label claim throughout the declared life of a food product, the food technologist needs to obtain a reasonably accurate estimation of the stability of each of the vitamins in the product. This has to be evaluated in the context of the food system (solid, liquid, etc.), the packaging and probable storage conditions and is achieved by conducting well-designed stability tests.

10.4 Fat-soluble vitamins

10.4.1 Vitamin A

Nutritionally, the human body can obtain its vitamin A requirements from two sources: from animal sources as forms of retinol, and from plant sources from β-carotene and related carotenoids. Both sources provide a supply of vitamin A, but by different metabolic pathways. In terms of stability the two sources are different from each other.

Vitamin A is one of the more labile vitamins and retinol is less stable than the retinyl esters. The presence of double bonds in its structure makes it subject to isomerisation, particularly in an aqueous medium at acid pH. The isomer with the highest biological activity is the all-*trans* vitamin A. The predominant *cis* isomer is 13-*cis* or neovitamin A which only has a biological activity of 75% of the all-*trans* isomer; and 6-*cis* and 2, 6-di-*cis* isomers which may also form during isomerisation have less than 25% of the biological activity of the all-*trans* form of vitamin A. The natural vitamin A sources usually contain about one-third neovitamin A while most synthetic sources generally contain considerably less. For aqueous products where isomerisation is known to occur, mixtures of vitamin A palmitate isomers at the equilibrium ratio have been produced commercially. Vitamin A is relatively stable in alkaline solutions.

Vitamin A is sensitive to atmospheric oxygen with the alcohol form being less stable than the esters. The decomposition is catalysed by the presence of trace minerals. As a consequence of its sensitivity to oxygen, vitamin A is normally available commercially as a preparation that includes an antioxidant and often a protective coating. While butylated hydroxyanisole (BHA) and butylated hydroxytoluene (BHT) are permitted in a number of countries for use as antioxidants in vitamin A preparations, the recent trend has been towards the use of tocopherols (vitamin E). Both retinol and its esters are inactivated by the ultraviolet component of light.

In general, vitamin A is relatively stable during food processing involving heating, with the palmitate ester more stable to heat than retinol. It is normally regarded as stable during milk processing, and food composition tables give only small differences between the retinol contents of fresh whole milk, sterilised and ultra high temperature (UHT) treated milk.[1] However, prolonged holding of milk or butter at high temperatures in the presence of air can be shown to result in a significant decrease in the vitamin A activity.

A provitamin is a compound that can be converted in the body to a vitamin and there are a number of carotenoids with provitamin A activity. Carotenoids are generally found as naturally occurring plant pigments that give the characteristic yellow, orange and red colours to a wide range of fruits and vegetables. Some can also be found in the liver, kidney, spleen and milk. The provitamin A with the greatest nutritional and commercial importance is β-carotene. The stability of the carotenoids is similar to vitamin A in that they are sensitive to oxygen, light and acid media.

It has been reported that treatment with sulphur dioxide reduces carotenoid destruction in vegetables during dehydration and storage. A study with model systems showed that the stability of β-carotene was greatly enhanced by sulphur dioxide added either as a sulphite solution to cellulose powder prior to β-carotene absorption or as a headspace gas in containers of β-carotene. While it was found that the β-carotene stability was improved by increasing the nitrogen levels in the containers, the stability was even greater when the nitrogen was replaced by sulphur dioxide. Comparative values for the induction period were 19 hours for β-carotene samples stored in oxygen only, 120 hours in nitrogen and 252 hours in sulphur dioxide.[2]

Investigations into the effect of sulphur dioxide treatment on the β-carotene stability in dehydrated vegetables have given varying results and it has been postulated that the effects of the drying and storage conditions on the stability of the sulphur dioxide has a consequential effect on the stability of the β-carotene in dehydrated products.[3] Studies on the heat stability of both α-carotene and β-carotene showed that the β-carotene was about 1.9 times more susceptible than α-carotene to heat damage during normal cooking and blanching processes.[4] Products containing β-carotene should be protected from light and headspace air kept to the minimum.

10.4.2 Vitamin E

A number of naturally occurring substances exhibit vitamin E activity, including the α, β, γ and δ tocopherols and α tocotrienols. Dietary sources of vitamin E are found in a number of vegetables and cereals, with some vegetable oils such as wheatgerm, sunflower seed, safflower seed and maize oils being particularly good sources. Both synthetic and naturally-sourced forms of vitamin E are available commercially. Whilst the natural sources of the tocopherols, which also have the highest biological activity, are in the d form, the synthetic versions can only be produced in the dl form. Both the d and dl forms are also commercially available as esters.

There is a considerable difference in the stability of the tocopherol forms of vitamin E and the tocopherol esters. While vitamin E is regarded as being one of the more stable vitamins, the unesterified tocopherol is less stable due to the free phenolic hydroxyl group.

Vitamin E is unusual in that it exhibits *reduced* stability at temperatures below freezing. The explanation given for this is that the peroxides formed during fat oxidation are degraded at higher temperatures but are stable at temperatures below 0°C and as a consequence can react with the vitamin E.[5] It has also been shown that α-tocopherol may function as a pro-oxidant in the presence of metal ions such as iron.

α-Tocopherol is readily oxidised by air. It is stable to heat in the absence of air but is degraded if heated in the presence of air and is readily oxidised during the processing and storage of foods. One of the most important naturally-occurring sources of tocopherols are the vegetable oils, particularly wheat germ and cotton-seed oils. While deep-frying of the oils may result in a loss of vitamin E of around 10%, it has been found that the storage of fried foods, even at temperatures as low as −12°C, can result in very significant losses.

DL-α-Tocopheryl acetate is relatively stable in air but is hydrolysed by moisture in the presence of alkalis or strong acids to free tocopherols.

10.4.3 Vitamin D

Present in nature in several forms, dietary vitamin D occurs predominantly in animal products with very little being obtained from plant sources. Vitamin D_3

or cholecalciferol is derived in animals, including man, from ultra-violet irradiation of 7-dehydrocholesterol found in the skin. Human requirements are obtained both from the endogenous production in the skin and from dietary sources. Vitamin D_2 (ergocalciferol) is produced by the ultraviolet irradiation of ergosterol, which is widely distributed in plants and fungi. Both vitamins D_2 and D_3 are manufactured for commercial use.

Both vitamins D_2 and D_3 are sensitive to light and can be destroyed relatively rapidly if exposed to light. They are also adversely affected by acids. Preparations of vitamin D in edible oils are more stable than the crystalline forms, and the vitamin is normally provided for commercial usage as an oil preparation or stabilised powder containing an antioxidant (usually tocopherol). The preparations are normally provided in lightproof containers with inert gas flushing.

The presence of double bonds in the structure of both forms of vitamin D can make them susceptible to isomerisation under certain conditions. Studies have shown that the isomerisation rates of ergocalciferol and cholecalciferol are almost equal. Isomerisation in solutions of cholecalciferol resulted in an equilibrium being formed between ergocalciferol and precalciferol with the ratios of the isomers being temperature dependent. The isomerisation of ergocalciferol has been studied in powders prepared with calcium sulphate, calcium phosphate, talc and magnesium trisilicate. It was found that the isomerisation was catalysed by the surface acid of these additives.[6]

Crystalline vitamin D_2 is sensitive to atmospheric oxygen and will show signs of decomposition after a few days storage in the presence of air at ambient temperatures. Crystalline cholecalciferol, D_3, is also destroyed by atmospheric oxygen but is relatively more stable than D_2, possibly due to the fact that it has one less double bond.

The vitamin D_3 naturally occurring in foods such as milk and fish, appears to be relatively stable to heat processing.

10.4.4 Vitamin K

Vitamin K occurs in a number of forms. Vitamin K_1 (phytomenadione or phylloquinone) is found in green plants and vegetables, potatoes and fruits, while vitamin K_2 (menaquinone) can be found in animal and microbial materials.

The presence of double bonds in both vitamins K_1 and K_2 makes them liable to isomerisation. Vitamin K_1 has only one double bond in the side chain in the 3-position whereas in K_2 double bonds recur regularly in the side chain. Vitamin K_1 exists in the form of both *trans* and *cis* isomers. The *trans* isomer is the naturally occurring form and is the one that is biologically active. The *cis* form has no significant biological activity.

The various forms of vitamin K are relatively stable to heat and are retained after most cooking processes. The vitamin is destroyed by sunlight and is decomposed by alkalis. Vitamin K_1 is only slowly decomposed by atmospheric oxygen.

Vitamin K is rarely added to food products and the most common commercially available form is K_1 (phytomenadione), which is insoluble in water. A water-soluble K_3 is available as menadione sodium bisulphite.

10.5 Water-soluble vitamins

The water-soluble vitamin group contains eight vitamins collectively known as the B-complex vitamins plus vitamin C (ascorbic acid).

10.5.1 Thiamin (vitamin B_1)

Thiamin is widely distributed in living tissues. In most animal products it occurs in a phosphorylated form, and in plant products it is predominantly in the non-phosphorylated form. Commercially it is available as either thiamin hydrochloride or thiamin mononitrate. Both these salts have specific areas of application and their use depends on the product matrix to which they are added.

A considerable amount of research has been carried out on the heat stability of thiamin and its salts, particularly in the context of cooking losses. Early work on thiamin losses during bread-making showed an initial cleavage of the thiamin to pyrimidine and thiazole.[7] The destruction of thiamin by heat is more rapid in alkaline media. Vitamin B_1 losses in milk, which has an average fresh content of 0.04 mg thiamin per 100 g, are normally less than 10% for pasteurised milk, between 5 and 15% for UHT milk and between 30 and 40% for sterilised milk.[7] Between 30 and 50% of the vitamin B_1 activity can be lost during the production of evaporated milk.

Losses of thiamin during the commercial baking of white bread are between 15 and 20%. Part of this loss is due to the yeast fermentation, which can convert thiamin to cocarboxylase, which is less stable than thiamin. Thiamin is very sensitive to sulphites and bisulphites as it is cleaved by sulphite. This reaction is rapid at high pH, and is the cause of large losses of the vitamin in vegetables blanched with sulphite, and in meat products such as comminuted meats where sulphites and bisulphites are used as preservatives. Where the pH is low, such as in citrus fruit juices, the bisulphite occurs mainly as the unionised acid, and thiamin losses in such systems are not significantly different from those in products not containing bisulphite.[8]

Studies on the rate of sulphite-induced cleavage of thiamin during the preparation and storage of minced meat showed that losses of thiamin were linear with sulphur dioxide concentrates up to 0.1%. The storage temperature did not have a significant effect on the losses. It has also been reported that thiamin is cleaved by aromatic aldehydes. Thiamin is decomposed by both oxidising and reducing agents. If it is allowed to stand in alkaline solution in air it is oxidised to the disulphide and small amounts of thiothiazolone.

A range of food ingredients has been shown to have an effect on the stability of thiamin. In general, proteins are protective of the vitamin, particularly food proteins such as egg albumin and casein. When heated with glucose, either as a dry mixture or in solution, a browning analogous to a Maillard reaction can occur. This reaction is similar to the reaction between sugars and amino acids and may be important in the loss of thiamin during heat processing. Work has shown that fructose, invertase, mannitol and inositol can actually retard the rate of destruction of thiamin.[9]

Thiamin is unstable in alkaline solutions and becomes increasingly unstable as the pH increases. The stability of the vitamin in low pH solutions such as fortified fruit drinks is very good. In common with that of some other vitamins, the stability of thiamin is adversely affected by the presence of copper ions. This effect can be reduced by the addition of metal-chelating compounds such as calcium disodium ethylenediamine tetra-acetate (EDTA). The heavy metals only appear to influence thiamin stability when they are capable of forming complex anions with constituents of the medium.

The enzymes, thiaminases, which are present in small concentrations in a number of animal and vegetable food sources, can degrade thiamin. These enzymes are most commonly found in a range of seafoods such as shrimps, clams and raw fish, but are also found in some varieties of beans, mustard seed and rice polishings. Two types of thiaminases are known and these are designated thiaminase I and thiaminase II. The former catalyses the decomposition of the thiamine by a base-exchange reaction, involving a nucleophilic displacement of the methylene group of the pyrimidine moiety. Thiaminase II catalyses a simple hydrolysis of thiamin.

A problem associated with the addition of vitamin B_1 to food products is the unpleasant flavour and odour of the thiamin salts.[10] The breakdown of thiamin, particularly during heating, may give rise to off-flavours, and the compounds derived from the degradation of the vitamins are believed to contribute to the 'cooked' flavours in a number of foods. However, both thiamin hydrochloride and mononitrate are relatively stable to atmospheric oxygen in the absence of light and moisture, and both are normally considered to be very stable when used in dry products with light and moisture-proof packaging.

10.5.2 Riboflavin (vitamin B_2)

Riboflavin is the most widely distributed of all the vitamins and is found in all plant and animal cells, although there are relatively few rich food sources. It is present naturally in foods in two bound forms, riboflavin mononucleotide and flavin adenine dinucleotide. Plants and many bacteria can synthesise riboflavin and it is also found in dietary amounts in dairy products. Riboflavin is available commercially as a crystalline powder that is only sparingly soluble in water. As a consequence, the sodium salt of riboflavin-5'-phosphate, which is more soluble in water, is used for liquid preparations.

The most important factor influencing the stability of this vitamin is light, with the greatest effect being caused by light in the 420 to 560 µm range. Fluorescent light is less harmful than direct sunlight, but products in transparent packaging can be affected by strip lighting in retail outlets. Riboflavin and riboflavin phosphate are both stable to heat and atmospheric oxygen, particularly in an acid medium. In this respect, riboflavin is regarded as being one of the more stable vitamins. It is degraded by reducing agents and becomes increasingly unstable with increasing pH. While riboflavin is stable to the heat processing of milk, one of the main causes of loss in milk and milk products is from exposure to light. Liquid milk exposed to light can lose between 20 and 80% of its riboflavin content in two hours, with the rate and extent of loss being dependent upon the light intensity, the temperature and the surface area of the container exposed. Although vitamin B_2 is sensitive to light, particularly in a liquid medium such as milk, it remains stable in white bread wrapped in transparent packaging and kept in a lit retail area.

10.5.3 Niacin

The term 'niacin' is generic for both nicotinic acid and nicotinamide (niacinamide) in foods. Both forms have equal vitamin activity, both are present in a variety of foods and both forms are available as commercial isolates. Niacin occurs naturally in the meat and liver of hoofed animals and also in some plants. In maize and some other cereals it is found in the form of niacytin, which is bound to polysaccharides and peptides in the outer layers of the cereal grains and is unavailable to man unless treated with a mild alkali.

Both forms of niacin are normally very stable in foods because they are not affected by atmospheric oxygen, heat and light in either aqueous or solid systems.

10.5.4 Pantothenic acid

In nature, pantothenic acid is widely distributed in plants and animals, but is rarely found in the free state as it forms part of the coenzyme A molecule. It is found in yeast and egg yolk, and in muscle tissue, liver, kidney and heart of animals. It is also found in a number of vegetables, cereals and nuts. Pantothenic acid is optically active and only its dextro-rotary forms have vitamin activity. Losses of pantothenic acid during the preparation and cooking of foods are normally not very large. Milk generally loses less than 10% during processing, and meat losses during cooking are not excessive when compared to those of the other B vitamins.

Free pantothenic acid is an unstable and very hygroscopic oil. Commercial preparations are normally provided as calcium or sodium salts. The alcohol form, panthenol, is available as a stable liquid but is not widely used in foods. The three commercial forms, calcium and sodium D-pantothenate and D-pantothenol, are moderately stable to atmospheric oxygen and light when protected from moisture. All three compounds are hygroscopic, especially sodium pantothenate. Aqueous solutions of both the salts and the alcohol form are thermolabile and will undergo hydrolytic cleavage, particularly at high or low pH. The compounds are unstable in both acid and alkaline solutions and maximum stability is in the pH range of 6 to 7. Aqueous solutions of D-panthenol are more stable than the salts, particularly in the pH range 3 to 5.

10.5.5 Folic acid/folates

Folic acid (pteroylglutamic acid) does not occur in nature but can be produced commercially. The naturally occurring forms are a number of derivatives collectively known as folates or folacin, which contain one or more linked molecules of glutamic acid. Polyglutamates predominate in fresh food, but on storage these can slowly break down to monoglutamates and oxidise to less biologically available folates. The folic acid synthesised for food fortification contains only one glutamic group.

Most of the stability studies have been carried out with the commercially available folic acid, which has been found to be moderately stable to heat and atmospheric oxygen. In solution it is stable at around pH 7 but becomes increasingly unstable in acid or alkali media, particularly at pH less than 5. Folic acid is decomposed by oxidising and reducing agents. Sunlight, and particularly ultraviolet radiation, has a serious effect on the stability of folic acid. Cleavage by light is more rapid in the presence of riboflavin, but this reaction can be retarded by the addition of the antioxidant BHA to solutions containing folic acid and riboflavin.[11]

The stability of the folates in foods during processing and storage is variable. Folic acid loss during the pasteurisation of milk is normally less than 5%. Losses in the region of 20% can occur during UHT treatment and about 30% loss is found after sterilisation. UHT milk stored for three months can lose over 50% of its folic acid. The extra heat treatment involved in boiling pasteurised milk can decrease the folic acid content by 20%. Losses of around 10% are found in boiled eggs, while other forms of cooking (fried, poached, scrambled) give between 30 and 35% loss. Total folic acid losses from vegetables as a result of heating and cooking processes can be very high.

A study carried out on the stability of folic acid in spinach during processing and storage showed major differences between water blanching and steam blanching, with a folate retention of 58% with steam blanching and only 17% with water. Frozen spinach was found to retain 72% folate after 3 months storage.[12]

10.5.6 Vitamin B_6 (pyridoxine)

Vitamin B_6 activity is shown by three compounds, pyridoxol, pyridoxal and pyridoxamine and these are often considered together as pyridoxine. Vitamin B_6 is found in red meat, liver, cod roe and liver, milk and green vegetables. The commercial form normally used for food fortification is the salt, pyridoxine hydrochloride.

Pyridoxine is normally stable to atmospheric oxygen and heat. Decomposition is catalysed by metal ions. Pyridoxine is sensitive to light, particularly in neutral and alkaline solutions. One of the main causes of loss of this vitamin in milk is sunlight with a 21% loss being reported after 8 hours exposure.[7] Pyridoxine is stable in milk during pasteurisation but about 20% can be lost during sterilisation. Losses during UHT processing are around 27%,[13] but UHT milk stored for 3 months can lose 35% of this vitamin. Average losses as a result of roasting or grilling of meat are 20%, with higher losses (30–60%) in stewed and boiled meat. Cooking or canning of vegetables results in losses of 20–40%.

10.5.7 Vitamin B_{12}

The most important compound with vitamin B_{12} activity is cyanocobalamin. This has a complicated chemical structure and occurs only in animal tissue and as a metabolite of certain microorganisms. The other compounds showing this vitamin activity differ only slightly from the cyanocobalamin structure. The central ring structure of the molecule is a 'corrin' ring with a central cobalt atom. In its natural form, vitamin B_{12} is probably bound to peptides or protein.

Vitamin B_{12} is commercially available as crystalline cyanocobalamin, which is a dark red powder. As human requirements of vitamin B_{12} are very low (about 1–2 µg a day), it is often supplied as a standardised dilution on a carrier.

Cyanocobalamin is decomposed by both oxidising and reducing agents. In neutral and weakly acid solutions it is relatively stable to both atmospheric oxygen and heat. It is only slightly stable in alkaline solutions and strong acids. It is sensitive to light and ultraviolet radiation, and controlled studies on the effect of light on cyanocobalamin in neutral aqueous solutions showed that sunlight at a brightness of 8.6×10^4 lux caused a 10% loss for every 30 minutes of exposure, but exposure to levels of brightness 3.2×10^3 lux had little effect.[5] Vitamin B_{12} is normally stable during pasteurisation of milk but up to 20% can be lost during sterilisation, and losses of 20–35% can occur during spray drying of milk. The stability of vitamin B_{12} is significantly influenced by the presence of other vitamins.

10.5.8 Biotin

The chemical structure of biotin is such that eight different isomers are possible and of these only the dextro-rotatory or D-biotin possesses vitamin activity. D-biotin is widely distributed, but in small concentrations, in animal and plant tissues. It can occur both in the free state (milk, fruit and some vegetables) and in a form bound to protein (animal tissues and yeast). It is commercially available as a white crystalline powder.

Biotin is generally regarded as having a good stability, being fairly stable in air, heat and daylight. It can, however, gradually be decomposed by ultraviolet radiation. Biotin in aqueous solutions is relatively stable if the solutions are either weakly acid or weakly alkaline. In strong acid or alkaline solutions the biological activity can be destroyed by heating.

Avidin, a protein complex, which is found in raw egg white, can react with biotin and bind it in such a way that the biotin is inactivated. Avidin is denatured by heat and biotin inactivation does not occur with cooked eggs.

10.5.9 Vitamin C

Although a number of compounds possess vitamin C activity, the most important is L-ascorbic acid. Vitamin C is widely distributed in nature and can occur at relatively high levels in some fruits and vegetables and is also found in animal organs such as liver and kidney. Small amounts can be found in milk and other meats.

Ascorbic acid is the enolic form of 3-keto-1-gulofuranolactone. The endiol groups at C-2 and C-3 are sensitive to oxidation and can easily convert into a diketo group. The resultant compound, dehydro-L-ascorbic acid, also has vitamin C activity. The D-isomers do not have vitamin activity.

The L-ascorbic acid in foods is easily oxidised to the dehydro-L-ascorbic acid. In fresh foods the reduced form normally predominates but processing, storage and cooking increase the proportions of the dehydro form. Commercially, vitamin C is available as L-ascorbic acid and its calcium, sodium and magnesium salts, the ascorbates. It is also available as ascorbyl palmitate and can be used in this form as an antioxidant in processed foods. Ascorbic acid and the ascorbates are relatively stable in dry air but are unstable in the presence of moisture. Ascorbic acid is readily oxidised in aqueous solutions, first forming dehydro-L-ascorbic acid which is then further and rapidly oxidised. Conversion to dehydroascorbic acid is reversible but the products of the latter stages of oxidation are irreversible.

Ascorbic acid is widely used in soft drinks and to restore manufacturing losses in fruit juices, particularly citrus juices. Research has shown that its stability in these products varies widely according to the composition and oxygen content of the solution. It is very unstable in apple juice but stability in blackcurrant juice is good, possibly as a result of the protective effects of phenolic substances with antioxidant properties.

The effect of dissolved oxygen is very significant. As 11.2 mg of ascorbic acid is oxidised by 1.0 mg of oxygen, 75–100 mg of ascorbic acid can be destroyed by one litre of juice. Vacuum treatment stages are normally added to the process to deaerate the solution to reduce the problem. It is also important to avoid significant head-spaces in containers of liquids with added ascorbic acid as 3.3 mg of ascorbic acid can be destroyed by the oxygen in 1 cm^3 of air.[14] Different production and filling processes can have a significant effect on the retention of vitamin C in drinks. For example, the ascorbic acid loss in a drink packed in a 0.7 litre glass bottle with a partial deaeration of the water and vacuum deaeration of the drink immediately before filling was 16% of the same product filled without any deaeration.

Traces of heavy metal ions act as catalysts to the degradation of ascorbic acid. Studies on the stability of pharmaceutical solutions of ascorbic acid showed that the order of the effectiveness of the metallic ions was $Cu^{+2} > Fe^{+2} > Zn^{+2}$.[5] A Cu^{+2}-ascorbate complex has been identified as being intermediate in the oxidation of the ascorbic acid in the presence of Cu^{+2} ions. Other work on model systems has shown that copper ion levels as low as 0.85 ppm was sufficient to catalyse oxidation, and that the reaction rate was approximately proportional to the square root of the copper concentration.

The stability of vitamins during food processing 259

Work with sequestrants has shown that ethylenediamine tetra-acetate (EDTA) has a significant effect on the reduction of ascorbic acid oxidation, with the optimal level of EDTA required to inhibit the oxidation of vitamin C in blackcurrant juice being a mole ratio of EDTA to [Cu + Fe] of approximately 2.3.[15,16] Unfortunately, EDTA is not a permitted sequestrant for fruit juices in many countries. The amino acid cysteine has also been found to inhibit ascorbic acid oxidation effectively.

Copper and iron ions play such a significant part in metal catalysed oxidation of ascorbic acid that the selection of process equipment can have a marked effect on the stability of vitamin C in food and drink products. Contact of product with bronze, brass, cold rolled steel or black iron surfaces or equipment should be avoided and only stainless steel, aluminium or plastic should be used.

The rate of ascorbic acid degradation in aqueous solutions is pH-dependent with the maximum rate at about pH 4. Vitamin C losses can occur during the frozen storage of foods, and work has shown that oxidation of ascorbic acid is faster in ice than in the liquid water. Frozen orange concentrates can lose about 10% of their vitamin C content during twelve months' storage at −23°C (−10°F).[17] Light, either in the form of sunlight or white fluorescent light, can have an effect on the stability of vitamin C in milk, with the extent of the losses being dependent on the translucency and permeability of the container and the length and conditions of exposure. Bottled orange drinks exposed to light have been found to lose up to 35% vitamin C in three months.[7]

The destruction of vitamin C during processing or cooking of foods can be quite considerable, with losses during pasteurisation being around 25%, sterilisation about 60% and up to 100% in UHT milk stored for three months. Milk boiled from pasteurised can show losses of between 30 and 70%. Large losses of vitamin C are also found after cooking or hot storage of vegetables and fruits. The commercial dehydration of potatoes can cause losses of between 35 and 45%. Destruction of vitamin C during the processing of vegetables depends on the physical processing used and the surface area of product exposed to oxygen. Slicing and dicing of vegetables will increase the rate of vitamin loss. Blanching of cabbage can produce losses of up to 20% of the vitamin C, whilst subsequent dehydration can account for a further 30%.

10.6 Vitamin–vitamin interactions

One of the least expected and less understood aspects of maintaining the stability of vitamins in foods is the detrimental interaction between vitamins. This can lead to the more rapid degradation of one or more of the vitamins in a food or beverage. These interactions should be taken into consideration when vitamins are used to restore or fortify products presented in the liquid (aqueous) phase such as soft drinks or fruit juices. Most of the work in the area of vitamin–vitamin interactions has been carried out by the pharmaceutical industry in relation to the development of liquid multivitamin preparations. Four of the thirteen vitamins

Table 10.3 Principal vitamin–vitamin interactions

Activator	Increased instability
Ascorbic acid	Folic acid
Ascorbic acid	Vitamin B_{12}
Thiamin	Folic acid
Thiamin	Vitamin B_{12}
Riboflavin	Thiamin
Riboflavin	Folic acid
Riboflavin	Ascorbic acid

have been identified as having interactions with each other with deleterious effects. These are ascorbic acid (vitamin C), thiamin (vitamin B_1), riboflavin (vitamin B_2) and vitamin B_{12}. The principal interactions are given in Table 10.3. Other interactions have been identified that can be advantageous, particularly in increasing the solubility of the less soluble vitamins in aqueous solutions. For example, niacinamide has been shown to act as a solubiliser for riboflavin and folic acid.

10.7 Vitamin loss during processing

As already discussed, all vitamins exhibit a degree of instability, the rate of which is affected by a number of factors. Naturally-occurring vitamins in foods are susceptible to many of these factors during the harvesting, processing and storage of the food and its ingredients. It is particularly important that the effects of processing are taken into consideration when assessing vitamin stability in foods, as the food may have been subjected to a number of adverse factors during processing. The most common factor during processing is the application of heat, which in some cases, such as canning, can be for a relatively long time. Most of the work on the stability of vitamins in fruits and vegetables during blanching and canning was carried out during the 1940s and 1950s. Although there have since been refinements both in processing and analytical techniques, many of the conclusions drawn from this research are still valid.

10.7.1 Blanching

In terms of blanching it was found that a high temperature–short time water blanch gave a better vitamin retention than a low temperature–long time blanch and that, overall, steam blanching was superior to water blanching. The addition of sulphite to the blanching water has been shown to affect significantly thiamin levels in fruits and vegetables. Beta carotene was found to be the best survivor during blanching. Riboflavin had retentions in the range 80 to 95%;

vitamin C was in the range 70 to 90% under optimum conditions and niacin 75 to 90%.[19]

10.7.2 Heat processing

Studies on the heat processing of fruits and vegetables in both tin and glass containers showed significant losses of both vitamin C and thiamin. In some cases, the vitamin C levels assayed immediately after the heat processing were between 15 and 45% of the fresh product and these values further reduced during storage.

Thiamin reduced by about 50% during heat processing and further declined to between 15 and 40% of the original level after 12 months' storage. Riboflavin losses were between 12 and 15% during processing but levels of about 50% of the original were observed after 12 months. Niacin was more stable with initial losses of 15 to 25% but with much less than riboflavin being lost during storage. Beta carotene was found to be relatively stable.

In milk, the fat soluble vitamins A and D are relatively stable to the heat treatments used for the processing of milk, as are the water soluble vitamins riboflavin, niacin, pantothenic acid and biotin. Vitamin C, thiamin, vitamin B_6, vitamin B_{12} and folic acid are all affected by the heat processing of milk, with the more severe the process, the greater the loss. With the exception of vitamin C, vitamin losses are generally less than 10% after pasteurisation of milk and between 10 and 20% after Ultra High Temperature (UHT) treatment. Average losses following sterilisation of milk are reported as 20% for thiamin, vitamin B_6 and vitamin B_{12} and 30% for folic acid. Studies have shown that the stability of vitamin C during the processing of milk is also affected by the oxygen content of the milk. Average losses for the vitamin C were 25% after pasteurisation, 30% after UHT and 60% after sterilisation. However, vitamin C appears to be particularly well retained in condensed full cream milk.[10]

B-vitamin stability during the heat processing and cooking of meats varies widely. Cooking conditions can have a marked effect on stability and the retention of thiamin in beef and pork is related to roasting temperatures. If the vitamin content of the drippings is taken into consideration, it is generally found that riboflavin, niacin and vitamin B_{12} are stable during the cooking of meat. Pantothenic acid losses in cooked meat are usually less than 10% although high losses of folate (both free and total) of over 50% have been found in pork, beef and chicken that had been boiled for 15 minutes. Post-mortem ageing of beef can result in up to a 30% loss of niacin over seven days, although the remaining niacin is relatively stable on cooking. The baking of bread can induce losses of about 20% for thiamin, up to 17% for vitamin B_6 and up to one third of the natural folate content. Niacin and pantothenic acid are normally stable during baking.

10.7.3 Freezing

Although most of the vitamins are stable in frozen fruits and vegetables for periods of up to a year, losses of vitamin C have been found to occur at temperatures as low as −23°C.

10.7.4 Dehydration

Studies on the dehydration of blanched vegetables show that the dehydration process can result in additional losses. The dehydration of blanched cabbage (unsulphited) gave an additional 30% reduction in vitamin C content, 5 to 15% in the niacin content and about 15% of the thiamin.

10.7.5 Effect of irradiation on vitamin stability in foods

The use of ionising radiation (irradiation) as a sterilisation technique for foods has been accepted in a number of countries, including the European Union. In many countries the foods and ingredients that are allowed to be irradiated are restricted by law and the process is normally only used for foods at risk of high levels of microbiological contamination.

It has been shown that vitamin levels in a food can be affected by irradiation and the losses can, in general, be related to the dose. At low doses (e.g. up to 1 kilogray), the losses for most vitamins are not significant. At higher doses (3–10 kGy) it has been shown that vitamin losses can occur in foods that are exposed to air during the irradiation and subsequent storage. At the highest permitted radiation doses, care has to be taken to protect the food by using packaging that excludes the air and by carrying out the irradiation process at a low temperature.

There is evidence that the fat-soluble vitamins A, E and K and the water-soluble thiamin are the most sensitive to irradiation, whereas niacin, riboflavin and vitamin D are relatively stable. There is conflicting evidence for vitamins with some foods showing significant losses and others almost none. If it is intended that nutrition claims are to be made for irradiated foods, it is essential that studies are carried out on the content and stability of the vitamins after the treatment with the ionising radiation.

10.8 Vitamins and food product shelf-life

As the tendency to include nutritional information on the labels of food products has increased, so have the liabilities of the manufacturers. For many, if not most, foods the inclusion of nutrition information is optional but any statements made on the label come under the force of law. A company making an inaccurate voluntary nutritional declaration can be subject to prosecution. Within a nutritional information statement, vitamins are the main category of declared nutrients where the quantities can significantly decrease during the shelf life of the food. The vitamin content of processed foods can decrease during storage and it has already been pointed out that losses of vitamin C can occur in frozen vegetables stored at −23°C (page 259).

If declarations of vitamin levels are required on the label, whether voluntary or statutory, the manufacturer needs to carry out suitable stability trials to determine the stability of each vitamin claimed on the label over the duration of the declared shelf life. The actual procedures used for the study will depend on the composition of the food, the processing and the form in which it is presented and stored. The type of packaging can have a significant effect on vitamin stability and the quality of the barriers to oxygen, moisture and light is very important. A requirement for label claims for vitamins can influence the selection of the form of packaging. The need to retain the vitamins often means that a compromise has to be achieved between the length of required shelf life and the barrier quality of the packaging.

Due to the wide variety of products, processes and packaging, it is not possible to give specific procedures for the determination of the shelf life of vitamins in a food. However, guidelines have been established for the determinations and predictions of shelf life.[20] The determination of the vitamin levels at each stage of the shelf life study should be built into the protocol. As the degradation of most of the vitamins follow 'first order' or 'zero order' kinetics, it is possible for shelf life predictions to be made using a classical Arrhenius model on the assumptions that the model holds for all the reactions being studied; that the same reaction mechanism occurs throughout the temperature range of the study; that the energy of activation is between 10 and 20 kcal/mole and that the effects of moisture at ambient temperature are equivalent to maintaining the same relative humidity at the higher temperatures.[18]

Where it is possible to add vitamins to a food either to restore losses during processing or to fortify the food, it is common practice to add an amount above the label claims to compensate for losses during storage. This additional amount is called an overage and is normally quoted as a percentage of the claimed level. For example, if a label claim is made for 60 mg/serving of vitamin C and it is determined that a 10% overage is required to achieve a stored shelf life of one year, the input of vitamin C would be 110% of label claim, or 66 mg/serving. The amount of overage added should be reasonable and well within any safety concerns for the vitamin.

10.9 Protection of vitamins in foods

For all products for which claims for vitamins are intended, it is essential that all stages of the processing, handling and storage of the product are evaluated to minimise the degradation of the vitamins. This can be accomplished by keeping residence times at high temperatures to a minimum and reducing or eliminating exposure to light and oxygen. For example, during the processing of fruit juices, fruit squashes and fruit drinks, the deaeration of the solution can have a protective effect on the vitamin C levels in the product by reducing or eliminating the oxygen.

Commercial sources of vitamins for addition to foods can be obtained in forms that have been encapsulated or coated to improve their stability.

10.10 References

1. *McCance and Widdowson's The Composition of Foods* (1991), 5 ed. (eds: Holland et al), London, The Royal Society of Chemistry/MAFF
2. BALOCH A K, BUCKLE K A and EDWARDS R A (1977), 'Stability of beta carotene in model systems containing sulphate', *J. Food Technol.*, **12**, 309–16
3. BALOCH A K (1976), *The stability of beta carotene in model systems*, PhD Thesis, University of New South Wales, Kensington, Australia
4. BALOCH A K, BUCKLE K A and EDWARDS R A (1977), 'Effect of processing on the quality of dehydrated carrot', *J. Food Technol.*, **12**, 285–7
5. INSTITUTE OF FOOD SCIENCE AND TECHNOLOGY UK (1997), *Addition of Micronutrients to Food*, London, IFST
6. DE RITTER M (1982), 'Vitamins in pharmaceutical formulations', *J. Pharm. Sci.*, **71**(10), 1073–96
7. RYLEY J and KAJDA P (1994), 'Vitamins in thermal processing', *Food Chem.*, **49**, 119–29
8. DWIVEDI B K and ARNOLD R G (1973), 'Chemistry of thiamin degradation in food products and model systems: a review,' *J. Agric. Food Chem.*, **21**(1), 54–60
9. BORENSTEIN B (1981), 'Vitamins and amino acids', in: *Handbook of Food Additives* Volume I. (ed.: Furia T), Boca Raton, Florida, CRC Press, 85–114
10. CLYDESDALE F M, HO C-T, LEE C Y, MONDY N I and SHEWFELT R L (1991), 'The effects of postharvest treatment and chemical interactions on the bioavailability of ascorbic acid, thiamin, vitamin A, carotenoids and minerals', *Crit. Rev. Food Sci. Nutr.*, **30**(6), 599–638
11. TANSEY R P and SCHNELLER G H (1955), 'Studies in the stabilisation of folic acid in liquid pharmaceutical preparations', *J. Am. Pharm. Assoc. (Sci. Ed.)*, **44**(1), 35–7
12. MORGAN W (1996), 'Effects of processing and preparation of foods on folate content', *Austral. J. Nutr. Dietetics*, **53**, S31–S35
13. SCOTT K J and BISHOP D R (1993), 'The influence of combined storage procedures of foods on B vitamin content demonstrated at the example of heat sterilisation and irradiation', *Nahrung*, **38**(4), 345–51
14. BENDER A E (1958), 'The stability of vitamin C in a commercial fruit squash', *J. Sci. Food Agric.*, **9**, 754–60
15. TIMBERLAKE C F (1960), 'Metallic components of fruit juices. III Oxidation and stability of ascorbic acid in model systems', *J. Sci. Food Agric.*, **11**, 258–68
16. TIMBERLAKE C F (1960), 'Metalic components of fruit juices. IV Oxidation and stability of ascorbic acid in blackcurrant juice', *J. Sci. Food Agric.*, **11**, 268–73
17. GRANT N H and ALBURN H E (1965), 'Fast reactions of ascorbic acid and hydrogen peroxide in ice,' *Science*, **150**, 1589–90
18. BERRY OTTAWAY P (1993), 'The stability of vitamins in food', in *The Technology of Vitamins in Food*, Chapter 5 (ed. Berry Ottaway P), Glasgow, Blackie Academic and Professional Press
19. MALLETTE M F, DAWSON C R, NELSON W L and GORTNER W A (1946), 'Commercially dehydrated vegetables, oxidative enzymes, vitamin content and other factors', *Ind. Eng. Chem.*, **38**, 437–41
20. LENZ M K and LUND D B (1980), 'Experimental procedures for determining destruction kinetics of food components', *Food Technol.*, **34**(2), 51–5

11

Thermal processing and nutritional quality

A. Arnoldi, University of Milan

11.1 Introduction

The taming of fire, permitting the thermal processing of vegetable foodstuffs in particular, extended enormously the number of natural products that could be used as foods by humans and gave a tremendous impulse to the extraordinary diffusion and development of the human population in almost every region of the world (De Bry, 1994). Foodstuffs can be roughly divided in two classes, those that are or are not edible in their raw form. The most important naturally edible foods are meat and milk, which are heated mainly for eliminating dangerous microorganisms, and some fruits, used by plants to attract animals for diffusing their seeds in the environment. In contrast, many plants protect themselves and especially their seeds and tubers from the consumption of insects and superior animals with several antinutritional components that may be deactivated only by thermal treatments. For this reason cereals, grain legumes, and vegetables, such as potatoes, although they are considered the base of a balanced diet in view of the most up-to-date dietary recommendations, are never consumed raw.

With the exception of milk, fruit juices, and some other foods, in which a fresh and natural appearance is required, thermal treatments have also relevant hedonistic consequences, as they confer the desired sensory and texture features to foods. Bread and baked products, or chocolate, coffee, and malt are well known products that are consumed world-wide; here thermal treatments produce the characteristic aroma, taste, and colour (Arnoldi, 2001). Such sensory characteristics have positive psychological effects that facilitate digestion and therefore contribute to an individual's well-being.

During thermal treatment many reactions take place at a molecular level:

- Denaturation of proteins, with the important consequence of the deactivation of enzymes that destabilise foods or decrease their digestibility, such as lipases, lipoxygenases, hydrolases, and trypsin inhibitors.
- Lipid autoxidation.
- Transformations of minor compounds, for example vitamins.
- Reactions involving free or protein-bound amino acids.

The last reactions belong essentially to four categories:

- breaking and/or recombination of intramolecular or intermolecular disulfide bridges;
- reactions of the basic and acidic side chains of amino acids to give isopeptides (for example Lys + Asp);
- reactions involving the side chains of amino acids and reducing sugars in a very complex process generally named as 'Maillard reaction' (MR);
- reactions involving the side chains of amino acids through leaving group elimination to give reactive dehydro intermediates, which can produce cross-linked amino acids.

The Maillard reaction is described in this chapter and some information given on those reactions involving the side chains of amino acids. The Maillard reaction, or non-enzymatic browning, is one of the most important processes involving on one hand amino acids, peptides and proteins, and on the other reducing sugars (Ledl and Schleicher, 1990; Friedman, 1996). The MR is a complex mixture of competitive organic reactions, such as tautomerisations, eliminations, aldol condensations, retroaldol fragmentations, oxidations and reductions. Their interpretation and control is difficult because they occur simultaneously and give rise to many reactive intermediates.

Soon after the discovery of the MR it became clear that it influences the nutritive value of foods. The loss in nutritional quality and, potentially, in safety is attributed to the destruction of essential amino acids, interaction with metal ions, decrease in digestibility, inhibition of enzymes, deactivation of vitamins and formation of anti-nutritional or toxic compounds. However, while the reaction has its negative effects, the positive effects are considerably greater.

11.2 The Maillard reaction

About 90 years ago Maillard (1912) observed a rapid browning and CO_2 development while reacting amino acids and sugars: he had discovered a new reaction that became known as the 'Maillard reaction' or non-enzymatic browning. Nineteen years later Amadori (1931) detected the formation of rearranged stable products from aldoses and amino acids that became known as the Amadori rearrangement products (ARPs). The development of industrial food processing, especially after World War II, gave a large impulse to research in this field and

Thermal processing and nutritional quality 267

after some years Hodge (1953) was able to propose an overall picture of the reactions of non-enzymatic browning in a review that, after almost 50 years, remains one of the most cited in food chemistry.

The mechanism of non-enzymatic browning is generally studied in simple model systems in order to control all the parameters and the results are extrapolated to foods quite efficiently.

The reactants include reducing sugars. Pentoses, such as ribose, arabinose or xylose are very effective in non-enzymatic browning, hexoses, such as glucose or fructose, are less reactive, and reducing disaccharides, such as maltose or lactose, react rather slowly. Sucrose as well as bound sugars (for example glycoproteins, glycolipids, and flavonoids) may give reducing sugars through hydrolysis, induced by heating or very often by yeast fermentation, as in cocoa bean preparation before roasting or dough leavening.

The other reactants are proteins or free amino acids; these may already be present in the raw material or they may be produced by fermentation. In some cases (e.g. cheese) biogenic amines can react as amino compounds. Small amounts of ammonia may be produced from amino acids during the Maillard reaction or large amounts added for the preparation of a particular kind of caramel colouring.

A very simplified general picture of the MR may be found in Fig. 11.1. Following the classical interpretation by Hodge (1953), the initial step is the condensation of the carbonyl group of an aldose with an amino group to give an unstable glycosylamine **1** which undergoes a reversible rearrangement to the ARP (Amadori, 1931), i.e. a 1-amino-1-deoxy-2-ketose **2** (Fig. 11.2). Fructose reacts in a similar way to give the corresponding rearranged product, 2-amino-2-deoxy-

Early stage ⟶ First interactions between sugars and amino groups, rearrangements

⇓

Intermediate stage ⟶ Fissions, cyclisations, dehydrations, condensations, oligomerisations

⇓

Advanced stage ⟶ Polymerisations

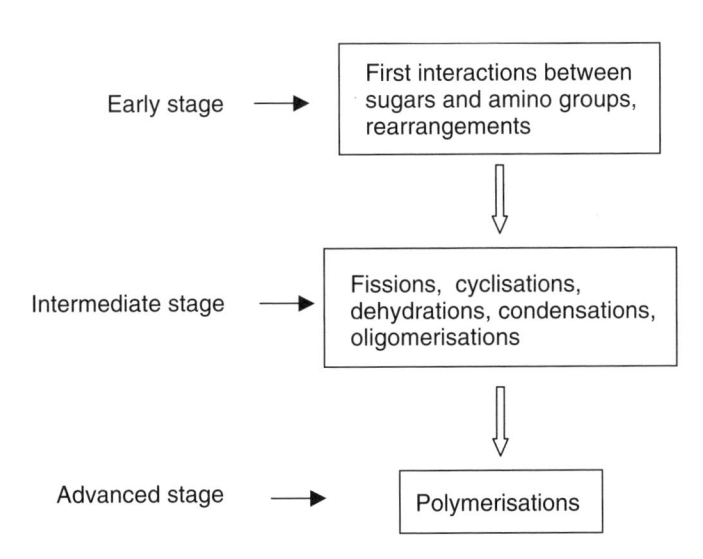

Fig. 11.1 Simplified scheme of the Maillard reaction.

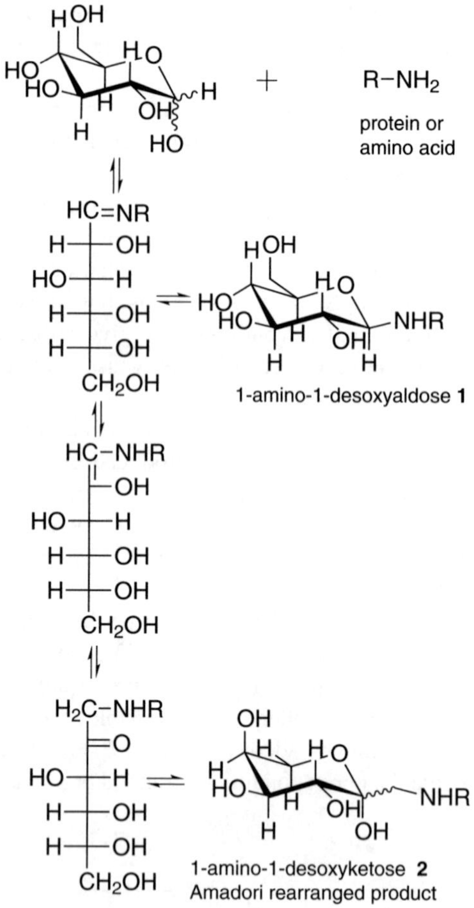

Fig. 11.2 Mechanism of the Amadori rearrangement.

2-aldose **3** (Fig. 11.3, Heyns, 1962). The formation of these compounds, that have been separated from model systems as well as from foods, takes place easily even at room temperature and is very well documented also in physiological conditions. Here long-lived body proteins and enzymes can be modified by reducing sugars such as glucose through the formation of ARPs (a process known as glycation) with subsequent impairment of many physiological functions. This takes place especially in diabetic patients and during aging (Baynes, 2000; Furth, 1997; James and Crabbe 1998; Singh et al, 2001; Sullivan, 1996). A detailed description of the synthetic procedures, physico-chemical characterisation, properties and reactivity of the ARPs may be found in an excellent review by Yaylayan and Huyggues-Despointes (1994).

Where the water content is low and pH values are in the range 3–6, ARPs are considered the main precursors of reactive intermediates in model systems.

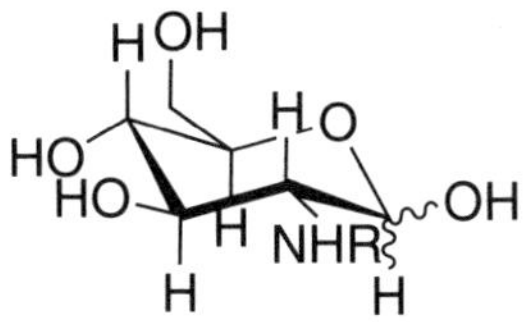

2-amino-2-desoxy-D-glucose **3**
Heyns rearranged product

Fig. 11.3 Heyns products.

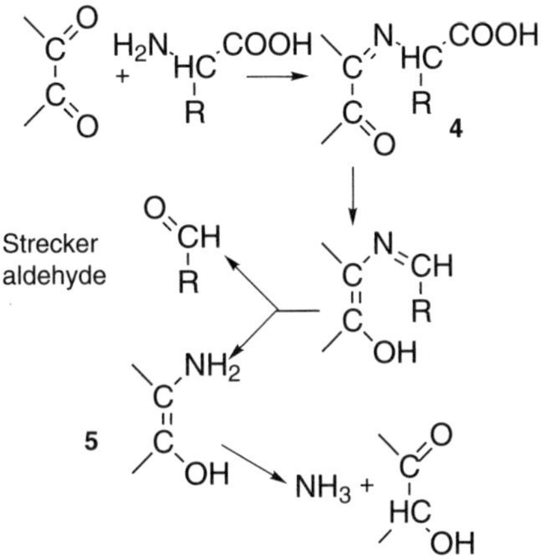

Fig. 11.4 Mechanism of the Strecker degradation of amino acids.

Below pH 3 and above pH 8 or at temperatures above 130°C (caramelisation), sugars will degrade in the absence of amines (Ledl and Schleicher, 1990). Ring opening followed by 1, 2 or 2, 3-enolisation are crucial steps in ARP transformation and are followed by dehydration and fragmentation with the formation of many very reactive dicarbonyl fragments. This complex of reactions is considered the intermediate stage of the MR.

Maillard observed also the production of CO_2, which is explained by a process named the Strecker degradation (Fig. 11.4). The mechanism involves the reaction of an amino acid with an α-dicarbonyl compound to produce an azovinylogous β-ketoacid **4**, that undergoes decarboxylation. In this way amino acids are converted to aldehydes containing one less carbon atom per molecule. These are very reactive and often have very peculiar sensory properties. The aldehydes that derive from cysteine and methionine degrade further to give hydrogen sulfide, 2-methylthio-propanal, and methanethiol: that means that the Strecker degradation is responsible for the incorporation of sulfur in some Maillard reaction products (MRPs). Another important consequence of the Strecker reaction is the incorporation of nitrogen in very reactive fragments deriving from sugars, such as **5**.

$$
\begin{array}{c}
\text{CHO} \\
|\\
\text{CHOH} \\
|\\
\text{CHOH} \\
|\\
\text{CHOH} \\
|\\
\text{R'}
\end{array}
\;+\text{RNH}_2\;
\xrightarrow{-\text{H}_2\text{O}}
\begin{array}{c}
\text{C=N-R} \\
|\\
\text{CHOH} \\
|\\
\text{CHOH} \\
|\\
\text{CHOH} \\
|\\
\text{R'}
\end{array}
\;\xrightarrow{\text{reverse aldol reaction}}\;
\begin{array}{c}
\text{CH-NH-R} \\
||\\
\text{CHOH} \quad 5\\
|\\
\text{CH=O} \\
|\\
\text{CHOH} \\
|\\
\text{R'}
\end{array}
$$

Fig. 11.5 Possible pathway for the formation of glycolaldehyde alkylimines proposed by Namiki and Hayashi (1986).

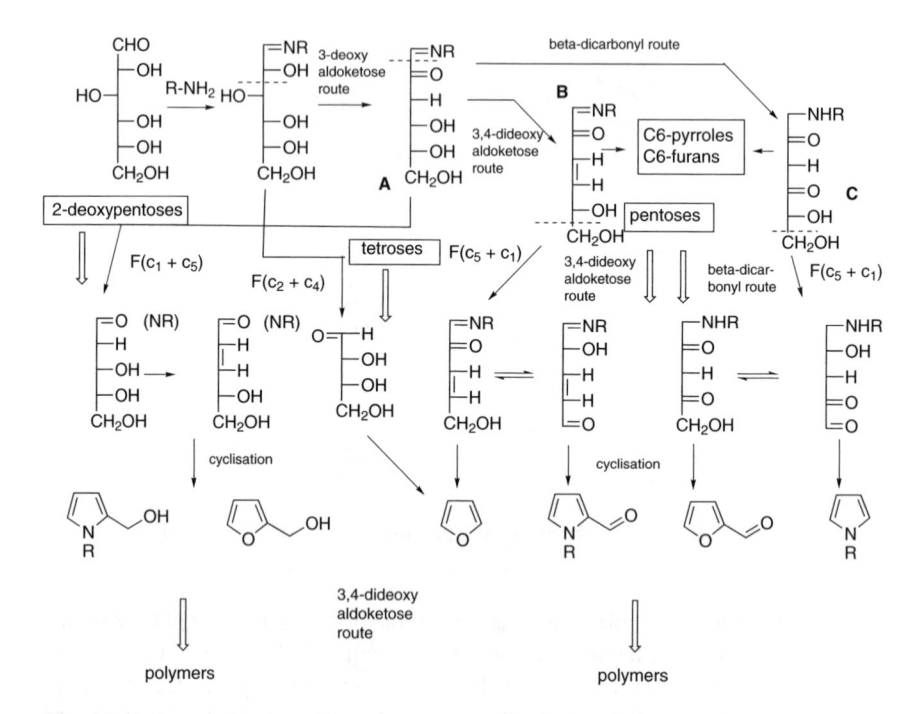

Fig. 11.6 Transformation of hexoses and pentoses to C_5- and C_4-pyrroles and -furans. (Reproduced with permission from Tressel et al, 1998a)

However, in the last two decades other mechanisms have been proposed. For example, starting from the experimental observation of free radical formation at the start of the MR, Hayashi and Namiki (1981; 1986) proposed a reducing sugar degradation pathway that produces glycolaldehyde alkylimines without passing through the formation of ARPs (Fig. 11.5).

Very recently, on the basis of extensive experiments with ^{13}C- and ^{2}H-labelled sugars, a detailed reaction scheme was proposed by Tressel et al (1995 and 1998a): the formation of various C_6-, C_5-, and C_4-pyrroles and furans from both intact and fragmented hexoses and amines could be unambiguously attributed to distinct reaction pathways via the intermediates **A–C** without involving the

Table 11.1 Composition of the primary fragmentation pools

Type of pool	Constituents
Amino acid fragmentation pool {A}	Amines Carboxylic acids Alkanes and aromatics Aldehydes Amino acid specific side chain fragments: H_2S (Cys), CH_3SH (Met), styrene (Phe)
Sugar fragmentation pool {S}	C1 fragments: formaldehyde, formic acid C2 fragments: glyoxal, glycoladehyde, acetic acid C3 fragments: glyceraldehyde, methylglyoxal, hydroxyacetone, dihydroxyacetone, etc. C4 fragments: tetroses, 2, 3-butanedione, 1-hydroxy-2-butanone, 2-hydroxybutanal, etc. C5 fragments: pentoses, pentuloses, deoxy derivatives, furanones, furans C6 fragments: pyranones, furans, glucosones, deoxyglucosones
Amadori and Heyns fragmentation pool {D}	C3-ARP/HRP derivatives: glyceraldehyde-ARP, amino acid-propanone, amino acid-propanal, etc. C4-ARP/HRP derivatives: amino acid-tetradiuloses, amino acid-butanones C5-ARP/HRP derivatives: amino acid-pentadiuloses C6-ARP/HRP derivatives: amino acid-hexadiuloses, pyrylium betaines
Lipid fragmentation pool {L}	Propanal, pentanal, hexanal, octanal, nonanal 2-Oxoaldehydes (C6–9) C2 fragments: glyoxal C3 fragments: $CHOCH_2CHO$, methylglyoxal Formic acid, acids

Amadori rearrangement (Fig. 11.6). These pyrroles and furans polymerise very easily to highly coloured compounds that may be involved in the formation of melanoidins.

By means of experiments showing that sugars and most amino acids also undergo independent degradation (Yaylayan and Keyhani, 1996), a new conceptual approach to the MR has been proposed recently by Yaylayan (1997). He suggested that in order to understand the MR better, it is more useful to define a sugar fragmentation pool {S}, an amino acid fragmentation pool {A}, and an interaction fragmentation pool {D}, deriving from the Amadori and Heyns compounds (Table 11.1). Together they constitute a primary fragmentation pool of building blocks that react to give a secondary pool of interaction intermediates and eventually a very complex final pool of stable end-products.

However, most foods contain also lipids that can degrade by autoxidation (Grosch, 1987) giving reactive intermediates, mainly saturated or unsaturated aldehydes or ketones and also glyoxal and methylglyoxal (in common with the

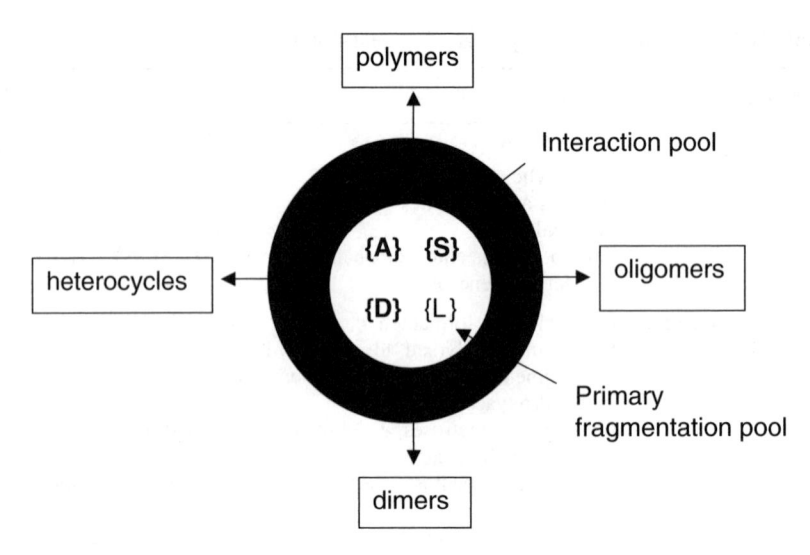

Fig. 11.7 Conceptual representation of the Maillard reaction: generalogy of primary fragmentation pools, interaction pools (containing self-interaction pools as well as mix-interaction pools) and end-products.

Maillard reaction) and malondialdehyde (Table 11.1). These belong to a fourth pool, the lipid fragmentation pool {L} (D'Agostina et al, 1998) and in this way the scheme proposed by Yaylayan (1997) was revised to include it (Fig. 11.7). Clear interconnections between the MR and lipid autoxidation have been extensively studied in the case of food aromas, where many end-products deriving from lipids and amino acids or sugars are very well documented (Whitfield, 1992), but certainly they may be relevant also for other sensory aspects, such as colour or taste, or for nutrition, although these research areas have been almost completely neglected until the present.

Depending on food composition and heating intensity applied, thousands of different end products may be formed in the advanced stage of the MR: they are classified here according to their functions in foods (Fig. 11.8). Very volatile compounds, such as pyrazines, pyridines, furans, thiophenes, thiazoles, thiazolines, and dithiazines are of interest, when considering aroma; some low molecular weight compounds relate to taste (Frank et al, 2001; Ottiger et al, 2001), others behave as antioxidants and a few are mutagenic. Polymers (melanoidins) that in sugar/amino acid model systems and some foods such as coffee, roasted malt, or chocolate are the major MRPs, and determine the colour of the food.

This review will discuss only the mechanism of formation of MRPs that have some nutritional significance or may be used as molecular markers for quantifying the MR in foods. A very detailed description of the pathways leading to most Maillard reaction products may be found in an excellent review by Ledl and Schleicher (1990).

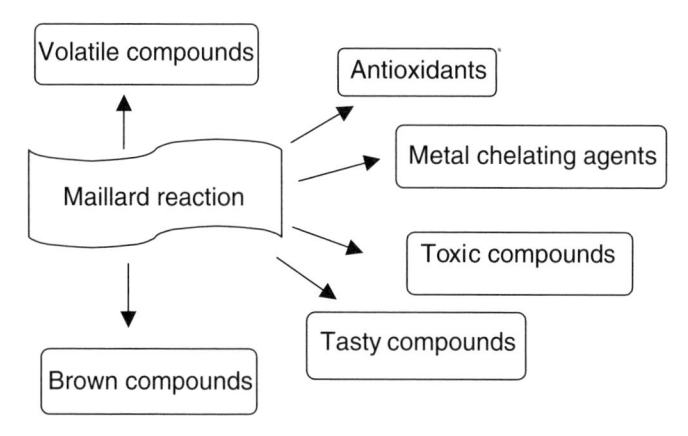

Fig. 11.8 Functional classification of Maillard reaction products.

11.3 Nutritional consequences and molecular markers of the Maillard reaction in food

As the MR involves some of the most important food nutrients, its nutritional consequences must be carefully considered. Researcher attention has previously been focused mainly on milk and milk products, where thermal treatments are necessary for obtaining microbial stabilisation and the preservation of high nutritional quality. Vegetable products, which become edible only after thermal treatments, have been relatively neglected so far.

The degradation of sugars *per se* is never considered a problem because it is only rarely they are lacking in diet. However, free or protein-bound essential amino acids may be damaged irreversibly; the amount of free amino acids in food is always very low and they are important as constituents of proteins. This means that the most relevant nutritional effect of the Maillard reaction is non-enzymatic glycosylation of proteins which involves mostly lysine, whose bioavailability may be drastically impaired. This should be distinguished very clearly from enzymatic glycosylation, a normal step in the biosynthesis of glycoproteins, in which oligosaccharides are bound to serine or asparagine through a glycosidic bond.

The first glycation products are then converted to the Amadori product, fructosyllysine, that eventually can cross-link with other amino groups intramolecularly or intermolecularly. The resulting polymeric aggregates are called advanced glycation end products (AGEs).

Lysine availability is an important nutritional parameter especially in foods for particular classes of consumers, such as infant formulas (Ferrer et al, 2000). Statistically significant losses of available lysine (about 20%) with respect to raw milk have been reported as a consequence of the thermal treatment applied in the preparation of these foods.

Because the reactions of lysine are so relevant in nutrition, over a period of time different MRPs have been proposed as markers of protein glycosylation.

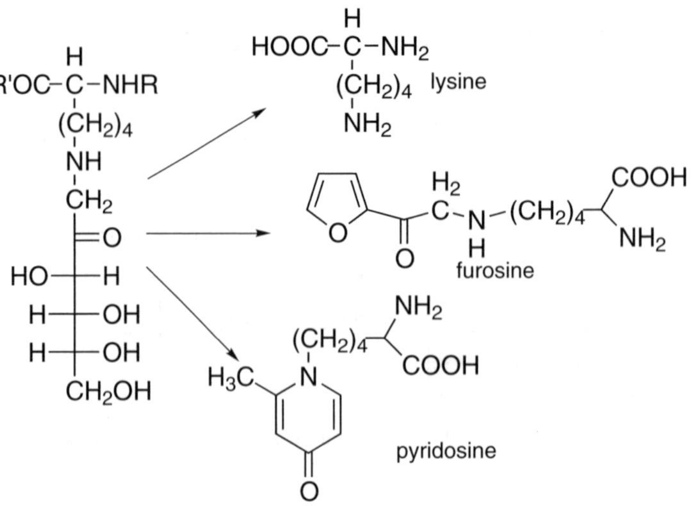

Fig. 11.9 Compounds derived from fructosyllysine decomposition.

Fructosyllysine is unstable in the acid conditions of protein hydrolysis, producing about 30% furosine, pyridosine (a minor cyclisation product) and about 50% lysine (Fig. 11.9). Furosine was first detected in foods by Erbersdobler and Zucker (1966) and can be easily analysed by HPLC: thus furosine quantification is considered a good estimate of nutritionally unavailable lysine. Milk proteins, owing to their nutritional relevance, have been considered with particular attention. Owing to the presence of lactose, the Amadori compound in this case is lactulosyllysine and furosine is again a useful marker of lysine unavailability. For this reason several authors have used the furosine method for determining the progress of the Maillard reaction in different foods (Chiang, 1983; Hartkopf and Erbersdobler, 1993 and 1994, Henle et al, 1995; Resmini et al, 1990). However, today very powerful analytical techniques are disclosing new possibilities, permitting, for example, the direct determination of fructosyllysine (Vinale et al, 1999) by the use of a stable isotope dilution assay performed in liquid chromatography – mass spectrometry (LC–MS). This method overcomes the problems of hydrolytic instability of the analyte and the incompleteness of the enzymatic digestion technique.

Other possible markers of lysine transformation are N-ε-carboxymethyllysine (CML) and 5-hydroxymethylfurfural (HMF) (Fig. 11.10). CML was detected for the first time in milk by Büser and Erbersdobler (1986) and an oxidative mechanism was proposed for its formation (Ahmed et al, 1986). The formation of HMF in foods has been explained in two ways: via the Amadori products through enolisation (in the presence of amino groups) and via lactose isomerisation and degradation, known as the Lobry de Bruyn-Alberda van Ekenstein transformation (Ames, 1992). Because of this, it has recently been proposed to measure separately the HMF formed only by the acidic degradation of Amadori products and

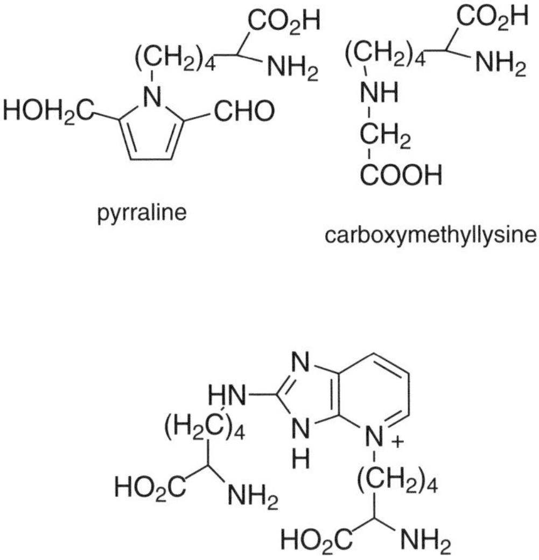

Thermal processing and nutritional quality 275

Fig. 11.10 Some possible markers of the Maillard reaction.

directly related to the MR, called bound HMF, and total HMF that also derives from the degradation of other precursors (Morales et al, 1997). This method is considered more reliable than the previous spectrophotometric one of Keeney and Bassette (1959).

Many authors have observed that the values of furosine, carboxymethyllysine, and HMF are very well correlated (Corzo et al, 1994; O'Brien, 1995). Hewedy et al (1991), however, comparing several damage indicators for the classification of UHT milk have shown that carboxymethyllysine is suitable only for monitoring very severe damage, because it is formed only in very small amounts, whereas furosine and HMF have a more general applicability. ε-Pyrrolelysine (known also as pyrraline, Fig. 11.10) is another substance that has been proposed to measure the MR in foods. It was observed for the first time in the reaction between glucose and lysine (Nakayama et al, 1980) and is particularly useful in dry foods because it is very stable: for example Resmini and Pellegrino (1994) have proposed a methodology for measuring protein-bound pyrraline in dried pasta. The formation of this MRP parallels very well the formation of furosine. Another useful substance for assessing protein damage is lysinoalanine (see section 11.7).

11.4 Melanoidins

The modifications of amino acids described in the preceding section take place also during either mild treatments or short duration treatments at high temperatures, where the changing of food appearance is hardly perceptible. However, many processes usually dealing with the processing of vegetables, such as bread baking, roasting of coffee and nuts, and kiln drying of malt as well as roasting of meat require severe thermal treatments. In these cases the Maillard reaction is responsible for colour formation, a very critical parameter in determining food quality. The most important contribution to colour comes from polymers, known as melanoidins that in some foods are the major MRPs. Their structure is still elusive but many methodological difficulties have slowed down the progress of knowledge in this field. Some attempts have been made to isolate melanoidins from such foods as soy sauce (Lee et al, 1987), dark beer (Kuntcheva and Obretenov, 1996), malt or roasted barley (Milic et al, 1975; Obretenov et al, 1991), coffee (Maier and Buttle, 1973; Steinhart and Packert, 1993; Nunes and Coimbra, 2001), but their very complex and probably non-repetitive structure has limited structural characterisation.

Studies on model systems have clearly indicated that reducing carbohydrates and compounds possessing a free amino group, such as amino acids, either in free or protein-bound form, are the basic material for their formation (Ledl and Scleicher, 1990). They are reported to have molecular weight up to 100 000 Da, and to possess structural features, elemental analysis and degrees of unsaturation depending on the reaction conditions.

As already indicated at the beginning of this review, the Maillard reaction is often studied through model systems; however, in the case of melanoidins this approach shows limitations. Many authors have used model systems to isolate and characterise low molecular weight coloured compounds (Rizzi, 1997; Arnoldi et al, 1997; Ravagli et al, 1999; Tressl et al, 1998a and 1998b; Wondrack et al, 1997). Currently the most active in this field are Hofmann (Hofmann, 1998a, b, c, d) and co-workers (Hofmann et al, 1999). However, it has been clearly demonstrated that completely different compounds are produced by reacting glucose with single amino acids or β-casein (Hofmann, 1998c). With amino acids the majority of coloured compounds have molecular weights below 1000 amu, whereas the reaction between glucose and casein gives rise to products with much higher molecular weights (Hofmann, 1998a). Moreover, only very rarely has it been demonstrated that the chromophores isolated from amino acids/sugars model systems may be incorporated in melanoidins, as in the case of the free radical chromophore named CROSSPY (Fig. 11.11), which was successfully identified in several processed foods, such as coffee and bread crusts by EPR (Hofmann et al, 1999).

However, the formation of melanoidins in real foods does not involve simply proteins and sugars: biopolymers (proteins in animal proteins, both proteins and polysaccharides in vegetables) probably act as a non-coloured skeleton bearing a variety of chromophoric substructures. Thus the melanoidins separated from coffee brews contain about 33% polysaccharides, 9% proteins, and 33% polyphenols (Nunes and Coimbra, 2001). The polyphenol substructures derive from chlorogenic acids (Heinrich and Baltes, 1987) that disappear during coffee roasting. Physico-chemical properties of melanoidins other than colour may be

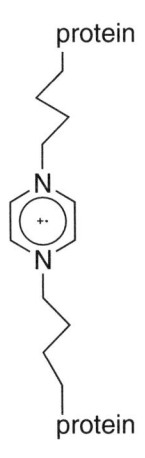

Thermal processing and nutritional quality   277

Fig. 11.11   Structure of the radical cation CROSSPY.

important in foods. For example, in *espresso* coffee brew, they may have foaming properties (Petracco, 1999) that stabilise the foamy layer on top of the beverage, which is well known by the Italian term *crema*.

Beside their obvious importance in determining the brown colour of roasted foods, in recent years great interest has developed around melanoidins for their possible role in physiology and in food stabilisation: in fact some authors (Anese et al, 1999; Nicoli et al, 1997) have demonstrated that they possess antioxidative activity. Antioxidants are able to delay or prevent oxidation processes, typically involving lipids, which greatly affect the shelf-life of foods. In coffee, the antioxidant activity (attributed to the development of Maillard reaction products) increases with roasting up to the medium-dark roasted stage, then decreases with further roasting (Nicoli et al, 1997), possibly indicating a partial decomposition in the antioxidative compounds.

11.5   Transformations not involving sugars: cross-linked amino acids

Another kind of transformation of the side chains of protein-bound amino acids induced by thermal treatments of foods, particularly in basic conditions, is the formation of cross-linked amino acids. A dehydroalanine residue may be formed through elimination of a leaving group from protein-bound serine, *O*-phosphorylserine, *O*-glycosylserine, or cystine, and may undergo Michael addition by another nucleophilic amino acid residue (Fig. 11.12). For example the ε-amino group of lysine may react to give a secondary amine, which is normally indicated with the trivial name of lysinoalanine (LAL) (Maga, 1984). Analogous reactions may involve ornithine to give ornithinoalanine (OAL), cysteine to give lanthionine (LAN), and histidine to produce histidinoalanine (HAL)

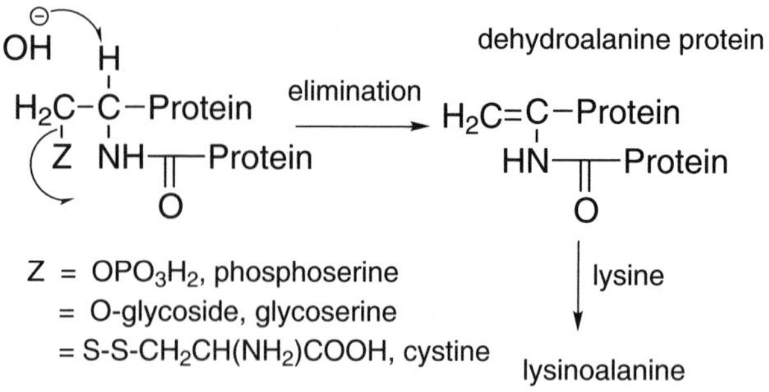

$$\underset{\text{OH}}{\ominus} \underset{\text{H}}{\overset{\text{H}}{|}} \quad \underset{\text{H}_2\text{C-C-Protein}}{\underset{|}{|}} \xrightarrow{\text{elimination}} \underset{\text{H}_2\text{C=C-Protein}}{\overset{\text{dehydroalanine protein}}{}}$$

(with Z = OPO$_3$H$_2$, phosphoserine; = O-glycoside, glycoserine; = S-S-CH$_2$CH(NH$_2$)COOH, cystine)

↓ lysine

lysinoalanine

Fig. 11.12 Mechanism of the formation of dehydroalanine residues in protein chains.

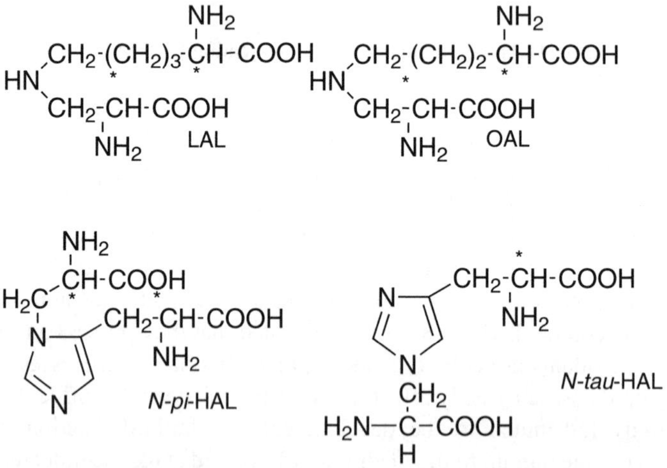

LAL, OAL, N-pi-HAL, N-tau-HAL structures

Fig. 11.13 Main cross-linker amino acids.

(Finley and Friedman, 1977). Both nitrogens of histidine may react, giving rise to the regioisomers N^π-HAL and N^τ-HAL (Fig. 11.13) (Henle et al, 1993).

The formation of cross-linked amino acids does not involve the participation of reducing sugars and is particularly extensive when proteins are submitted to aqueous alkali treatments. Such treatments include those used in the preparation of soy protein concentrates and in the recovery of proteins from cereal grains, milling by-products, and oilseeds, such as cottonseeds, peanuts, safflower seeds and flaxseeds, and in the separation of sodium caseinate. Other alkali procedures are commonly used for destroying microorganisms, preparing peeled fruits, and inducing fiber-forming properties in textured soybean proteins, used, for example, in the preparation of meat substitutes. A recent review lists the processes and foods that have been studied for the formation of cross-linked amino acids (Friedman, 1999). The main feature of these compounds is that they are stable during acidic protein hydrolysis and are relatively easy to analyse when other compounds that derive from modification of the amino acid side chains in proteins, such as isopeptides, must be considered. This makes them useful in quality control as molecular markers of the processes applied in food preparation (Pellegrino et al, 1996).

LAL is certainly the most frequently studied cross-linked amino acid. Many investigations have been devoted to investigating the effects of its presence on protein functionality and nutritional value, because LAL acts as a bridge or a cross-linker between two different parts of the protein chain (Pellegrino et al, 1998). It can thus impair the approach of the enzymes and consequently decrease protein digestibility (Anantharaman and Finot, 1993; Savoie et al, 1991). The nutritional consequences of LAL formation in foods have been extensively reviewed (Karayiannis et al, 1980; Maga, 1984; Friedman, 1999), adverse effects on growth, protein digestibility, protein quality, and mineral bioavailability and utilisation were observed (Sarwar et al, 1999).

There are also some concerns about toxicity; LAL has been shown to provoke lesions in rat kidney cells causing nephrocitomegaly (Friedman et al, 1984; Friedman and Pearce, 1989). Although these effects seem very species specific, such observations promoted investigation on humans, in particular on preterm infants (Langhendries et al, 1992). The higher level of Maillard reaction products and LAL in infant formulas compared to breast milk had no influence on creatinine clearance or electrolyte excretion and there was no evidence of tubular damage as determined by the urinary excretion of four kidney-derived enzymes. Feeding with formulas, however, did result in a general increase in urinary microprotein levels.

Some authors have investigated the presence of LAL in infant formulas in the 1980s (Fritsch and Klostermeyer, 1981; de Koning and van Rooijen, 1982; Bellomonte et al, 1987): the data were in the range of 150–2120 µg/g protein. Some dried and liquid samples have been analysed very recently by us (D'Agostina et al, 2002): the LAL contents in dried formulas were negligible, whereas in liquid samples they were lower than 80 µg/g protein in adapted formulas, 80–370 µg/g protein in follow-on formulas, and about 500 µg/g protein in growing milk, indicating that current products are much better than older ones and that producers have made considerable efforts to improve the manufacturing procedures especially in adapted formulas. In particular, the replacement of in-bottle sterilisation by UHT treatments can reduce the thermal damage in liquid samples (Rennen and Vetter, 1988). LAL contents ranging from 150 to 800 µg/g protein were observed in liquid samples for enteral nutrition, which are mainly based on casein, a protein more sensitive than lactalbumin to this reaction (Boschin et al, 2002).

Some studies were focused also on histidinoalanine, that was detected for the first time by Finley and Friedman (1977) in soybean protein isolates treated with alkali. The HAL content of several proteins (bovine serum albumin, bovine tendon collagen, and casein) heated in neutral pH buffer was greater than their LAL content (Fujimoto, 1984). This probably derives from the lower pKa of the NH group of histidine ($pK_a = 5.5$) in respect to $\varepsilon\text{-NH}_3^+$ of lysine ($pK_a = 10$).

Analysis of various milk-protein containing foods, such as heated skim milk, sterilised milk, and baby formulas, permitted detection of amounts of HAL between 50 and 1800 µg/g protein, comparable to LAL amounts (Henle et al, 1993; Henle et al, 1996). However, no toxicological effects have been reported for HAL.

11.6 Metabolic transit and *in vivo* effects of Maillard reaction products

These topics are considered in detail in an excellent review by Faist and Erbersdobler (2001) that has been used extensively to prepare this section. The two authors suggest dividing MRPs into three classes: melanoidin precursors (reactive low molecular weight compounds), premelanoidins (non-polymeric end products), and melanoidins. At the outset, it is important to underline that most data have been obtained by feeding experiments in rats, whereas only the Amadori compound fructosyllysine has been administered to humans (Erbersdobler et al, 1986; Lee and Erbersdobler, 1994).

11.6.1 Absorption

The intestinal absorption of the Amadori compounds occurs by passive diffusion (Faist and Erbersdobler, 2001). Amounts varying from 60 to 80% of ingested fructosyllysine is excreted in the urine, whereas only 1–3% undergoes faecal excretion (Faist and Erbersdobler, 2001). In humans trials (Erbersdobler et al, 1986; Lee and Erbersdobler, 1994) about 3% of orally administered casein-bound fructosyllysine is excreted in urine, and only 1% via the faeces. Higher transit rates have been reported for infants (Niederweiser et al, 1975), as 16 and 55% of casein-bound fructosyllysine ingested from glucose-containing formula were excreted in the urine and faeces, respectively. The fate of most protein-bound fructosyllysine in humans remains completely obscure, indicating that its fate is probably metabolisation, degradation by intestinal microorganisms, or accumulation in different tissues. Microbiological degradation up to 80% has been demonstrated by Erbersdobler et al (1970).

Consistent amounts of CML are formed in foods containing milk protein which are severely treated and very small amounts of CML, detectable in the urine of human infants, are now considered normal constituents of urine (Wadman et al, 1975). Among the few other premelanoidins that have been investigated, furans and pyrroles are known to inhibit intestinal carboxypeptidases and aminopeptidases (Öste et al, 1986). HMF, by radio-labelling experiments, has been demonstrated to accumulate mainly in the kidney and less in the bladder and liver (Germond, 1987).

In conclusion, taking into account the data collected to date, it can be said that three different mechanisms are likely to be involved in the metabolic transit of early and advanced MRPs: (1) intestinal degradation by digestive or microbial enzymes and subsequent adsorption of the MRPs or their degradation products;

(2) metabolisation of MRPs themselves or their degradation products, probably neither acting as metabolically inert substance; (3) different retention mechanisms in various tissues and organs (Faist and Erbersdobler, 2001).

In the case of melanodins, studies indicate that they are partially absorbed in the intestine; the level is low for high molecular weight fractions, and high for low molecular weight fractions. Specific transport mechanisms are still unknown. It is speculated that the fractions absorbed are not used by the organism and are excreted slightly modified or unmodified with the urine. Kidneys retain these compounds more than do other organs, such as liver. For the nonabsorbable low molecular weight fractions, intestinal degradation by digestive or microbial enzymes may be postulated while the high molecular weight fraction is not degraded (O'Brien and Morrissey, 1989).

11.6.2 Antioxidant activity

In vivo effects of MRPs and melanoidins may be classified as primary, attributed to specific actions, and secondary, based on interaction with other nutrients (Faist and Erbersdobler, 2001). Most of the secondary nutritional effects may be corrected with a suitable dietary supplementation.

An important primary effect of browning is the formation of antioxidants, compounds that are able to delay or prevent oxidation processes, typically involving lipids. Such antioxidants greatly affect the shelf-life of foods but may also benefit health (Halliwel, 1996), especially in the prevention of cancer (Kim and Mason, 1996), cardiovascular disease (Maxwell and Lip, 1997) and ageing (Deschamps et al, 2001).

The formation of antioxidants in browning has been observed in several different systems, for example sugar/amino acids model systems (Lignert and Eriksson, 1981), model melanoidins (Hayase et al, 1990), and honey/lysine model systems (Antony et al, 2000). They have also been seen in heated or roasted foods, such as coffee brews (Nicoli et al, 1997). However, the processing conditions should be chosen very carefully: in coffee, for example, the antioxidant activity increases with roasting up to the medium-dark roasted stage, then decreases with further roasting (Nicoli et al, 1997). This experimental observation is explained by the partial decomposition of the antioxidant compounds.

11.6.3 Activation of xenobiotic enzymes

Much interest has been raised also by the possible activation of xenobiotic enzymes by MRPs. Induction of detoxifying enzymes, either by natural or synthetic substances, is still a promising chemopreventive strategy (Faist and Erbersdobler, 2001). Naturally occurring substances in foods have been shown to serve as antimutagens, which may function as chemical inactivators, enzymatic inducers, scavengers and antioxidants. The modulators can act through enzyme systems by inducing phase-I and phase-II enzymes or by altering the balance of different enzyme activities.

Phase-I metabolic transformations include reduction, oxidation and hydrolytic reactions in order to release or induce functional or reactive groups from or into the xenobiotic substances. Phase-II transformations are mostly conjugation reactions of the parent xenobiotics, or phase-I metabolites, with sulphur-containing amino acids or glutathione. The conjugation reactions facilitate transport and hence elimination. Thus the balance between phase-I and phase-II enzymes is very critical (Prochaska and Talalay, 1988). The most potent inducers of these enzymes in foods are phenolic compounds and antioxidants. Antimutagenic properties of MRPs have been noted by Kim et al (1986) and are attributed to the inhibition of mutagenic activation through enhanced detoxification of reactive intermediates (Kitts et al, 1993; Pintauro and Lucchina, 1987). Because several MPRs or melanoidins exhibit antioxidant properties, they may inhibit phase-I mutagenic activating enzymes and may induce detoxifying phase-II enzymes. CML-casein increases significantly the activity of phase-II glutathione-S-transferase in kidney isolates, whereas LAL-casein has no effect (Faist et al, 1998; Wenzel et al, 2000).

11.6.4 Other activities

Melanodins possess the ability to bind metals, such as copper and zinc (O'Brien and Morrissey, 1989; Andrieux et al, 1980 and 1984; Furniss et al, 1986).

Some antibiotic activity against both pathogenic or spoilage organisms, including *Lactobacillus*, *Proteus*, *Salmonella* and *Streptococcus faecalis* and others, has been observed in mixtures obtained by heating arginine and xylose or histidine and glucose (Einarsson et al, 1983, 1988).

An interesting topic, still to be investigated in detail, is the relationship of MRPs with products that derive from physiological protein glycation, especially in diabetic patients and that are involved in ageing and act as promoting agents in Alzheimer's disease. However, it has been suggested that dietary restriction of food MRPs may be useful to reduce the burden of AGEs in diabetic patients and possibly improve the prognosis of the disease (Koschinsky et al, 1997).

11.7 Formation of toxic compounds

Epidemiological studies indicate that diet is an important factor in human cancer. In this respect, the negative consequence of thermal processing is the possible formation of highly mutagenic heterocyclic amines (HAs), that have attracted a growing interest since their discovery about 25 years ago (Sugimura et al, 1977). HAs include about 20 different derivatives that are found at ppb level in cooked muscle foods and can be divided in two classes: the amino-carbolines and the amino-imidazo-azaarenes (AIAs).

Amino-carbolines are sometimes called pyrolysis products, because they were first isolated from smoke condensates collected from cigarettes or from pyrolysed single amino acids or proteins. Figure 11.14 shows the structures of

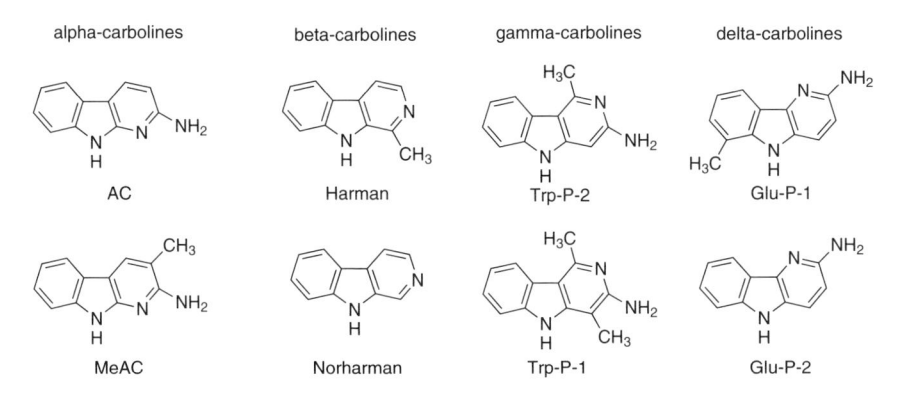

Fig. 11.14 Structures and trivial names of amino-carbolines.

the carbolines that have been detected in food or model systems. A typical feature is the presence of an exocyclic amino group on the pyridine ring, with the exception of β-carbolines (harman and norharman) that do not have the amino group and are not mutagenic, but have been demonstrated to be comutagenic (Hatch, 1986). They are assumed to be formed by a free-radical mechanism, but the pathways of their formation are still rather obscure. The α- and β-carbolines are formed by pyrolysis of animal proteins, such as albumin and casein, as well as of vegetable proteins, for example soy protein isolates. They are formed in model systems at temperatures similar to those applied to food cooking (Jägerstad et al, 1998). β-Carboline concentration in foods is generally 10–100 times greater than in that of other more mutagenic congeners.

AIAs are also referred to as thermic mutagens because they are formed at temperatures used during ordinary cooking and were first isolated from cooked meat and fish. Since they are very mutagenic, much attention has been applied to their determination in foods. They are characterised by the presence of a 2-amino-imidazo group, indispensable for genotoxic/mutagenic activity, and derive from the condensation of creatine with an aldehyde, coming from the Strecker degradation, and a pyrazine or pyridine. There are indications that free radicals may be involved (Pearson et al, 1992). Phenylalanine and creatine are the precursors of PhIP (Felton and Knize, 1991).

The number and position of the methyl groups on each ring contributes to a wide number of congeners (Fig. 11.15): the 2-amino-imidazo group is indispensable for mutagenic activity, but the number and position of the methyl groups determine the genotoxic potential of each congener (Benigni et al, 2000). They are fairly stable under ordinary cooking conditions, but start to degrade under prolonged heating (Arvidsson et al, 1997). A very detailed recent review (Jägerstad et al, 1998) contains a complete list of these toxic compounds and of the foods where they may be encountered. Minimising their formation requires knowledge of precursors, cooking conditions, reaction mechanisms and kinetics as well as information that the food industry needs to choose optimal

Structures (Fig. 11.15)

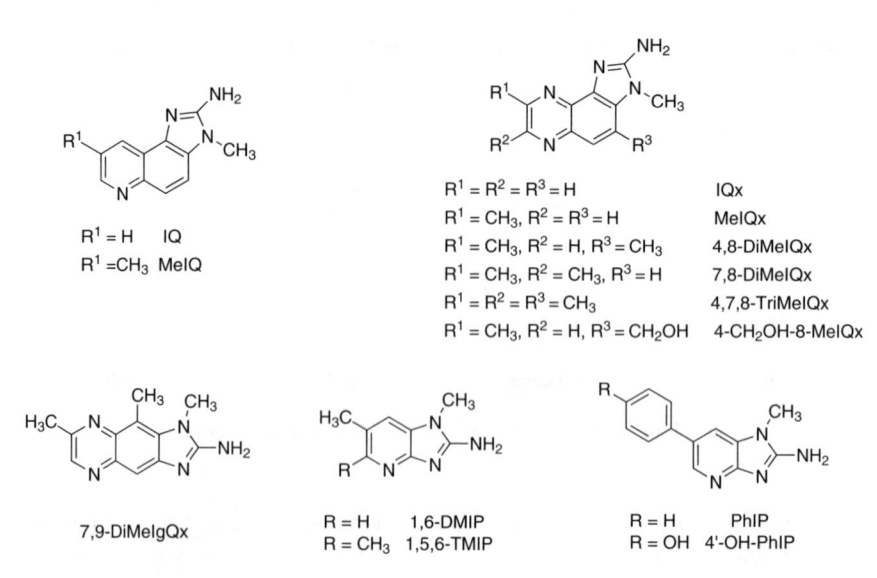

Structure 1 (quinoline-imidazole):
- $R^1 = H$ IQ
- $R^1 = CH_3$ MeIQ

Structure 2 (quinoxaline-imidazole):
- $R^1 = R^2 = R^3 = H$ — IQx
- $R^1 = CH_3, R^2 = R^3 = H$ — MeIQx
- $R^1 = CH_3, R^2 = H, R^3 = CH_3$ — 4,8-DiMeIQx
- $R^1 = CH_3, R^2 = CH_3, R^3 = H$ — 7,8-DiMeIQx
- $R^1 = R^2 = R^3 = CH_3$ — 4,7,8-TriMeIQx
- $R^1 = CH_3, R^2 = H, R^3 = CH_2OH$ — 4-CH$_2$OH-8-MeIQx

7,9-DiMeIgQx

1,6-DMIP / 1,5,6-TMIP:
- $R = H$ 1,6-DMIP
- $R = CH_3$ 1,5,6-TMIP

PhIP / 4′-OH-PhIP:
- $R = H$ PhIP
- $R = OH$ 4′-OH-PhIP

Fig. 11.15 Structures and trivial names of aminoimidazo-azaarenes.

conditions for designing food processes and food processing equipment. Temperature and cooking time are relevant parameters in determining their amount, and of the two temperature is the more critical (Knize et al, 1994). A kinetic model for the formation of polar HAs in a meat model system has been proposed (Arvidsson et al, 1998) and a detailed discussion of the selection of conditions and additives that may minimise their formation may be found in Jägerstad et al (1998).

HAs are found mostly in the crust of grilled and fried meat and fish and in the pan residue and, to a much lesser extent, in the interior of meat (Skog et al, 1995). In some countries pan residues are used to make gravy, which may result in a substantial contribution of HAs to the diet; to discard the pan residue is certainly a highly recommended habit.

The low concentration of HAs and the complex sample matrix of cooked foods make the analysis of these compounds very difficult (Pais and Knize, 2000). Most data reported in the literature refer to polar HAs in cooked muscle foods that are found at low ng/g level (for reviews see Skog, 1993; Layton et al, 1995). An improved method for the determination of non-polar HAs has been published more recently (Skog et al, 1998).

Many HAs have been shown to be carcinogenic in mice, rats, and non-human primates. However, epidemiological studies show conflicting data: some have shown an association between cooked meat and fish intake and cancer development and others no significant relationship (Sugimura et al, 1993; Steineck et al, 1993). Human liver metabolically activates some HAs through cytochrome P450 mediated N-oxidation and subsequent esterification reactions to produce the ultimate carcinogenic metabolites (Friedman, 1996). This metabolic activation leads to DNA adducts (Schut and Snyderwine, 1999).

The International Agency for Research on Cancer (IARC) regards some HAs as possibly or probably carcinogenic to humans and recommends to minimise exposure to them (IARC, 1993). Data suggest that HAs are the only known animal colon carcinogens that humans other than vegetarians consume every day and, although very difficult, it would be desirable to control their level in food. A detailed overview of the risk assessment can be found in a review by Friedman (1996).

11.8 Future trends

From the point of view of nutrition the two most important areas of research are either the toxicological aspects, principally related to the formation in particular conditions of mutagenic heterocyclic amines, or the positive nutritional features of some MRPs. In this sense most of the efforts are toward a better comprehension of the role of melanoidins in health, especially in relation to their antioxidant properties.

In fact, in recent years, nutritionists have dedicated much interest to the presence of antioxidants in vegetable foods. Some traditional products, such as extra virgin olive oil, red wine and tomato, have received great promotion from a better comprehension of their beneficial role in diet. Tomato is an interesting case because it has been demonstrated that in contrast to what one might superficially expect processing enhances the antioxidant activity (Anese et al, 1999). This fact has opened completely new scenarios to the possibilities offered in this field by processed foods.

The European Commission is financing a European cooperation in the field of scientific and technical research: COST Action 919 'Melanoidins in Food and Health', which aims to promote research on melanoidins both in food and health. The two work packages of greatest interest are WP4 'Antioxidant and other properties related to food shelf-life', and WP5 'Effects on health as assessed by *in vitro* and *in vitro* studies'. The results are being published in a series of books (Ames, 2001).

11.9 Sources of further information and advice

The reader will find useful discussion about the thermal treatment of food in Belitz and Grosch (1999). Every three to four years researchers working on the MR both in food science and medicine meet for an extremely important international symposium, whose proceedings are a very useful source of multidisciplinary information (Waller and Feather, 1983; Fujimaki et al, 1986; Finot et al, 1990; Labuza et al, 1994; O'Brien et al, 1998).

11.10 References

AHMED M U, THORPE S R and BAYNES J W (1986), 'Identification of N-ε-carboxymethyllysine as a degradation product of fructoselysine in glycated protein', *J Biol Chem*, **61**, 4889–94

ALAIZ M, HIDALGO F J and ZAMORA R (1997), 'Antioxidative activity of non-enzymatically browned proteins produced in oxidised lipid/protein reaction', *J Agric Food Chem*, **45**, 3250–4

AMADORI M (1931), 'Condensation products of glucose with *p*-toluidine', *Atti R Accad Naz Lincei Mem Cl Sci Fis Mat Nat*, **13**, 72

AMES J M (1992), 'The Maillard reaction', in Hudson B J F (ed), *Biochemistry in Food Proteins*, London, Elsevier, 99–153

AMES J M (2001), COST *Action 919. Melanoidins in Food and Health. Vol. 1. Food Science and Technology.* EUR 19 684, Brussels, European Commission

ANANTHARAMAN K and FINOT P A (1993), 'Nutritional aspects of food proteins in relation to technology', *Food Rev Int*, **9**, 629–55

ANDRIEUX C and SACQUET E (1984), 'Effects of Maillard's reaction products on apparent mineral absorption in different parts of the digestive tract. The role of microflora', *Reprod Nutr Develop*, **24**, 379–82

ANDRIEUX C, SACQUET E and GUEGUEN L (1980), 'Interactions between Maillard's reaction products, the microflora of the digestive tract and mineral metabolism', *Reprod Nutr Develop*, **20**, 1061–9

ANESE M, MANZOCCO L, NICOLI M C and LERICI C R (1999), 'Antioxidant activity of tomato juice as affected by heating', *J Sci Food Agric*, **79**, 750–4

ANTONY S M, HAN I Y, RIECK J R and DAWSON P L (2000), 'Antioxidative effect of Maillard reaction products formed from honey at different reaction times', *J Agric Food Chem*, **48**, 3985–9

ARDVIDSSON P, VAN BOEKEL M A J S, SKOG K and JÄGERSTAD M (1997), 'Kinetics of formation of polar heterocyclic amines in a meat model system', *J Food Sci*, **62**, 911–16

ARDVISSON P, VAN BOEKEL M A J S, SKOG K and JÄGERSTAD M (1998), 'Analysis of non-polar heterocyclic amines in cooked foods and meat extracts using gas chromatography-mass spectrometry', *J Chromat A*, **803**, 227–33

ARNOLDI A (2001), 'Thermal processing and food quality: analysis and control', in Richardson P, *Thermal Technologies in Food Processing*, Cambridge, UK, Woodhead Publishing Ltd., 138–59

ARNOLDI A, CORAIN E A, SCAGLIONI L and AMES J M (1997), 'New coloured compounds from the Maillard reaction between xylose and lysine', *J Agric Food Chem*, **45**, 650–5

BAYNES J W (2000), 'From life to death – the struggle between chemistry and biology during aging: the Maillard reaction as an amplifier of genomic damage', *Biogerontology*, **1**, 235–46

BELITZ H-D and GROSCH W (1999), *Food Chemistry*, Berlin Springer

BELLOMONTE G, BONIGLIA C, CARRATÙ B and FILESI C (1987), 'Lisinoalanina, presenza nei latti adattati per la prima infanzia', *Riv Soc It Sci Alim*, **16**, 459–64

BENIGNI R, GIULIANI A, FRANKE R and GRUSKA A (2000), 'Quantitative structure-activity relationships of mutagenic and carcinogenic aromatic amines', *Chem Rev*, **100**, 3697–714

BOSCHIN G, D'AGOSTINA, RINALDI A and ARNOLDI A (2002), 'Lysinoalanine content of formulas for enteral nutrition', *J Dairy Sci*, in press

BÜSER W and ERBERSDOBLER H F (1986), 'Carboxymethyllysine, a new compound of heat damage in milk products', *Milchwissenschaft*, **41**, 780–5

CHIANG G H (1983), 'A simple and rapid high-performance liquid-chromatography procedure for determination of furosine lysine-reducing sugar derivative', *J Agric Food Chem*, **31**, 1373–4

CODEX ALIMENTARIUS COMMISSION (1982), CX/VP 82/5 *Lysinoalanine Toxicity*. Ottawa 1–5 March
CORZO N, DELGADO T, TROYANO E and OLANO A (1994), 'Ratio of lactulose to furosine as indicator of quality of commercial milks', *J Food Prot*, **57**, 737–9
D'AGOSTINA A, BOSCHIN G, RINALDI A and ARNOLDI A (2002), 'Updating on the lysinoalanine content of infant formulae and beicost products', *Food Chem*, in press
D'AGOSTINA A, NEGRONI M and ARNOLDI A (1998), 'Autoxidation in the formation of volatiles from glucose-lysine', *J Agric Food Chem*, **46**, 2554–9
DE BRY L (1994), 'Antropological implications of the Maillard reaction: an insight', in Labuza T P, Reineccius G A, Monnier V M, O'Brien J, Baynes J W, *Maillard Reaction in Chemistry Food and Health*, Cambridge UK, The Royal Society of Chemistry, 28–36
DE KONING P J and VAN ROOIJEN P J (1982), 'Aspects of the formation of lysinoalanine in milk and milk products', *J Dairy Res*, **49**, 725–36
DESCHAMPS V, BARBERGER-GATEAU P, PEUCHANT E and ORGOGOZO J M (2001), 'Nutritional factors in cerebral aging and dementia: epidemiological arguments for a role of oxidative stress', *Neuroepidemiology*, **20**, 7–15
EINARSSON H, GORAN S, SNYGG B G and ERIKSSON C (1983), 'Inhibition of bacterial growth by Maillard reaction products', *J Agric Food Chem*, **31**, 1043–7
EINARSSON H, EKLUND T and NES I F (1988), 'Inhibitory mechanisms of Maillard reaction products', *Microbios*, **53**, 27–36
ERBERSDOBLER H F and ZUCKER H (1966), 'Untersuchungen zum gehalt an lysin und verfügbarem lysin in trockenmagermilch', *Milchwissenschaft*, **21**, 564–8
ERBERSDOBLER H F, GUSSNER I and WEBER G (1970), 'Abbau von fruktoselysin durch die Darmflora', *Zentralb Vet Med*, **A17**, 573–5
ERBERSDOBLER H F, PURWING U, BOSSEN M and TRAUTWEIN E A (1986), 'Urinary excretion of fructoselysine in human volunteers and diabetic patients', in Fujimaki M, Namiki M, Kato H, *Amino-carbonyl Reactions in Food and Biological Systems. Developments in Food Science 13*, Tokyo, Elsevier, 503–8
FAIST V and ERBERSDOBLER H F (2001), 'Metabolic transit and *in vivo* effects of melanoidins and precursor compounds deriving from the Maillard reaction', *Ann Nutr Metab*, **45**, 1–12
FAIST V, WENZEL E, TASTO S, MÜLLER C and ERBERSDOBLER H F (1998), 'Tissue specific induction of phase I and phase II xenobiotic enzymes and oxygen free radical metabolism in rats fed alkali treated protein containing high level of lysinoalanine', *FASEB J*, A1268
FELTON J S and KNIZE M G (1991), 'Occurrence, identification and bacterial mutagenicity of heterocyclic amines in cooked foods', *Mutant Res*, **259**, 205–17
FERRER E, ALEGRÌA A, FARRÈ R, ABELLÀN P and ROMERO F (2000), 'Effects of thermal processing and storage on available lysine and furfural compounds contents of infant formulas', *J Agric Food Chem*, **48**, 1817–22
FINLEY J and FRIEDMAN M (1977), 'New amino acid derivatives formed by alkaline treatment of proteins', *Adv Exp Med Biol*, **86B**, 123–30
FINOT P A, AESCHBACKER H U, HURRELL R F and LIARDON R (1990), *The Maillard Reaction in Food Processing, Human Nutrition and Physiology. Adv. Life Science*, Basel, Birkhäuser
FRANK O, OTTIGER H and HOFMANN T (2001), 'Characterisation of an intense bitter-tasting 1H,4H-quinolizinium-7-olate by application of the taste dilution analysis, a novel bioassay for the screening and identification of taste-active compounds in foods', *J Agric Food Chem*, **49**, 231–8
FRIEDMAN M (1996), 'Browning and its prevention: an overview', *J Agric Food Chem*, **44**, 631–53
FRIEDMAN M (1999), 'Chemistry, biochemistry, nutrition, and microbiology of lysinoalanine, lanthionine, and histidinoalanine in food and other proteins', *J Agric Food Chem*, **47**, 1295–319

FRIEDMAN M and PEARCE K N (1989), 'Copper (II) and cobalt (II) affinities of LL- and LD-lysinolanine diastereomers: implications for food safety and nutrition', *J Agric Food Chem*, **37**, 123–7

FRIEDMAN M, GUMBMANN M R and MASTERS P M (1984), 'Protein-alkali reactions: chemistry, toxicology, and nutritional consequences', *Adv Exper Med Biol*, **177**, 367–412

FRITSCH R J and KLOSTERMEYER H (1981), 'Improved method for the determination of lysinoalanine in foods', *Z Lebensm-Untersch Forsch*, **172**, 435–439

FUJIMAKI M, NAMIKI M and KATO H (1986), *Amino-carbonyl reactions in food and biological systems*, Tokyo, Elsevier

FUJIMOTO D (1984), 'Formation of histidinolanine crosslinks in heated proteins', *Experientia*, **40**, 832–33

FURNISS D E, HURRELL R F and FINOT P A (1986), 'Modification of urinary zinc excretion in the rat associated with the feeding of Maillard reaction products', *Acta Pharmacol Toxicol*, **59**, 188–90

FURTH A J (1997), 'Glycated proteins in diabetes', *Brit J Biomed Sci*, **54**, 192–200

GERMOND J E, PHILIPPOSSIAN G, RICHLI U, BRACCO I and ARNAUD M J (1987), 'Rapid and complete urinary elimination of [^{14}C]-5-hydroxymethyl-2-furaldehyde administered orally or intravenously to rats', *J Environm Health*, **22**, 79–89

GROSCH W (1987), 'Reaction of hydroperoxides – products of low molecular weight', in Chang H W-S, *Autoxidation of Unsaturated Lipids*, London, Academic Press, 95–140

GUMBMANN M R, FRIEDMAN M and SMITH G A (1993), 'The nutritional values and digestibilities of heat damaged casein and casein-carbohydrates mixtures', *Nutr Rep Int*, 355–61

HALLIWELL B (1996), 'Antioxidants in human health and disease', *Ann Rev Nutr*, **16**, 33–50

HARTKOPF J and ERBERSDOBLER H F (1993), 'Stability of furosine during ion-exchange chromatography in comparison with reverse-phase HPLC', *J Chromatogr*, **635**, 151–4

HARTKOPF J and ERBERSDOBLER H F (1994), 'Model studies of conditions for the formation of N-ε-carboxymethyllysine in food', *Z Lebensm Unters Forsch*, **198**, 15–19

HATCH F T (1986), 'A current genotoxicity database for heterocyclic amines food mutagens I. Genetically relevant endpoints', *Environ Health Perspect*, **67**, 93–103

HAYASE F, HIRASHIMA S, OKAMOTO G and KATO H (1990), 'Scavenging of active oxygen by melanoidins', in Finot P A, Aeschbacker H U, Hurrell R F, Liardon R (1990), *The Maillard Reaction in Food Processing, Human Nutrition and Physiology. Adv. Life Science*, Basel, Birkhäuser, 361–6

HAYASHI T and NAMIKI M (1981), 'On the mechanism of free radical formation during browning reaction of sugars with amino compounds', *Agric Biol Chem*, **45**, 933–9

HAYASHI T and NAMIKI M (1986), 'Role of sugar fragmentation in early stage browning of amino-carbonyl reaction of sugars with amino acids', *Agric Biol Chem*, **50**, 1965–70

HEINRICH L and BALTES W (1987), 'Occurrence of phenols in coffee melanoidins', *Z Lebensm Untersch*, **185**, 366–70

HENLE T, WALTER A W and KLOSTERMEYER H (1993), 'Detection and identification of the cross-linking amino acids N^τ- and N^π-(2'-amino-2'-carboxy-ethyl)-L-histidine ("histidinoalanine", HAL) in heated milk products', *Z Lebensm Unters Forsch*, **197**, 114–17

HENLE T, ZEHTNER G and KLOSTERMEYER H (1995), 'Fast and sensitive determination of furosine in food', *Z Lebensm Unters Forsch*, **200**, 235–7

HENLE T, SCHWARZENBOLZ U and KLOSTERMEYER H (1996), 'Irreversible cross-linking of casein during storage of UHT-treated skim milk', *Int. Dairy Fed. (Spec. issue) S.I. 9602 (Heat Treatments & Alternative Methods)*, 290–8

HEWEDY M, KIESNER C, MEISSNER K, HARTKOPF J and ERBERSDOBLER H F (1991), 'Effect of UHT heating milk in an experimental plant on several indicators of heat treatment', *J Dairy Res*, **61**, 304–9

HEYNS K and NOACK H (1962), 'Die Umzetzung von d-fructose mit L-Lysine and L-Arginin und deren Beiziehung zu nichtenenzymatischen Bräunungsreaktionen', *Chem Ber*, 720–7

HODGE J E (1953), 'Chemistry of browning reactions in model systems', *J Agric Food Chem*, **1**, 928–43
HOFMANN T (1998a), 'Characterization of the most intensely coloured compounds from Maillard reactions of pentoses by application of colour dilution analysis', *Carbohydr Res*, **313**, 203–13
HOFMANN T (1998b), 'Characterization of precursors and elucidation of the reaction pathway leading to a novel coloured 2*H*,7*H*,8a*H*-pyrano[2,3-*b*]pyran-3-one from pentoses by quantitative studies and application of ^{13}C-labelling experiments', *Carbohydr Res*, **313**, 215–24
HOFMANN T (1998c), 'Studies on the relationship between molecular weight and colour potency of fractions obtained by thermal treatment of glucose/amino acid and glucose/protein solutions by using ultracentrifugation and colour dilution techniques', *J Agric Food Chem*, **46**, 3891–5
HOFMANN T (1998d), 'Identification of novel colored compounds containing pyrrole and pyrrolinone structures formed by Maillard Reactions of pentoses and primary amino acids', *J Agric Food Chem*, **46**, 3902–11
HOFMANN T, BORS W and STETTMAIER K (1999), 'On the radical-assisted melanoidin formation during thermal processing of foods as well as under physiological conditions', *J Agric Food Chem*, **47**, 391–6
IARC (1993), *Monographs on the Evaluation of Carcinogenic Risk to Humans: Vol. 56. Some Naturally Occurring Aromatic Amines and Mycotoxins*, Lyon, International Agency for Research on Cancer, 163–242
JÄGERSTAD M, SKOG K, ARVIDSSON P and SOLYAKOV A (1998), 'Chemistry, formation, and occurrence of genotoxic heterocyclic amines identified in model systems and cooked foods', *Z Lebensm Unters Forsch A*, **207**, 419–27
JAMES M and CRABBE C (1998), 'Cataract as a conformational disease – the Maillard reaction, α-crystalline and chemotherapy', *Cell Molec Biol*, **44**, 1047–50
KARAYIANNIS N I, MACGREGOR J T and BJELDANES L F (1980), 'Biological effects of alkali-treated soy protein and lactalbumin in the rat and mouse', *Food Cosmet Toxicol*, **18**, 333–46
KEENEY M and BASSETTE R (1959), 'Detection of intermediate compounds in the early stages of browning reaction in milk products', *J Dairy Sci*, **42**, 945–60
KIM S B, HAYASE F and KATO H (1986), 'Desmutagenic effects of melanoidins against amino acid and protein pyrolisates', in Fujimaki M, Namiki M, Kato H (eds), *Amino-carbonyl Reactions in Food and Biological Systems. Developments in Food Science 13*, Tokyo, Elsevier, 383–92
KIM Y I and MASON J B (1996), 'Nutrition chemoprevention of gastrointestinal cancers – a critical review', *Nutr Rev*, **54**, 259–79
KITTS D D, WU C H and POWRIE W D (1993), 'Effect of glucose-lysine Maillard reaction products fractions on tissue xenobiotic enzyme systems', *J Agric Food Chem*, **41**, 2359–63
KNIZE M G, CUNNINGHAM P L, AVILA J R, GRIFFIN E A JR and FELTON J S (1994), 'Formation of mutagenic activity from amino acids heated at cooking temperatures', *Food Chem Toxicol*, **32**, 55–60
KOSCHINSKY T, HE C J, MITSUHASHI T, BUCALA R, LIU C, BUENTING C, HEITMANN K and VLASSARA H (1997), 'Orally adsorbed reactive glycation products (glycotoxins): an environmental risk factor in diabetic retinopathy', *Proc Natl Acad Sci USA*, **94**, 6474–9
KUNTCHEVA M J and OBRETENOV T D (1996), 'Isolation and characterization of melanoidins from beer', *Z Lebensm Untersch*, **202**, 238–43
LABUZA T P, REINECCIUS G A, MONNIER V M, O'BRIEN J and BAYNES J W (1994), *Maillard Reaction in Chemistry Food and Health*, Cambridge UK, The Royal Society of Chemistry, 28–36
LANGHENDRIES J P, HURRELL R F, FURNISS D E, HISCHENHUBER C, FINOT P A, BERNARD A, BATTISTI O, BERTRAND J M and SENTERRE J (1992), 'Maillard reaction products and

lysinoalanine: urinary excretion and the effects on kidney function of preterm infants fed heat-processed milk formula', *J Pediatr Gastroenter Nutr*, **14**, 62–70

LAYTON D W, BOGEN K T, KNIZE M G, HATCH F T, JOHNSON V M and FELTON J S (1995), 'Cancer risk of heterocyclic amines in cooked foods; an analysis and implications for research', *Carcinogenesis*, **16**, 39–52

LEDL F and SCHLEICHER E (1990), 'New aspects of the Maillard reaction in foods and in the human body', *Angew Chem Int Ed*, **29**, 565–706

LEE K and ERBERSDOBLER H F (1994), 'Balance experiments on human volunteers with fructoselysine (FL) and lysinoalanine (LAL)', in Labuza T P, Reineccius G A, Monnier V M, O'Brien J, Baynes J W (eds), *Maillard Reaction in Chemistry Food and Health*, Cambridge UK, The Royal Society of Chemistry, 358–63

LEE Y S, HOMMA S and AIDA K (1987), 'Characterisation of melanoidins in soy sauce and fish sauce by electrofocusing and high performance gel permeation chromatography', *J Jap Soc Food Sci Technol*, **34**, 313–19

LIGNERT H and ERIKSSON C E (1981), 'Antioxidative effect of Maillard reaction products', *Prog. Food Nutr Sci*, **5**, 453–66

MAGA J A (1984), 'Lysinoalanine in foods', *J Agric Food Chem*, **32**, 955–64

MAIER H G and BUTTLE H (1973), 'Isolation and characterization of brown compounds of coffee' (in German), *Z Lebensm Untersch*, **150**, 331–4

MAILLARD A C (1912), 'Action des acides amines sur les sucres. Formation des melanoidines par voie methodologique', *C R Acad Sci*, **154**, 66–8

MAXWELL S R J and LIP G Y H (1997), 'Free radicals and antioxidants in cardiovascular disease', *Brit J Clinic Pharmac*, **44**, 307–17

MILIC B LJ, GRUJIC INJAC B, PILETIC M V, LAJSIC S and KOLAROV LJ A (1975), 'Melanoidins and carbohydrates in roasted barley', *J Agric Food Chem*, **23**, 960–3

MORALES F, ROMERO C and JIMENEZ-PEREZ S (1997), 'Chromatographic determination of bound hydroxymethylfurfural as an index of milk protein glycosylation', *J Agric Food Chem*, **45**, 1570–3

NAKAYAMA T, HAYASE F and KATO H (1980), 'Formation of ε-(2-formyl-4-hydroxymethyl-pyrrol-1-yl)-L-norleucine in the Maillard reaction between D-glucose and L-lysine', *Agric Biol Chem*, **44**, 1201–1201

NICOLI M C, MARZOCCO L, LERICI C R and ANESE M (1997), 'Antioxidant properties of coffee-brews in relation to roasting', *Lebensm Wiss U-Technol*, **30**, 292–7

NIEDERWEISER A, GILIBERTI P and MATASOVIC A (1975), 'Nε-L-deoxyfructosyl-lysine in urine after ingestion of a lactose-free, glucose containing milk formulas', *Pediatr Res*, **9**, 867–72

NUNES F M and COIMBRA M A (2001), 'Chemical characterisation of the high molecular weight material extracted with hot water from green and roasted arabica coffee', *J Agric Food Chem*, **49**, 1773–82

OBRETENOV T D, KUNTCHEVA M J, MANTCHEV S C and VALKOVA G D (1991), 'Isolation and characterization of melanoidins from malt and malt roots', *J Food Biochem*, **15**, 279–94

O'BRIEN J (1995), 'Heat induced changes in lactose: isomerisation, degradation, Maillard browning', in Fox R F, *Heat Induced Changes in Milk*. 2 ed., London, International Dairy Federation, Elsevier, 134–70

O'BRIEN J and MORRISSEY P A (1989), 'Nutritional and toxicological aspects of the Maillard browning reaction in foods', *Crit Rev Food Nutr*, **28**, 211–48

O'BRIEN J, NURSTEN H E, CRABBE M J C and AMES J M (1998), *The Maillard Reaction in Foods and Medicine*, Cambridge UK, The Royal Society of Chemistry

ÖSTE R E, DAHLQUIST A, SJÖSTRÖM H, NORÉN O and MILLER R (1986), 'Effect of Maillard reaction products on protein digestion: *in vitro* studies', *J Agric Food Chem*, **34**, 354–8

OTTIGER H, BARETH A and HOFMANN T (2001), 'Characterization of natural "cooling" compounds formed from glucose and L-proline in dark malt by application of taste dilution analysis', *J Agric Food Chem*, **49**, 1336–44

PAIS P and KNIZE M G (2000), 'Chromatographic and related techniques for the determination of aromatic heterocyclic amines in foods', *J Chromat B*, **747**, 139–69

PEARSON A M, CHEN C, GRAY J L and AUST S D (1992), 'Mechanism(s) involved in meat mutagen formation and inhibition', *Free Rad Biol Med*, **13**, 161–7

PELLEGRINO L, RESMINI P, DE NONI I and MASOTTI F (1996), 'Sensitive determination of lysinoalanine for distinguishing natural from imitation mozzarella cheese', *J Dairy Sci*, **79**, 725–34

PELLEGRINO L, VAN BOEKEL M A J S, GRUPPEN H and RESMINI P (1998), 'Maillard compounds as crosslinks in heated β-casein-glucose systems', in O'Brien J, Nursten H E, Ames J M (eds), *The Maillard Reaction in Food and Medicine*, Cambridge UK, The Royal Society of Chemistry, 100–1

PETRACCO M, NAVARINI L, ABATANGELO A, GOMBAC V, D'AGNOLO E and ZANETTI F (1999), 'Isolation and characterisation of a foaming fraction from hot water extracts of roasted coffee', *Colloq Sci Int Cafè 18th*, 95–105

PINTAURO S J and LUCCHINA L A (1987), 'Effects of Maillard browned egg albumin on drug-metabolizing enzyme systems in the rat', *Food Chem Toxicol*, **25**, 369–72

PROCHASKA H J and TALALAY P (1988), 'Regulatory mechanisms of monofunctional and bifunctional anticarcinogenic enzyme inducers in murine liver', *Cancer Res*, **48**, 4776–82

RAVAGLI A, BOSCHIN G, SCAGLIONI L and ARNOLDI A (1999), 'Reinvestigation of the reaction between 2-furan-carbaldehyde and 4-hydroxy-5-methyl-3(2H)-furanone', *J Agric Food Chem*, **47**, 4962–9

RENNER E and VETTER M (1988), 'Formation of lactulose and lysinoalanine in milk-based infant formulae', *J Dairy Sci*, **71**, Suppl. 1, 79

RESMINI P and PELLEGRINO L (1994), 'Occurence of protein-bound lysylpyrrolealdehyde in dried pasta', *Cereal Chem*, **71**, 254–62

RESMINI P, PELLEGRINO L and BATTELLI G (1990), 'Accurate quantification of furosine in milk and dairy products by a direct HPLC method', *Ital J Food Sci*, **3**, 173–83

RIZZI G P (1997), 'Chemical structure of coloured Maillard reaction products', *Food Rev Int*, **13**, 1–28

SARWAR G, L'ABBE M R, TRICK K, BOTTIG H G and MA C Y (1999), 'Influence of feeding alkaline heat treated processed proteins on growth and protein and mineral status of rats', *Adv Exp Med Biol*, **459**, 161–77

SAVOIE L, PARENT G and GALIBOIS I (1991), 'Effects of alkali treatment on the *in-vitro* digestibility of proteins and the release of amino acids', *J Sci Food Agric*, **56**, 363–72

SCHUT H A J and SNYDERWINE E G (1999), 'DNA adducts of heterocyclic amine food mutagens: implications for mutagenesis and carcinogenesis', *Carcinogenesis*, **20**, 353–68

SINGH R, BARDEN A, MORI T and BEILIN L (2001), 'Advanced glycation end-products: a review', *Diabetologia*, **44**, 129–46

SKOG K (1993), 'Cooking procedures and food mutagens: a literature review', *Food Chem Toxicol*, **31**, 655–75

SKOG K, STEINECK G, AUGUSTSSON K and JÄGERSTAD M (1995), 'Effect of cooking temperature on the formation of heterocyclic amines in fried meat products and pan residues', *Carcinogenesis*, **16**, 861–7

SKOG K, SOLYAKOV A, ARDVISSON P and JÄGERSTAD M (1998), 'Analysis of non polar heterocyclic amines in cooked foods and meat extracts using gas chromatography-mass spectrometry', *J Chromat A*, **803**, 227–33

STEINECK G, GERHARDSSON DE VERDIER M and ÖVERVIK E (1993), 'The epidemiological evidence concerning intake of mutagenic activity from fried surface and the risk of cancer cannot justify preventive measures', *Eur J Cancer Prev*, **2**, 293–300

STEINHART H and PACKERT A (1993), 'Melanoidins in coffee. Separation and characterization by different chromatographic procedures', *Colloq. Sci. Int. Café 15th*, 593–600

SUGIMURA T, NAGAO M, KAWACHI T, HONDA M, YAHAGI T, SEINO Y, SATO S, MATSUKARA

N, SHIRAI A, SAWAMURA M and MATSUMOTO H (1977), 'Mutagens–carcinogens in food, with special reference to highly mutagenic pyrolytic products in boiled foods', in Hiatt H H, Watson J D, Winsten J A (eds), *Origins of Human Cancer*, Cold Spring Harbor Laboratory, 1561–77

SUGIMURA T, WAKABAYASHI K, NAGAO M and ESUMI H (1993), 'A new class of carcinogens: heterocyclic amines in cooked food', in Parke D V, Ioannides C, Walker R (eds), *Food, Nutrition and Chemical Toxicity*, London, Smith-Gordon and Company, 259–76

SULLIVAN R (1996), 'Contributions to senescence-non-enzymatic-glycosylation of proteins', *Arch Physiol Biochem*, **104**, 797–806

TRESSL R, NITTKA C H, KERSTEN E and REWICKI D (1995), 'Formation of isoleucine specific Maillard products from [1-^{13}C]-D-glucose and [1–^{13}C]-D-fructose', *J Agric Food Chem*, **43**, 1163–9

TRESSL R, WONDRACK G, KRUGER R-P, REWICKI D and GARBE L-A (1998a), 'Pentoses and hexoses as source of new melanoidin-like Maillard-polymers', *J Agric Food Chem*, **46**, 1756–76

TRESSL R, WONDRACK G T, KRÜGER R P and REWICKI D (1998b), 'New melanoidin-like Maillard polymers from 2-deoxypentoses', *J Agric Food Chem*, **46**, 104–10

VINALE F, FOGLIANO V, SCHIERBERLE P and HOFMANN T (1999), 'Development of a stable isotope dilution assay for an accurate quantification of protein-bound Nε-(1-deoxy-D-fructos-1-yl)-L-lysine using a ^{13}C-labeled internal standard', *J Agric Food Chem*, **47**, 5084–92

WADMAN S K, DE BREE P K, VAN SPRANG F J, KAMERLING J P, HAVERKAMP J and VLIEGENTHART J F G (1975), 'Nε-carboxymethyllysine, a constituent of human urine', *Clin Chim Acta*, **59**, 313–20

WALLER G R and FEATHER M S (1983), *The Maillard Reaction in Foods and Nutrition, ACS Symposium Ser. 215*, Washington DC, American Chemical Society

WENZEL E, FAIST V, TASTO S and ERBERSDOBLER H F (2000), 'Einfluss von freiem und Proteingebundenem Nε-Carboxymethyllysine auf die NADPH-cytochrom c-Reduktase und die Glutathion-*S*-Transferase *in vitro* und *in vivo*', *Proc Germ Nutr Soc*, **2**, 18

WHITFIELD F B (1992), 'Volatiles from the interactions of the Maillard reaction and lipids', *Crit Rev Food Sci Nutr*, **31**, 1–58

YAYLAYAN V A (1997), 'Classification of the Maillard reaction: a conceptual approach', *Trends Food Sci Technol*, **8**, 13–18

YAYLAYAN V A and HUYGGUES-DESPOINTES A (1994), 'Chemistry of Amadori rearrangement products', *Crit Rev Food Sci Nutr*, **34**, 321–69

YAYLAYAN V A and KEYHANI A (1996), 'Py/GC/MS analysis of non-volatile flavor precursors: Amadori compounds', in Pickenhagen W, Ho C-T, Spanier A M (eds), *Contribution of Low and Non-volatile Materials to the Flavor of Food*, Carol Stream IL, USA, Allured Publishing Company, 13–26

YEBOAH F K and YAYLAYAN V A (2001), 'Analysis of glycated proteins by mass spectrometric techniques: qualitative and quantitative aspects', *Nahrung-Food*, **45**, 164–71

12

Frying

J. Pokorný, Prague Institute of Chemical Technology

12.1 Introduction

Frying, especially deep fat frying, has become the most popular food preparation technology during the last five decades. The reason is that the preparation is easy even for less experienced cooks, the procedure is rapid, and the finished product is highly palatable. In the frying procedure, fat is the medium of heat transfer. Two main frying methods exist, namely shallow frying and deep frying.

In case of shallow frying, the layer of frying oil is about 1–10 mm thick in a pan and the fried food is only partially immersed; it has to be turned during the process to obtain an evenly cooked product. The frying takes about 5–10 min, and frying oil is used for greasing the food as it is cooking. The oil is not reused.

In case of deep frying, the layer of frying oil is 20–200 mm thick or greater and the fried material is immersed in oil or floats on the surface. The frying again takes about 5–10 min, depending on the dimensions of the food being fried and on the temperature. After frying, the food is removed and the frying oil is used again for the next frying. The duration of use depends mainly on the frying medium, the technical equipment and on the food.

The increasing consumption of fried foods contributes to a high intake of fats and oils. Because consumers wish to reduce their consumption of fats and oils pans are offered on the market that do not require any fat. When these are used the heat transfer medium is not oil and therefore the process should not be regarded as frying but as roasting. During frying, fat or oil is preheated to temperatures of 150–180 °C. In contact with oil, fried food is heated rapidly in the surface layers to the temperature of the frying oil. The temperature reaches only 80–100 °C in inner layers.

12.2 Changes in frying oil

12.2.1 Types of reaction

The oil is subject to three types of reaction during deep frying:

- hydrolytic reactions;
- oxidation reactions;
- pyrolysis of oxidation products.

Triacylglycerols in frying oil are hydrolysed by steam produced from water in the fried product when it is in contact with the hot frying oil. As the two reacting partners are not miscible, the reaction is relatively slow, resulting in the formation of diacylglycerols and free fatty acids. Diacylglycerols are more polar and therefore their contact with water vapour is better; monoacylglycerols and free fatty acids are formed by further hydrolysis. Monoacylglycerols are rapidly hydrolysed into fatty acid and glycerol. Under deep frying conditions, glycerol is dehydrated into acrolein, which is very volatile and its vapours irritate the eyes and mucosa.

The rate of oxidation reactions depends on the concentration of oxygen. Oxygen present in the original frying oil is rapidly consumed, usually before the temperature of oil reaches the frying temperature. Additional oxygen can enter frying oil only through diffusion from air (Fujisaki et al, 2000). When contact with air is moderate the oxidation of the frying oil is slow. It is consumed for the destruction of natural antioxidants, and only when they are destroyed, triacylglycerols are oxidised, too. Hydroperoxides are formed as primary reaction products, but they are very unstable at high temperature so that their content rarely exceeds 1%.

Some components present in fried food affect the oxidation rate of frying oil (Pokorný, 1998). The oxidation rate could be reduced by addition of antioxidants even when they are less efficient than under storage conditions. Most synthetic antioxidants, such as BHT and BHA, are too volatile under frying so that they have only moderate activity. Gallates are more efficient in frying oils. Currently it is considered preferable to use natural antioxidants. Tocopherols are present in most frying oils, and their addition is efficient (Gordon and Kourimska, 1995). Ascorbyl palmitate, citric acid and its esters are useful as synergists. Rosemary and sage resins were also found to be active in frying oils (Che Man and Tan, 1999). Oxidation reactions can be inhibited by polysiloxanes, which form a very thin layer on the surface of the frying oil, preventing the access of oxygen (Ohta et al, 1988). Because they are not resorbed in the intestines they are considered safe for human consumption.

The third group of reactions are secondary reactions of hydroperoxides. They are decomposed in three ways during frying:

- Decomposition into nonvolatile products with the same number of carbon atoms, such as epoxides, ketones or hydroxylic compounds. When the concentration of these products (known as polar products) exceeds 25–27%, the frying oil has to be replaced by fresh oil. At still higher levels of polar products, foaming takes place, which increases the contact area of oil with air, and thus the rate of oxidation.

- Decomposition into volatile low-molecular weight compounds, such as aldehydes, alcohols, ketones or hydrocarbons. Some products possess a typical fried flavour, e.g. 2,4-decadienals or unsaturated lactones. They are formed from linoleic acid bound in frying oil.
- Decomposition into high molecular weight compounds, usually dimers or trimers with fatty acid chains bonded by C–C, C–O–C or C–O–O–C bonds. The content of polymers is a good indicator of the degree of frying oil degradation. When their content reaches 10%, used oil should be replaced by fresh oil.

Several methods are used for monitoring oil degradation during frying (Wu and Nawar, 1986). Used oil can be analysed with use of HPLC (for polar compounds) or HPSEC (for polymers); this is best done in combination with column chromatography (Sánchez-Muniz et al, 1993). Among other methods, the spectrophotometry, determination of permittivity (dielectric constant), specific gravity or different colour tests can be used (Xu, 2000).

Frying oil can be used for a longer time if it is purified from insoluble particles and polar substances by using a suitable adsorbent, such as magnesium silicate (Perkins and Lamboni, 1998). Commercial products for this pupose are available (Gertz et al, 2000). Their combination with antioxidants is recommended (Kochhar, 2000). Membrane processes have been proposed for purification of frying oil (Miyagi et al, 2001).

12.2.2 Choice of frying oil

Frying oil should contain some bound linoleic acid to generate a fried flavour (Warner et al, 1997). Some oils, such as soybean, sunflower or rapeseed oils are rich in linoleic acid, but are rather unstable under frying conditions and should be replaced very often by fresh oil, which is expensive (Gertz et al, 2000). Low polyunsaturated oils, such as olive oil, are highly priced. Hydrogenated vegetable oils are more stable but are objectionable because of the content of *trans*-unsaturated fatty acids. Pork lard is an excellent frying medium from the standpoint of sensory value, but there are objections because of its high content of saturated fatty acids and of cholesterol. The best choice are high-oleic low-polyenoic modified vegetable oils, such as fractionated palm oil, i.e. the palm olein fraction (Che Man and Hussin, 1998), modified soybean, sunflower, rapeseed, peanut, and even linseed oil. If they contain 3–10% linoleic acid, they still produce an attractive fried flavour and are sufficiently stable on frying. A problem is their availability on the market.

12.3 Impact of deep frying on nutrients

The following main changes occur in the frying process (Fillion and Henry, 1998):

- Mass transfer between frying oil and fried food;
- Thermal decomposition of nutrients and antinutritional substances in fried food;
- Interaction between fried food components and oxidation products of fried oil (Dobarganes et al, 2000).

12.3.1 Impact of frying on main nutrients

The main change in the food composition during frying is the loss of water and its replacement with frying oil. Most foods (other than nuts) contain water as their major component. In contact with hot frying oil, water is rapidly converted into steam, at least in the surface layer of fried material. The temperature of inner layers does not exceed the boiling point of water so that water losses are only moderate.

Spaces left in fried food after water evaporation are filled with frying oil (Pinthus et al, 1995). This process increases the available energy content of the product and because the energy intake in the diet is too high in many countries, it is desirable to reduce the absorption of frying oil. This may be achieved by drying pieces of food on the surface before immersion into oil (Baumann and Escher, 1995). Another way is to produce a crust on the surface of fried pieces, which prevents water losses and oil uptake, and preserves juiciness in fried material (Ateba and Mittal, 1994). It is possible to cover the surface with batter or various other preparations, such as cellulose derivatives (Priya et al, 1996). The oil absorption can be reduced by half using these procedures. The oil removed by absorption into fried food should be replenished by fresh oil from time to time in order to keep the volume of frying oil constant.

Changes in nutritional value depend not only on the amount of absorbed frying oil, but also on its composition. If fresh edible oil is used, the contents of essential fatty acids and tocopherols in fried food rise. If food is fried in oil used for a longer time, the content of essential fatty acids and tocopherols becomes low, so that the increase in nutritional value, due to absorbed oil, is not significant. On the contrary, such antinutritional products as polar lipids and polymers are absorbed with used frying oil.

If fried food is stored, even under refrigeration, the thin layer of frying oil on the surface is autoxidized, especially in case of oil rich in polyunsaturated fatty acids (Warner et al, 1994). Fried food should be stored either in vacuum or an inert gas or protected by antioxidants.

If fat-rich food is fried, such as bacon, sausages or fat fishes, some fat originally present in food is released into frying oil. Eicosapentaenoic and docosahexaenoic acids were detected in oils used for frying fish like sardines (Sánchez-Muniz et al, 1992). Cholesterol may also be extracted into frying oil.

If plant foods are subsequently fried in the same oil, cholesterol or fish fatty acids may be absorbed.

Lipids present in food are decomposed only to a small extent, including high unsaturated fish oils. It is due to short frying time and limited access of oxygen. Based on dry matter content, the concentration of most nutrients is reduced during frying, as the original nutrients are diluted with absorbed frying oil. Starch and non-starch carbohydrates are partially destroyed during frying, and starch-lipid complexes are formed (Thed and Phillips, 1995). The fraction of resistant (undigestible) starch changes during the operation (Parchure and Kulkarni, 1997). Sucrose is hydrolysed into glucose and fructose, which are destroyed by heating, mostly by Maillard or caramelisation reactions.

Proteins are rapidly denatured in surface layers of food particles, more slowly in inner layers than on the surface. Enzymes get nearly completely deactivated. The availability of proteins in humans is usually reduced by frying (Fukuda et al, 1989), especially on the surface (Pokorný et al, 1992). Some essential amino acids are destroyed, such as lysine or tryptophan (Ribarova et al, 1994). If protein comes into contact with the hot walls of the frying pan above the oil level, it is dehydrated and pyrolysed into polycyclic aromatic compounds (Övervik et al, 1989).

12.3.2 Impact of frying on micronutrients

Vitamins are relatively labile substances. Tocopherols are decomposed by oxidation reactions so that frying oil used for repeated frying contains only traces of tocopherols. Ascorbic acid is also destroyed by mechanisms similar to those of reducing sugars. The Vitamin B complex is also substantially damaged by frying (Kimura et al, 1991; Olds et al, 1993). Carotenes and carotenoid pigments are easily oxidised and polymerised (Speek et al, 1988), which is visible from colour changes.

Mineral components are also affected. Iron and other heavy metals are mostly bound in complexes, which are partially decomposed during frying, and metal ions may contaminate frying oil by decreasing its resistance to oxidation. Ferric ions are less digestible than iron in haem complexes. Sodium and potassium chlorides present in food are very slightly dissociated, and sodium and potassium ions react with free fatty acids forming soaps (Blumenthal and Stockler, 1986). Soaps are surface active agents, increasing foaming and thus accelerating oxidation. Volatile mineral components, such as selenium or mercury derivatives, are partially lost at high frying temperatures. Many foods contain antinutritional or even toxic substances, which are often partially decomposed or evaporated during frying.

12.3.3 Changes in sensory characteristics

Frying imparts a distinctive flavour to fried products; some flavours are common to all fried foods and some are additional and, specific for particular products, e.g. french fries (Wagner and Grosch, 1998).

The colour of the fried product often differs substantially from that of the original food material. The most important reactions are nonenzymic browning reactions between reducing sugars and free amino acids, called Maillard reactions. Colourless premelanoidins are a group of intermediary products with very low nutritional value. They are rapidly polymerised into macromolecular deep brown melanoidins, which are completely unavailable for human nutrition. To obtain light-coloured potato chips, it is necessary to adjust the concentration of reducing sugars to low values (Califano and Calvelo, 1987). A side reaction is the Strecker degradation of free amino acids under attack of dicarbonylic sugar degradation products. Heterocyclic products, such as pyrazines or furans, have typical fried or roasted flavour notes (Chun and Ho, 1997). Similar browning reactions are caused by interactions of frying oil oxidation products (mostly hydroperoxides or unsaturated aldehydes) with the free amine group of bound lysine (Pokorný, 1981). Lysine thus becomes unavailable for human nutrition.

Oxidised frying oil also contributes in significant degree to the flavour of fried food (Chang et al, 1978). Moderate amounts are necessary to produce the typical fried flavour but greater amounts are objectionable. For this reason the frying oil should not be too fresh for high quality fried foods. The flavour improves by repeated use for frying, but if use is too long then products are of lower quality. The producer's aim is to maintain frying oil for the longest time possible at the stage of optimum performance (Blumenthal and Stier, 1991).

12.4 Future trends

Deep frying will probably become an even more important process of food preparation, and its conditions and the equipment will be improved gradually. Fried foods contain high amounts of fat, and are therefore rich in available energy. Since energy intake is too high in most countries, frying technology will be modified in order to reduce the absorption of frying oil during the operation; however, the intensity and pleasantness of fried food should remain unaffected.

Frying oil is oxidised during heating. Criteria for replacing used oil by fresh oil are arbitrary (Firestone, 1993), e.g. 25% polar products and 10% polymers, and are not based on experimental evidence. The composition of oxidation products and their impact on food safety should be determined more precisely. Frying oil deterioration depends on its degree of unsaturation and on the content of natural and/or added antioxidants. New oils will be introduced on the market with better stability during frying and intervals between necessary replacing of used oil will get longer. The flavour quality of fried products should not be affected by new, more stable frying oils. New flavourings will be developed for flavouring products fried in oils free of polyunsaturated fatty acids, or obtained by heating in pans designed for frying without oil. The flavour of such products should be that of deep fried products.

12.5 Sources of further information and advice

BLUMENTHAL M M (1987), *Optimum frying: theory and practice*, Piscataway, NJ, Libra Laboratories
BOSKOU D and ELMADFA I (1999), *Frying of food*, Lancaster, PA, Technomic Publishing
PERKINS E G and ERICKSON M D (1996), *Deep frying: chemistry, nutrition and practical application*, Champaign, IL, AOCS
POKORNÝ J (1989), 'Flavor chemistry of deep fat frying in oil', in Min D B, Smouse T H, (eds), *Flavour Chemistry of Lipid Foods*, Champaign, IL, AOCS, 113–55
A special issue on deep frying (1998), *Grasas Aceites*, **49**, No. 3/4
A special issue on deep frying (2000), *Eur J Lipid Sci Technol*, **102**, No. 8/9

12.6 References

ATEBA P and MITTAL G S (1994), 'Dynamics of crust formation and kinetics of quality changes during frying of meatballs', *J Food Sci*, **59**, 1275–8, 1290
BAUMANN B and ESCHER F (1995), 'Mass and heat transfer during deep-fat frying of potato slices, I. Rate of drying and oil uptake', *Lebensm Wiss Technol*, **28**, 395–403
BLUMENTHAL M M and STOCKLER J R (1986), 'Isolation and detection of alkaline contaminant materials in used frying oils', *J Am Oil Chem Soc*, **63**, 687–8
BLUMENTHAL M M and STIER R F (1991), 'Optimization of deep-fat frying operations', *Trends Food Sci Technol*, **2**, 144–8
CALIFANO A N and CALVELO A (1987), 'Adjustment of surface concentration of reducing sugars before frying of potato strips', *J Food Process Preserv*, **12**, 1–9
CHANG S S, PETERSON R J and HO C T (1978), 'Chemical reactions involved in the deep-fat frying of foods', *J Am Oil Chem Soc*, **55**, 718–27
CHE MAN Y B and HUSSIN W R W (1998), 'Comparison of the frying performance of refined, bleached and deodorized palm olein and coconut', *J Food Lipids*, **5**, 197–210
CHE MAN Y B and TAN C P (1999), 'Effects of natural and synthetic antioxidants on changes in refined, bleached and deodorized palm olein during deep-fat frying of potato chips', *JAOCS*, **76**, 331–9
CHUN H K and HO C T (1997), 'Volatile nitrogen-containing compounds generated from Maillard reactions under simulated frying conditions', *J Food Lipids*, **4**, 239–44
DOBARGANES C, MÁRQUEZ-RUIZ G and VELASCO J (2000), 'Interactions between fat and food during deep frying', *Eur J Lipid Sci Technol*, **102**, 521–8
FILLION L and HENRY C J K (1998), 'Nutrient losses and gains during frying', *Int J Food Sci Nutr*, **49**, 157–68
FIRESTONE D (1993), 'Worldwide regulation of frying fats and oils', *INFORM*, **4**, 1366–71
FUJISAKI M, MORI S, ENDO Y and FUJIMOTO K (2000), 'The effect of oxygen concentration on oxidative deterioration in heated high-oleic safflower oil', *JAOCS*, **77**, 231–4
FUKUDA M, KUMISADA Y and TOYOSAWA I (1989), 'Some properties and *in vitro* digestibility of fried and roasted soybean proteins', *Nihon Eiyo Shokuryo Gakkaishi*, **42**, 305–11
GERTZ C, KLOSTERMANN S and KOCCHAR S P (2000), 'Testing and comparing oxidative stability of vegetable oils and fats at frying temperature', *Eur J Lipid Sci Technol*, **102**, 543–51
GORDON M H and KOURIMSKA L (1995), 'Effect of antioxidants on losses of tocopherols during deep-fat frying', *Food Chem*, **52**, 175–77
KIMURA M, ITOKAWA Y and FUJISAWA M (1991), 'Cooking losses of thiamin in food and its nutritional significance', *J Nutr Sci Vitaminol Suppl*, **36**, 17–24
KOCHHAR S P (2000), 'Stabilization of frying oils with natural antioxidative components', *Eur J Lipid Sci Technol*, **102**, 552–9

MIYAGI A, NAKAJIMA M, NABETANI H and SUBRAMANIAN R (2001), 'Feasibility of recycling used frying oil using membrane process', *Eur J Lipid Sci Technol*, **103**, 208–15

OHTA S, NAGANO S, YASUSHI A, HONDA K and HARA Y (1988), 'Preventive effects of silicone oil on the thermal deterioration of oils heated at wide surface', *Yukagaku*, **37**, 185–9

OLDS S I, VANDERSLICE J T and BROCHETTI D (1993), 'Vitamin B_6 in raw and fried chicken by HPLC', *J Food Sci*, **58**, 505–7, 561

ÖVERVIK E, KLEMAN M, BERG I and GUSTAFSSON J A (1989), 'Influence of creatine, amino acids and water on the formation of the mutagenic heterocyclic amines found in cooked meat', *Carcinogenesis*, **10**, 2293–301

PARCHURE A A and KULKARNI P R (1997), 'Effect of food processing treatments on generation of resistant starch', *Int J Food Sci Nutr*, **48**, 257–60

PERKINS E G and LAMBONI C (1998), 'Magnesium silicate treatment of dietary heated fats: effects on rat liver enzyme activity', *Lipids*, **33**, 683–7

PINTHUS E J, WEINBERG P and SAGUY I S (1995), 'Oil uptake in deep fat frying as affected by porosity', *J Food Sci*, **60**, 767–9

POKORNÝ J (1981), 'Browning from lipid-protein interactions', *Proc Food Nutr Sci*, **5**, 421–8

POKORNÝ J (1998), 'Substrate influence on the frying process', *Grasas Aceites*, **49**, 265–70

POKORNÝ J, RÉBLOVÁ Z, KOUŘIMSKÁ L, PUDIL F and KWIATKOWSKA A (1992), 'Effect of interactions with oxidized lipids on structure change and properties of food proteins', in Schwenke K D, Mothes R, (eds), *Food Proteins*, Weiheim, Chemie, 232–5

PRIYA R, SINGHAL R S and KULKARNI P R (1996), 'Carboxymethylcellulose and hydroxypropylmethylcellulose as additives in reduction of oil content in batter based deep-fat fried boondies', *Carbohydrate Polymers*, **29**, 333–5

RIBAROVA F, YURUKOV H and SHISHKOV S (1994), 'Stability of tryptophan during heat treatment of meat products', *Hranit Prom*, **43**, 9–11

SÁNCHEZ-MUNIZ F J, VIEJO J M and MEDINA R (1992), 'Deep frying of sardines in different culinary fats. Changes in the fatty acid composition of sardines and frying fats', *J Agric Food Chem*, **40**, 2252–6

SÁNCHEZ-MUNIZ F J, CUESTA C and GARRIDO-POLONIO C (1993), 'Sunflower oil used for frying: Combination of column, gas and HPSEC for its evaluation', *JAOCS*, **70**, 235–40

SPEEK A J, SPEEK-SAICHUA S and SCHREURS W H P (1988), 'Total carotenoid and β-carotene contents in Thai vegetables and the effect of processing', *Food Chem*, **27**, 245–57

THED S T and PHILLIPS R D (1995), 'Changes of dietary fiber and starch composition of processed potato products during domestic cooking', *J Food Sci*, **52**, 301–4

WAGNER R K and GROSCH W (1998), 'Key odorants of french fries', *JAOCS*, **75**, 1385–92

WARNER K, ORR P, PARROTT L and GLYNN M (1994), 'Effects of frying oil composition on potato chip stability', *JAOCS*, **71**, 1117–21

WARNER K, ORR P and GLYNN M (1997), 'Effect of fatty acid composition of oils on flavor and stability of fried foods', *JAOCS*, **74**, 347–56

WU P F and NAWAR W W (1986), 'A technique for monitoring the quality of used frying oil', *J Am Oil Chem Soc*, **63**, 1363–7

XU X Q (2000), 'A new spectrophotometric method for the rapid assessment of deep frying oil quality', *JAOCS*, **77**, 1083–6

13

The processing of cereal foods

A. J. Alldrick, Campden and Chorleywood Food Research Association; and M. Hajšelová, Consultant

13.1 Introduction

The domestication of different grasses, all members of the monocotyledonous family Gramineae, was a seminal event in the history of mankind. The cultivation of these plants led to the generation of agricultural surpluses. These in turn enabled societies in different parts of the world to make the transition from a nomadic or semi-nomadic lifestyle to one based on communities living in permanent settlements, forming the basis of civilisation as we now know it (discussed by Roberts, 1988).

The principal cereal crops grown in the world are maize, wheat, barley, rice, oats, rye and sorghum. Current estimates of world production, together with the major producing areas, are detailed in Table 13.1. It is estimated that for wheat alone, approximately 250 thousand hectars were planted world-wide during the 1998 growing season (International Grains Council, 2000).

Essentially, the cereal grain comprises the embryo plant for the next generation plus nutrients for its germination and initial growth. These in turn are surrounded by a protective seed coat. Kent and Evers (1994) described a 'generalised' model for all cereal grains. In this model, the cereal grain comprises an embryo that divides into the embryonic axis (the proto-plant) surrounded by the scutellum, which provides secretory and absorptive functions during the germination process. Around the embryo is the endosperm, most of which is referred to as the starchy endosperm. This consists of cells containing nutrients (in particular starch) that support growth following germination. The starchy endosperm is surrounded by the aleurone layer, which is mainly comprised of protein and lipids. Enclosing the endosperm and embryo is the protective seed coat. It contains substantial amounts of protein as well as dietary fibre.

Table 13.1 World cereal production (1998/99 estimates)

Grain	Production volume (million tonnes)	Principal producing areas (by tonnage)
Maize	602.9	USA, China, EU, Brazil
Wheat	586.6	China, EU, USA, India, CIS
Rice (milled basis)	385.0	China, India, Indonesia,
Barley	135.7	EU, CIS, Canada, USA
Sorghum	61.9	USA, India, Nigeria, China
Oats	26.5	EU, CIS, Canada, USA
Rye	21.2	EU, Poland, CIS

Data adapted from International Grains Council (2000) and United States Department of Agriculture (1998).

13.2 The nutritional significance of cereals and cereal processing

Cereals are nutritionally dense. They supply carbohydrate and protein as well as a variety of micronutrients; in particular certain B vitamins, vitamin E and minerals such as iron, in the case of wheat. In addition, cereal-based foods can also supply significant amounts of dietary fibre. Dietary studies, such as those of Gregory et al (1990) in the UK suggest that cereal-based foods contribute approximately 30% of dietary energy, over 20% of protein and approximately 45% of dietary fibre to the adult diet. Additionally, cereals are an important component of animal feed. It has been estimated, using 1990 figures (Cook and Hill, 1994), that within the European Union, 81.5 million tonnes or 59% of the cereal crop was used for animal feed purposes. This compares with 36.3 million tonnes, or 27% of the crop used for direct human consumption. Cereals therefore make a major contribution to both human and animal nutrition.

Although cereals are an excellent source of nutrients, they have two key limitations.

1. In terms of the amino acid composition of their proteins, cereals tend to have reduced levels of some of the indispensable amino acids, in particular lysine and threonine. While this is of significance to livestock nutrition, in human terms this only has relevance in societies where levels and diversity of protein intakes are limited.
2. Cereals have to be processed in order to maximise the bioavailability of the nutrients. The bioavailability of a nutrient can best be defined as the amount of nutrient present in a food, which is eventually absorbed from the gastro-intestinal (GI) tract of the consuming organism.

Cereal processing takes two basic forms: mechanical (e.g. milling) and thermal (e.g. baking). These can be performed separately, for example in converting the grain to a meal and subsequently cooking it, or almost simultaneously, as in a puffing process. The principal nutritional benefit of processing is to increase the bioavailability of the nutrients present in the grain. Essentially this is brought about by making the cereal grain a better substrate for digestive enzymes. This is achieved at both a physical (increased surface area) and/or a chemical (more random molecular structures) level.

Mechanical processes, such as milling, assist bioavailability in two ways: firstly, by breaking and often removing the outer seed coat; and secondly, by converting the grain to smaller particles thereby effectively increasing the surface area available to attack by digestive enzymes. While thermal processing can also in part contribute to the physical reduction of the grain, in terms of its primary nutritional benefit, the role of thermal processing is to disrupt the highly organised three-dimensional structures of both the starch and protein components. This generally leads to them being better substrates for the digestive enzymes within the GI tract.

In terms of foods for human use in particular, the consequences of processing on nutritional parameters have to be considered in combination with customer satisfaction. This includes both food safety and sensory aspects. However, the nutritional role of processing should not be underestimated. Developments in our understanding of nutrition and its role in health all indicate that the diversity of processing technologies can make significant contributions to the nutritional qualities of the grain as it is consumed. The sources of this understanding take many forms. These range from the bases of nutrient deficiency diseases such as beriberi (thiamin deficiency) through the role of diet in the aetiology of chronic diseases such as diabetes, cardiovascular disease and certain cancers, to developments in animal feed technology. A more detailed analysis of the significance of the role of technology follows in the next section.

13.3 Mechanical processing

As briefly discussed above, the primary outcome of cereal processing is to increase the bioavailability of nutrients within the cereal grain to the consumer, be they human or animal. Mechanical processing can be divided into three broad categories: abrasive, reductive or a combination of the two.

13.3.1 Abrasive processes

At their simplest, abrasive processes remove the outer seed coat and aleurone layers (often referred to as the bran layers) from the kernel leaving the starchy endosperm exposed and more susceptible to the effects of cooking. Two of the principal grains processed in this way are rice and barley, yielding white rice or pearled barley respectively. Production of white rice also leads to the removal of the embryo. In terms of nutrition, one of the principal challenges with abrasive and other methods, which lead to the removal of the bran layers, is the corresponding loss of some B-vitamins (e.g. thiamin). Kik (1943) reported losses of between 5- and 10-fold when comparing the thiamin contents of milled, polished rice with those of paddy rice. Historically, this only presented a problem in societies with a restricted food supply, leading to the vitamin deficiency disease beriberi (summarised by Bender and Bender, 1997). Despite improvements in the quality of the food supply, both in terms of quantity and diversity, sociological changes can contribute to reoccurrence of the disease, where it was once thought to have been eliminated. Kawai et al (1980) reported the reappearance of shoshin (acute) beriberi in Japanese adolescents consuming a diet made up predominantly of high carbohydrate, low nutrient density foods such as carbonated soft drinks, polished rice and 'instant' noodles.

13.3.2 Reductive processes

Most cereals are converted to smaller particles before processing and consumption. At the very basic level, this can involve simply cutting the grain into large fragments, for example in the manufacture of maize grits. Alternatively, grain can be reduced to a powder form which may or may not be fractionated into different components of the kernel. This can lead to the separation of the bran, aleurone and embryo from the starchy endosperm.

Most modern industrial flour production involves a progressive reduction process using a system of roller mills (discussed by Kent and Evers, 1994). In summary, wheat grains are adjusted to an appropriate moisture content and pass through a system whereby they are first fragmented (*Break Release*) and the starchy endosperm is removed from the bran. This in itself is a progressive process, involving a number of break mills. Grain particles are separated on the basis of size by a sieve process and either re-enter the break operation or pass on to the second stage of the process (*Reduction*). 'Break Release' leads to the production of two fractions, bran (seed coats) and the starchy endosperm, referred to as semolina in the UK. Particles of bran still attached to endosperm and which have not been reduced by the break system pass into the *Scratch* system, which effects a separation between the seed coat and the endosperm.

The coarse semolina is ground to a flour of desired particle size through a further system of roller mills (between 8 and 16 grinding stages). Whereas the rollers used in the break process are fluted, those for the size reduction process are usually smooth or matt. The process not only brings about the generation of a flour with the desired particle size, but also effects a separation of the starchy endosperm from the embryo and any remaining bran. The proportion of the original wheat that is ultimately converted to flour is referred to as the extraction rate. Typical values for white flours are between 72 and 80%, between 85 and 98% for brown flours and 100% for wholemeal flour (referred to as 'wholewheat' or 'Graham' flour in the USA).

13.3.3 Regulatory control of flour and its nutritional significance

As indicated above, modern milling techniques not only achieve the mechanical reduction of the cereal grain, but also separate the starchy endosperm from the bran and embryo. Both the bran and embryo of cereal grains contain significant quantities of essential nutrients. Even in recent times, their removal has had potentially deleterious consequences with regard to public health. In many countries, therefore, the composition of flour is regulated by law. This is not only with regard to technical aspects, for example purity, but also to its nutritional composition. In the United Kingdom these are detailed within the Bread and Flour Regulations 1998.

In nutritional terms these regulations are of importance in that they specify certain nutrient contents for all flours. Flours with extraction rates of less than 100% must be supplemented with the vitamins niacin and thiamin and also with iron to make up for losses during the milling process as well as being fortified with calcium (in the form of calcium carbonate). Analysis of studies such as those by Gregory et al (1990), looking at the dietary habits of the UK adult population, shows that cereal-based foods make a significant contribution to the nation's calcium intake. In the case of the UK this was approximately 25%. A substantial proportion (in excess of 50%) of this figure would be as a direct consequence of mandatory calcium carbonate fortification of low extraction rate flours. The separation of the bran layers from the endosperm also leads to significant reductions in the amount of dietary fibre present within the resultant flour. Thus while wholemeal flour has been reported as having a dietary fibre content expressed as nonstarch polysaccharide (NSP) of 5.8 g per 100 g, white flour has a corresponding dietary fibre content of 1.5 g per 100 g (Holland et al, 1991).

13.4 Thermal processing

Livestock can be fed cereals or by-products from cereal processing without any thermal processing (cooking). In contrast, cereal-based foods intended for human consumption almost inevitably undergo some form of cooking. The cooking processes can be as simple as boiling the grain or its meal in water. Alternatively, they can be complex systems involving mixing with other ingredients to form a dough, followed by mechanical processing and subsequent cooking (e.g. baking, as in the case of bread). Processed cereal products are many and diverse. This is reflected in the different technologies used and how the products are finally consumed. As discussed below, the technology used to make a particular product can be as nutritionally important as the ingredients themselves. In terms of nutrition, two of the most significant effects of mechanical and thermal processing concern the vitamin content and the physico-chemical structure of the complex carbohydrates present in the finished product.

13.4.1 Vitamins

A number of the vitamins associated with cereals or which are added during the manufacture of cereal-based products are thermally unstable. This is particularly true of the water-soluble vitamins (B vitamins and vitamin C). Cooking therefore leads to the destruction of a proportion of the vitamins present. The degree of destruction is dependent on the ingredient, recipe and the method of cooking of food. Nutritional databases, such as *McCance and Widdowson's The Composition of Foods* (Holland et al, 1991), detail typical correction factors for vitamin losses during cooking. In the case of baking, one might expect reductions of: between 15% (bread) and 25% for thiamin; 15% for riboflavin; 25% for both vitamin B_6 and pantothenate and 50% for folate values.

The phenomenon of thermal destruction is particularly important with regard to those products which are marketed (in part) on the basis of their vitamin content, for example breakfast cereals. This is usually addressed by one or a combination of two approaches: recipe formulation, where an increased amount of vitamin is incorporated to allow for thermal destruction or spray application to the cooled intermediate or finished product. Irrespective of the method of application, appropriate QC systems must be in place. These include monitoring the rate of application of vitamin mixes into the ingredients' mix or sprayed onto the product, as well as verification of the vitamin content in both intermediate and finished products by laboratory analysis.

13.4.2 Complex carbohydrates

Cereal-based foods account for approximately 30% of the energy intake of the UK adult population (Gregory et al, 1990). This figure includes the energy contribution from other ingredients, for example fat in pastry products. In terms of the cereal itself, the primary energy source is complex carbohydrate. Complex carbohydrates have been defined as carbohydrate molecules that contain twenty or more monosaccharide residues (British Nutrition Foundation, 1990). In the case of cereals, interest has focused on two forms of complex carbohydrate: starch and non-starch polysaccharide (NSP). NSP can be considered to be the principal component of dietary fibre.

Complex carbohydrates are believed to make a beneficial contribution towards a healthy diet. Changes in demography and public health have seen the development of longer-lived populations, increasingly suffering and/or dying from chronic diseases, in particular diabetes, cardiovascular disease and cancer. Numerous groups have proposed that diet makes a contribution to the incidence of these diseases and dietary guidelines such as the USDA Food Guide Pyramid (United States Department of Agriculture, 1992) have recommended substantial intakes of complex carbohydrates.

Processing can lead to significant differences in the effects of these dietary components on physiological function. For reasons of convenience, the effect of processing on the physiological properties of starch will be discussed here, while those for dietary fibre (including NSP) in section 13.5.

At a basic level, thermal treatment of a cereal-based raw material leads to substantial changes in the physico-chemical structure of the starch within the endosperm. This expresses itself by the irreversible disruption of the starch granules (gelatinisation) and, in most cases, the formation by the starch molecules present of more random structures. At a nutritional level, gelatinisation of starch renders it far more susceptible to breakdown by the α-amylase enzymes present in the GI tract. What has become increasingly apparent since the late 1970s is that the situation is complex and that the combination of thermal and mechanical processing can lead to foods with starches of differing relative starch digestibilities.

Foods containing starch that are digested at different rates can be classified in terms of their, 'glycaemic index' (Jenkins et al, 1981). This parameter is a measure of the rate of uptake of glucose into the blood stream from a carbohydrate-rich food compared with that of a reference meal (often a glucose solution) containing the equivalent amount of carbohydrate. A glycaemic index of 100% indicates that the carbohydrate in a food is digested and absorbed as glucose into the blood stream at the same rate as the reference meal. Similarly, a value of 50% for a food indicates that the carbohydrate present is digested and absorbed into the blood stream at half the rate of that seen with the reference meal. Generally speaking, white bread has a glycaemic index of approximately 100%, whole grain breads between 35 and 90% and pasta between 40 and 70% (Bjørck and Asp, 1994). Bjørck and Asp summarised the nutritional benefits of low glycaemic index foods as including: improved metabolic control for diabetics; lower blood lipid concentrations; improved glucose tolerance; prolonged satiety; improved performance during endurance exercise and reduced cariogenic potential.

Differences in glycaemic index relate in one degree to the physical accessibility of the starch molecules to the intestinal α-amylase enzymes. At its simplest, this could be by virtue of using whole or crudely milled (kibbled) grains. This explanation, however, cannot apply to pasta, which although made from semolina, involves particle sizes much smaller than those associated with kibbled grains. Yokoyama et al (1994) made bread and pasta from the same type of flour and demonstrated that, under *in vitro* conditions, starch in white bread was digested by α-amylase approximately four times faster than starch in cooked fettuccine. This difference is probably attributable to the pasta manufacture process. Pasta production involves the preparation of a semolina/water dough, which is either kneaded into sheets and cut or extruded at relatively low temperatures which do not facilitate starch gelatinisation. The finished product may or may not be dried. During this process the starch granules are enrobed with protein which entraps the starch granules once they have been gelatinised during the final cooking process (Feillet, 1984). Protein enrobement of the gelatinised starch molecules restricts their accessibility to digestive enzymes in the GI tract.

The underlying food technology used to prepare the food product can also modify starch structure leading to the generation of 'resistant starch' (RS). RS was described by Berry (1986), when he identified starch fractions that were resistant to α-amylase breakdown during dietary fibre determinations. It was put into a physiological context by Englyst and Cummings (1987), who used the term to describe a starch fraction which was resistant to digestion by secreted α-amylases within the GI tract, and which passed into the large intestine undigested. Three types of RS were originally identified (Englyst et al, 1992):

- RS$_1$ Physically inaccessible starch, found in partly milled grains or seeds.
- RS$_2$ Resistant starch granules, starches of a particular crystalline form that are refractory to breakdown by α-amylases.
- RS$_3$ Retrograded starch, in other words gelatinised starch which has recrystallised to an indigestible form.

Brown et al (1995) extended this list to include:

- RS$_4$ Chemically modified starches (e.g. esters and ethers).

Of particular interest to the cereal foods industry is RS$_3$ (retrograded starch). This is often formed during the production of cereal-based foods. The amount produced is in part determined by the product and the processes used in its manufacture. For example, breakfast cereals produced by methods such as flaking tend to have higher amounts of RS compared to products made by alternative technologies. The quantity of retrograded starch produced is not only determined by the processes but also by how much starch is present in the form of amylose. The higher the amylose content, the greater the amount of retrograded starch produced (Brown et al, 1995). At a physiological level, resistant starch, in particular RS$_3$, is interesting, since it appears to behave in many ways like dietary fibre (reviewed by Annison and Topping, 1994) and a proportion of it can be detected as such in the AOAC dietary-fibre assay.

13.5 Developing nutritionally-enhanced cereal-based foods

13.5.1 Current status

Reference has already been made to the role that diet plays in the incidence of chronic disease (section 13.4.2). One of the major challenges to face the modern food industry is the need to develop products that can contribute to the customers' desire for a healthy diet and the additional benefits such a diet provides. Alldrick (1998, 2001) has previously discussed the general principles underlying the design and marketing of these types of products both in general terms and with specific regard to cereal products.

A number of foods designed to meet the consumers' aspiration of improving their health through diet might be described as 'Functional Foods'. Ichikawa (1994) defined these products as: 'Processed foods containing ingredients that aid specific bodily functions in addition to being nutritious.' A key point to remember about functional foods is that they are not medicines. Thus while health claims (e.g. 'as part of a low fat diet our product may help to reduce blood cholesterol concentrations') might be permitted, medical claims, in other words claims to the effect that the food could cure, prevent or alleviate a disease, are generally prohibited.

Over the last few years, an increasing number of cereal-based products have come onto the functional-foods market. Some have been marketed on the basis of elevated vitamin or mineral content. What has been more novel is the development of products containing pharmacologically active compounds. One group of compounds that has attracted interest is the phyto-oestrogens. These are plant compounds which bear a structural similarity to the female sex hormone oestradiol and fall into three broad chemical categories: isoflavones, coumestans and lignans. They are thought to have beneficial health effects with regard to cardiovascular disease, certain cancers and the menopause (Bingham et al, 1998). A number of baked products, for example breads containing soya, linseed and/or flax and with high contents of phyto-oestrogens, have been released (Dalais et al, 1998; Payne, 2000). These have sometimes been referred to as 'Sheila' breads, reflecting their Australian origin.

Arguably, however, the key growth area has been fibre-enriched products. These products may be enriched with cereal-based dietary fibre or fibre derived from other plants, for example psyllium. As discussed in more detail elsewhere in this book, dietary fibre has been shown, or is thought to be, beneficial in managing the risk of a number of diseases. From classical times (British Nutrition Foundation, 1990) the beneficial effects of cereal fibre and in particular insoluble fibre on colonic function have been known. More recent work, such as the meta-studies of Ripsin et al (1992) have demonstrated that soluble fibres may have beneficial blood cholesterol lowering effects, particularly when eaten as part of a reduced fat diet.

13.5.2 Design considerations

Within the context of this chapter, a fundamental aspect that must be addressed in the design, development and manufacture of any nutritionally enhanced cereal food, is that of functionality. Here the term functionality not only applies to achieving the desired physiological consequences of eating the food in question, but also to the way ingredients behave during processing, together with their effects on product attributes. In developing this type of product, therefore, two questions need to be addressed.

- Can the product deliver the desired amount of the physiologically active ingredient and, where necessary, the desired physiological consequences, without adverse side effects?
- What effect does the physiologically active ingredient have on the technological functionality of other ingredients in the recipe with regard to giving an acceptable product?

These questions can be best examined looking at specific examples using one particular physiologically active dietary component. Here the component discussed is dietary fibre.

Physiological functionality
The two questions raised above can be intimately linked, and in unexpected ways. For example, the introduction by the animal feed industry of 'High Temperature Short Time' (HTST) processing (e.g. use of expanders), particularly for poultry

feed, in the early 1990s led to a reduction in feed efficiencies. This was related to an increase in the proportion of soluble dietary fibre in the feed and consequent increased viscosity of the animal's digesta (Sundberg et al, 1995). In the previous decade, it had been demonstrated that processing cereals in equipment such as expanders led to a solubilisation of the fibre component (Ralet et al, 1990). The degree to which this occurred was dependent on the energy input. The problem was overcome eventually by the addition of appropriate dietary-fibre degrading enzymes (Sundberg et al, 1995).

Although extreme, the above example does highlight the need to consider other physiological effects that may impact on the consumer. This can be in the form of unpleasant side effects, such as, in the case of dietary fibre, large bowel complaints such as flatulence (Bolin and Stanton, 1998) or impaired eating qualities in certain subgroups of the population, such as the elderly (Laurin et al, 1994). A simple moral can be derived from these examples. Failing to have a detailed understanding of both the links between the effects of food processing on the physiologically functional ingredient and all of the roles played by that ingredient on the consumer's physiology and/or sensory expectations can be prejudicial to the product's commercial success.

Technological functionality
In addition to the needs of the customer, any new product design process must also take into account the need for the product to be compatible with existing manufacturing technology. This is particularly true for high dietary fibre products. One such example is the manufacture of wholemeal (100% extraction) flour bread using 'no-time' dough making processes (e.g. Chorleywood Bread Making Process). Studies performed at the Flour Milling and Baking Research Association (Collins and Hook, 1991) have demonstrated that production of a loaf with those characteristics preferred by the consumer is dependent on a number of parameters. Particle size distribution within the flour was important not only for baking quality but also for the overall appearance of the crust and crumb. Addition of dried gluten protein was found to be a suitable method for improving hedonic parameters including loaf volume and crumb-score.

Increasing the content of a physiologically desirable component within an existing product can have consequences with regard to the behaviour of intermediate products and/or the appearance of the finished product. Work with bread containing elevated amounts of dietary fibre has shown that the addition of extra dietary fibre could lead to changes in dough rheology and handling characteristics as well as product appearance and texture (Pomeranz et al, 1977; Laing et al, 1990).

13.5.3 Marketing
In marketing any cereal product with enhanced physiological benefits, it will be necessary to ensure that the product contains sufficient active ingredients to meet

local regulatory requirements. However, it will also be important to ensure that the food is physiologically functional and has acceptable sensorial properties. Any advertising campaign for the product should be, 'legal, honest and truthful' (Advertising Standards Authority, 1999). Enthusiasm for the product should not be allowed to diminish the accuracy of advertisements. The functional foods area is a growing market. Young (1999) valued the European market at USD 1.24 billion in 1997, with bakery and cereal products commanding a 9% share. Consequently, functional foods also attract attention from consumer protection groups. Winkler (1998) reported that during the period 1994–1997, the UK Advertising Standards Authority upheld 21 complaints concerning advertisements for functional foods.

13.6 Conclusions

Cereals have been, and continue to be, a staple foodstuff. What has changed and what is expected to change further is the type of food products they are presented as. For example, in the United Kingdom bread consumption has halved during the last 50 years, while breakfast cereal consumption has tripled (Griffiths, 1999). These changes have been brought about, in no small part, by the tremendous socio-economic changes experienced in the Western world, which have led to the consumerist society. The demands of this society plus the consequences of demographic changes, together with the identification of the significant role that diet plays in the incidences of a wide number of chronic diseases have become key motivators in the design of new food products. Cereal foods are well placed to meet these challenges. This can take many forms, including capitalising on existing nutritional attributes (e.g. insoluble fibre in wholemeal flour products) to new functional foods. One example of functional high fibre foods is a range of products (e.g. pasta, breakfast cereals and snack bars) supplemented with psyllium fibre. Psyllium fibre has been demonstrated to be capable of reducing blood cholesterol concentrations (Roberts et al, 1994). Developing such foods is not necessarily a guarantee for commercial success, persuasive and ethical marketing is also required. There has been a number of well published cases (e.g. Buss, 2000), where cereal-based functional foods have failed by virtue of inadequate market research and poor sales strategies rather than by a defective product *per se.*

13.7 Sources of further information and advice

BENDER D A and BENDER A E (1997), *Nutrition, A Reference Handbook*, Oxford, Oxford University Press
KENT N L and EVERS A D (1994), *Kent's Technology of Cereals* (4 ed.), Oxford, Elsevier
MCCLEARY B V and PROSKY L (eds.) *Advanced Dietary Fibre Technology*, Oxford, Blackwell Science

13.8 References

ADVERTISING STANDARDS AUTHORITY (1999), *The British codes of advertising and sales promotion*, www.asa.org.uk
ALLDRICK A J (1998), 'Functional foods, assuring quality', in Sadler, M J and Saltmarsh, M (eds.), *Functional Foods – The Consumer, The Products, The Evidence*, Cambridge, Royal Society of Chemistry, 135–42
ALLDRICK A J (2001), 'Developing fibre-rich foods in the twenty-first century', in McCleary, B V and Prosky, L (eds.), *Advanced Dietary Fibre Technology*, Oxford, Blackwell Science, 239–47
ANNISON G and TOPPING D L (1994), 'Nutritional role of resistant starch: chemical structure vs. physiological function', *Annual Review of Nutrition*, **14**, 297–320
BENDER D A and BENDER A E (1997), *Nutrition, a Reference Handbook*, Oxford, Oxford University Press
BERRY C S (1986), 'Resistant starch: formation and measurement of starch that survives exhaustive digestion with amylolytic enzymes during the determination of dietary fibre', *Journal of Cereal Science*, **4**, 301–14
BINGHAM S A, ATKINSON C, LIGGINS J, BLUCJ L and COWARD A (1998), 'Phyto-oestrogens: where are we now?', *British Journal of Nutrition*, **79**, 393–406
BJØRCK I and ASP N-G (1994), 'Controlling the nutritional properties of starch in foods – a challenge to the food industry', *Trends in Food Science & Technology*, **5**, 213–18
BOLIN T D and STANTON R A (1998), 'Flatus emission patterns and fibre intake', *European Journal of Surgery*, **582** (suppl.), 115–18
Bread and Flour Regulations 1998, Statutory Instrument (SI) 1998, No. 141, London, HMSO
BRITISH NUTRITION FOUNDATION (1990), *Complex Carbohydrates in Foods: the Report of the British Nutrition Foundation's Taskforce*, London, Chapman & Hall
BROWN I L, MCNAUGHT K J and MALONEY E (1995), 'Hi-maize™ new directions in starch technology and nutrition', *Food Australia*, **47**, 272–5
BUSS D (2000), 'Kellogg bids farewell to much hyped Ensemble', *New Nutrition Business*, **5**, 11
COLLINS T H and HOOK S C W (1991), 'Milling, analysis and baking of wholemeal flour', *Flour Milling and Baking Research Association Report* No. 148, FMBRA Chorleywood
COOK E and HILL B (1994), *Economic Aspects of Cereal Production in the EC*, Luxembourg, Eurostat
DALAIS F S, WAHLQVIST M L and RICE G E (1998), 'Phytoestrogens – health significance and the food industry', *Food Australia*, **50**, 494–5
ENGLYST H N and CUMMINGS J H (1987), 'Resistant starch, a "new" food component: a classification of starch for nutritional purposes', in: Morton, I D (ed.), *Cereals in a European Context*, Chichester, Ellis Horwood, 221–33
ENGLYST H N, KINGMAN S M and CUMMINGS J H (1992) 'Classification and measurement of nutritionally important starch fractions', *European Journal of Clinical Nutrition* **46** (suppl.2), S33–S50
FEILLET P (1984), 'Present knowledge on biochemical basis of pasta cooking quality, consequences for wheat breeders', *Science Alimentaire*, **4**, 551–66
GREGORY J, FOSTER K, TYLER H and WISEMAN M (1990), *The Dietary and Nutritional Survey of British Adults*, London, HMSO
GRIFFITHS J (ed.) (1999), *UK food market: 1999 market review*, Hampton, Key Note
HOLLAND B, WELCH A A, UNWIN I D, BUSS D H, PAUL A A and SOUTHGATE D A T (1991), *McCance and Widdowson's The Composition of Foods*, (5 ed.) Cambridge, Royal Society of Chemistry and Ministry of Agriculture, Fisheries and Foods
ICHIKAWA T (1994), 'Functional foods in Japan', in Goldberg, I (ed.) *Functional Foods*, New York, Chapman & Hall, 453–67

INTERNATIONAL GRAINS COUNCIL (2000), *World Grain Statistics*, London, International Grain Council
JENKINS D J A, WOLEVER T M S, TAYLOR R H, BARKER H, FIELDEN H, BALDWIN J M, BOWLING A C, NEWMAN H C, JENKINS A L and GOFF D (1981), 'Glycaemic index of food: a physiological basis for carbohydrate exchange', *American Journal of Clinical Nutrition* **34**, 302–6
KAWAI C, WAKAYBAYASHI A, MATSUMURA T and YUI Y (1980), 'Reappearance of beriberi heart disease in Japan: a study of 23 cases', *American Journal of Medicine*, **69**, 383–6
KENT N L and EVERS A D (1994), *Kent's Technology of Cereals* (4 ed.), Oxford, Elsevier
KIK M C (1943), 'Thiamin in products of commercial rice milling', *Cereal Chemistry*, **20**, 563–9
LAING C E, NEUFELD K J and WALKER C J (1990), 'Effect of fiber on dough rheology', *American Institute of Baking Technical Bulletin. Bull.* XII (11)
LAURIN D, BRODEUR J M, BOURDRAGES J, VALL'EE R and LACHAPPELLE D (1994), 'Fibre intake in elderly individuals with poor masticatory performance', *Journal of the Canadian Dental Association*, **60**, 443–6
PAYNE T J (2000), 'Promoting better health with flax seed in bread', *Cereals Food World*, **45**, 102–4
POMERANZ Y, SHOGREN M D, FINNEY K F and BEEHTEL D B (1977), 'Fibre in bread making – effects on functional properties', *Cereal Chemistry*, **54**, 25–41
RALET M-C, THIBAULT J-F and DELLA VALLE G (1990), 'Influence of extrusion cooking on the physico-chemical properties of wheat bran', *Journal of Cereal Science*, **11**, 249–59
RIPSIN C M, KEENAN J M, JACOBS D R, ELMER P J, WELCH R R, VAN HORN L, LIU K, TURNBULL W H, THYE F W and KESTIN M (1992), 'Oat products and lipid lowering', *Journal of the American Medical Association*, **267**, 3317–25
ROBERTS J M (1988), *The Pelican History of The World* (rev. ed.), London, Penguin Group
ROBERTS D C, TRUSWELL A S, BENCKE A, DEWAR H M and FARMAKALIDIS E (1994), 'The cholesterol lowering effect of a breakfast cereal containing psyllium fibre', *Medical Journal of Australia*, **161**, 660–4
SUNDBERG B, PETTERSON D and AMAN P (1995), 'Nutritional properties of fiber-rich barley products fed to broiler chickens', *Journal of Food Science and Agriculture*, **67**, 469–76
UNITED STATES DEPARTMENT OF AGRICULTURE (1992), *Food Guide Pyramid*, www.usda.gov
UNITED STATES DEPARTMENT OF AGRICULTURE (1998), *World Agricultural Supply and Demand Estimates (WASDE-344). 10th November 1998*, www.usda.gov
WINKLER J T (1998), 'The future of functional foods', in Sadler, M J and Saltmarsh, M (eds.) *Functional Foods – The Consumer, The Products, The Evidence*, Cambridge, Royal Society of Chemistry, 184–95
YOKOYAMA W H, HUDSON C A, CHIU M M and BETSCHART A A (1994), 'Effect of formulation and processing on the enzymatic digestion of common cereal products', *Cereal Foods World*, **39**, 439–43
YOUNG J (1999), 'The influence of scientific research, market developments and regulatory issues on the future development of nutraceuticals and functional foods – a global overview', *Leatherhead Food RA Food Industry Journal*, **2**, 100–13

14

Extrusion cooking

M. E. Camire, University of Maine

14.1 Introduction

Extrusion cooking is a relatively recent form of food processing. Forcing material through a hole is the process of extrusion. Sausage extruders were developed in the nineteenth century as simple forming machines. Eventually pasta was produced in extruders. Flour and water were added at one end of the machine, and a screw mixed and compressed the dough before extruding it through numerous holes or dies that gave the pasta its shape. During the 1930s heat was added to the barrel containing the screw; puffed corn curl snacks resulted. The pressure developed as the dough moved along the screw; this, together with the heat under pressure, caused the corn to puff upon exiting the dies. As extrusion cooking processed more types of food, extruders became more specialised for food applications. Twin-screw extruders containing two screws were adapted from the polymer industry, and these machines are considerably more versatile than are single screw extruders. Extruded products are often subjected to further processing, such as frying, baking, and rolling.

The improved mixing ability of these extruders provided impetus for further product development. Table 14.1 lists major food categories produced by extrusion cooking. Extrusion cooking can be performed as either a batch or continuous operation, offering many advantages over conventional food processing methods (Table 14.2) (Harper, 1981). Several manufacturers produce cooking extruders. Laboratory-size extruders have screw diameters of 10–30 mm and throughputs of up to a few hundred kilogram per hour. The length of the barrels for these research extruders, which are the most common machines cited in the literature, varies from about one to two meters. Production-sized extruders can create thousands of kilogram of product per hour.

Table 14.1 Common food products prepared by extrusion cooking

Category	Examples
Ready-to-eat breakfast cereals	Puffed cereals
	Flaked cereals
	High-fiber strands
Snacks	Puffed snacks
	Half-products or pellets (third generation snacks)
	Crispbreads
Confections	Licorice
	Chocolate
Texturised protein	Soy meat analogues
	Restructured seafood
	Processed cheese
Infant foods	Biscuits
	Weaning cereals

Table 14.2 Unique advantages of extrusion cooking[a]

Batch or continuous processing
High throughput
Low labor and energy costs
Variety of products produced and types of ingredients that can be processed
Control of thermal/mechanical environment
Negligible effluent

[a] Adapted from Harper (1981).

14.1.1 Unique aspects of extrusion cooking

Most extruders act as heat exchangers, and they also shape and form food products. Mixing, dehydration, and pasteurisation and sterilisation are other unit operations that typically occur during extrusion. Aside from thermal destruction of nutrients, the shear that develops within the extruder barrel can damage food chemicals. Temperature can be controlled by many means including limiting direct heating, adding water, and increasing throughput. Shear may be reduced by using low-shear screw elements, increasing water or lipid content, modifying screw speed (based on other parameters), and by reducing pressure at the die.

Extrusion research often focuses upon one to four variables, although screening studies should be performed to identify key factors. Extruder operators may select parameters such as screw speed, feed moisture, and barrel temperature as primary factors, that in turn determine a secondary set of factors: specific mechanical energy (SME), product or mass temperature (PT) and pressure (Meuser and van Lengerich, 1984). These factors influence the viscosity of the food within the extruder barrel, the residence time of the material in the extruder, and the shear applied to the food (Fig. 14.1). Variations caused by feed composition

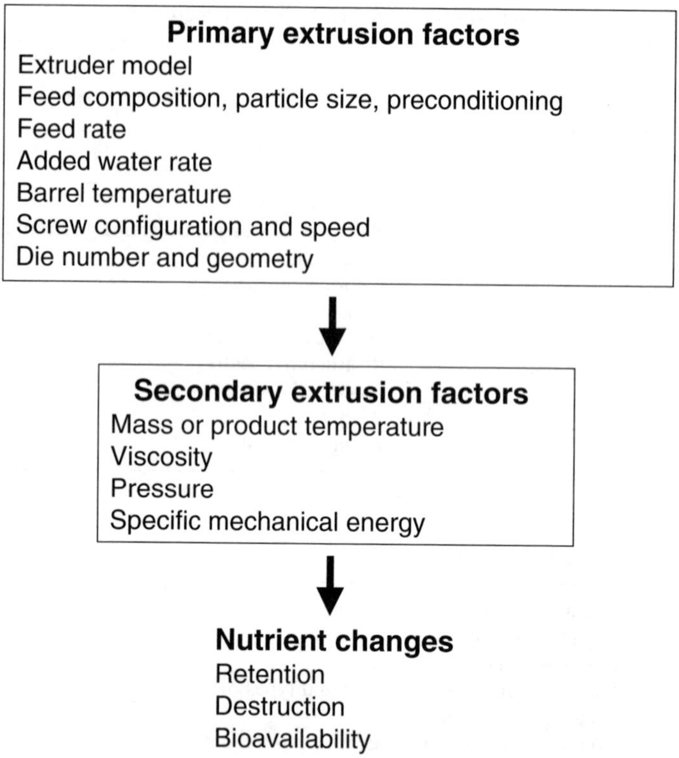

Primary extrusion factors
Extruder model
Feed composition, particle size, preconditioning
Feed rate
Added water rate
Barrel temperature
Screw configuration and speed
Die number and geometry

↓

Secondary extrusion factors
Mass or product temperature
Viscosity
Pressure
Specific mechanical energy

↓

Nutrient changes
Retention
Destruction
Bioavailability

Fig. 14.1 Interrelationships of extruder variables and their potential effects on nutrients.

and prior processing of the feed materials are important sources of experimental variation.

Extrusion can produce safe, lightweight, shelf-stable foods that can be stored for use during famines and natural disasters. Simple single screw extruders are fairly inexpensive and simple to maintain so these machines can be used in less-developed nations to produce weaning and other foods. Harper and Jansen (1985) have reviewed advantages and limitations of extrusion for weaning foods. Friction from the rotation of the screw can cook the food thoroughly, reducing production costs for fuel sources. Extruders can blend diverse ingredients, permitting government and relief agencies to use donated foods such as dried milk as well as indigenous crops such as beans, millet, and cassava. Extruded pellets can be ground, then mixed with milk or water as needed to form gruel for infants.

Functional ingredients such as soy and botanicals that are relatively unpalatable alone can be incorporated into new food items by extrusion. Traditional foods such as rye crispbread can be further enhanced by addition of extra dietary fiber or other ingredients during extrusion. A relatively new form of extrusion known as wet extrusion operates at higher moisture contents (>40%) and lower barrel temperatures (Akdogan, 1999). These conditions permit extrusion and texturisation of high-protein materials since protein denaturation is limited. Very little has yet been published on the effects of wet extrusion on nutrient retention, but nutrient destruction should be considerably less than in conventional extrusion cooking.

14.2 Impact on key nutrients: carbohydrates

Reducing sugars such as glucose and lactose participate in Maillard reactions, which will be discussed further in section 14.3. The shear forces during extrusion can also create reducing sugars from complex carbohydrates as well as from sucrose and other sugars. Sucrose losses of up to 20% were found in protein-enriched biscuits (Noguchi and Cheftel, 1983). While sucrose loss may affect product color and flavor, there is an opportunity to reduce the content of indigestible oligosaccharides that can cause flatulence. Sucrose, raffinose and stachyose decreased significantly in extruded pinto bean high-starch fractions (Borejszo and Khan, 1992). Corn-soy snacks had lower levels of both stachyose and raffinose compared to unextruded soy grits and flour, but values were not corrected for the 50–60% corn present (Omueti and Morton, 1996). Starch and stachyose were lower in extruded peas compared to raw peas (Alonso et al, 2000), but an increase in total free sugars did not fully account for these losses (Fig. 14.2).

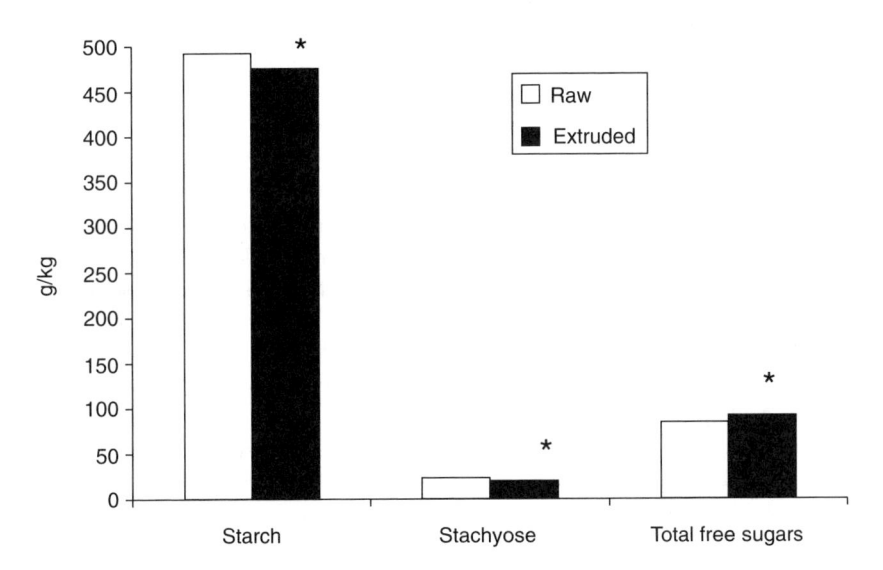

Fig. 14.2 Carbohydrate changes (g/kg dry matter) due to extrusion of peas (*Pisum sativum* L) at an exit temperature of 145 °C and 25% feed moisture. (Adapted from Alonso et al, 2000)

Starch is usually the major food constituent in extruded foods such as breakfast cereals, snacks and weaning foods. Humans and other monogastric species do not readily digest native or ungelatinised starch. Unlike many thermal processes, extrusion cooking gelatinises starch at fairly low (12–22%) moisture levels. Removal of cooking water is not a problem, and leaching of water-soluble nutrients is avoided. Increased temperature, shear, and pressure during extrusion increase the rate of gelatinisation, but lipids, sucrose, dietary fiber and salts can retard gelatinisation (Jin et al, 1994). While full gelatinisation may not occur during extrusion, digestibility is often improved (Wang, S et al, 1993).

During extrusion, starch molecules can be physically broken into smaller, more digestible fragments. For example, amylopectin branches can be sheared off the main molecule, with larger molecules experiencing the greatest effect (Politz et al, 1994b). Both amylose and amylopectin molecules may be affected, however. Molecular weight in extruded wheat starch was retained better under processing conditions of higher die temperature (185 °C) and feed moisture (20%) (Politz et al, 1994a). Screw configurations using more reverse and high-shear elements favor starch breakdown (Gautam and Choudhoury, 1999).

Lower molecular weight starch fragments may be sticky, thereby increasing the risk for dental caries, since bacteria in the mouth rapidly ferment these dextrins. Toothpack, the amount of material retained on teeth, has been used as an indication of the severity of extrusion processing. Björck and co-workers (1984) found that white wheat flour extruded under 'mild' and 'severe' conditions caused drops in dental plaque pH comparable to those obtained with glucose.

While easily-digested starch is desirable for infants and invalids, the resulting rapid post-prandial rise in blood sugar and insulin levels is thought to be a risk factor for development of insulin insensitivity and Type II, or adult-onset, diabetes. Extrusion offers the ability to reduce the high glycemic index (GI) of some foods by converting starch to digestion-resistant starch (RS). Theander and Westerlund (1987) reported transglycosidation in extruded wheat flour, presumably from attachment of sheared amylopectin branches to other reactive sites. The resulting novel bonds would be resistant to digestion by enzymes. Addition of high amylose starch also reduces digestibility. As much as 30% resistant starch was reported when high amylose starch was reacted with pullulanase prior to extrusion (Chiu et al, 1994). Extruded high amylose rice noodles had lower starch digestibility and reduced GI (Panlasigui et al, 1992).

An evolving area of research involves the use of additives to promote RS formation. Adding 30% corn, potato or wheat starch did not increase RS values in cornmeal, but RS and fiber values more than doubled when 7.5% citric acid was used, and 30% high-amylose cornstarch with 5 or 7.5% citric acid resulted in values of 14%, compared with slightly more than 2% in 100% cornmeal (Unlu and Faller, 1998). Polydextrose may have been formed during extrusion. Limitations to this approach would be the expenses of the additives and sour taste of the extrudates. Yields of up to 93.7% oligosaccharides and polydextrose were reported when glucose-citric acid mixtures were extruded at different barrel temperatures (Hwang et al, 1998).

Longer cellulose fibers added to cornstarch decreased starch solubility (Chinnaswamy and Hanna, 1991). Removal of insoluble dietary fiber from wheat flour in combination with 20% protein addition resulted in pasta with significantly delayed dextrin release under *in vitro* digestion conditions (Fardet et al, 1999), possibly due to enhanced protein–starch interactions. Amylose forms complexes with lipids during extrusion, thereby reducing both starch and lipid availability. This phenomenon will be addressed in section 14.4.

The term dietary fiber is used to describe nondigestible carbohydrates and associated compounds such as lignin. Although a global definition of dietary fiber does not yet exist, there is a consensus that adequate fiber consumption is essential for good health. Analytical methods for quantitating dietary fiber vary considerably. The AOAC total dietary fiber method used for US nutritional labeling does not measure compounds that are soluble in 80% aqueous ethanol such as certain fructans and polydextrose, and this procedure does not detect changes in extruded fiber solubility. If different dietary fiber fractions are not analysed separately, it is possible to overlook important changes in dietary fiber composition and functionality caused by extrusion.

Like starch, branched dietary fiber molecules are susceptible to shear. The smaller fragments may be soluble in water. Fragments may also combine to form large insoluble complexes that may be analysed as lignin. Although extrusion did not affect pectin, both soluble and insoluble nonstarch polysaccharides (NSP) were increased in extruded oatmeal and potato peels (Camire and Flint, 1991). Corn meal fiber was unaffected by extrusion under the same conditions as the other foods. Extruded beans (*Phaseolus vulgaris* L) had total fiber values comparable to those before extrusion, but a redistribution of insoluble to soluble fiber occurred (Martín-Cabrejas et al, 1999). Sugar beet pectin and hemicellulose molecular weight decreased with extrusion, and water solubility of those compounds increased by 16.6 to 47.5% (Ralet et al, 1991). Extrusion increased the solubility of beta-glucans in regular and waxy barley cultivars (Gaosong and Vasanthan, 2000).

Does the 'soluble' fiber created during extrusion have the same health benefits as natural forms such as pectin and β-glucan? Viscous gels formed in the small intestine trap bile acids and thus may contribute to lower serum cholesterol levels; the soluble fiber matrix is also thought to slow glucose absorption from the small intestine. Extrusion increased the viscosity of aqueous suspensions of wheat, oats and barley (Wang and Klopfenstein, 1993). Although increased *in vitro* viscosity was correlated with higher levels of soluble citrus peel fiber after extrusion (Gourgue et al, 1994), *in vitro* starch digestion and glucose diffusion were unaffected. Extrusion of wheat flakes containing guar gum did not reduce the guar gum's ability to lower post-prandial blood glucose and insulin in healthy adults (Fairchild et al, 1996). In an intervention study involving middle-aged men with hyperlipidemia, baked goods fortified with 92 g/day extruded dry white beans did not lower serum lipoproteins (Oosthuizen et al, 2000).

14.3 Proteins

Two reviews of protein extrusion have been published (Camire, 1991; Arêas, 1992). The effects of extrusion on protein nutrition have been studied extensively for animal feeds and for human weaning foods. Total protein changes very little during most extrusion operations. Changes in nutritional quality may be overlooked if only total nitrogen is assayed; animal feeding studies or *in vitro* protein digestibility testing should be performed on products that are designed to provide significant amounts of high-quality protein. Disulfide and other covalent cross-linking, aggregation and fragmentation are among reactions reported in the literature. Free radical reactions are significant during wheat flour extrusion (Schaich and Rebello, 1999).

Excessive Maillard browning can result in losses of lysine up to approximately 50% (de la Gueriviere et al, 1985). High barrel temperature, low moisture, and high shear promote Maillard reactions. Browning may occur even when reducing sugars are excluded from formulations because new reducing sugars may be formed from hydrolysis of sucrose, starch, and other polysaccharides. In a model system of wheat starch, glucose and lysine, low pH increased Maillard reactions (Bates et al, 1994). Lysine can be preserved, however, if extruder operating conditions and formulations are carefully balanced. Corn-soy blends extruded for reconstitution as porridge or gruel had good lysine retention (Konstance et al, 1998).

Extrusion may improve protein digestibility by denaturating proteins, exposing enzyme-accessible sites. Enzymes and enzyme inhibitors generally lose activity due to denaturation. Reductions in protease inhibitors can contribute to better plant protein utilisation. Although a single test for protein denaturation is not used internationally, protein solubility in water or aqueous solutions is commonly used to assess the extent of denaturation. High shear extrusion conditions in particular promote denaturation (Della Valle et al, 1994), although mass temperature and moisture are also important factors. Protein solubility is reduced in pasta despite the low process temperatures used in pasta making (Ummadi et al, 1995).

The mechanism for cholesterol lowering by a diet with soy protein is not well understood, but the lysine/arginine ratio may play an important role. Health effects of food proteins could be significantly affected by extrusion cooking if lysine is selectively lost via Maillard reactions. Extrusion-texturised soy isolate fed to rats had similar effects as nonextruded soy on serum cholesterol, cholesterol and steroid fecal excretion, or protein nutrition (Fukui et al, 1993). In another rat study, amino acid-supplemented extruded pea (*Pisum sativum* L., cv. Ballet) seed meal lowered total and LDL cholesterol as well as did supplemented raw seeds compared with a control diet (Alonso et al, 2001). The peas were extruded under fairly mild conditions (145 °C exit temperature and feed moisture of 25%), but antinutritional factors were adequately inactivated, as evidenced by lower pancreatic weights in rats fed the extruded peas. Amaranth protein has a lysine/arginine ratio similar to soy. LDL cholesterol in rabbits fed an extruded amaranth diet for 21 days was less than half that in animals fed a casein control diet (Plate and Areâs, 2002).

14.4 Lipids

Extruded foods are generally low in lipid content, but fat is often added post-extrusion by frying or spraying of lipids to hold seasonings. Generally, foods containing less than 10% lipids are extruded because greater quantities of lipids reduce slip within the extruder barrel, making extrusion difficult, particularly for expanded products. Single screw extruders can process lipid levels of 12–17%, while twin screw extruders with proper screw configurations can handle feed lipid contents as high as 22% (Riaz, 2001). Extruders are used in oilseed extraction because the heat and shear disrupt cellular tissue and free oil (Nelson et al, 1987).

An early problem in extrusion was the apparent disappearance of lipids during processing. Starch–lipid complexes formed during extrusion are resistant to some lipid extraction procedures. Lipid recovery is higher when extruded foods are first digested with acid or amylase, then extracted with ether or another organic solvent. While total fat was not significantly changed in extruded whole wheat, just half of ether-extractable lipids were detected (Wang, W-M et al, 1993). In the same study, wheat bran had more free lipids after extrusion. Cornmeal extruded at lower barrel temperatures (50–60 °C or 85–90 °C) had greater than 75% of its lipids bound, but extrusion at 120–125 °C bound 70% of the lipids (Guzman et al, 1992).

Other nutritional aspects of lipids before and after extrusion have been studied very little. Both docosahexaenoic (DHA) and eicosapentaenoic (EPA) acids were retained in extruded chum salmon muscle with 10% wheat flour (Suzuki et al, 1988). Unlike other processing methods, extrusion cooking does not promote significant *cis-trans* isomerisation of unsaturated lipids. Corn and soy blends had 1.5% more *trans*-fatty acids after extrusion (Maga, 1978). Formation of free radicals and subsequent lipid oxidation could have nutritional implications. Artz et al (1992) reviewed extrusion factors affecting lipid oxidation. Screw and barrel wear raise levels of pro-oxidant minerals in extruded foods. For example, iron and peroxide values were higher in extruded rice and dhal compared to dried products (Semwal et al, 1994). Increased surface area in expanded products is another factor increasing oxidation. Factors that retard oxidation in extruded foods include denaturation of lipolytic enzymes, formation of starch-lipid complexes, and creation of antioxidant Maillard compounds.

14.5 Vitamins

Killeit (1994) reviewed vitamin retention in extruded foods. More research on the bioavailability of added and endogenous vitamins is needed, particularly in light of fortification programs for folate and other vitamins. Concerns of reduced vitamin levels prompt some manufacturers to apply vitamins post-extrusion as a spray. More recent research has focused on vitamin stability in feeds. Fat-coated ascorbic acid, menadione, pyridoxine and folic acid were retained better than were crystalline forms in extruded fish feed (Marchetti et al, 1999).

Although many extruded foods do not naturally have high levels of lipid-soluble vitamins, stability of these nutrients is a concern for fortified foods. Over 50% of all *trans*-beta-carotene in wheat flour were destroyed when barrel temperature increased from 125 to 200 °C (Guzman-Tello and Cheftel, 1990). The degradation process is not straightforward. Fifteen degradation products of all *trans*-beta-carotene dispersed in corn starch were recovered after twin-screw extrusion (Marty and Berset, 1988). Retention of retinyl palmitate in tapioca snacks mixed with either fish or protein flour was 52% and 73%, respectively after extrusion (Suknark et al, 2001).

Vitamins D and K are fairly stable during food processing, but are not used in many extruded human foods. Vitamin E and related tocopherols function as both vitamin and antioxidant. Gamma and delta tocopherols underwent greater losses (~40%) during extrusion than did alpha and beta forms (23–28%) (Suknark et al, 2001). Rice bran tocopherol decreased as extrusion temperature increased; bran extruded at 120–140 °C lost more tocopherols over a year's storage than did bran extruded at 110 °C (Shin et al, 1997). Less than 20% of vitamin E was retained in extruded and drum-dried wheat flour (Wennermark, 1993). The stability of lipid-soluble vitamins is shown in Table 14.3.

Ascorbic acid (vitamin C) decreased in wheat flour when extruded at higher barrel temperatures at fairly low moisture (10%) (Andersson and Hedlund, 1991). Blueberry concentrate appeared to protect 1% added vitamin C in an extruded breakfast cereal compared to a product containing just corn, sucrose, and ascorbic acid (Chaovanalikit, 1999). When ascorbic acid was added to cassava starch

Table 14.3 Stability of lipid-soluble vitamins during the production of tapioca–peanut flour snacks

Processing step	Vitamin content (g/100 g), fat- and moisture-free basis	
	Total tocopherols	Retinyl palmitate
Raw material	14.44[b]	2.74[a]
Extrusion	10.55[c]	2.19[b]
Drying to form half-product	10.36[c]	1.92[c]
Frying	43.18[a]	2.00[c]

Different letters within columns indicate statistically significant differences.
Adapted from Suknark et al, 2001.

to increase starch conversion, retention of over 50% occurred at levels of 0.4–1.0% addition (Sriburi and Hill, 2000).

Thiamine is the water-soluble vitamin most susceptible to thermal processing. Thiamine destruction in extruded wheat flour is a first-order reaction (Guzman-Tello and Cheftel, 1987). Killeit (1994) summarised thiamine losses as ranging from 5 to 100%. Thiamine retention in potato flakes decreased under extrusion conditions of lower moisture and higher barrel temperature; sulfites in the potato flakes may have also contributed to vitamin destruction (Maga and Sizer, 1978). Large losses of thiamine occurred when no water was added during extrusion, but riboflavin (B_2) and niacin were not affected (Andersson and Hedlund, 1991). Using low-cost single screw extruders, Lorenz and Jansen (1980) found retention of over 90% for thiamin, riboflavin, vitamin B_6 and folic acid in corn-soy blends processed at 171 °C.

14.6 Minerals

Mineral content and bioavailability are generally retained well during extrusion. Abrasive foods, such as brans rich in dietary fiber, or with low lipid and moisture content, gradually wear away metal from the extruder screws and barrel. The equipment must be replaced or refurbished periodically due to this wear, as the metal accumulates in the extruded food. As barrel temperature increased during single screw extrusion of potato flakes, iron content also increased (Maga and Sizer, 1978). Total iron increased by as much as 38% due to extrusion (Camire et al, 1993). On the other hand, cornmeal, which has a low dietary fiber content, had no changes in total, elemental, or soluble iron after twin screw extrusion (Camire and Dougherty, 1998).

Although iron from screw wear is typically in the elemental form, the bioavailability appears adequate as long as excessive amounts of iron and related metals are not present. Rats fed extruded corn and potato absorbed iron well (Fairweather-Tait et al, 1987). Utilisation of iron and zinc from wheat bran and wheat in adult human volunteers was not affected by extrusion (Fairweather-Tait et al, 1989). Extrusion slightly increased iron availability in corn snacks under *in vitro* digestion followed by dialysis (Hazell and Johnson, 1989). Low-shear extrusion retained dialysable iron in navy beans, lentils, chickpeas and cowpeas better than did high-shear extrusion (Ummadi et al, 1995). Weaning food blends of pearl millet, cowpea and peanut had greater iron availability and protein digestibility compared to similar foods processed by roasting (Cisse et al, 1998). None of the processed blends provided adequate iron to meet infant needs, however. Zinc bioavailability of semolina and soy protein concentrate blends (85:15) (Kang, 1996) was unaffected by extrusion.

Mineral bioavailability may be improved in extruded foods if mineral-binding phytate is reduced during processing. Published research has had mixed results. Extrusion reduced phytate levels in wheat flour (Fairweather-Tait et al, 1989), possibly due to inactivation of phytases during extrusion. Although phytic acid was reduced under all processing conditions, total phytate was not affected. Legume phytate was not affected by extrusion (Lombardi-Boccia et al, 1991; Ummadi et al,1995).

While screw speed had no effect on phytate in wheat, rice and oat brans, insoluble fiber decreased in all but wheat bran after extrusion (Gualberto et al, 1997). After phytate was removed, extruded rice and oat brans bound more calcium and zinc, but not copper, *in vitro* (Bergman et al, 1997). Comparable results were found with a high-fiber cereal fed to seven persons with ileostomies (Sandberg et al, 1986; Kivistö et al, 1986). Dietary fiber and phytate values in the cereals were not affected by extrusion, but nonetheless mineral availability was reduced. Despite the formation of phytate complexes with protein and starch in rice bran, over 90% of the phytate could still be extracted (Fuh and Chiang, 2001).

Mineral fortification has become common, especially in ready-to-eat breakfast cereals. Calcium hydroxide added at levels of 0.15–0.35% to corn reduced expansion and increased lightness in color (Martínez-Bustos, et al, 1998); bioavailability was not determined. Snacks made from blue maize on a small single screw extruder had acceptable textural characteristics with added calcium hydroxide levels of 0.02–0.078% (Zazueta-Morales et al, 2001). Since dark color can result when some iron salts react with phenolics, Kapanidis and Lee (1996) recommended ferrous sulfate heptahydrate as an added iron source in a simulated rice product.

14.7 Other nutritional changes

14.7.1 Antinutrients

Extrusion cooking also improves the nutritional quality of foods by destroying many natural toxins and antinutrients (Table 14.4). A dilemma exists as to whether it is desirable to remove these compounds. Enzyme inhibitors, hormone-like compounds, saponins and other compounds could impair growth and development in children, but these same compounds may offer protection against chronic diseases in adults. Allergens and mycotoxins are very resistant to thermal

Table 14.4 Antinutrients and toxins affected by extrusion cooking

Compound	Foods	Factors favoring reduction
Allergens	Peanut, soy	Increased shear; added starch
Glucosinolates	Canola	Added ammonia
Glycoalkaloids	Potato	Added thiamine
Gossypol	Cottonseed	Higher feed moisture
Mycotoxins	Grains	Increased mixing, lower temperatures; added amine sources
Protease inhibitors	Legumes, potato	Higher extrusion temperatures

processing, but extrusion in combination with chemical treatment via reactive extrusion may effectively reduce these compounds to safe levels.

Glucosinolates found in many commercially important *Brassica* species might protect against certain forms of cancer (Van Poppel et al, 1999). Extrusion alone does not affect glucosinolates (Fenwick et al, 1986), but extrusion plus ammonia decreased glucosinolates in canola (Darroch, et al, 1990). Although extrusion with ammonium carbonate did not result in glucosinolate-free rapeseed meal, the process did improve nutritional parameters in a rat-feeding study (Barrett et al, 1997).

14.7.2 Phenolic compounds

The health benefits of phenolic acids and flavonoids are being actively studied today. Potato peels free phenolics, primarily chlorogenic acid, were reduced by extrusion (unpublished data, Camire and Dougherty), with improved retention at higher barrel temperature and feed moisture. Blueberry and grape anthocyanins were significantly reduced by extrusion and by ascorbic acid in sweetened corn breakfast cereals (Chaovanalikit, 1999).

14.7.3 Phytohormones

Phytoestrogens in soy and other foods may protect post-menopausal women from osteoporosis and heart disease and protect men against prostate and other testosterone-dependent cancers. Extrusion can transform soy into food products with broad appeal for consumers, but processing effects on soy isoflavones and other phytoestrogens should be evaluated for any products for which health effects are intended. Blends of soy protein concentrate and cornmeal (20:80) were processed under different extrusion conditions (Mahungu et al, 1999). Increasing barrel temperature caused decarboxylation of isoflavones, with increased proportions of acetyl derivatives, but total isoflavones also decreased.

Extrusion decreased the aglycone (genistein) of okara, a tofu by-product, mixed with wheat flour (Rinaldi et al, 2000). Glucosides of daidzin and genistin increased, but acetyl and malonyl forms decreased in the mixtures. Total isoflavone values were reduced in 40% okara samples extruded at high-temperature. Aglycones did not change in extruded corn-soy blends, but they were less effective in preventing proliferation of breast cancer cells *in vitro* (Singletary et al, 2000).

14.8 Future trends

Many opportunities exist for product development research in extrusion. Very little has been published on the effects of extrusion on phytochemicals and other healthful food components, in part due to the need for identification of active principles and suitable analytical procedures. Evaluations of nutrient retention by either high-moisture extrusion or by supercritical fluid extrusion have yet to be published.

Improved understanding of scaled-up issues in extrusion is necessary for valid interpretation of studies conducted using laboratory-scale and pilot plant extruders. Few universities possess extruders, and those that do typically own small models that are inexpensive to acquire and operate. Long-term animal and feeding studies are tedious and costly, yet essential for demonstrating safety and efficacy of extruded foods.

14.9 Sources of further information and advice

Among the books published on extrusion cooking are those by Guy (2001), Frame (1994), Harper (1981), Hayakawa (1992), Kokini et al (1992), Mercier et al (1989), O'Connor (1987) and Riaz (2000). Chemical and nutritional changes in extruded foods have been the subject of review articles as well (Björck and Asp, 1983; Camire, 1998; Camire et al, 1990; Cheftel, 1986; de la Gueriviere et al, 1985). As yet there is no journal focused on food extrusion. Relevant articles may be found in *Cereal Chemistry, Journal of Agricultural and Food Chemistry, Journal of Cereal Science, Journal of Food Engineering,* and *Journal of Food Science.* Short courses on extrusion are offered by the American Association of Cereal Chemists, several universities, as well as extruder manufacturers.

14.10 References

AKDOGAN H (1999), 'High moisture food extrusion', *Intl J Food Sci Technol*, **34**(3), 195–207

ALONSO R, GRANT G, DEWEY P and MARZO F (2000), 'Nutritional assessment *in vitro* and *in vivo* of raw and extruded peas (*Pisum sativum* L)', *J Agric Food Chem*, **48**(6), 2286–90

ALONSO R, GRANT G and MARZO F (2001), 'Thermal treatment improves nutritional quality of pea seeds (*Pisum sativum* L) without reducing their hypocholesterolemic properties', *Nutr Res*, **21**(7), 1067–77

ANDERSSON Y and HEDLUND B (1991), 'Extruded whey flour: correlation between processing and product quality parameters', *Food Quality and Preference*, **2**(3), 201–16

ARÊAS J A G (1992), 'Extrusion of food proteins', *Crit Rev Food Sci Nutr*, **32**(4), 365–92

ARTZ W E, RAO S K and SAUER R M (1992), 'Lipid oxidation in extruded products during storage as affected by extrusion temperature and selected antioxidants', in Kokini J L, Ho C-T and Karwe M V (eds), *Food Extrusion Science and Technology*, New York, Marcel Dekker

BARRETT J E, KLOPFENSTEIN C F and LEIPOLD H W (1997), 'Detoxification of rapeseed meal by extrusion with an added basic salt', *Cereal Chem*, **74**(2), 168–70

BATES L, AMES J M and MACDOUGALL D B (1994), 'The use of a reaction cell to model the development and control of colour in extrusion cooked foods', *Lebensm-Wiss u-Technol*, **27**(4), 375–9

BERGMAN C J, GUALBERTO D G and WEBER C W (1997), 'Mineral binding capacity of dephytinized insoluble fiber from extruded wheat, oat and rice brans', *Plant Foods Hum Nutr*, **51**(4), 295–310

BJÖRCK I and ASP N-G (1983), 'The effects of extrusion cooking on nutritional value – a literature review', *J Food Engin*, **2**(4), 281–308
BJÖRCK I, ASP N-G, BIRKHED D and LUNDQUIST, I (1984), 'Effects of processing on availability of starch for digestion *in vitro* and *in vivo*; I. extrusion cooking of wheat flours and starch', *J Cereal Sci*, **2**(2), 91–103
BOREJSZO Z and KHAN K (1992), 'Reduction of flatulence-causing sugars by high temperature extrusion of pinto bean high starch fractions', *J Food Sci*, **57**(3), 771–2 and 777
CAMIRE M E (1991), 'Protein functionality modification by extrusion cooking', *J Am Oil Chem Soc*, **68**(3), 200–5
CAMIRE M E (1998), 'Chemical changes during extrusion cooking. process-induced chemical changes in food', in Shahidi F, Ho C-T and van Chuyen H (eds), *Process-induced Chemical Changes in Food*, New York, Plenum Press
CAMIRE M E and FLINT S I (1991), 'Thermal processing effects on dietary fiber composition and hydration capacity in corn meal, oat meal and potato peels', *Cereal Chem*, **68**(6), 645–7
CAMIRE M E and DOUGHERTY M P (1998), 'Added phenolic compounds enhance lipid stability in extruded corn', *J Food Sci*, **63**(4), 516–18
CAMIRE M E, CAMIRE A and KRUMHAR K (1990), 'Chemical and nutritional changes in foods during extrusion', *Crit Rev Food Sci Nutr*, **29**(1), 35–57
CAMIRE M E, ZHAO J and VIOLETTE D A (1993), '*In vitro* binding of bile acids by extruded potato peels', *J Agric Food Chem*, **41**(12), 2391–4
CHAOVANALIKIT A (1999), 'Anthocyanin stability during extrusion cooking', M.S. Thesis, Univ. of Maine, Orono ME
CHEFTEL J C (1986), 'Nutritional effects of extrusion cooking', *Food Chem*, **20**, 263–83
CHINNASWAMY R and HANNA M A (1991), 'Physicochemical and macromolecular properties of starch-cellulose fiber extrudates', *Food Structure*, **10**(3), 229–39
CHIU C W, HENLEY M and ALTIERI P (1994), 'Process for making amylase resistant starch from high amylose starch', United States Patent. Patent No: 5 281 276. Date of Patent: Jan. 25, 1994
CISSE D, GUIRO A T, DIAHAM B, SOUANE M, DOUMBOUYA N T and WADE S (1998), 'Effect of food processing on iron availability of African pearl millet weaning foods', *Intl J Food Sci Nutr*, **49**(5), 375–81
DARROCH C S, BELL J M and KEITH M O (1990), 'The effects of moist heat and ammonia on the chemical composition and feeding value of extruded canola screenings for mice', *Can J Anim Sci*, **70**, 267–77
DE LA GUERIVIERE J F, MERCIER C and BAUDET L (1985), 'Incidences de la cuisson-extrusion sur certains parametres nutritionnels de produits alimentaires notamment céréaliers', *Cah Nutr Diet*, **20**(3), 201–10
DELLA VALLE G, QUILLIEN L and GUEGUEN J (1994), 'Relationships between processing conditions and starch and protein modifications during extrusion-cooking of pea flour', *J Sci Food Agric*, **64**(4), 509–17
FAIRCHILD R M, ELLIS P R, BYRNE A J, LUZIO S D and MIR M A (1996), 'A new breakfast cereal containing guar gum reduces postprandial plasma glucose and insulin concentrations in normal-weight human subjects', *Brit J Nutr*, **46**(1), 63–73
FAIRWEATHER-TAIT S J, SYMSS L L, SMITH A C and JOHNSON I T (1987), 'The effect of extrusion cooking on iron absorption from maize and potato', *J Sci Food Agric*, **39**(4), 341–8
FAIRWEATHER-TAIT S J, PORTWOOD D E, SYMSS L L, EAGLES J and MINSKI M J (1989), 'Iron and zinc absorption in human subjects from a mixed meal of extruded and non-extruded wheat bran flour', *Am J Clin Nutr*, **49**(1), 151–5
FARDET A, ABECASSIS J, HOEBLER C, BALDWIN P M, BULEON A, BEROT S and BARRY J L (1999), 'Influence of technological modifications of the protein network from pasta on *in vitro* starch degradation', *J Cereal Sci*, **30**(2), 33–145
FENWICK G R, SPINKS E A, WILKINSON A P, HEANEY R K and LEGOY M A (1986), 'Effect of processing on the antinutrient content of rapeseed,' *J Sci Food Agric*, **37**(8), 735–41

FRAME N D (1994), *The Technology of Extrusion Cooking*, Glasgow, Blackie Academic and Professional

FUH W-S and CHIANG B-H (2001), 'Dephytinisation of rice bran and manufacturing a new food ingredient', *J Sci Food Agric*, **81**(15), 1419–25

FUKUI K, AOYAMA T, HASHIMOTO Y and YAMAMOTO T (1993), 'Effect of extrusion of soy protein isolate on plasma cholesterol level and nutritive value of protein in growing male rats', *J Jap Soc Nutr Food Sci*, **46**(3), 211–16

GAOSONG J and VASANTHAN T (2000), 'Effect of extrusion cooking on the primary structure and water solubility of beta-glucans from regular and waxy barley', *Cereal Chem*, **77**(3), 396–400

GAUTAM A and CHOUDHOURY G S (1999), 'Screw configuration effects on starch breakdown during twin screw extrusion of rice flour', *J Food Process Preserv*, **23**(4), 355–75

GOURGUE C, CHAMP M, GUILLON F and DELORT-LAVAL J (1994), 'Effect of extrusion-cooking on the hypoglycaemic properties of citrus fibre: an *in vitro* study', *J Sci Food Agric*, **64**(4), 493–9

GUALBERTO D G, BERGMAN C J, KAZEMZADEH M and WEBER C W (1997), 'Effect of extrusion processing on the soluble and insoluble fiber, and phytic acid contents of cereals bran', *Plant Foods Human Nutrition*, **51**(3), 187–98

GUY, R (2001), *Extrusion Cooking*, Cambridge, Woodhead Publishing Ltd.

GUZMAN L B, LEE T-C and CHICHESTER C O (1992), 'Lipid binding during extrusion cooking', in Kokini J L, Ho C-T and Karwe M V (eds), *Food Extrusion Science and Technology*, New York, Marcel Dekker

GUZMAN-TELLO R and CHEFTEL J C (1987), 'Thiamine destruction during extrusion cooking as an indicator of the intensity of thermal processing', *Intl J Food Sci Technol*, **22**(5), 549–62

GUZMAN-TELLO R and CHEFTEL J C (1990), 'Colour loss during extrusion cooking of beta-carotene–wheat flour mixes as an indicator of the intensity of thermal and oxidative processing', *Intl J Food Sci Technol*, **25**(4), 420–34

HARPER J M (1981), *Extrusion of Foods*, Boca Raton, FL, CRC Press

HARPER J M and JANSEN G R (1985), 'Production of nutritious precooked foods in developing countries by low-cost extrusion technology', *Food Reviews Intl*, **1**(1), 27–97

HAYAKAWA I (1992), *Food Processing by Ultra High Pressure Twin Screw Extrusion*, Lancaster, PA, Technomic Publ

HAZELL T and JOHNSON I T (1989), 'Influence of food processing on iron availability *in vitro* from extruded maize-based snack food', *J Sci Food Agric*, **46**(3), 365–74

HWANG J-K, KIM C-J and KIM C-T (1998), 'Production of glucooligosaccharides and polydextrose by extrusion reactor', *Starch*, **50**(2–3), 104–7

JIN Z, HSIEH F and HUFF H E (1994), 'Extrusion cooking of corn meal with soy fiber, salt, and sugar', *Cereal Chem*, **71**(3), 227–34

KANG S-Y (1996), *Zinc bioavailability in a semolina/soy protein mixture was not affected by extrusion processing*, M.S. Thesis, East Lansing, MI, Michigan State University

KAPANIDIS A N and LEE T-C (1996), 'Novel method for the production of color-compatible ferrous sulfate-fortified simulated rice through extrusion', *J Agric Food Chem*, **44**(2), 522–5

KILLEIT U (1994), 'Vitamin retention in extrusion cooking', *Food Chem*, **49**(2), 149–55

KIVISTÖ B, ANDERSSON H, CEDERBLAD G, SANDBERG A-S and SANDSTROM B (1986), 'Extrusion cooking of a high-fiber cereal product. 2: effects on apparent absorption of zinc, iron, calcium, magnesium and phosphorus in humans', *British J Nutr*, **55**(2), 255–60

KOKINI J L, HO C-T and KARWE M V (1992), *Food Extrusion Science and Technology*, New York, Marcel Dekker

KONSTANCE R P, ONWULATA C I, SMITH P W, LU D, TUNICK M H, STRANGE E D and HOLSINGER V H (1998), 'Nutrient-based corn and soy products by twin-screw extrusion', *J Food Sci*, **63**(5), 864–8

LOMBARDI-BOCCIA G, DI LULLO G and CARNOVALE E (1991), '*In vitro* iron dialysability from legumes: influence of phytate and extrusion cooking', *J Sci Food Agric*, **55**(4), 599–605

LORENZ K and JANSEN G R (1980), 'Nutrient stability of full-fat soy flour and corn-soy blends produced by low-cost extrusion', *Cereal Foods World*, **25**(4), 161–2, 171–2

MAGA J A (1978), '*Cis-trans* fatty acid ratios as influenced by product and temperature of extrusion cooking', *Lebensm-Wiss u-Technol*, **11**(4), 183–4

MAGA J A and SIZER C E (1978), 'Ascorbic acid and thiamin retention during extrusion of potato flakes', *Lebensm-Wiss u-Technol*, **11**(4), 192–4

MAHUNGU S M, DIAZ-MERCADO S, LI J, SCHWENK M, SINGLETARY K and FALLER J (1999), 'Stability of isoflavones during extrusion processing of corn/soy mixture', *J Agric Food Chem*, **47**(1), 279–84

MARCHETTI M, TOSSANI N, MARCHETTI S and BAUCE G (1999), 'Stability of crystalline and coated vitamins during manufacture and storage of fish feeds', *Aquaculture Nutr*, **5**(2), 115–20

MARTIN-CABREJAS M A, JAMIE L, KARANJA C, DOWNIE A J, PARKER M L, LOPEZ-ANDREU F J, MAINA G, ESTEBAN R M, SMITH A C and WALDRON K W (1999), 'Modifications to physicochemical and nutritional properties of hard-to-cook beans (*Phaseolus vulgaris* L) by extrusion cooking', *J Agric Food Chem*, **47**(3), 1174–82

MARTINEZ-BUSTOS F, CHANG Y K, BANNWART A C, RODRIGUEZ M E, GUEDES P A and GAIOTTI E R (1998), 'Effects of calcium hydroxide and processing conditions on corn meal extrudates', *Cereal Chem*, **75**(6), 796–801

MARTY C and BERSET C (1988), 'Degradation products of *trans*-beta-carotene produced during extrusion cooking', *J Food Sci*, **53**(6), 1880–6

MERCIER C, LINKO P and HARPER J M (1989), *Extrusion Cooking*, St. Paul, MN, Am Assoc Cereal Chem

MEUSER F and VAN LENGERICH B (1984), 'Systems analytical model for the extrusion of starches', in Zeuthen P, Cheftel J C, Eriksson C, Jul M, Leniger H, Linko P, Varela G and Vos G (eds), *Thermal Processing and Quality of Foods*, London, Elsevier Applied Sci, 175–9

NELSON A I, WIJERATNE W B, YEH S W, WEI T M and WEI L S (1987), 'Dry extrusion as an aid to mechanical expelling of oil from soybeans', *J Am Oil Chem Soc*, **64**(9), 1341–7

NOGUCHI A and CHEFTEL J-C (1983), 'Extrusion-cooking of protein-enriched cookies', *Nippon Shokuhin Kogyo Gakkai Shi*, **30**(2), 114–24

O'CONNOR C (1987), *Extrusion Technology for the Food Industry*, London, Elsevier Applied Sci Publ

OMUETI O and MORTON I D (1996), 'Development by extrusion of soyabari snack sticks: a nutritionally improved soya-maize product based on the Nigerian snack (kokoro)', *Intl J Food Sci Nutr*, **47**(1), 5–13

OOSTHUIZEN W, SCHOLTZ C S, VORSTER H H, JERLING J C and VERMAAK W J H (2000), 'Extruded dry beans and serum lipoprotein and plasma haemostatic factors in hyperlipidaemic men', *Eur J Clin Nutr*, **54**(5), 373–9

PANLASIGUI L N, THOMPSON L U, JULIANO B O, PEREZ C M, JENKINS D J A and YIU S H (1992), 'Extruded rice noodles: starch digestibility and glycemic response of healthy and diabetic subjects with different habitual diets', *Nutr Res*, **12**(10), 1195–204

PLATE Y A and AREÂS J A G (2002), 'Cholesterol-lowering effect of extruded amaranth (*Amaranthus caudatus* L) in hypercholesterolemic rabbits', *Food Chem*, **76**(1), 1–6

POLITZ M L, TIMPA J D, WHITE A R and WASSERMAN B P (1994a), 'Non-aqueous gel permeation chromatography of wheat starch in dimethylacetamide (DMAC) and LiCl: extrusion-induced fragmentation', *Carbohydrate Polymers*, **24**(2), 91–9

POLITZ M L, TIMPA J D and WASSERMAN B P (1994b), 'Quantitative measurement of extrusion-induced starch fragmentation products in maize flour using nonaqueous automatic gel-permeation chromatography', *Cereal Chem*, **71**(6), 532–6

RALET M-C, THIBAULT J-F and DELLA VALLE G (1991), 'Solubilization of sugar-beet pulp cell wall polysaccharides by extrusion-cooking', *Lebensm-Wiss u-Technol*, **24**(2), 107–12

RIAZ M N (2000), *Extruders in Food Applications*, Lancaster PA, Technomic Publ

RIAZ M N (2001), 'Selecting the right extruder', in Guy R, *Extrusion Cooking*, Cambridge, Woodhead Publishing Ltd., 29–50

RINALDI V E A, NG P K W and BENNICK M R (2000), 'Effects of extrusion on dietary fiber and isoflavone contents of wheat extrudates enriched with wet okara', *Cereal Chem*, **77**(2), 237–40

SANDBERG A S, ANDERSSON H, KIVISTÖ B and SANDSTROM B (1986), 'Extrusion cooking of a high-fibre cereal product. 1. Effects on digestibility and absorption of protein, fat, starch, dietary fibre and phytate in the small intestine', *Br J Nutr*, **55**(2), 245–54

SCHAICH K M and REBELLO C A (1999), 'Extrusion chemistry of wheat flour proteins. I. Free radical formation', *Cereal Chem*, **76**(5), 748–55

SEMWAL A D, SHARMA G K and ARYA S S (1994), 'Factors influencing lipid autooxidation in dehydrated precooked rice and bengalgram dhal', *J Food Sci Technol*, **31**(4), 293–7

SHIN T S, GODBER J S, MARTIN D E and WELLS J H (1997), 'Hydrolytic stability and changes in E vitamers and oryzanol of extruded rice bran during storage', *J Food Sci*, **62**(4), 704–8

SINGLETARY K, FALLER J, LI J Y and MAHUNGU S (2000), 'Effect of extrusion on isoflavone content and antiproliferative bioactivity of soy/corn mixtures', *J Agric Food Chem*, **48**(8), 3566–71

SRIBURI P and HILL S E (2000), 'Extrusion of cassava starch with either variations in ascorbic acid concentration or pH', *Intl J Food Sci Technol*, **35**(2), 141–54

SUKNARK K, LEE J, EITENMILLER R R and PHILLIPS R D (2001), 'Stability of tocopherols and retinyl palmitate in snack extrudates', *J Food Sci*, **66**(6), 897–902

SUZUKI H, CHUNG B S, ISOBE S, HAYAKAWA S and WADA S (1988), 'Changes in ω(omega)-3 polyunsaturated fatty acids in the chum salmon muscle during spawning migration and extrusion cooking', *J Food Sci*, **53**(6), 1659–61

THEANDER O and WESTERLUND E (1987), 'Studies on chemical modifications in heat-processed starch and wheat flour', *Starch/Stärke*, **39**(3), 88–93

UMMADI P, CHENOWETH W L and NG P K W (1995), 'Changes in solubility and distribution of semolina proteins due to extrusion processing,' *Cereal Chem*, **72**(6), 564–7

UNLU E and FALLER J F (1998), 'Formation of resistant starch by a twin-screw extruder', *Cereal Chem*, **75**(3), 346–50

VAN POPPEL G, VERHOEVEN D T, VERHAGEN H and GOLDBOHM R A (1999), '*Brassica* vegetables and cancer prevention. Epidemiology and mechanisms', *Adv Exp Med Biol*, **472**, 159–68

WANG S, CASULLI J and BOUVIER J M (1993), 'Effect of dough ingredients on apparent viscosity and properties of extrudates in twin-screw extrusion cooking', *Intl J Food Sci Technol*, **28**(5), 465–79

WANG W-M and KLOPFENSTEIN C F (1993), 'Effect of twin-screw extrusion on the nutritional quality of wheat, barley, and oats', *Cereal Chem*, **70**(6), 712–5

WANG W-M, KLOPFENSTEIN C F and PONTE J G (1993), 'Effects of twin-screw extrusion on the physical properties of dietary fiber and other components of whole wheat and wheat bran and on the baking quality of the wheat bran', *Cereal Chem*, **70**(6), 707–11

WENNERMARK B (1993), *Vitamin E retention during processing of cereals*, FILDR Thesis, Lund, Lunds Universistet

ZAZUETA-MORALES J J, MARTINEZ-BUSTOS F, JACOBO-VALENZUELA N, ORDORICA-FALOMIR C and PAREDES-LÓPEZ O (2001), 'Effect of the addition of calcium hydroxide on some characteristics of extruded products from blue maize (*Zea mays* L) using response surface methodology', *J Sci Food Agric*, **81**(14), 1379–86

ZIELINSKI H, KOZLOWSKA H and LEWCZUK B (2001), "Bioactive compounds in the cereal grains before and after hydrothermal processing', *J Food Processing Preserv*, **23**(3), 177–91

15

Freezing

J. M. Fletcher, Unilever R & D Colworth

15.1 Introduction

The modern frozen food industry was started by Clarence Birdseye in America in 1925. As a fur trader in Labrador Birdseye had noticed that fillets of fish left by the natives to freeze rapidly in arctic winters retained the taste and texture attributes of fresh fish better than fillets frozen in milder temperatures at other times of the year. Frozen foods were available before Birdseye's pioneering innovations, but they were of poor and uncertain quality. Birdseye's insight was that speed of freezing is crucial to retain quality and he was the first to develop machinery that could freeze foods rapidly on an industrial scale. Quick freezing allowed the transport of produce over long distances and the year-round consumption of seasonal produce that was of very superior quality compared with alternative preservation methods such as canning and drying. Although Birdseye was probably unaware of this particular advantage, quick freezing, if combined with appropriate treatments prior to freezing, also has the potential to ensure excellent preservation of nutritional value for a wide range of foods. In the context of the nutritional value of vegetables and fruits, the US Food and Drug Administration has recently (1998) approved frozen produce to be labelled as healthy. Based on presented data the Food and Drug Administration concluded that '... because frozen fruits or vegetable products are nutritionally comparable to the raw versions, they would likely have the same inherent beneficial effects as the raw version'.

In the years since 1925 the application of freezing has become globally an important aspect of food processing technology. In the year 2000 total world wide sales of frozen foods (excluding ice cream) was estimated as 13.6 million tonnes with a retail value of US$ 58.5 billion (Euromonitor). The process of quick freezing was first applied to a limited range of fish, meat, fruits and vegetables; today, in addition to these still important basics there is a very wide range of processed foods, meal components and whole meals available in the frozen format. Currently, the sectors of red meat, poultry, fish/seafood and vegetables make up approximately 10% each of the total tonnage of the total frozen food market as well as frozen potatoes at 15% and ready meals at 20% (Euromonitor). As might be expected, there are considerable geographical differences between regions and countries in usage of frozen food. Whereas in the US and in Europe approximately 13 kg and 10 kg of frozen food are consumed per capita per year, in Africa and Asia the amounts consumed are only 0.3 kg and 0.9 kg respectively. In the future it is anticipated that freezing as a processing option will take an increasing share of the food market. In both developed and undeveloped nations the increased demand for frozen foods will come from consumers' wishes for high convenience, high organoleptic quality and high nutritional value.

Although freezing on its own has a negligible impact on nutrient levels in food, the associated pre-freezing processing, storage in the frozen state and structural damage evident in some thawed frozen foods may have significant detrimental effects. The early literature describing the effects of freezing and associated processing on nutrient content and nutritional value has been reviewed by Bender in 1978, and more recently in 1993. This chapter will summarise the key principles, review newer findings and highlight areas of continuing uncertainty in assessing the nutritional impact of freezing.

15.2 Change and stability in frozen foods

The defining step in freezing is the removal of heat. This lowers the temperature of foods so that microbial and chemical changes are prevented or minimised. By storing in the frozen state it is possible to prolong greatly the length of time that many foods may be maintained with an excellent sensory and nutritional value. It is, however, important to realise that at the typical temperatures used for industrial and domestic storage of frozen foods (typically $-24°C$ and $-18°C$ respectively), chemical reactions that can lead to a reduction of quality and nutrient loss may continue to occur. Many of these reactions take place in solution and even at $-24°C$, natural foods such as fruit, vegetables and meats may still contain 2–5% of their total water content in the liquid phase. As the temperature of natural foods is reduced below $0°C$ ice crystals begin to form and the solutes present in intra- and extra-cellular fluids become more concentrated in the remaining liquid water, thereby lowering the freezing point of this water. Therefore, although the rates of most reactions will be substantially reduced by the lower temperature of frozen foods, the increased solute concentration may to some extent counteract this effect. Another effect of the increased solute concentration is to move water by osmosis between compartments. The formation of ice may also rupture cell structures causing mixing and reactions between components previously held apart. The complex nature of the changes that take place when foods are frozen makes it difficult to predict effects on quality and stability.

Probably the most important reaction leading to both quality and nutrient losses in frozen foods is oxidation. The consequences of oxidative instability are the key factors that limit the storage life of frozen foods. Just as in foods kept at more normal ambient temperatures, unless they are stored in a vacuum, or in an inert gas, atmospheric oxygen will diffuse through frozen food and may react with many of the soluble and insoluble components. One consequence of oxidation on sensory quality is the development of 'off flavours' and rancidity, usually caused by oxidative breakdown of membrane and storage lipids (Erickson, 1997). Other adverse consequences of oxidation may include colour loss and/or change, and in fish and meat foods a toughening of muscle structures. Although macromolecular components such as carbohydrates and protein may undergo limited oxidation, any influence on nutritional value is likely to be small. However, several vitamins such as ascorbate and folates are particularly susceptible to oxidative damage.

A feature of the quick freezing of foods is the formation of a large number of relatively small ice crystals that cause minimal damage to cellular and tissue structures but on prolonged frozen storage, and particularly in conditions where temperatures fluctuate, crystals of ice grow in size. Although at any temperature below 0°C, the total amount of ice in a food will remain constant, large crystals grow instead of a larger number of smaller crystals, a process known as Ostwald ripening. The growth of larger ice crystals may break delicate food structures and compress others. On thawing of frozen foods these changes may have serious effects on texture leading to poor sensory quality; vegetables and fruits may lose their characteristic crispness and meat or fish may become tougher and drier. An adverse consequence for nutritional value is the reduced water-holding capacity of structurally damaged foods, leading to increased 'drip loss'. Significant amounts of water-soluble nutrients may be discarded if this drip loss is not incorporated into the food to be consumed.

15.3 Vegetables and fruits

There are several factors that potentially contribute to differences in nutrient levels between vegetables and fruits in the frozen format and those supplied as fresh or preserved by other processes. Any differences are likely to be in the loss and preservation of vitamins; it has been shown that compared with fresh vegetables, there are negligible differences between the mineral and fibre contents of equivalent frozen vegetables (Polo et al, 1992; Nyman, 1995).

15.3.1 Selection of cultivar and time of harvesting

Particular cultivars and harvest times are chosen to optimise sensory quality and these may differ between those selected for freezing and those that are consumed in fresh, canned or dried formats. The cultivar and harvest time may have some effects on nutritional value (Shewfelt, 1990); for example peas selected for

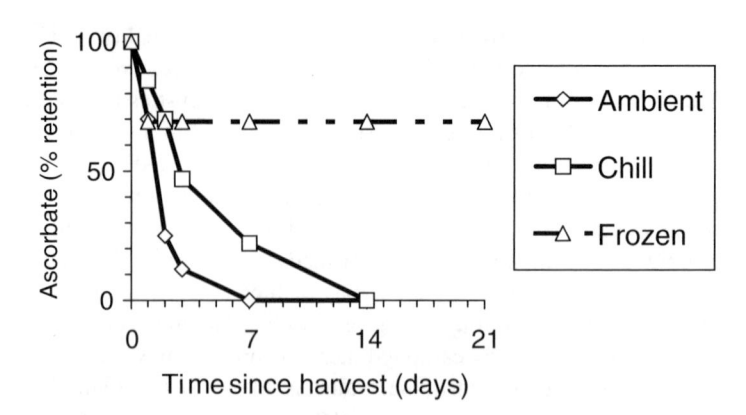

Fig. 15.1 Effects of storage and freezing on ascorbate retention in spinach: typical values for retention of ascorbate in spinach stored at either ambient or chill temperature (4°C) compared with blanched and frozen spinach. All samples were taken from the same field and time zero levels were obtained from freshly harvested spinach. Blanching and freezing were carried out in a commercial factory. (from Favell, 1998)

canning are usually harvested at a more mature stage than those selected for freezing and consequently have approximately 10% lower ascorbate concentration. The type of cultivar may also influence the amount of nutrient lost during processing, reflecting differences between culitvars in morphology and mechanical strength.

15.3.2 Storage after harvest

Many vegetables, and to a lesser extent fruits, are relatively unstable after harvesting and undergo rapid chemical changes that result in significantly reduced levels of some nutrients. For example, concentrations of ascorbate in spinach may fall to 50% of their initial, pre-harvest level, after two days of storage as shown in Fig. 15.1 (Favell, 1998). The magnitude of nutrient losses during storage prior to freezing is highly variable and depends on the crop, the method of harvesting and the duration and conditions of storage. To preserve the nutritional value of fresh vegetables and fruits it is clearly desirable to minimise the time in blanching and freezing and to cause minimal mechanical damage.

15.3.3 Washing and blanching

The need for washing of vegetables and fruits may cause some loss of water-soluble nutrients, particularly from cut surfaces. As noted above, oxidation is a key factor influencing stability in the frozen state and this is particularly a concern with vegetables and fruits because they contain many enzyme systems that give rise to reactive oxygen species. It is to prevent enzyme-mediated oxidation reactions that most vegetables and fruits are blanched before freezing. Another reason is to ensure microbiological safety but this can be achieved by other means. The advantages of blanching can be illustrated with reference to cauliflower and spinach. If they are frozen without blanching they become unpalatable after only a few months due to the development of 'off' flavours and odours caused primarily by oxidation of membrane lipids. If these vegetables are blanched before freezing they have a storage life of 18–24 months. Commercial blanching conditions typically involve heating in water or steam at 95–100°C for 3–10 minutes, depending on the type and size of material to be blanched. The conditions are chosen so as to ensure inactivation of the enzymes responsible for oxidation. During blanching, nutrients may be lost by leaching and by chemical degradation. A great deal of information has been published on losses of labile nutrients during blanching (for review see Clydesdale et al, 1991). Ascorbate is often used as an indicator of potential nutrient loss because of its high solubility, sensitivity to heat and ease of measurement. Typical losses of ascorbate from vegetables during blanching are of the order 5–40% (Favell, 1998; Bender, 1993). In general, it may be concluded that nutrient losses are minimised if the raw material is as little damaged as possible during handling and if processing conditions are chosen that keep the temperature, duration of heat exposure and product to water ratio as low as is consistent with denaturing the enzymes responsible for oxidative spoilage.

15.3.4 Frozen storage

Bender (1993) has summarised the contradictory results of published studies designed to estimate the magnitude of vitamin loss during frozen storage of vegetables and fruits. Even for a particular vegetable, processed and stored under apparently similar conditions, the extent of ascorbate loss has been reported as negligible, or up to 40% after a year of frozen storage (Bender, 1993). As Bender comments, there are many possible sources of experimental variation that may lead to these different conclusions, most notably incomplete denaturation of oxidative enzymes during blanching. Since the review by Bender no large scale systematic study addressing this issue has been published. It may be concluded that if vegetables and fruits are adequately blanched and stored at conventional freezer temperatures without undue temperature fluctuations they will still possess valuable levels of potentially labile nutrients for a period of at least 12–18 months.

15.3.5 Cooking

When comparing the nutritional value of different processing methods it is also necessary to consider the ways in which consumers handle these different products. Cooking methods may have important effects on the quantity of nutrients within a food. Because frozen vegetables have already been blanched, they require less cooking time than fresh vegetables to reach the same levels of palatability. This means that while frozen vegetables may have lost some nutrients during blanching they will probably suffer reduced losses during cooking.

It is increasingly recognised that regular consumption of vegetables and fruits significantly reduces the risk of some cancers and of cardiovascular disease. Although it is by no means certain, it appears likely that these beneficial effects are not just a consequence of consuming the recognised nutrients found in vegetables and fruits. A large number of potentially beneficial compounds, the so called phyto-nutrients, or non-nutrient phyto-chemicals are found in vegetables and fruits. It is not yet clear which particular compounds, or even which group of phytochemicals may be responsible for the health benefits, but if and when the protective agents are identified it will be necessary to ascertain the effects of freezing and associated processes on their retention in frozen vegetables and fruits.

15.4 Meat and fish

Quick freezing is extensively used to preserve a wide range of raw and cooked meat and fish. Freezing and frozen storage does not significantly affect the nutritional value of meat and fish proteins. However, as pointed out above, on thawing frozen meat and fish substantial amounts of intra- and extra-cellular fluids and their associated water-soluble proteins and other nutrients may be lost ('drip-loss'). The volume of drip-loss on thawing of meat and fish is highly variable, usually of the order of 2–10% of wet weight but in exceptional circumstances up to 15% of the weight of the product may be lost.

Many factors influence the amount of drip loss and not all are related to freezing:

- Variables influencing the raw material – The age, the species and the variety of the animal may have important effects. Additional factors may include the diet fed to the animal, the method of slaughter, and the pre- and post-slaughter handling.
- Water-binding chemicals – A variety of chemicals are often used as additives to meat and fish before freezing, e.g. polyphosphates. These chemicals penetrate muscle fibres and they associate with proteins where they serve to protect the texture and succulence of meat and fish and to reduce drip loss.
- Freezing and frozen storage – The rate of freezing, the temperature of frozen storage and temperature fluctuations during storage.
- Thawing – The rate of thawing from the frozen state and the holding temperature before cooking.

In the frozen state meat and fish are generally less susceptible to oxidative spoilage than are vegetables and fruits and they are not subjected to the equivalent of blanching. On prolonged storage, however, oxidation may lead to significant chemical changes and loss of labile vitamins. The poly-unsaturated fatty acids in meat and fish are particularly susceptible to oxidation. As with vegetables and fruits, it is the products of fatty acid oxidation that give rise to characteristic 'off' and rancid flavours and aromas. The recommended storage lives of frozen meat and fish products are chosen to be within the period before 'off' and rancid flavours and aroma are detectable. In general, those meat and fish products that contain a larger amount of poly-unsaturated fatty acids are least stable and have shorter storage lives. For example, oily fish have a typical frozen shelf life in the region of 6–9 months at −18°C whereas white fish have a frozen shelf life of 12–24 months. Equivalent cuts of pork and beef have frozen shelf lives of 10–12 months and 18–24 months respectively (International Institute of Refrigeration, 1986).

A particular nutritional advantage of fish, and especially of oily fish, is as a dietary source of long chain n-3 poly-unsaturated fatty acids (docosahexanoic acid and eicosapentanoic acid; DHA and EPA respectively). Intake of these fatty acids has been implicated in many health benefits and as noted above they are particularly susceptible to oxidation. Several recent studies have been carried out to determine the effects of freezing and frozen storage on their levels in fish. A significant reduction in the total n-3 PUFA content was reported in saithe (a lean fish) fillets stored at −20°C for six months (Dulavik et al, 1998). Similarly, levels of total n-3 PUFA were reduced in salmon fillets stored at −20°C (Refsgaard et al, 1998) and levels of DHA and EPA were reduced in sardine and mackerel fillets stored for 24 months (Rougerou and Person, 1991). In contrast to these reports of PUFA loss, Polvi et al (1991) found no difference in total n-3 PUFA levels when salmon fillets were stored at the relatively high temperature of −12°C for three months. Xing et al (1993) also failed to see any losses of DHA and EPA in mackerel and cod fillets stored frozen at −20°C for 28 weeks.

As with many aspects of nutrient stability, the extent of n-3 PUFA loss from frozen fish by oxidation will depend on several factors, e.g. access of oxygen to the muscle, handling before freezing and the type of muscle (dark fish muscle suffers higher rates of iron-catalysed oxidation than does white muscle). Although loss of nutritionally important n-3 PUFAs from frozen fish may undoubtedly occur on prolonged frozen storage, in practice this is not likely to be a serious cause for concern. The threshold for sensory detection of rancidity is very low and therefore if frozen fish are consumed within the recommended period of storage, significant proportions of their original content of n-3 PUFAs will not have been lost to oxidation.

15.5 Nutritional implications of new developments in freezing

In considering the introduction of new developments in the freezing of foods and in associated technologies it is clear that they are unlikely to be driven solely by the motivation to improve nutritional value. If processed according to current good practice and consumed within their recommended storage lives, frozen foods already often have a nutritional value equivalent to foods available as fresh in the retail supply chain. Nevertheless, new developments designed to improve the organoleptic properties of frozen foods or to reduce the costs of production may have significance for nutrient retention.

15.5.1 Developments in blanching of vegetables and fruits

More rapid blanching of vegetables and fruits, and alternatives that do not use hot water immersion would be expected to preserve labile nutrients from leaching and chemical destruction. Alternative heating systems have been developed, such as those using steam and microwaves. However, as pointed out by Bender (1993), consistent evidence for nutritional benefits from these alternative blanching procedures has not been observed. Part of the reason lies in the inherent variability in plant raw materials. For example, ascorbate levels may differ by as much as two-fold in freshly harvested vegetables and the improved ascorbate retention to be achieved by alternative methods to conventional blanching may be only within the order of 5–10%.

15.5.2 Frozen storage in the glassy state

As pointed out above, natural foods stored at $-18°C$ to $-24°C$ contain significant amounts of liquid water in which reactions leading to quality and nutrient loss may occur. If the temperature of foods is further lowered, the remaining liquid eventually enters a so-called 'glassy state', i.e. a non-crystalline solid (for reviews, see Levine and Slade, 1989; Goff, 1997). In this state, rates of reaction, including enzyme mediated reactions become insignificant or greatly reduced. This gives rise to the possibility of storing frozen foods for longer periods than currently used without the risk of significant oxidation. There is also the possibility of freezing vegetables and fruits without the need for blanching and suffering the associated nutrient losses. The effects on ascorbate retention of storing unblanched peas at different temperatures compared with conventionally blanched and frozen peas are shown in Fig. 15.2. The temperature at which peas

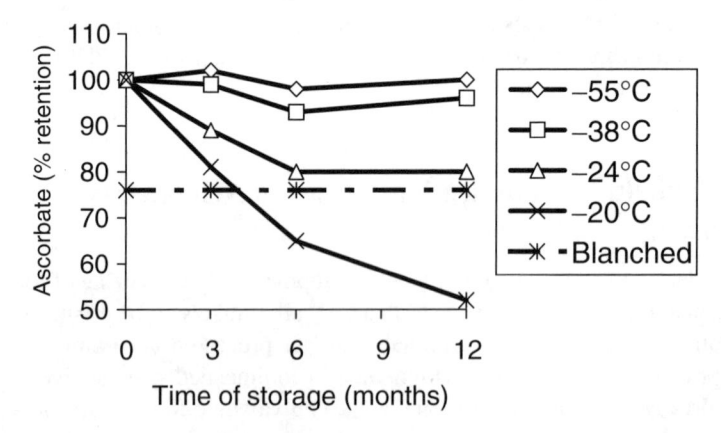

Fig. 15.2 Effects of frozen storage temperature on ascorbate retention of peas: Ascorbate retention in unblanched peas stored frozen at different temperatures compared with commercially blanched and frozen peas stored at $-24°C$. (from Sharp, unpublished)

are estimated to be in the glassy state is approximately −30°C and below this temperature they do not lose significant amounts of ascorbate. The temperature at which foods enter the glassy state varies and depends on the type and concentration of molecules in solution. Generally, the glassy state transition temperatures for foods are well below those used in the commercial supply chain and the costs entailed in modification of freezer operation would delay widespread uptake of this procedure.

15.5.3 Use of anti-freeze peptides

Anti-freeze peptides (AFP) are a class of compound that both depress the freezing point of water and prevent ice crystal enlargement during frozen storage (Lillford and Holt, 1994; Griffith and Ewart, 1995). If incorporated into frozen foods they may potentially prevent the structural and mechanical damage caused by ice crystal enlargement, thereby improving the sensory properties of food and potentially reducing drip loss from frozen food when it is thawed. This is illustrated by the finding that fish naturally containing AFPs suffer a lower amount of drip loss on freezing and thawing than those without such peptides (Payne and Wilson, 1994). Widespread applications of AFPs in frozen foods are currently limited by their cost and the need to produce them on any commercially relevant scale by using biotechnology.

15.6 Sources of further information and advice

15.6.1 Literature

- For an extensive review of the effects of freezing on the chemical and physical properties of foods see *Low temperature preservation of foods and living matter* (1973), edited by Fennema OR, Powrie WD and Marth EH, published by Marcel Dekker, New York.
- For details of industry standards and procedures relating to frozen food see *Recommendations for the Processing and Handling of Frozen Foods* (1986), published by the International Institute of Refrigeration, Paris.
- For a description of the effects of blanching, freezing and other processing steps on the nutritional value of individual vegetables see *Handbook of vegetable science and technology* (1998), edited by Salunkhe DK and Kadam SS, published by Marcel Dekker, New York.
- For a summary of modern frozen food theory and practice see *Maximising quality and stability of frozen foods* (1999), edited by Kennedy CJ and Archer GP, published by the EU Concerted Action CT96–1180.
- For more comprehensive reviews of frozen food theory and practice (including a review on nutritional aspects by Bender 1993, see references) see 'Frozen Foods Technology' (1993) edited by Mallett CP and published by Blackie Academic and Professional and 'Quality in Frozen Food' (1997), edited by Erickson MC and Hung Y-C, published by Chapman & Hall.

15.6.2 Trade organisations

Below are listed the trade organisations that are sources of general information on frozen food and the frozen food industry:

- The British Frozen Food Federation at 3rd Floor, Springfield House, Springfield Business Park, Springfield Road, Grantham, Lincolnshire, NG31 7BG. Email on http://www.bfff.co.uk
- The (US based) National Frozen and Refrigerated Foods Association, at 4755 Linglestown Rd., Suite 300, P.O. Box 6069, Harrisburg, PA 17112. Email on http://www.nfraweb.org
- The American Frozen Food Institute at 2000 Corporate Ridge, Suite 1000, McLean, Virginia 22102. Email on http://info@affi.com

15.7 References

BENDER A E (1978), *Food Processing and Nutrition*, Academic Press
BENDER A E (1993), 'Nutritional aspects of frozen foods,' in *Frozen Food Technology*, ed Mallett CP, Blackie Academic and Professional, 123–40
CLYDESDALE F M, HO C T, LEE C Y, MONDY N I and SHEWFELT R L (1991), 'Effects of post-harvest treatment and chemical interaction on the bioavailability of ascorbic acid, thiamine, vitamin A carotenoids and other minerals,' Critical reviews in *Food Science and Nutrition* **30**, 599–638
DULAVIK B, SORENSEN N K, BARSTAD H, HORVLI O and OLSEN R L (1998), 'Oxidative stability of frozen light and dark muscles of saithe (*Pollachius virens*),' *Journal of Food Lipids* **5**, 233–45
ERICKSON M C (1997), 'Lipid oxidation: flavour and nutritional quality deterioration in frozen foods,' in *Quality in Frozen Food*, eds Erickson MC and Hung Y-C. Chapman & Hall, 141–73
FAVELL D J (1998), 'A comparison of the vitamin C content of fresh and frozen vegetables,' *Food Chemistry* **62**, 59–64
GOFF H D (1997), 'Measurement and interpretation of the glass transition in frozen foods,' in *Quality in Frozen Food*, eds Erickson MC and Hung Y-C, Chapman & Hall, 29–50
GRIFFITH M and EWART K V (1995), 'Antifreeze proteins and their potential use in frozen foods,' *Biotechnol. Adv.*, **13**, 375–402
International Institute of Refrigeration (1986), Recommendations for the Processing and Handling of Frozen Foods, Paris.
LEVINE H and SLADE L (1989), 'A food polymer science approach to the practice of cryostabilisation technology: comments,' *Agric. and Food Chemistry*, **1**, 315–96
LILLFORD P J and HOLT C B (1994), 'Antifreeze Proteins, *Journal of Food Engineering*, **22**, 475–82
NYMAN M (1995), 'Effects of processing on dietary fibre in vegetables,' *European Journal of Clinical Nutrition*, **49**, S215–S218
PAYNE S R and WILSON P W (1994), 'Comparison of the freeze/thaw characteristics of Antarctic cod (*Dissostichus mawsoni*) and black cod (*Paranotohenia augustata*),' *J. Muscle Foods*, **5**, 233–44
POLO M V, LAGARDA M J and FARRE R (1992), 'The effect of freezing on mineral element content of vegetables,' *Journal of Food Composition and Analysis*, **5**, 77–83
POLVI S M, ACKMAN R G, LALL S P and SAUNDERS R L (1991), 'Stability of lipids and omega-3 fatty acids during frozen storage of Atlantic salmon,' *Journal of Food Processing and Preservation*, **15**, 167–81

REFSGAARD H H F, BROCKHOFF P B and JENSEN B (1998), 'Sensory and chemical changes in farmed Atlantic salmon (*Salmo salar*) during frozen storage,' *Journal of Agricultural and Food Chemistry*, **46**, 3473–9

ROUGEROU A and PERSON O (1991), 'Influence of preservation method on unsaturated fatty acids of nutritional interest in sardines and mackerels,' *Medicine et Nutrition*, **27**, 353–8

SHEWFELT R L (1990), 'Sources of variation in the nutrient content of agricultural commodities from the farm to the consumer,' *Journal of Food Quality*, **13**, 37–54

XING Y, YOO Y, KELLEHER S D, NAWAR W W and HULTIN H O (1993), 'Lack of changes in fatty acid composition of mackerel and cod during iced and frozen storage,' *Journal of Food Lipids*, **1**, 1–14

16

Modified atmosphere packaging (MAP)

F. Devlieghere, Ghent University; M. I. Gil, CEBAS-CSIC, Spain; and J. Debevere, Ghent University

16.1 Introduction

Modified atmosphere packaging (MAP) may be defined as 'the enclosure of food products in gas-barrier materials, in which the gaseous environment has been changed' (Young et al, 1988). Because of its substantial shelf-life extending effect, MAP has been one of the most significant and innovative growth areas in retail food packaging over the past two decades. The potential advantages and disadvantages of MAP have been presented by both Farber (1991) and Parry (1993), and summarised by Davies (1995) in Table 16.1.

There is considerable information available regarding suitable gas mixtures for different food products. However, there is still a lack of scientific detail regarding many aspects relating to MAP. These include:

- Mechanism of action of carbon dioxide (CO_2) on microorganisms.
- Safety of MAP packaged food products.
- Interactive effects of MAP and other preservation methods.
- The influence of CO_2 on the microbial ecology of a food product.
- The effect of MAP on the nutrional quality of packaged food products.

16.2 Principles of MAP

16.2.1 General principles

Modified atmosphere packaging can be defined as packaging a product in an atmosphere that is different from air. This atmosphere can be altered in four different ways:

Table 16.1 The potential positive and negative effects MAP has on the food industry

		Benefits	Disadvantages
1.	Product packaging	A centralised packaging system incorporating portion control Clear, all-round visibility of the product, improving its presentation characteristics	Increased package volume, adds to the transport costs and affects area required for retail display Benefits are lost when the package leaks or is opened
2.	Product quality	Overall product quality is high Sliced products are much easier to separate Shelf life increases by 50–400%	Product safety has not yet been fully established
3.	Special features	Use of chemical preservatives can be reduced or discontinued	Temperature control is essential Different products require their own specific gas formulation Speciality equipment and associated training is required
4.	Economics	Improved shelf life decreases financial losses Distribution costs are reduced due to fewer deliveries being necessary over long distances	Increased costs

after Davies, 1995.

1. Vacuum packaging.
2. Passive MAP.
3. Introduction of a gas at the moment of packaging.
4. Active packaging. In passive MAP, the modified atmosphere is created by the packaged commodity that continues its respiration after packaging. Active packaging systems alter the atmosphere using packaging materials or inserts absorbing and/or generating gases. Typical examples are oxygen absorbers and CO_2 emitting films or sachets.

The gases that are applied in MAP today are basically O_2, CO_2 and N_2. The last has no specific preservative effect but functions mainly as a filler gas to avoid the collapse that takes place when CO_2 dissolves in the food product. The functions of CO_2 and O_2 will be discussed in more detail.

16.2.2 Carbon dioxide as anti-microbial gas

CO_2, because of its antimicrobial activity, is the most important component in applied gas mixtures. When CO_2 is introduced into the package, it is partly dissolved in the water phase and the fat phase of the food. This results, after equilibrium, in a certain concentration of dissolved CO_2 ($[CO_2]_{diss}$) in the water phase of the product. Devlieghere et al (1998) have demonstrated that the growth inhibition of microorganisms in modified atmospheres is determined by the concentration of dissolved CO_2 in the water phase.

The effect of the gaseous environment on microorganisms in foods is not as well understood by microbiologists and food technologists as are other external factors, such as pH and a_w. Despite numerous reports of the effects of CO_2 on microbial growth and metabolism, the 'mechanism' of CO_2 inhibition still remains unclear (Dixon and Kell, 1989; Day, 2000). The question of whether any specific metabolic pathway or cellular activity is critically sensitive to CO_2 inhibition has been examined by several workers. The different proposed mechanisms of action are:

1. Lowering the pH of the food.
2. Cellular penetration followed by a decrease in the cytoplasmic pH of the cell.
3. Specific actions on cytoplasmic enzymes.
4. Specific actions on biological membranes.

When gaseous CO_2 is applied to a biological tissue, it first dissolves in the liquid phase, where hydration and dissociation lead to a rapid pH decrease in the tissue. This drop in pH, which depends on the buffering capacity of the medium (Dixon and Kell, 1989), is not large in food products. In fact, the pH drop in cooked meat products only amounted to 0.3 pH units when 80% of CO_2 was applied in the gas phase with a gas/product volume ratio of 4:1 (Devlieghere et al, 2000b). Several studies have proved that the observed inhibitory effects of CO_2 could not solely be explained by the acidification of the substrate (Becker, 1933; Coyne, 1933).

Many researchers have documented the rapidity with which CO_2 in solution penetrates into the cell. Krogh (1919) discovered that this rate is 30 times faster than for oxygen (O_2), under most circumstances. Wolfe (1980) suggested the inhibitory effects of CO_2 are the result of internal acidification of the cytoplasm. Eklund (1984) supported this idea by pointing out that the growth inhibition of four bacteria obtained with CO_2 had the same general form as that obtained with weak organic acids (chemical preservatives), such as sorbic and benzoic acid. Tan and Gill (1982) also found that the intracellular pH of *Pseudomonas fluorescens* fell by approximately 0.03 units for each 1 mM rise in extracellular CO_2 concentration.

CO_2 may also exert its influence upon a cell by affecting the rate at which particular enzymatic reactions proceed. One way this may be brought about is to cause an alteration in the production of a specific enzyme, or enzymes, via induction or repression of enzyme synthesis (Dixon, 1988; Dixon and Kell, 1989; Jones, 1989). It was also suggested (Jones and Greenfield, 1982; Dixon and Kell, 1989) that the primary sites where CO_2 exerts its effects are the enzymatic carboxylation and decarboxylation reactions, although inhibition of other enzymes has also been reported (Jones and Greenfield, 1982).

Another possible factor contributing to the growth-inhibitory effect of CO_2 could be an alteration of the membrane properties (Daniels et al, 1985; Dixon and Kell, 1989). It was suggested that CO_2 interacts with lipids in the cell membrane, decreasing the ability of the cell wall to uptake various ions. Moreover, perturbations in membrane fluidity, caused by the disordering of the lipid bilayer, are postulated to alter the function of membrane proteins (Chin et al, 1976; Roth, 1980).

Studies examining the effect of a CO_2 enriched atmosphere on the growth of microorganisms are often difficult to compare because of the lack of information regarding the packaging configurations applied. The gas/product volume ratio and the permeability of the applied film for O_2 and CO_2 will influence the amount of dissolved CO_2 and thus the microbial inhibition of the atmosphere. For this reason, the concentration of dissolved CO_2 in the aqueous phase of the food should always be measured and mentioned in publications concerning MAP (Devlieghere et al, 1998).

Only a few publications deal with the effect of MAP on specific spoilage microorganisms. Gill and Tan (1980) compared the effect of CO_2 on the growth of some fresh meat spoilage bacteria at 30°C. Molin (1983) determined the resistance to CO_2 of several food spoilage bacteria. Boskou and Debevere (1997;1998) investigated the effect of CO_2 on the growth and trimethylamine production of *Shewanella putrifaciens* in marine fish, and Devlieghere and Debevere (2000) compared the sensitivity for dissolved CO_2 of different spoilage bacteria at 7°C. In general, Gram-negative microorganisms such as *Pseudomonas*, *Shewanella* and *Aeromonas* are very sensitive to CO_2. Gram-positive bacteria show less sensitivity and lactic acid bacteria are the most resistant. Most yeasts and moulds are also sensitive to CO_2. The effect of CO_2 on psychrotrophic food pathogens is discussed in section 16.5.

16.3 The use of oxygen in MAP

16.3.1 Colour retention in fresh meat products

The colour of fresh meat is determined by the condition of myoglobin in the meat. When an anaerobic atmosphere is applied, myoglobin (purplish-red) will be transformed to metmyoglobin, producing a brown colour, which is an undesirable trait for European consumers. It is therefore essential that O_2 is included (e.g. 40%) into the applied gas atmosphere when fresh meat, destined for the consumer, is packaged. This will ensure the myoglobin is oxygenated, resulting in an attractive bright red colour. However, by doing this, the microbial shelf life of the packaged meat is decreased compared with meat that is packaged in an O_2 free atmosphere.

16.3.2 Inhibition of the reduction of trimethylamineoxide (TMAO) in marine fish

Marine fish contain TMAO, which is an osmo-regulator. In O_2 poor conditions (e.g. when stored in ice), TMAO is used by spoilage organisms (e.g. *Shewanella putrifaciens*) as a terminal electron-acceptor, and is reduced to trimethylamine

(TMA). TMA is the main active component responsible for the unpleasant 'fishy' odour. However, by introducing high levels of O_2 in the gas atmosphere, the TMAO-reduction can be retarded, and consequently the shelf-life of the fish is increased. This was clearly demonstrated by Boskou and Debevere (1997, 1998). Therefore, packaging atmospheres for lean marine fish should contain oxygen levels of at least 30%.

16.3.3 Avoiding anaerobic respiration of fresh produce

When fresh produce is packaged in a closed packaging system, it continues to respire. It is of great importance to avoid anaerobic conditions in the package of fresh produce because anaerobic respiration of the plant tissue will result in the production of off-odour compounds such as ethanol and acetaldehyde. The techniques applied to maintain an aerobic atmosphere in the packaging of fresh produce are discussed in detail in section 16.4.2.

16.4 Applications of MAP in the food industry

16.4.1 Non-respiring products

Non-respiring food products do not consume any oxygen during further storage. When such food products are packaged in a modified atmosphere, the aim is to retain the introduced atmosphere during the storage period. Therefore, high barrier films are used which are most often composed out of different layers of materials. Typical O_2 and CO_2 barrier materials are PA (polyamide), PVDC (polyvinylidenechloride) and EVOH (ethylenevinyl alcohol). Depending on the intended storage time, the O_2-permeability of the applied films should be <2 ml O_2/m^2.24h.atm determined at 75% relative humidity at 23 °C for products with a long shelf life and <10 ml O_2/m^2.24h.atm determined at the same conditions for products with a limited shelf life (<1 week).

One of the bottlenecks in modified atmosphere packaging lies in defining the optimal gas atmosphere for a food product in a specific packaging design. This optimal atmosphere depends on the intrinsic parameters of the food product (pH, water activity, fat content, type of fat) and the gas/product volume ratio in the chosen package type. The intrinsic parameters determine the sensitivity of the product for specific microbial, chemical and enzymatic degradation reactions. Products that are susceptible to microbial spoilage due to the development of Gram-negative bacteria (e.g. fresh meat and fish) and yeasts (salads) should be packaged in a CO_2 enriched atmosphere because the growth of those microorganisms is significantly retarded by CO_2. In general, oxygen is excluded from the gas mixture. For prolonging the shelf life of products which are spoiled by mould growth (e.g. hard cheeses) or by oxidation, it is essential to package in O_2 free atmospheres. In some cases, O_2 will be included for the reasons previously mentioned in section 16.3.

The use of CO_2 is however limited due to its solubility in water and fat. This

Table 16.2 Recommended gas regimes for MAP of various non-respiring foods

Food type	Gas composition (%)			Purpose
	CO_2	N_2	O_2	
Fresh meat				
retail	15–40	0	60–85	↔ Gram⁻ organisms (CO_2) &
	20	10	70	Colour (O_2)
industrial packages	50–100	0–50	0	↔ Gram⁻ organisms
Poultry	70	20	10	↔ Gram⁻, colour
Fish				
lean, marine	50–60	0–20	30–40	↔ Gram⁻, ↔ TMA production
fatty or fresh water	40–65	35–60	0	↔ Gram⁻, ↔ oxidation
Meat and fish products				
$a_w > 0.94$	50–70	30–50	0	↔ Gram⁺
$a_w < 0.94$	10–20	80–90	0	↔ Yeasts and moulds
Shrimps	35	65		↔ Gram⁻ & Gram⁺
Cheese				
hard	0–70	0–30	0	
	0	100	0	↔ Moulds, ↔ oxidation
soft	0	100	0	
Bakery products	20–70	30–80	0	↔ Yeasts & moulds
Dry products ($a_w < 0.60$)	0	100	0	↔ Oxidation

high solubility can cause collapsing of the package when the concentrations of CO_2 are too high. This will especially be the case for food products containing high amounts of unsaturated fat such as smoked salmon and salads that contain mayonnaise. The influence of pH, temperature, fat content, water activity and gas/product ratio on the CO_2 solubility has been quantified by Devlieghere et al (1998). Moreover, too high CO_2 concentrations in the atmosphere can lead to an increased drip loss during storage. This can be explained by the pH drop induced by CO_2 dissolving in the water phase of the product, causing a decrease in the water binding capacity of the proteins. Table 16.2 gives an overview of the recommended gas regimes for different non-respiring food products and the specific purpose of the gas mixture.

16.4.2 Respiring products (Equilibrium Modified Atmosphere Packaging)

In contrast to other types of food, fruits and vegetables continue to respire actively after harvesting. A packaging technology, used for prolonging the shelf life of respiring products, is Equilibrium Modified Atmosphere Packaging (EMAP). The air around the commodity is replaced by a gas combination of 1–5% O_2 and 3–10% CO_2 with the balance made up of N_2. Inside the package, an equilibrium becomes established, when the O_2 transmission rate (OTR) of the packaging film is matched by the O_2 consumption rate of the packaged commodity. The respiration of the living plant tissue also results in the production of CO_2, which diffuses through the packaging film, depending on the film's CO_2 transmission rate

(CO_2TR). The type of packaging film selected is based on the film OTR and CO_2TR, which is required to obtain a desirable equilibrium modified atmosphere. For packaging fruits, the film also needs to have a certain permeability for ethylene (C_2H_4), which prevents an accumulation of the ripening hormone and prolongs fruit shelf life (Kader et al, 1989).

The modified atmosphere not only reduces the respiration rate and the ripening behaviour of fruit, but it also maintains the general structure and turgidity of the plant tissue for a much longer period, which results in better protection against microbial invasion. This atmosphere is also thought to inhibit the growth of spoilage microorganisms (Farber, 1991), which is mostly due to the low O_2 concentration, because the elevated CO_2 concentration (<10%) inside the package is not sufficiently high enough to act as an antimicrobial (Bennik et al, 1998). The shelf life is also prolonged by the suppression of the enzymatic browning reactions on cut surfaces (Kader et al, 1989, Jacxsens et al, 1999a).

Regarding the relatively short shelf life of fruits, raw vegetables, and fresh-cut vegetables, an active modification of the atmosphere is preferred, compared to a passive modification, which is caused by the produce respiring. Form-Fill-Seal (FFS) machines are used with a flushing system to obtain the optimal modified atmosphere for packaging this type of product.

The attained EMAs are influenced by produce respiration (which in turn is affected by product type, temperature, variety, size, maturity, and processing method), packaging film permeability (OTR, CO_2TR, and C_2H_4TR), package dimensions, and fill weight. Consequently, it is a very complex procedure to establish an optimal EMA for different items of produce. The current knowledge of EMAP of fruits and vegetables is mainly empirical, but a systematic approach for designing optimal EMA packages for minimally processed fruits and vegetables is proposed by a number of different authors (Exama et al, 1993; Peppelenbos, 1996; Jacxsens et al, 1999b; Jacxsens et al, 2000). Several mathematical models have been published that predict the OTR and CO_2TR of the packaging film, which is necessary to obtain the desired equilibrium gas atmosphere (Mannaperuma and Singh, 1994; Solomos, 1994; and Talasila et al, 1995). However, in these models an unrealistic constant storage temperature is assumed. Two important parameters in EMAP of fresh-cut produce, respiration rate and permeability of the packaging film are temperature dependent. The respiration rate is less affected by the temperature change (Q_{10}^R = 2–3) than is the permeability of the packaging film (Q_{10}^P = 1–2) (Exama et al, 1993; Jacxsens et al, 2000), as is illustrated in Fig. 16.1.

When temperature increases, a larger volume of O_2 will be consumed by the fresh-cut produce than is diffused through the packaging film, resulting in a shift of the EMA towards an anaerobic atmosphere (<1% O_2 and >10% CO_2). Anaerobic atmospheres must be avoided in EMAP of respiring products because the shift towards anaerobic respiration will cause the formation of ethanol, acetaldehyde, off-flavours, and off-odours. At lower temperatures, the O_2 level will increase (>5%) in the EMA package and the benefits of EMA are lost. Changing temperatures during the transport, distribution, or storage of EMA packages will

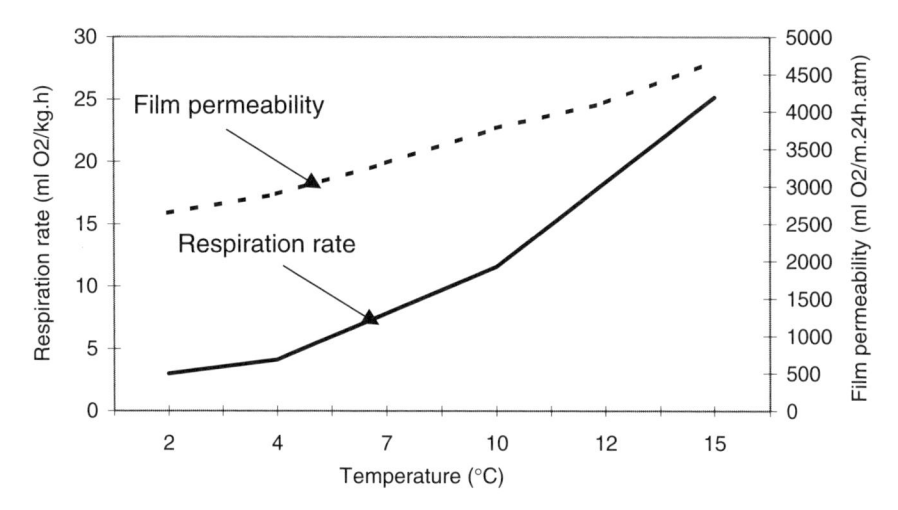

Fig. 16.1 Temperature dependence of the oxygen permeability and the respiration rate of shredded chicory. (Devlieghere et al, 2000c)

result in an equilibrium O_2 level inside the packages that differs from the optimal 3%. A lack of OTR and CO_2TR of commercial films adapted to the needs of middle and high respiring products can result in undesirable anaerobic atmospheres. When both gas fluxes cannot be matched, the O_2 flux should take priority because it is the limiting factor in EMA packaging. A decreased O_2 content is more effective in inhibiting respiration rate and decay than is a decreased CO_2 concentration (Kader et al, 1989; Bennik et al, 1995). New types of packaging films, with an OTR that is adaptable to the needs of fresh cut packaged produce, offer new possibilities in replacing OPP (oriented polypropylene), BOPP (biaxially oriented polypropylene), or LDPE (low density polyethylene) that are currently used in the industry and from which the OTR is not high enough for packaging products with medium or high respiration rates (Exama et al, 1993).

Jacxsens et al (2000) proposed an integrated model in which the design of an optimal EMA package for fresh-cut produce and fruits is possible, taking into consideration the changing temperatures and O_2/CO_2 concentrations inside the package. A prediction of the equilibrium O_2 concentration inside the packages, designed to obtain 3% O_2 at 7°C, could be conducted between a temperature range of 2 to 15°C. These packages (3% O_2 at 7°C) had acceptable O_2 concentrations between 2 and 10°C. However, above 10°C an increase in the growth of spoilage microorganisms and a sharp decrease in sensorial quality were noticed.

The application of high O_2 concentrations (i.e. >70% O_2) could overcome the disadvantages of low O_2 modified atmosphere packaging (EMA) for some ready-to-eat vegetables. High O_2 was found to be particularly effective in inhibiting enzymatic discolouration, preventing anaerobic fermentation reactions and inhibiting microbial growth (Day, 1996; Day, 2000; Day, 2001). Amanatidou et al (1999) screened microorganisms associated with the spoilage and safety of minimally processed vegetables. In general, exposure to high oxygen alone (80 to 90% O_2, balance N_2) did not inhibit microbial growth strongly and was highly variable. A prolongation of the lag phase was more pronounced at higher O_2 concentrations. Amanatidou et al, (1999) as well as Kader and Ben-Yehoshua (2000) suggested that these high O_2-levels could lead to intracellular generation of reactive oxygen species (ROS, O_2^-, H_2O_2, OH*), damaging vital cell components and thereby reducing cell viability when oxidative stresses overwhelm cellular protection systems. Combined with an increased CO_2 concentration (10 to 20%), a more effective inhibitory effect on the growth of all microorganisms was noticed in comparison with the individual gases alone (Gonzalez Roncero and Day, 1998; Amanatidou et al, 1999; Amanatidou et al, 2000). Wszelaki and Mitcham (1999) found that 80–100% O_2 inhibited the *in vivo* growth of *Botrytis cinerea* on strawberries. Based on practical trials (best benefits on sensory quality and antimicrobial effects), the recommended gas levels immediately after packaging are 80–95% O_2 and 5–20% N_2. Carbon dioxide level increases naturally due to product respiration (Day, 2001; Jacxsens et al, 2001a). Exposure to high O_2 levels may stimulate, have no effect on or reduce rates of respiration of produce depending on the commodity, maturity and ripeness stage, concentrations of O_2, CO_2 and C_2H_4 and time and temperature of storage (Kader and Ben-Yehoshua, 2000). Respiration intensity is directly correlated to the shelf life of produce (Kader et al, 1989). Therefore, the quantification of the effect of high O_2 levels on the respiratory activity is necessary (Jacxsens et al, 2001a). To maximise the benefits of a high O_2 atmosphere, it is desirable to maintain levels of >40% O_2 in the headspace and to build up CO_2 levels to 10–25%, depending on the type of packaged produce. These conditions can be obtained by altering packaging parameters such as storage temperature, selected permeability for O_2 and CO_2 of the packaging film and reducing or increasing gas/product ratio (Day, 2001).

High O_2 MAP of vegetables is only commercialised in some specific cases, probably because of the lack of understanding of the basic biological mechanisms involved in inhibiting microbial growth, enzymatic browning and concerns about possible safety implications. Concentrations higher than 25% O_2 are considered to be explosive and special precautions have to be taken on the work floor (BCGA, 1998). In order to keep the high oxygen inside the package, it is advised to apply barrier films or low permeable OPP films (Day, 2001). However, for high respiring products, such as strawberries or raspberries, it is better to combine high O_2 atmospheres with a permeable film for O_2 and CO_2, as applied in EMA packaging, in order to prevent a too high accumulation of CO_2 (Jacxsens et al, 2001b).

16.5 The microbial safety of MAP

Modified atmospheres containing CO_2 are effective in extending the shelf life of many food products. However, one major concern is the inhibition of normal aerobic spoilage bacteria and the possible growth of psychrotrophic food pathogens, which may result in the food becoming unsafe for consumption before it appears to be organoleptically unacceptable. Most of the pathogenic bacteria can be inhibited by low temperatures (<7°C). At these conditions, only psychrotrophic pathogens can proliferate. The effect of CO_2 on the different psychrotrophic foodborne pathogens is described below.

16.5.1 *Clostridium botulinum*

One major concern is the suitability of MAP in the food industry. This is mainly due to the possibility that psychrotrophic, non-proteolytic strains of *C. botulinum* types B, E, and F are able to grow and produce toxins under MAP conditions. Little is known about the effects of modified atmosphere storage conditions on toxin production by *C. botulinum*. The possibility of inhibiting *C. botulinum* by incorporating low levels of O_2 in the package does not appear to be feasible. Miller (1988, cited by Connor et al, 1989) reported that psychrotrophic strains of *C. botulinum* are able to produce toxins in an environment with up to 10% O_2. Toxin production by *C. botulinum* type E, prior to spoilage, has been described in 3 types of fish, at O_2 levels of 2% and 4% (O'Connor-Shaw and Reyes, 2000). Dufresne et al (2000) also proposed that additional barriers, other than headspace O_2 and film, need to be considered to ensure the safety of MAP trout fillets, particularly at moderate temperature abuse conditions.

The probability of one spore of non-proteolytic *C. botulinum* (types B, E, and F) being toxicogenic in rock fish was outlined in a report by Ikawa and Genigeorgis (1987). The results showed that the toxigenicity was significantly affected ($P < 0.005$) by temperature and storage time, but not by the used modified atmosphere (vacuum, 100% CO_2, or 70% CO_2/30% air). In Tilapia fillets, a modified atmosphere (75% CO_2/25% N_2), at 8°C, delayed toxin formation by *C. botulinum* type E, from 17 to 40 days, when compared to vacuum packaged fillets (Reddy et al, 1996). Similar inhibiting effects were recorded for salmon fillets and catfish fillets, at 4°C (Reddy et al, 1997a and 1997b). Toxin production from non-proteolytic *C. botulinum* type B spores was also retarded by a CO_2 enriched atmosphere (30% CO_2/70% N_2) in cooked turkey at 4°C but not at 10°C nor at 15°C (Lawlor et al, 2000). Recent results in a study by Gibson et al (2000) also indicated that 100% CO_2 slows the growth rate of *C. botulinum*, and that this inhibitory effect is further enhanced with appropriate NaCl concentrations and chilled temperatures.

16.5.2 *Listeria monocytogenes*

Listeria monocytogenes is considered a psychrotrophic foodborne pathogen. Growth is possible at 1°C (Varnam and Evans, 1991) and has even been reported at temperatures as low as −1.5°C (Hudson et al, 1994). The growth of *L. monocytogenes* in food products, packaged under modified atmospheres, has been the focus of several, although in some cases contradicting, studies (Garcia de Fernando et al, 1995). In general, *L. monocytogenes* is not greatly inhibited by

CO_2 enriched atmospheres (Zhao et al, 1992) although when combined with other factors such as low temperature, decreased water activity and the addition of Na lactate the inhibiting effect of CO_2 is significant (Devlieghere et al, 2001). *Listeria* growth in anaerobic CO_2 enriched atmospheres has been demonstrated in lamb in an atmosphere of 50:50 CO_2/N_2, at 5 °C (Nychas, 1994); in frankfurter type sausages in atmospheres of distinct proportions of CO_2/N_2, at 4, 7, and 10 °C (Krämer and Baumgart, 1992) and in pork in an atmosphere of 40:60 CO_2/N_2, at 4 °C (Manu-Tawiah et al, 1993). However, other authors have not detected growth in chicken anaerobically packaged in 30:70 CO_2/N_2, at 6 °C (Hart et al, 1991); in 75:25 CO_2/N_2 at 4 °C (Wimpfheimer et al, 1990) and at 4 °C in 100% CO_2 in raw minced meat (Franco-Abuin et al, 1997) or in buffered tryptose broth (Szabo and Cahill, 1998). Several investigations demonstrated possible growth of *L. monocytogenes* on modified atmosphere packaged fresh-cut vegetables, although the results depended very much on the type of vegetables and the storage temperature (Berrang et al, 1989a; Beuchat and Brackett, 1990; Omary et al, 1993; Carlin et al, 1995; Carlin et al, 1996a and 1996b; Zhang and Farber, 1996; Juneja et al, 1998; Bennik et al, 1999; Jacxsens et al, 1999a; Liao and Sapers, 1999; Thomas et al, 1999; Castillejo-Rodriguez et al, 2000).

There is no agreement about the effect of incorporating O_2 in the atmosphere on the antimicrobial activity of CO_2 on *L. monocytogenes* (Garcia de Fernando et al, 1995). However, this effect could be very important in practice, as the existence of residual O_2 levels after packaging, and the diffusion of O_2 through the packaging film, can result in substantial O_2 levels during the storage of industrially 'anaerobically' modified atmosphere packaged food products. Most publications suggest there is a decrease in the inhibitory effect of CO_2 on *L. monocytogenes* when O_2 is incorporated into the atmosphere. Experiments on raw chicken showed *L. monocytogenes* failed to grow at 4, 10, and 27 °C, in an anaerobic atmosphere containing 75% CO_2 and 25% N_2 (Wimpfheimer et al, 1990). However, an aerobic atmosphere containing 72.5% CO_2, 22.5% N_2, and 5% O_2 did not inhibit the growth of *L. monocytogenes*, even at 4 °C. *L. monocytogenes* was also only minimally inhibited on chicken legs, in an atmosphere containing 10% O_2 and 90% CO_2 (Zeitoun and Debevere, 1991). There was no significant difference in the inhibitory effect of CO_2 between the range of 0% and 50%, when 1.5% O_2, or 21% O_2 was present in the atmosphere of gas packaged brain heart infusion agar plates (Bennik et al, 1995). When *L. monocytogenes* was cultured in buffered nutrient broth, at 7.5 °C, in atmospheres containing 30% CO_2, with four different O_2 concentrations (0, 10, 20, and 40%), the results showed that bacterial growth increased with the increasing O_2 concentrations (Hendricks and Hotchkiss, 1997).

16.5.3 *Yersinia enterocolitica*

Yersinia enterocolitica is generally regarded as one of the most psychrotrophic foodborne pathogens. Growth of *Y. enterocolitica* was reported in vacuum packaged lamb at 0 °C (Doherty et al, 1995; Sheridan and Doherty, 1994; Sheridan

Table 16.3 Growth of *Yersina enterocolitica* in different atmospheres

Product type	pH	Temp. (°C)	Storage time (days)	Atmosphere (%O_2/CO_2/N_2)	Increase (log cfu/g)	Reference
Beef	>6.0	−2	126	0/100/0	0	Gill and Reichel (1989)
			63	vacuum	2.4	
		0	98	0/100/0	0	
			49	vacuum	4.1	
		2	42	0/100/0	0	
			35	vacuum	5.1	
		5	35	0/100/0	1.9	
			17	vacuum	5.5	
		10	10	0/100/0	3.4	
			5	vacuum	4.0	
Sliced roast beef	6.1	−1.5	112	0/100/0	0	Hudson et al (1994)
			56	vacuum	4.2	
		3	70	0/100/0	3.8	
			21	vacuum	4.7	
Pork	5.57 (normal)	4	30	0/100/0	0	Bodnaruk and Draughon (1998)
			25	vacuum	1.7	
	6.21 (high)		30	0/100/0	1.7	
			25	vacuum	2.6	
Pork chops	6.0	4	35	0/20/80	4.1	Manu-Tawiah et al (1993)
			35	0/40/60	4.0	
			35	10/40/50	4.0	
			35	vacuum	4.1	
Lamb	5.4–5.8	0	28	80/20/0	1.2	Doherty et al (1995)
			28	0/50/50	3.9	
			28	0/100/0	1.6	
			28	vacuum	5.9	
		5	28	80/20/0	6.8	
			28	0/50/50	8.5	
			28	0/100/0	5.6	
			28	vacuum	8.1	

et al, 1992), beef at −2 °C (Gill and Reichel, 1989), pork at 4 °C (Bodnaruk and Draughon, 1998; Manu-Tawiah et al, 1993), fresh chicken breasts (Özbas et al, 1997) and roast beef at 3 °C but not at −1.5 °C (Hudson et al, 1994).

CO_2 retards the growth of *Y. enterocolitica* at refrigerated temperatures. The effect of CO_2 on the growth of *Y. enterocolitica* has been described by several authors. Some of the results are shown in Table 16.3. Oxygen also seems to play an inhibiting role on the growth of *Y. enterocolitica* (Garcia de Fernando et al, 1995). To ensure total inhibition of *Y. enterocolitica* in O_2 poor atmospheres and at realistic temperatures throughout the cooling chain, high CO_2 concentrations in the headspace are necessary.

16.5.4 Aeromonas spp.

Aeromonas species are able to multiply in food products stored in refrigerated conditions. Growth of A. hydrophila has been detected at low temperatures in a variety of vacuum packaged fresh products, such as chicken breasts at 3 °C (Özbas et al, 1996), lamb at 0 °C under high pH conditions (Doherty et al, 1996), and at −2 °C (Gill and Reichel, 1989), and in sliced roast beef at −1.5 °C (Hudson et al, 1994). Devlieghere et al (2000a) developed a model, predicting the influence of temperature and CO_2 on the growth of A. hydrophila. Proliferation of A. hydrophila is greatly affected by CO_2 enriched atmospheres. Some reports regarding the effect of CO_2 on the growth of A. hydrophila on meat are summarised in Table 16.4.

In a study by Berrang et al (1989b), regarding controlled atmosphere storage of broccoli, cauliflower and asparagus stored at 4 °C and 15 °C, fast proliferation of A. hydrophila was observed at both temperatures, but growth was not significantly affected by gas atmosphere. Garcia-Gimeno et al (1996) published the survival of A. hydrophila on mixed vegetable salads (lettuce, red cabbage and carrots) packaged under MA (initial 10% of O_2–10% CO_2, after 48h 0% O_2–18% CO_2) and stored at 4 °C while at 15 °C a fast growth was noticed (5 log units in 24 h). The combination of high CO_2 concentration and low temperature were revealed as responsible for the inhibition of growth. Bennik et al (1995) concluded from their solid-surface model that at MA-conditions, generally applied for minimally processed vegetables (1–5% O_2 and 5–10% CO_2), growth of A. hydrophila is possible. Growth was virtually the same under 1.5% and 21% O_2. The behaviour of a cocktail of A. caviae (HG4) and A. bestiarum (HG2) in air or in low O_2–low CO_2 atmosphere was investigated in fresh-cut vegetables: no difference between both atmospheres was observed on grated carrots, a decreased growth on shredded Belgian endive and Brussels sprouts in MA but an increased growth on shredded iceberg lettuce in MA storage (Jacxsens et al, 1999a).

16.6 The effect of MAP on the nutritional quality of non-respiring food products

Because by using modified atmosphere packaging, the shelf-life of the packaged products can be extended by 50–200% questions could arise regarding the nutritional consequences of MAP on the packaged food products. This section will discuss the effect of MAP on the nutritional quality of non-respiring food products while the effect of MAP on the nutritional value of respiring products, such as fresh fruits and vegetables, will be discussed in detail in section 16.7.

Very little information is available about the influence of MAP on the nutritional quality of non-respiring food products. In most cases, for packaging non-respiring food products, oxygen is excluded from the atmosphere and therefore one should expect a retardation of oxidative degradation reactions. Moreover, modified atmosphere packaged food products should be stored under refrigera-

Table 16.4 Growth of *Aeromonas hydrophila* in different atmospheres

Product type	pH	Temp (°C)	Storage time (days)	Atmosphere (%O_2/CO_2/N_2)	Increase (log cfu/g)	Reference
Beef	>6.0	−2	126	0/100/0	0	Gill and Reichel (1989)
			63	vacuum	1.0	
		0	98	0/100/0	0	
			49	vacuum	3.1	
		2	42	0/100/0	0	
			35	vacuum	3.0	
		5	35	0/100/0	0	
			17	vacuum	3.0	
		10	10	0/100/0	3.8	
			5	vacuum	5.8	
Sliced roast beef	6.1	−1.5	112	0/100/0	0	Hudson et al (1994)
			56	vacuum	4.3	
		3	70	0/100/0	3.1	
			21	vacuum	4.6	
Lamb	5.4–5.8	0	45	80/20/0	0	Doherty et al (1996)
			45	0/50/50	0	
			45	0/100/0	0	
			45	vacuum	0	
		5	45	80/20/0	0	
			45	0/50/50	0	
			45	0/100/0	0	
			45	vacuum	0	
Lamb	>6.0	0	42	80/20/0	0	Doherty et al (1996)
			42	0/50/50	0	
			42	0/100/0	0	
			42	vacuum	4.1	
		5	42	80/20/0	4.2	
			42	0/50/50	1.7	
			42	0/100/0	0	
			42	vacuum	4.0	

tion to allow CO_2 to dissolve and perform its antimicrobial action. At these chilled conditions, chemical degradation reactions have only a limited importance.

No information is available regarding the nutritional consequences of enriched oxygen concentrations in modified atmospheres which can be applied for packaging fresh meat and marine fish. Some oxidative reactions can occur with nutritionally important compounds such as vitamins and polyunsaturated fatty acids. However, no quantitative information is available about these degradation reactions in products packaged in O_2 enriched atmospheres.

16.7 The effect of MAP on the nutritional quality of fresh fruits and vegetables

During the last few years many studies have demonstrated that fruit and vegetables are rich sources of micronutrients and dietary fibre. They also contain an immense variety of biologically active secondary metabolites that provide the plant with colour, flavour and sometimes antinutritional or toxic properties (Johnson et al, 1994). Among the most important classes of such substances are vitamin C, carotenoids, folates, flavonoids and more complex phenolics, saponins, phytosterols, glycoalkaloids and the glucosinolates.

The nutrient content of fruit and vegetables can be influenced by various factors such as genetic and agronomic factors, maturity and harvesting methods, and postharvest handling procedures. There are some postharvest treatments which undoubtedly improve food quality by inhibiting the action of oxidative enzymes and slowing down deleterious processes. Storage of fresh fruits and vegetables within the optimum range of low O_2 and/or elevated CO_2 atmospheres for each commodity reduces their respiration and C_2H_4 production rates (Kader, 1986; Kader, 1997). Optimum CA retards loss of chlorophyll, biosynthesis of carotenoids and anthocyanins, and biosynthesis and oxidation of phenolic compounds. In general, CA influences flavour quality by reducing loss of acidity, starch to sugar conversion, and biosynthesis of aroma volatiles, especially esters. Retention of ascorbic acid and other vitamins results in better nutritional quality, including antioxidant activity, of fruits and vegetables when kept in their optimum CA (Kader, 2001). However, little information is available on the effectiveness of controlled atmospheres or modified atmosphere packaging (CA/MAP) on the nutrient retention during storage. The influence of CA/MAP on the antioxidant constituents related to nutritional quality of fruits and vegetables, including vitamin C, carotenoids, phenolic compounds, as well as glucosinolates will be reviewed here.

16.7.1 Vitamin C

Vitamin C is one of the most important vitamins in fruits and vegetables for human nutrition. More than 90% of the vitamin C in human diets is supplied by the intake of fresh fruits and vegetables. Vitamin C is required for the prevention of scurvy and maintenance of healthy skin, gums and blood vessels. Vitamin C, as an antioxidant, reduces the risk of arteriosclerosis, cardiovascular diseases and some forms of cancer (Simon, 1992). Ascorbate oxidase has been proposed as the major enzyme responsible for enzymatic degradation of L-ascorbic acid (AA). The oxidation of AA, the active form of vitamin C, to dehydroascorbic acid (DHA) does not result in loss of biological activity since DHA is readily reconverted to L-AA *in vivo*. However, DHA is less stable than AA and may be hydrolysed to 2,3-diketogulonic acid, which does not have physiological activity (Klein, 1987) and it has therefore been suggested that measurements of vitamin C in fruits and vegetables in relation to their nutritional value should include both AA and DHA.

The vulnerability of different fruits and vegetables to oxidative loss of AA varies greatly, as indeed do general quality changes. Low pH fruits (citrus fruits) are relatively stable, whereas soft fruits (strawberries, raspberries) undergo more rapid changes. Leafy vegetables (e.g. spinach) are very vulnerable to spoilage and AA loss, whereas root vegetables (e.g. potatoes) retain quality and AA for many months (Davey et al, 2000). Fruits and vegetables undergo changes from the moment of harvest and since L-AA is one of the more reactive compounds it is particularly vulnerable to treatment and storage conditions. In broad terms, the milder the treatment and the lower the temperature the better the retention of vitamin C, but there are several interacting factors which affect AA retention (Davey et al, 2000). The rate of postharvest oxidation of AA in plant tissues has been reported to depend upon several factors such as temperature, water content, storage atmosphere and storage time (Lee and Kader, 2002).

The effect of controlled atmospheres on the ascorbate content of intact fruit has not been extensively studied. The results vary among fruit species and cultivars, but the tendency is for reduced O_2 and/or elevated CO_2 levels to enhance the retention of ascorbate (Weichmann, 1986; Kader et al, 1989). A reduction in temperature and of O_2 concentration in the storage atmosphere have been described as the two treatments which contribute to preserve vitamin C in fruits and vegetables (Watada, 1987) and so Delaporte (1971) and others observed that loss of AA can be reduced by storing apples in a reduced oxygen atmosphere. However, Haffner et al (1997) have shown than AA levels in various apple cultivars decreased more under ultra low oxygen (ULO) compared to air storage. On the other hand, increasing CO_2 concentration above a certain threshold seems to have an adverse effect on vitamin C content in some fruits and vegetables. It has been reported that the effect of elevated CO_2 on AA content varied among commodities and was dependent on CO_2 level and storage temperature and duration (Weichmann, 1986). Bangerth (1977) observed accelerated AA losses in apples and red currants stored in elevated CO_2 atmospheres. Vitamin C content was reduced by high CO_2 concentrations (10–30% CO_2) in strawberries and blackberries and only a moderate to negligible effect was found for black currants, red currants and raspberries (Agar et al, 1997). Storage of sweet pepper for 6 days at 13 °C in CO_2 enriched atmospheres resulted in a reduction in AA content (Wang, 1977). Wang (1983) noted that 1% O_2 retarded AA degradation in Chinese cabbage stored for 3 months at 0 °C. He observed that treatments with 10 or 20% CO_2 for 5 or 10 days produced no effect, and 30 or 40% CO_2 increased AA decomposition. Veltman et al (1999) have observed a 60% loss in AA content of 'Conference' pears after storage in 2% O_2 + 10% CO_2. There were no data available to show whether a parallel reduction in O_2 concentration alleviates the negative CO_2 effect. Agar et al (1997) proposed that reducing O_2 concentration in the storage atmosphere in the presence of high CO_2 had little effect on the vitamin C preservation. The only beneficial effect of low O_2 alleviating the CO_2 effect could be observed when applying CO_2 concentrations lower than 10%.

In fresh-cut products, high CO_2 concentration in the storage atmosphere has also been described to cause degradation of vitamin C. Thus, concentration of 5,

10, or 20% CO_2 caused degradation of vitamin C in fresh-cut kiwifruit slices (Agar et al, 1999). Enhanced losses of vitamin C in response to CO_2 higher than 10% may be due to the stimulating effects on oxidation of AA and/or inhibition of DHA reduction to AA (Agar et al, 1999). In addition, vitamin C content decreased in MAP-stored Swiss chard (Gil et al, 1998a) as well as in potato strips (Tudela et al, 2002). In contrast, MAP retarded the conversion of AA to DHA that occurred in air-stored jalapeno pepper rings (Howard et al, 1994; Howard et al, 1998). Wright and Kader (1997a) found no significant losses of vitamin C occurred during the post cutting life of fresh-cut strawberries and persimmons for 8 days in CA (2% O_2, air + 12% CO_2, or 2% O_2 + 12% CO_2) at 0°C. In studies of cut broccoli florets and intact heads of broccoli CA/MAP resulted in greater AA retention and shelf-life extension in contrast to air-stored samples (Barth et al, 1993; Paradis et al, 1996). Retention of AA was found in fresh-cut lettuce packaged with nitrogen (Barry-Ryan and O'Beirne, 1999). They suggest that high levels of CO_2 (30–40%) increased AA losses by conversion into DHA due to availability of oxygen in lettuce (Barry-Ryan and O'Beirne, 1999). This fact has also been shown in sweet green peppers (Petersen and Berends, 1993). The reduction of AA and the relative increase in DHA could be an indication that high CO_2 stimulates the oxidation of AA, probably by ascorbate peroxidase as in the case of strawberries (Agar et al, 1997) and of spinach (Gil et al, 1999). Mehlhorn (1990) demonstrated an increase in ascorbate peroxidase activity in response to ethylene. High CO_2 at injurious concentrations for the commodity may reduce AA by increasing ethylene production and therefore the activity of ascorbate peroxidase. Ascorbate oxidase from green zucchini fruit, which catalyses the oxidation of AA to DHA, has been found to be unstable and to lose activity below pH 4 (Maccarrone et al, 1993). This could partially explain the lower DHA content of the strawberries (pH 3.4–3.7) and the higher DHA content of the persimmons (pH 5.4–6.0) (Wright and Kader, 1997a) as well as the tendency of some vegetables at pH near to neutral to lose AA during storage (Gil et al, 1998b).

In conclusion, the loss of vitamin C after harvest can be reduced by storing fruits and vegetables in atmospheres of reduced O_2 and/or up to 10% CO_2 as Lee and Kader (2002) have reported. CA conditions do not have a beneficial effect on vitamin C if high CO_2 concentrations are involved, although the concentrations above which CO_2 affects the loss of AA must be estimated for each commodity (Kader, 2001).

16.7.2 Carotenoids

Carotenoids form one of the most important classes of plant pigments and play a crucial role in defining the quality parameters of fruit and vegetables. Their role in the plant is to act as accessory pigments for light harvesting and in the prevention of photo-oxidative damage, as well as acting as attractants for pollinators. The best documented and established function of some of the carotenoids is their provitamin A activity, especially of β-carotene. α-Carotene and β-crytoxanthin also possess provitamin A activity, but to a lesser extent than does β-carotene. Many yellow, orange or red fruit and root vegetables contain large amounts of carotenoids, which accumulate in the chloroplast during ripening or maturation. In some cases, the carotenoids present are simple, e.g. β-carotene in carrot or lycopene in tomato, but in other cases complex mixtures of unusual structures are found, e.g. in *Capsicum*. Carotenoids are found in membranes, as microcrystals, in association with proteins or in oil droplets. *In vivo*, carotenoids are stabilised by these molecular interactions, that are also important in determining the bioavailability of the carotenoids. Plant materials do not contain vitamin A, but provide carotenoids that are converted to vitamin A after ingestion. Provitamin A carotenoids found in significant quantities in fruits may have a role in cancer prevention by acting as free radical scavengers (Britton and Hornero-Mendez, 1997). Lycopene, although it has no provitamin A activity, has been identified as a particularly effective quencher of singlet oxygen *in vitro* (Di Mascio et al, 1989) and as an anticarcinogenic (Giovannucci, 1999). Carotenoids are unstable when exposed to acidic pH, oxygen or light (Klein, 1987). The effect of controlled and modified atmospheres on the carotenoid content of intact fruits has not been well studied. Modified atmospheres including either reduced O_2 or elevated CO_2 are generally considered to reduce the loss of provitamin A, but also to inhibit the biosynthesis of carotenoids (Kader et al, 1989). Reducing O_2 to lower concentrations enhanced the retention of carotene in carrots (Weichmann, 1986). The carotene content of leeks was found to be higher after storage in 1% O_2 + 10% CO_2 than after storage in air (Weichmann, 1986).

Few studies on the effect of CA storage on the provitamin A carotenoid content of fresh-cut products have been published. Wright and Kader (1997b) found for sliced peaches and persimmons, that the limit of shelf life was reached before major losses of carotenoids occurred. Low changes in carotenoids have been observed in minimally processed pumpkin stored for 25 days at 5°C in MAP (Baskaran et al, 2001). Petrel et al (1998) found no changes on the carotenoid content of ready to eat oranges after 11 days at 4°C in MAP (19% O_2 + 5% CO_2 and 3% O_2 + 25% CO_2). In addition, the content of β-carotene in broccoli florets increased at the end of CA storage (2% O_2 + 6% CO_2) and remained stable after returning the samples to ambient conditions for 24 h (Paradis et al, 1996). Lutein, the major carotenoid in green bean tissue, also showed an accumulation after 13 days of CA storage (1% O_2 + 3% CO_2) and in these conditions retained carotenoids up to 22 days at 8°C (Cano et al, 1998). However, Sozzi et al (1999) have observed that CA of 3% O_2 and 20% CO_2 both alone and together with ethylene prevented total carotenoid and lycopene biosynthesis on tomato. After exposing the fruits to air, total carotenoids and lycopene increased but were in all cases significantly lower than those which were held in air.

16.7.3 Phenolic compounds

There is a considerable evidence for the role of antioxidant constituents of fruits and vegetables in the maintenance of health and disease prevention (Ames et al,

1993). Epidemiological studies show that consumption of fruits and vegetables with high phenolic content correlates with reduced cardio- and cerebrovascular diseases and cancer mortality (Hertog et al, 1997). Recent work is also beginning to highlight the relation of flavonoids and other dietary phenolic constituents to these protective effects. They act as antioxidants by virtue of the free radical scavenging properties of their constituent hydroxyl groups (Kanner et al, 1994; Vinson et al, 1995). The biological properties of phenolic compounds are very variable and include anti-platelet action, antioxidant, antiinflamatory, antitumoral and oestrogenic activities, which might suggest their potential in the prevention of coronary heart diseases and cancer (Hertog et al, 1993; Arai et al, 2000).

In the last few years there has been an increasing interest in determining relevant dietary sources of antioxidant phenolics and red fruits such as strawberries, cherries, grapes and pomegranates have received considerable attention due to their antioxidant activity. However, storage under CA/MAP conditions has been focused on keeping the visual properties and few studies have been made on the effect on the nutritional quality. Generally an increase in phenolics is considered a positive attribute and enhances the nutritional value of plant product. However, many secondary metabolites typical of wild species of fruits or vegetables have toxic effects although they are not considered here. In addition, the organoleptic and nutritional characteristics of fruit and vegetables are strongly modified by the appearance of brown pigments. Oxidative browning is mainly due to the enzyme polyphenol oxidase (PPO) which catalyses the hydroxylation of monophenols to o-diphenols and, in a second step, the oxidation of colourless o-diphenols to highly coloured o-quinones (Vámos-Vigyázó, 1981). The o-quinones non-enzymatically polymerise and give rise to heterogeneous black, brown or red pigments called melanins decreasing the organoleptic and nutritional qualities (Tomás-Barberán et al, 1997; Tomás-Barberán and Espin, 2001).

Controlled atmospheres and modified atmosphere packaging (MAP) can directly influence the phenolic composition as reflected in the changes observed in anthocyanins. Carbon dioxide-enriched atmospheres (>20%) used to reduce decay and extend the postharvest life of strawberries induced a remarkable decrease in anthocyanin content of internal tissues compared with the external ones (Gil et al, 1997). Holcroft and Kader (1999) related the decrease in strawberry colour under CO_2 atmosphere, with a decrease of important enzyme activity involved in the biosynthesis of anthocyanins, phenylalanine ammonialyase (PAL; EC 4.3.1.5) and glucosyltransferase (GT; EC 2.4.1.91). A moderated CO_2 atmosphere (10%) prolongs the storage life and maintains quality and adequate red colour intensity of pomegranate arils (Holcroft et al, 1998). However, the arils of pomegranates stored in air were deeper red than were those of the initial controls and of those stored in a CO_2 enriched atmosphere.

Modified atmospheres can also have a positive effect on phenolic-related quality, as in the case of the prevention of browning of minimally processed lettuce (Saltveit, 1997; Gil et al, 1998b). In addition, modified atmosphere packaging of minimally processed red lettuce (2–3% O_2 + 12–14% CO_2) decreased the content of flavonol and anthocyanins of pigmented lettuce tissues when compared to air storage (Gil et al, 1998b). The increase of soluble phenylpropanoids observed in the midribs of minimally processed red lettuce after storage in air was avoided under MAP. When minimally processed Swiss chard was stored in MAP (7% O_2 + 10% CO_2), no effect was observed on flavonoid content after 8 days cold storage when compared to that stored in air (Gil et al, 1998b). In addition, the total flavonoid content of fresh-cut spinach remained quite constant during storage in both air and MAP atmosphere (Gil et al, 1999).

Abnormal browning frequently occurs when fruits are stored in very low oxygen atmospheres. Extended treatment in pure nitrogen enhances the appearance of brown surfaces in fruits, which then rot rapidly when they are returned to air (Macheix et al, 1990). These observations are probably the result of cell disorganisation under anaerobiosis, but may also be related to variations in phenolic metabolism.

There is a decrease in all phenolic compounds (e.g. anthocyanins, flavonols, and caffeoyl tartaric and *p*-coumaroyl tartaric acids) in both skin and pulp of grape berries rapidly brought under anaerobiosis in CO_2 enriched atmosphere (Macheix et al, 1990). Anaerobiosis generally appears to be harmful for the fruit products formed, with the frequent appearance of unwanted browning or loss of anthocyanins. In contrast, this treatment becomes necessary in the case of removal of astringency from persimmom fruit by means of an atmosphere of CO_2 or N_2. These treatments result in the production of acetaldehyde, and deastringency is due to the insolubilisation of kaki-tannin by reaction with the acetaldehyde (Haslam et al, 1992).

16.7.4 Glucosinolates

Brassica vegetables, such as cabbage, Brussels sprouts, broccoli and cauliflower are an important dietary source for a group of secondary plant metabolites known as glucosinolates. The sulphur-containing glucosinolates are present as glucosides and can be hydrolysed by the endogenous plant enzyme myrosinase (thioglucoside glucohydrolase EC 3.2.3.1). Myrosinase and the glucosinolates are physically separated from each other in the plant cell and therefore hydrolysis can only take place when cells are damaged, e.g. by cutting or chewing (Verkerk et al, 2001). The hydrolysis generally results in further breakdown of glucosinolates into isothiocyanates, nitriles, thiocyanates, indoles and oxazolidinethiones. Glucosinolate degradation products contribute to the characteristic flavour and taste of *Brassica* vegetables. Glucosinolates and their biological effects have been reviewed in detail (Rosa et al, 1997). Indol-3-ylmethylglucosinolates, which occur in appreciable amounts in several *Brassica* vegetables, are of interest for their potential contribution of anticarcinogenic compounds to the diet (Loft et al, 1992) and so broccoli has been associated with a decreased risk of cancer based on several beneficial properties such as the level of vitamin C, fibre and glucosinolates. The glucosinolate content in *Brassica* vegetables can vary depending on the variety, cultivation conditions, harvest time and climate. Storage and processing of the vegetables can also greatly affect the glucosinolate content.

Processes such as chopping, cooking and freezing influence the extent of hydrolysis of glucosinolates and the composition of the final products (Verkerk et al, 2001).

There are a few reports describing the effects of storage on the glucosinolate content; for instance the storage of white and red cabbage for up to five months at 4°C which does not seem to affect the levels of glucosinolates (Berard and Chong, 1985). However, there is still little information about the influence of CA/MAP on total or individual glucosinolate content of *Brassica* vegetables but an increase in total glucosinolate content was reported in broccoli florets when stored in air or CA while the absence of O_2 with a 20% CO_2 resulted in total loss (Hansen et al, 1995).

16.8 References

AGAR I T, STREIF J and BANGERTH F (1997), 'Effect of high CO_2 and controlled atmosphere on the ascorbic and dehydroascorbic acid content of some berry fruits', *Postharvest Biol Technol*, **11**, 47–55

AGAR I T, MASSANTINI R, HESS-PIERCE B and KADER A A (1999), 'Postharvest CO_2 and ethylene production and quality maintenance of fresh-cut kiwifruit slices', *J Food Sci*, **64**, 433–40

AMANATIDOU A, SMID E and GORRIS L (1999), 'Effect of elevated oxygen and carbon dioxide on the surface growth of vegetable-associated micro-organisms', *Journal of Applied Microbiology*, **86**, 429–38

AMANATIDOU A, SLUMP R, GORRIS L and SMID E (2000), 'High oxygen and high carbon dioxide modified atmospheres for shelf life extension of minimally processed carrots', *Journal of Food Science*, **65**, 61–6

AMES B M, SHIGENA M K and HAGEN T M (1993), 'Oxidants, antioxidants and the degenerative diseases of aging', *Proc Natl Acad Sci USA*, **90**, 7915–22

ARAI Y, WATANABE S, KIMIRA M, SHIMOI K, MOCHIZUKI R and KINAE N (2000), 'Dietary intakes of flavonols, flavones and isoflavones by Japanese women and the inverse correlation between quercetin intake and plasma LDL cholesterol', *J Nutr*, **130**, 2378–83

BANGERTH F (1977), 'The effect of different partial pressures of CO_2, C_2H_4, and O_2 in the storage atmosphere on the ascorbic acid content of fruits and vegetables', *Qual Plant*, **27**, 125–33

BARRY-RYAN C and O'BEIRNE D (1999), 'Ascorbic acid retention in shredded iceberg lettuce as affected by minimal processing', *J Food Sci*, **64**, 498–500

BARTH M M, KERBEL E L, PERRY A K and SCHMIDT S J (1993), 'Modified atmosphere packaging affects ascorbic acid, enzyme activity and market quality of broccoli', *J Food Sci*, **57**, 954–7

BASKARAN R H, PRASAD R and SHIVAIAH K M (2001), 'Storage behaviour of minimally processed pumpkin (*Cucurbiat maxima*) under modified atmosphere packaging conditions', *Eur Food Res Technol*, **212**, 165–9

BCGA (1998), *The Safe Application of Oxygen enriched Atmospheres when Packaging Food*, Hampshire, UK, British Compressed Gases Association, 39p

BECKER Z E (1933), 'A comparison between the action of carbonic acid and other acids upon the living cell', *Protoplasma*, **25**, 161–75

BENNIK M, VORSTMAN W, SMID E J and GORRIS L M G (1998), 'The influence of oxygen and carbon dioxide on the growth of prevalent *Enterobacteriaceae* and *Pseudomonas* species isolated from fresh and controlled-atmosphere-stored vegetables', *Food Microbiol*, **15**, 459–69

BENNIK M, VAN OVERBEEK W, SMID E and GORRIS L (1999), 'Biopreservation in modified atmosphere stored mungbean sprouts: the use of vegetable-associated bacteriogenic lactic acid bacteria to control the growth of *Listeria monocytogenes*', *Letters in Applied Microbiology*, **28**, 226–32

BENNIK M H J, SMID E J, ROMBOUTS F M and GORRIS L G M (1995), 'Growth of psychrotrophic foodborne pathogens in a solid surface model system under the influence of carbon dioxide and oxygen', *Food Microbiol*, **12**, 509–19

BERARD L and CHONG C (1985), 'Influences of storage on glucosinolate fluctuations in cabbage', *Acta Hort*, **157**, 29–44

BERRANG M, BRACKETT R and BEUCHAT L (1989a), 'Growth of *Listeria monocytogenes* on fresh vegetables stored under a controlled atmosphere', *J Food Prot*, **52**(10), 702–5

BERRANG M, BRACKETT R and BEUCHAT L (1989b), 'Growth of *Aeromonas hydrophila* on fresh vegetables stored under a controlled atmosphere', *Applied and Environmental Microbiology*, **55**, 2167–71

BEUCHAT L and BRACKETT R (1990), 'Survival and growth of *L. monocytogenes* on lettuce as influenced by shredding, chlorine treatment, modified atmosphere packaging and temperature', *Journal of Food Science*, **55**(3), 755–8, 870

BODNARUK P W and DRAUGHON F A (1998), 'Effect of packaging atmosphere and pH on the virulence and growth of *Yersinia enterocolitica* on pork stored at 4 degrees', *Food Microbiol*, **15**(2), 129–36

BOSKOU G and DEBEVERE J (1997), 'Reduction of trimethylamine oxide by *Shewanella* spp. under modified atmospheres *in vitro*', *Food Microbiol*, **14**, 543–53

BOSKOU G and DEBEVERE, J (1998), '*In vitro* study of TMAO reduction by *Shewanella putrefaciens* isolated from cod fillets packed in modified atmosphere', *Food Additives and Contaminants*, **15**(2), 229–36

BRITTON G and HORNERO-MÉNDEZ D (1997), 'Carotenoids and colour in fruit and vegetables', in *Phytochemistry of Fruit and Vegetables*, FA Tomás-Barberán, RJ Robins (eds), Oxford, Oxford University Press

CANO P, MONREAL M, DE ANCOS B and ALIQUE R (1998), 'Effects of oxygen levels on pigment concentrations in cold-stored green beans (*Phaseolus vulgaris* L. Cv Perona)', *J Agric Food Chem*, **46**, 4164–70

CARLIN F, NGUYEN-THE C and ABREU DA SILVA A (1995), 'Factors affecting the growth of *L. monocytogenes* on minimally processed fresh endive', *Journal of Applied Bacteriology*, **78**, 636–46

CARLIN F, NGUYEN-THE C, ABREU DA SILVA A and COCHET C (1996a), 'Effects of carbon dioxide on the fate of *L. monocytogenes*, of aerobic bacteria and on the development of spoilage in minimally processed fresh endive', *International Journal of Food Microbiology*, **32**, 159–72

CARLIN F, NGUYEN-THE C and MORRIS C (1996b), 'The influence of the background microflora on the fate of *Listeria monocytogenes* on minimally processed fresh broad leaved endive', *Journal of Food Protection*, **59**(7), 698–703

CASTILLEJO-RODRIGUEZ A, BARCO-ALCALA E, GARCIA-GIMENO R and ZURERA-COSANO G (2000), 'Growth modelling of *Listeria monocytogenes* in packaged fresh green asparagus', *Food Microbiology*, **17**, 421–7

CHIN J H, TRUDELL J R and COHEN E N (1976), 'The compression-ordering and solubility-disordering effects of high pressure gases on phospholipid bilayers', *Life Sciences*, **18**, 489–98

CONNOR D E, SCOTT V N and BERNARD D T (1989), 'Potential *Clostridium botulinum* hazards associated with extended shelf life refrigerated foods: a review', *J Food Safety*, **10**, 131–53

COYNE F P (1933), 'The effect of carbon dioxide on bacterial growth with special reference to the preservation of fish. Part II', *J Soc Chem Ind* (London), **52**, 19–24

DANIELS J A, KRISHNAMURTHI R and RIZVI S S H (1985), 'A review of effects of carbon dioxide on microbial growth and food quality', *J Food Prot*, **48**, 532–7

DAVEY, M W, VAN MONTAGU M, INZÉ D, SANMARTIN M, KANELLIS A, SMIRNOFF N, BENZIE I J J, STRAIN J J, FAVELL D and FLETCHER J (2000), 'Plant L-ascorbic acid: chemistry, function, metabolism, bioavailability and effects of processing', *J Sci Food Agri*, **80**, 825–60

DAVIES A R (1995), 'Advances in modified-atmosphere packaging', in *New Methods in Food Preservation*, GW Gould (ed), London, Blackie Academic and Professional, 304–20

DAY B (2001), *Fresh prepared produce: GMP for high oxygen MAP and non-suphite dipping. Guidelines* No. 31, Campden & Chorleywood Food Research Association Group, Chipping Campden, UK, 76p

DAY B P F (1996), 'High oxygen modified atmosphere packaging for fresh prepared produce', *Postharv News Inform*, **7**, 31–4

DAY B P F (2000), 'Chilled storage of foods, principles', in *Encyclopedia of Food Microbiology*, RK Robinson, CA Batt and PD Patel (eds), San Diego, Academic Press, 403–10

DELAPORTE N (1971), 'Effect of oxygen content of atmosphere on ascorbic acid content of apple during controlled atmosphere storage', *Lebens Wiss Technol*, **4**, 106–12

DEVLIEGHERE F and DEBEVERE J (2000), 'Influence of dissolved carbon dioxide on the growth of spoilage bacteria', *Lebens Wiss Technol*, **33**, 531–7

DEVLIEGHERE F, DEBEVERE J and VAN IMPE J (1998), 'Concentration of carbon dioxide in the water-phase as a parameter to model the effect of a modified atmosphere on microorganisms', *Int J Food Microbiol*, **43**, 105–13

DEVLIEGHERE F, VAN BELLE B and DEBEVERE J (1999), 'Shelf life of modified atmosphere packaged cooked meat products: a predictive model', *Int J Food Microbiol*, **46**, 57–70

DEVLIEGHERE F, LEFEVERE I, MAGNIN A and DEBEVERE J (2000a), 'Growth of *Aeromonas hydrophila* on modified atmosphere packaged cooked meat products', *Food Microbiol*, **17**, 185–96

DEVLIEGHERE F, GEERAERD A H, VERSYCK K J, BERNAERT H, VAN IMPE J H and DEBEVERE J (2000b), 'Shelf life of modified atmosphere packaged cooked meat products: addition of Na-lactate as a fourth shelf life determinative factor in a model and product validation', *Int J Food Microbiol*, **58**, 93–106

DEVLIEGHERE F, JACXSENS L and DEVLIEGHERE F (2000c), Modified atmosphere packaging: state-of-the-art. IFIS-webside: http://www.ifis.org/

DEVLIEGHERE F, GEERAERD A H, VERSYCK K J, VANDEWAETERE B, VAN IMPE J and DEBEVERE J (2001), 'Growth of *Listeria monocytogenes* in modified atmosphere packed cooked meat products: a predictive model', *Int J Food Microbiol*, **18**, 53–66

DI MASCIO P, KAISER S and SIES H (1989), 'Lycopene as the most efficient biological carotenoid singlet oxygen quencher', *Arch Biochem Biophys*, **274**, 532–8

DIXON N M (1988), *Effects of CO_2 on Anaerobic Bacterial Growth and Metabolism*, PhD thesis, University College of Wales, Aberystwyth

DIXON N M and KELL D B (1989), 'The inhibition by CO_2 of the growth and metabolism of micro-organisms', *J Appl Bacteriol*, **67**, 109–36

DOHERTY A, SHERIDAN J J, ALLEN P, MC DOWELL D A, BLAIR I S and HARRINGTON D (1995), 'Growth of *Yersinia enterocolitica* O:3 on modified atmosphere packaged lamb', *Food Microbiol*, **12**(3), 251–7

DOHERTY A, SHERIDAN J J, ALLEN P, MC DOWELL D A, BLAIR I S and HARRINGTON D (1996), 'Survival and growth of *Aeromonas hydrophila* in modified atmosphere packaged normal and high pH lamb', *Int J Food Microbiol*, **28**(3), 379–92

DUFRESNE I, SMITH J P, JIUN-NI-LIU and TARTE I (2000), 'Effect of headspace oxygen and films of different oxygen transmission rate on toxin production by *Clostridium botulinum* type E in rainbow trout fillets stored under modified atmospheres', *J Food Safety*, **20**(3), 157–75

EKLUND T (1984), 'The effect of carbon dioxide on bacterial growth and on uptake processes in bacterial membrane vesicles', *Int J Food Microbiol*, **1**, 179–85

EXAMA A, ARUL J, LENCKI R W, LEE L Z and TOUPIN C (1993), 'Suitability of plastic films for modified atmosphere packaging of fruits and vegetables', *J Food Sci*, **58**, 1360–70

FARBER J M (1991), 'Microbiological aspects of modified atmosphere packaging technology – a review', *J Food Prot*, **54**, 58–70

FARBER J M, CAI Y and ROSS W H (1996), 'Predictive modelling of the growth of *Listeria monocytogenes* in CO_2 environments', *Int J Food Microbiol*, **32**, 133–44

FRANCO-ABUIN C M, ROZAS-BARRERO J, ROMERO-RODRIGUEZ M A, CEPEDA-SAEZ A and FENTE-SAMPAYO C (1997), 'Effect of modified atmosphere packaging on the growth and survival of *Listeria* in raw minced beef', *Food Sci and Technol Int*, **3**, 285–90

GARCIA DE FERNANDO G D, NYCHAS G J E, PECK M W and ORDONEZ J A (1995), 'Growth/survival of psychrotrophic pathogens on meat packaged under modified atmospheres', *Int J Food Microbiol*, **28**, 221–31

GARCIA-GIMENO R, SANCHEZ-POZO M, AMARO-LOPEZ M and ZURERA-COSANO G (1996), 'Behaviour of *Aeromonas hydrophila* in vegetables salads stored under modified atmosphere at 4 and 15°C', *Food Microbiol*, **13**, 369–74

GIBSON A M, ELLIS-BROWNLEE R C L, CAHILL M E, SZABO E A, FLETCHER G C and BREMER P J (2000), 'The effect of 100% CO_2 on the growth of non-proteolytic *Clostridium botulinum* at chill temperatures', *Int J Food Microbiol*, **54**, 39–48

GIL M I, HOLCROFT D M and KADER A A (1997), 'Changes in strawberry anthocyanins in response to carbon dioxide treatments', *J Agric Food Chem*, **45**, 1662–7

GIL M I, FERRERES F and TOMÁS-BARBERÁN F A (1998a), 'Effect of modified atmosphere packaging on the flavonoids and vitamin C content of minimally processed Swiss chard (*Beta vulgaris* subsp. cycla)', *J Agric Food Chem*, **46**, 2007–12

GIL M I, CASTAÑER M, FERRERES F, ARTÉS F and TOMÁS-BARBERÁN F A (1998b), 'Modified-atmosphere packaging of minimally processed Lollo Rosso (*Lactuca sativa*)', *Z Lebensm Unters Forsch*, **206**, 350–4

GIL M I, FERRERES F and TOMÁS-BARBERÁN F A (1999), 'Effect of postharvest storage and processing on the antioxidant constituents (flavonoids and vitamin C) of fresh-cut spinach', *J Agric Food Chem*, **47**, 2213–17

GILL C O (1988), 'The solubility of carbon dioxide in meat', *Meat Sci*, **22**, 65–71

GILL C O and TAN K H (1980), 'Effect of carbon dioxide on growth of meat spoilage bacteria', *Appl Environ Microbiol*, **39**, 317–19

GILL C O and REICHEL M P (1989), 'Growth of the cold-tolerant pathogens *Yersinia enterocolitica*, *Aeromonas hydrophila* and *Listeria monocytogenes* on high-pH beef packaged under vacuum or carbon dioxide', *Food Microbiol*, **6**, 223–30

GIOVANNUCCI E (1999), 'Tomatoes, tomato-based products, lycopene and cancer: review of the epidemiologic literature', *J Natl Cancer Inst*, **91**, 317–31

GONZALEZ RONCERO G and DAY B (1998), 'The effects of novel MAP on fresh prepared microbial growth', *Proceedings of the Cost 915 Conference*, Ciudad Universitaria, Madrid, Spain, 15–16 October

HAFFNER K, JEKSRUD W K and TENGESDAL G (1997), 'L-ascorbic acid contents and other quality criteria in apples (*Malus domestica* Borkh.) after storage in cold store and controlled atmosphere', *Postharvest Horticultural Series* No **16**, University of California, EJ Micham (ed)

HANSEN M, MOLLER P, SORENSEN H and CANTWELL M (1995), 'Glucosinolates in broccoli stored under controlled atmosphere', *J Amer Soc Hort Sci*, **120**, 1069–74

HART C D, MEAD G C and NORRIS A P (1991), 'Effects of gaseous environment and temperature on the storage behaviour of *Listeria monocytogenes* on chicken breast meat', *J Appl Bacteriol*, **70**, 40–6

HASLAM E, LILLEY T H, WARMINSKI E, LIAO H, CAI Y, MARTIN R, GAFFNEY S H, GOULDING P N and LUCK G (1992), 'Polyphenol complexation', in *Phenolic Compounds in Food and Their Effects on Health I*, CT Ho, CY Lee, MT Huang (eds), Washington, DC, American Chemical Society

HENDRICKS M T and HOTCHKISS J H (1997), 'Effect of carbon dioxide on the growth of *Pseudomonas fluorescens* and *Listeria monocytogenes* in aerobic atmospheres', *J Food Prot*, **60**, 1548–52

HERTOG M G L, FESKENS E J M, HOLLMAN P C H, KATAN M B and KROMHOUT D (1993), 'Dietary antioxidant flavonoids and risk of coronary heart disease: the Zutphen elderly study', *The Lancet*, **342**, 1007–11

HERTOG M G L, SWEETNAM P M, FEHILY A M, ELWOOD P C and KROMHOUT D (1997), 'Antioxidant flavonols and ischaemic heart disease in a Welsh population of men. The Caerphilly study', *Am J Clin Nutr*, **65**, 1489–94

HOLCROFT D M, GIL M I and KADER A A (1998), 'Effect of carbon dioxide on anthocyanins, phenylalanine ammonia lyase and glucosyltransferase in the arils of stored pomegranates', *J Amer Soc Hort Sci*, **123**, 136–40

HOLCROFT D M and KADER A A (1999), 'Carbon dioxide-induced changes in color and anthocyanin synthesis of stored strawberry fruit', *HortSci*, **34**, 1244–8

HOWARD L R and HERNANDEZ-BRENES C (1998), 'Antioxidant content and market quality of jalapeno pepper rings as affected by minimal processing and modified atmosphere packaging', *J Food Quality*, **21**, 317–27

HOWARD L R, SMITH R T, WAGNER A B, VILLALON B and BURNS E E (1994), 'Provitamin A and ascorbic acid content of fresh pepper cultivars (*Capsicum annuum*) and processed jalapenos', *J Food Sci*, **59**, 362–5

HUDSON J A, MOTT S J and PENNEY N (1994), 'Growth of *Listeria monocytogenes*, *Aeromonas hydrophila* and *Yersinia enterocolitica* on vacuum and saturated carbon dioxide controlled atmosphere packaged sliced roast beef', *J Food Prot*, **57**(3), 204–8

IKAWA J Y and GENIGEORGIS C (1987), 'Probability of growth and toxin production by non-proteolitic *Clostridium botulinum* in rockfish fillets stored under modified atmospheres', *Int J Food Microbiol*, **4**, 167–81

JACXSENS L, DEVLIEGHERE F, FALCATO P and DEBEVERE J (1999a), 'Behaviour of *Listeria monocytogenes* and *Aeromonas* spp. on fresh cut produce packaged under equilibrium modified atmosphere', *J Food Prot*, **62**, 1128–35

JACXSENS L, DEVLIEGHERE F and DEBEVERE J (1999b), 'Validation of a systematic approach to design equilibrium modified atmosphere packages for fresh cut produce', *Food Sci Techn*, **32**, 425–32

JACXSENS L, DEVLIEGHERE F, DE RUDDER T and DEBEVERE J (2000), 'Designing EMAP for fresh-cut vegetables subjected to changes in temperature', *Food Sci Technol*, **33**, 178–87

JACXSENS L, DEVLIEGHERE F, VAN DER STEEN C and DEBEVERE J (2001a), 'Effect of high oxygen modified atmosphere packaging on microbial growth and sensorial qualities of fresh-cut produce', *Int J Food Microbiol*, **71**, 194–210

JACXSENS L, DEVLIEGHERE F, VAN DER STEEN C, SIRO I and DEBEVERE J (2001b), 'Application of ethylene adsorbers in combination with high oxygen atmospheres for the storage of strawberries and raspberries', *Proceedings CA2001, 8th International Conference of Controlled Atmosphere*, 8–13th July 2001, Rotterdam, the Netherlands

JOHNSON I T, WILLIAMSON G M and MUSK S R R (1994), 'Anticarcinogenic factors in plant foods: a new class of nutrients?', *Nutr Res Rev*, **7**, 175–204

JONES M V (1989), 'Modified atmospheres', in *Mechanisms of Action of Food Preservation Procedures*, GW Gould (ed), Elsevier Science, 247–84

JONES R P and GREENFIELD P F (1982), 'Effect of carbon dioxide on yeast growth and fermentation', *Enzyme & Microbial Technol*, **4**, 210–23

JUNEJA V, MARTIN S and SAPERS G (1998), 'Control of *L. monocytogenes* in vacuum-packaged pre-peeled potatoes', *J Food Sci*, **63**, 911–14

KADER A and BEN-YEHOSHUA S (2000), 'Effects of superatmospheric oxygen levels on postharvest physiology and quality of fresh fruits and vegetables', *Postharvest Biology and Technology*, **20**, 1–13

KADER A A (1986), 'Biochemical and physiological basis for effects of controlled and modified atmospheres on fruits and vegetables', *Food Technol*, **40**, 99–100, 102–4

KADER A A (1997), 'Biological bases of O_2 and CO_2 effects on postharvest-life of horticultural perishables', *Postharvest Horticultural Series* No **18**, University of California, ME Saltveit (ed)

KADER A A (2001), 'Physiology of CA treated produce', *8th International Controlled Atmosphere Research Conference*, Rotterdam, Oosterhaven

KADER A A, ZAGORY D and KERBEL E L (1989), 'Modified atmosphere packaging of fruit and vegetables', *Crit Rev Food Sci Nutr*, **28**, 1–30

KANNER J, FRANKEL E, GRANIT R, GERMAN B and KINSELLA J E (1994), 'Natural antioxidants in grapes and wines', *J Agric Food Chem*, **42**, 64–9

KLEIN B P (1987), 'Nutritional consequences of minimal processing fruits and vegetables', *J Food Qual*, **10**, 179–83

KRÄMER K H and BAUMGART J (1992), 'Brühwurstaufschnitt hemmung von *Listeria monocytogenes* durch eine modifizierte atmosphäre', *Fleischwirtschaft*, **72**, 666–8

KROGH A (1919), 'The rate of diffusion of gases through animal tissues with some remarks on the coefficient of invasion', *J Physiol*, **52**, 391–408

LAWLOR K A, PIERSON M D, HACKNEY C R, CLAUS J R and MARCY J E (2000), 'Non-proteolytic *Clostridium botulinum* toxigenesis in cooked turkey stored under modified atmospheres', *J Food Prot*, **63**, 1511–16

LEE S K and KADER A A (2002), 'Preharvest and postharvest factors influencing vitamin C content of horticultural crops', *Postharvest Biol Technol*, **20**, 207–20

LIAO C and SAPERS G (1999), 'Influence of soft rot bacteria on growth of *Listeria monocytogenes* on potato slices', *J Food Prot*, **62**, 343–8

LOFT S, OTTE J, POULSEN H E and SORENSEN H (1992), 'Influence of intact and myrosinase-treated indolyl glucosinolates on the metabolism *in vivo* of metronidazole and antipyrine in rat', *Food Chem Toxicology*, **30**, 927–35

MACCARRONE M, D'ANDREA G, SALUCCI M L, AVIGLIANO L and FINAZZI-AGRO A (1993), 'Temperature, pH, and UV irradation effects on ascorbate oxidase', *Phytochemistry*, **35**, 795–8

MACHEIX J J, FLEURIET A and BILLOT J (1990), *Fruit Phenolics*, Boca Raton, Florida, CRC Press

MANNAPERUMA J D and SINGH R P (1994), 'Modelling of gas exchange in polymeric packages of fresh fruits and vegetables', in *Minimal processing of foods and process optimalisation: an interface*, P Singh, F Oliveira (eds), Boca Raton, Florida, CRC Press, 437–58

MANU-TAWIAH W, MYERS D J, OLSON D G and MOLINS R A (1993), 'Survival and growth of *Listeria monocytogenes* and *Yersinia enterocolitica* in pork chops packaged under modified gas atmospheres', *J Food Sci*, **58**, 475–9

MEHLHORN H (1990), 'Ethylene-promoted ascorbate peroxidase activity protects plants against hydrogen peroxide, ozone and paraquat', *Plant Cell Environ*, **13**, 971–6

MILLER A J, CALL J E and WHITING R C (1993), 'Comparison of organic acid salts for *Clostridium botulinum* control in an uncured turkey product', *J Food Prot*, **56**, 958–62

MOLIN G (1983), 'The resistance to carbon dioxide of some food related bacteria', *European J Appl Microbiol Biotechnol*, **18**, 214–17

NYCHAS G J E (1994), 'Modified atmosphere packaging of meats', in *Minimal Processing of Foods and Process Optimization, an Interface*, RP Singh, FAR Oliveira (eds), London CRC Press, 417–36

O'CONNOR-SHAW R E and REYES V G (2000), 'Use of modified-atmosphere packaging', in

Encyclopedia of Food Microbiology, RK Robinson, CA Batt, PD Patel (eds), San Diego, Academic Press, 410–15

OMARY M, TESTIN R, BAREFOOT S and RUSHING J (1993), 'Packaging effects on growth of *Listeria innocua* in shredded cabbage', *Journal of Food Science*, **58**, 623–6

ÖZBAS Z Y, VURAL H and AYTAC S A (1996), 'Effect of modified atmosphere and vacuum packaging on the growth of spoilage and inoculated pathogenic bacteria on fresh poultry', *Z Lebensm Unters Forsch*, **203**, 326–32

ÖZBAS Z Y, VURAL H and AYTAC S A (1997), 'Effects of modified atmosphere and vacuum packaging on the growth of spoilage and inoculated pathogenic bacteria on fresh poultry', *Fleischwirtschaft*, **77**, 1111–16

PARADIS C, CASTAIGNE F, DESROSIERS T, FORTIN J, RODRIGUE N and WILLEMOT C (1996), 'Sensory, nutrient and chlorophyll changes in broccoli florets during controlled atmosphere storage', *J Food Qual*, **19**, 303–16

PARRY R T (1993), 'Introduction', in *Principles and Applications of Modified Atmosphere Packaging of Food*, RT Parry (ed), Glasgow, Blackie Academic and Professional, 1–18

PEPPELENBOS H W (1996), *The use of Gas Exchange Characteristics to Optimize CA Storage and MA Packaging of Fruits and Vegetables*, PhD thesis, University of Wageningen, the Netherlands, 157p

PETERSEN M A and BERENDS H (1993), 'Ascorbic acid and dehydroascorbic acid content of blanched sweet green pepper during chilled storage in modified atmospheres', *Z Lebens Unters Forsch*, **197**, 546–9

PETREL M T, FERNÁNDEZ P S, ROMOJARO F and MARTÍNEZ A (1998), 'The effect of modified atmosphere packaging on ready-to-eat oranges', *Lebensm Wiss Technol*, **31**, 322–8

REDDY N R, PARADIS A, ROMAN M G, SOLOMON H M and RHODEHAMEL E J (1996), 'Toxin development by *Clostridium botulinum* in modified atmosphere-packaged fresh Tilapia fillets during storage', *J Food Sci*, **61**, 632–5

REDDY N R, ROMAN M G, VILLANUEVA M, SOLOMON H M, KAUTTER D A and RHODEHAMEL E J (1997a), 'Shelf life and *Clostridium botulinum* toxin development during storage of modified atmosphere-packaged fresh catfish fillets', *J Food Sci*, **62**, 878–84

REDDY N R, SOLOMON H M, YEP H, ROMAN M G and RHODEHAMEL E J (1997b), 'Shelf life and toxin development by *Clostridium botulinum* during storage of modified-atmosphere-packaged fresh aquacultured salmon fillets', *J Food Prot*, **60**, 1055–63

ROSA E A S, HEANEY R K, FENWICK G R and PORTAS C A (1997), 'Glucosinolate in crop plants', *Hort Rev*, **19**, 99–215

ROTH S H (1980), 'Membrane and cellular actions for anesthetic agents', *Federation Proceedings*, **39**, 1595–9

SALTVEIT M E (1997), 'Physical and physiological changes in minimally processed fruits and vegetables', in *Phytochemistry of Fruit and Vegetables*, FA Tomás-Barberán, RJ Robins (eds), Oxford, Oxford University Press

SHERIDAN J J and DOHERTY A (1994), 'Growth of *Yersinia enterocolitica* on modified atmosphere packaging lamb', *Proceedings 40th International S.IIa.13. Congress on Meat Science Technology*, The Hague, Holland

SHERIDAN J J, DOHERTY A and ALLEN P (1992), *Improving the Safety and Quality of Meat and Meat Products by Modified Atmosphere and Assessment by Novel Methods*, FLAIR 89055 Interim. 2nd year report, EEC SGXII, Brussels

SIMON J A (1992), 'Vitamin C and cardiovascular disease: a review', *J Am Coll Nutr*, **11**, 107–25

SOLOMOS T (1994), 'Some biological and physical principles underlying modified atmosphere packaging', in *Minimally processed refrigerated fruits and vegetables*, RC Wiley (ed), New York, Chapman & Hall, 183–225

SOZZI G, TRINCHERO G D and FRASCHINA A A (1999), 'Controlled-atmosphere storage of tomato fruit: low oxygen or elevated carbon dioxide levels alter galactosidase activity and inhibit exogenous ethylene action', *J Sci Food Agric*, **79**, 1065–70

SZABO E A and CAHILL M E (1998), 'The combined affects of modified atmosphere, temperature, nisin and ALTA-T-M 2341 on the growth of *Listeria monocytogenes*', *Int J Food Microbiol*, **43**(1/2), 21–31

TALASILA P C, CHAU K V and BRECHT J K (1995), 'Design of rigid modified atmosphere packages for fresh fruits and vegetables', *J Food Sci*, **60**, 758–61

TAN K H and GILL C O (1982), 'Physiological basis of CO_2 inhibition of a meat spoilage bacterium, *Pseudomonas fluorescens*', *Meat Sci*, **7**, 9–17

THOMAS C, PRIOR O and O'BEIRNE D (1999), 'Survival and growth of *Listeria* species in a model ready-to-use vegetable product containing raw and cooked ingredients as affected by storage temperature and acidification', *International Journal of Food Science and Technology*, **34**, 317–24

TOMÁS-BARBERÁN F A and ESPÍN J C (2001), 'Phenolic compounds and related enzymes as determinants of quality in fruit and vegetables', *J Sci Food Agric*, **81**, 853–76

TOMÁS-BARBERÁN F A, GIL M I, CASTAÑER M, ARTÁS F and SALTVEIT M E (1997), 'Effect of selected browning inhibitors on harvested lettuce stem phenolic metabolism', *J Agric Food Chem*, **45**, 583–9

TUDELA J A, ESPÍN J C and GIL M I (2002), 'Vitamin C retention in fresh-cut potatoes', *Postharvest Biol Technol*, in press

VÁMOS-VIGYÁZÓ L (1981), 'Polyphenol oxidase and peroxidase in fruits and vegetables', *CRC Crit Rev Food Sci Nutr*, **15**, 49–127

VARNAM A H and EVANS M G (1991), *Foodborne pathogens: an Illustrated Text*, London, Wolfe Publishing

VELTMAN R H, SANDERS M G, PERSIJN S T, PEPPELENBOS H W and OOSTERHAVEN J (1999), 'Decreased ascorbic acid levels and brown core development in pears (*Pyrus communis* L. cv. Conference)', *Physiol Plant*, **107**, 39–45

VERKERK R, DEKKER M and JONGEN W M F (2001), 'Postharvest increase of indolyl glucosinolates in response to chopping and storage of *Brassica* vegetables', *J Sci Food Agric*, **81**, 953–8

VINSON J A and HONTZ B A (1995), 'Phenol antioxidant index: comparative antioxidant effectiveness of red and white wines', *J Agric Food Chem*, **43**, 401–3

WANG C Y (1977), 'Effects of CO_2 treatment on storage and shelf life of sweet pepper', *J Amer Soc Hortc Sci*, **102**, 808–12

WANG C Y (1983), 'Postharvest responses of Chinese cabbage to high CO_2 treatment or low O_2 storage', *J Amer Soc Hortc Sci*, **108**, 125–9

WATADA A E (1987), *Vitamins*, New York, Marcel Dekker

WEICHMANN J (1986), 'The effect of controlled-atmosphere storage on the sensory and nutritional quality of fruits and vegetables', *Hort Rev*, **8**, 101–27

WIMPFHEIMER L, ALTMAN N S and HOTCHKISS J H (1990), 'Growth of *Listeria monocytogenes* Scott A, serotype 4 and competitive spoilage organisms in raw chicken packaged under modified atmospheres and in air', *Int J Food Microbiol*, **11**, 205–14

WOLFE S K (1980), 'Use of CO and CO_2 enriched atmospheres for meats, fish and produce', *Food Technol*, **34**, 55–8

WRIGHT K P and KADER A A (1997a), 'Effect of slicing and controlled-atmosphere storage on the ascorbate content and quality of strawberries and persimmons', *Postharvest Biol Technol*, **10**, 39–48

WRIGHT K P and KADER A A (1997b), 'Effect of controlled-atmosphere storage on the quality and carotenoid content of sliced persimmons and peaches', *Postharvest Biol Technol*, **10**, 89–97

WSZELAKI A and MITCHAM E (1999), 'Elevated oxygen atmospheres as a decay control alternative on strawberry', *Hort Science*, **34**, 514–15

YOUNG L L, REVERIE R D and COLE A B (1988), 'Fresh red meats: a place to apply modified atmospheres', *Food Technol*, **42**(9), 64–6, 68–9

ZEITOUN A A M and DEBEVERE J M (1991), 'Inhibition, survival and growth of *Listeria monocytogenes* on poultry as influenced by buffered lactic acid treatment and modified atmosphere packaging', *Int J Food Microbiol*, **14**, 161–70

ZHANG S and FARBER J (1996), 'The effects of various disinfectants against *L. monocytogenes* on fresh-cut vegetables', *Food Microbiol*, **13**, 311–21

ZHAO Y, WELLS J H and MARSHALL D L (1992), 'Description of log phase growth for selected microorganisms during modified atmosphere storage', *J Food Proc Engin*, **15**, 299–317

17

Irradiation

D. A. E. Ehlermann, Federal Research Centre for Nutrition, Germany

17.1 Introduction

'Genetically modified food' has become the object of a heated debate by consumer activists and replaced irradiation's leading role as a target. In this debate the term *irradiation* is frequently confused with *radioactive contamination*, especially after the Chernobyl accident. The allegation is made that the nuclear industry needs food irradiation badly in order to find some use for the waste from nuclear power stations. In addition, the historical involvement of the US Army in research on food irradiation is used as proof of its link to nuclear weapons and military purposes.

However, this chapter on the radiation processing of food by ionising energy, i.e. on food irradiation, highlights the history of the subject which extends over a hundred years. It elaborates the peaceful background, emphasises that radiation processing is a non-nuclear technology and elucidates the physical principles of the interaction between ionising radiation and matter. This basic information is then used to elaborate the beneficial effects of ionising radiation by describing its chemical, biological and microbiological action in the food environment.

These two sections will lead to the radiological and toxicological safety of food processed by ionising radiation. The aim of the *Nutrition Handbook for Food Processors* is covered in a section on nutritional adequacy and is followed by a section summarising the evaluation of overall safety by national and international expert groups.

Radiation processing has already found its area of commercial application, governments have approved the process, the food industry is using it and where the irradiated product is available on the market consumers respond favourably. Under the WTO-agreement with the associated Codex Alimentarius standards

(1984) and recommended by the WHO*, it is a tool that helps resolve several recent problems of food production, manufacturing and marketing. It can greatly support food safety and environment conservation and therefore serve the consumer. In conclusion, there is a list of sources of further information; for detailed literature the reader is referred to the monographs referenced.

Several concerns have been voiced, for instance about nutritional quality, radiolytic products, toxicology, microbiology, occupational safety, environmental side-effects, deception of consumers, consumer acceptance, substitution for good manufacturing practice, negligent hygienic practice, misuse and increased prices. These are the main arguments of certain consumer organisations against the legal clearance of this technology. They still influence the officials and politicians who are responsible for the regulation of food technologies. However, with the information available in this chapter readers should be able to make their own informed decisions. References given are restricted to textbooks, monographs and survey or review articles only, but interested readers will use them to lead to more detailed information.

17.2 The history of food irradiation

As early as in 1885 and 1886 ionising radiation was discovered and in subsequent years its bactericidal effects were described. The purpose of the first patent on food irradiation (Appleby and Banks, 1905) was to bring about an improvement in food and its general keeping quality. It was followed by an invention of an 'Apparatus for preserving organic materials by the use of X-rays' (Gillett, 1918). However, radiation sources strong enough for industrial exploitation were not available before the 1950s. The following five decades were devoted to the development of this technology to a state where it could be applied both commercially and industrially as well as to an investigation into the health aspects of food treated by ionising radiation.

This was done in a world-wide, concerted effort; the US Army and the US Atomic Energy Commission were involved and stimulated by Eisenhower's initiative 'Atoms for Peace'. The academia were led by the Massachusetts Institute of Technology and followed by university and government research establishments in many countries. Details are given by Diehl (1995). Radiation sources, such as radioactive isotopes and machines, became available and were strong enough for treating food at commercial throughput. A radiation processing industry developed so that everyday goods could be produced by using ionising radiation. Floor-heating pipes, automobile tyres, car parts, electrical wires and cables, shrinkable food packaging, medical disposables (syringes, implants, compresses, bandaging material, blood transfusion equipment) – all are manufactured using ionising radiation. Even astronauts prefer irradiated food in their diets.

---

* The WHO Golden Rules for Safe Food Preparation list under 'Rule 1 "Chose foods processed for safety": . . . if you have the choice, select fresh or frozen poulty treated with ionizing radiation . . .

The world-wide first food irradiation facility became operational in Germany in 1957 for spices, but had to be dismantled in 1959 when Germany banned food irradiation. In 1974 in Japan the Shapiro Potato Irradiator was commissioned and is the oldest food irradiation facility still in operation today. When in 1980 the JECFI made a landmark decision and declared irradiated foods as safe and wholesome for human consumption, it led many governments to permit the radiation processing of food. This did not result in commercial application of the process in all countries. Nevertheless, the total amount of food treated by ionising radiation is increasing, about 200 000 tonne per annum at the time of writing, but is still a very small volume compared to the total amount consumed. However, food irradiation is a niche application, supplementing traditional methods of food processing and serving specific purposes.

Two important classes of application, sanitary and phytosanitary, are increasingly recognised.

As recently as 1993, children died tragically after eating undercooked ('rare') hamburgers. This was caused by *Escherichia coli* type O157:H7 (EHEC), an emerging pathogen microorganism which is now considered to be ubiquitous. There is always the threat of such emerging hazards in modern, industrial food production. Such risks can only be fought by further improvement of good manufacturing practices and the application of 'Hazard Analysis and Critical Control Point (HACCP)'. Adherence to such procedures and improvement of hygienic concepts can only reduce or limit the hazard but never eliminate it. For this reason, supplementary methods, in addition to good practices, help suppress such residual risks to a tolerable, acceptable level. Ionising radiation is such a tool, now legal in the USA and helping to make hamburgers, fresh or deep-frozen, far safer for the consumer. Many other pathogen microorganisms are a threat to society, causing death and illness, damages and economic losses. Other examples are *Campylobacter* and *Salmonella* in poultry, *Salmonella* in eggs, *Listeria* in cheese and sprouts. Governments increasingly recognise the value of radiation processing of food in fighting such threats to health and hygiene.

The threat to plant production (i.e. phytosanitary aspects) is less widely feared but many areas that are very productive in fruit and vegetables have suppressed several of the original pests. Such areas have strict quarantine controls on imports that might carry insects or pests capable of proliferation. The USA is the leading country in exploitation of ionising radiation for insect elimination: an X-ray facility for treating fruit on Hawaii is now operational and allows for the direct transport of fruit to mainland areas such as California. Also, other countries have strict quarantine regulations; they include Australia, Japan and South Africa where ionising radiation can play a valuable role. Certification systems presently under development will help facilitate international trade.

17.3 The principles of irradiation

Processing by ionising radiation is a particular kind of energy transfer: the portion of energy transferred per transaction is high enough to cause ionisation. This kind

Table 17.1 Types of particle

Particle	Description
electron	An elementary corpuscle carrying one unit of positive or negative electrical charge. The positively charged electron is called a positron.
alpha	A charged particle, identical to the nucleus of a helium atom, composed of two neutrons and two protons. It carries two positive elementary units of charge.
beta	A charged particle, identical to an electron or a positron but emitted from a radioactive nucleus.
gamma	A particle or photon emitted from a radioactive nucleus.
X	Fast-moving charged particles in an electric or magnetic field, usually generated by high-energy electrons impinging on a high-atomic-number absorber (e.g. tungsten); also called Röntgen-rays. They are generated by braking radiation (bremsstrahlung).

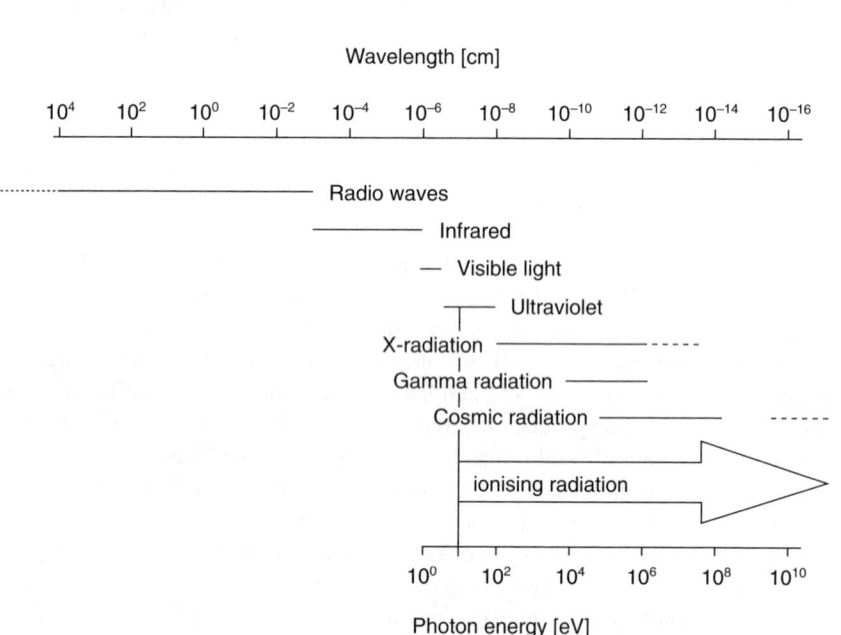

Fig. 17.1 Range of energies (electromagnetic spectrum): ionising radiation is characterised by the ability to split molecular bonds and to transfer electrons; this energy limit is indicated by the vertical, dashed line beginning in the range of ultraviolet light.

of radiation was discovered because the emitting radioactive material caused ionisation in the surrounding air. From the multitude of atomic particles known, only gamma rays from nuclear disintegration and accelerated electrons are useful for food processing (Table 17.1). Electrons may be converted into X-rays by stopping them in a converter or target (Fig. 17.1). Other particles such as neutrons

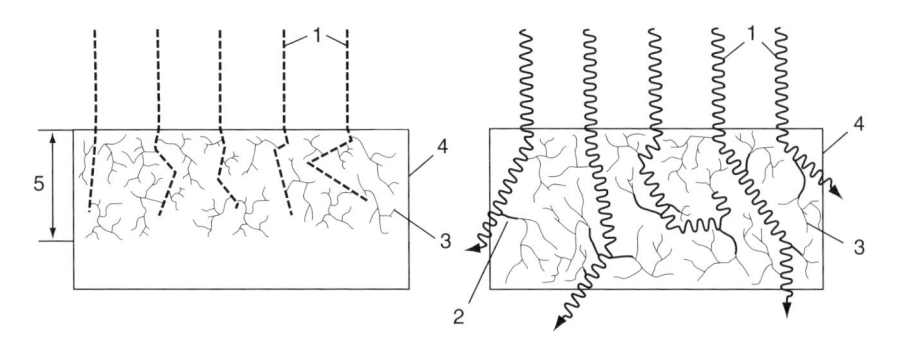

Fig. 17.2 Interaction with matter (photon versus electron): 1) primary incident radiation, 2) Compton electrons caused by photon interaction, 3) secondary electrons and final energy transfer, 4) irradiated medium, 5) finite depth of penetration for electrons.

are unsuitable because induced radioactivity is produced. The same may occur at elevated energy levels with electrons and X-rays; for this reason the electron energy is limited to a maximum of 10 MeV and the nominal energy of X-rays is limited to 5 MeV. Gamma rays of cobalt-60 have photon energies of 1.17 MeV and 1.33 MeV and cannot induce radioactivity; caesium-137 is not available in commercial quantities but gamma rays of 0.66 MeV are emitted from it. This means that gamma rays from available isotope sources are incapable of inducing radioactivity.

Whether in the form of particles or as electromagnetic waves, the primary high energy is broken into smaller portions and converted into a 'shower' of secondary electrons (Fig. 17.2). These electrons finally interact with other atoms and molecules knocking out electrons from their orbits or transferring them to other positions (Fig. 17.3). This means that an elementary negative charge is removed and a positively charged atom or molecule, i.e. an ion, is left behind. If an electron has been transferred then orbital electrons are no longer paired and free radicals are created. Both ions and free radicals are very reactive, in particular in an aqueous medium such as in food, leading finally to chemical reaction products that are stable. The effects caused by corpuscular or electromagnetic radiation are essentially equal; the difference is in the dose distribution along the penetration line into matter. Corpuscles have a definite physical range in matter, they are slowed down by several processes of collision and finally stopped. They have no energy beyond their range. Electromagnetic waves are attenuated exponentially and do not have a defined physical range.

A schematic diagramme of irradiation facilities (Fig. 17.4) helps to understand the simplicity of the irradiation process: the goods are brought by a transport system into the irradiation cell which essentially is a concrete bunker shielding

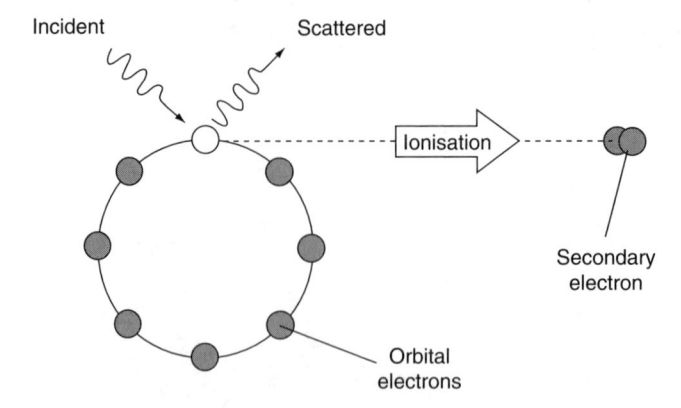

Fig. 17.3 Principal diagram of 'ionisation': whether photon or electron, the incident particles interact with the orbital electrons and are scattered, an orbital electron is removed gaining kinetic energy as a secondary electron; in this way an ionised atom/molecule is left behind and a cascade of secondary electrons causes further ionisation or formation of free radicals.

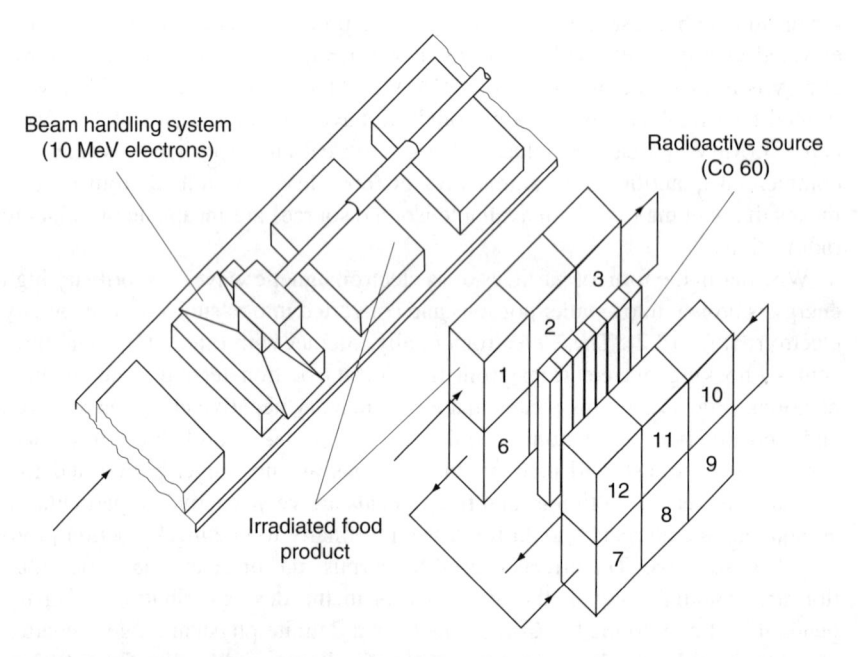

Fig. 17.4 Schematic diagram of irradiation facilities: the product to be irradiated has to pass through the irradiation zone; the design details largely depend on the physical properties of the type of radiation used and may be adapted to the packaging and handling requirements of the goods.

the environment and the workers from the radiation. A tunnel system allows free access for the goods but prevents radiation leakage; fences and detectors prevent unintentional access of anything or anyone when the radiation is 'on'. Machine sources (accelerators) emit the radiation uni-directionally, gamma sources (radioactive isotopes) emit it in all directions. This means that for electron and X-ray processing the goods pass just before the beam exit window and for gamma processing the goods are piled and moved around the source to absorb as much as possible of the emitted energy. When it is not needed a machine source is simply switched off; for radioactive isotopes the frame with the source must be moved to a safe position which is usually a deep water pool. The design of irradiation facilities is widely standardised; the safety-features are offically approved and authoritative control is well established.

17.4 The effects of irradiation on food

There is a vast literature on the effects of ionising radiation on food and food components; for the nutritional aspects of the subject a very few references are sufficient (Diehl, 1995; Molins, 2001). Early textbooks even today are still relevant (Elias and Cohen, 1977, Josephson and Peterson, 1983) and in later years there has been an updating of details (WHO, 1994).

The interaction of ionising radiation with matter takes place by means of a cascade of secondary electrons carrying enough kinetic energy to cause ionisation of atoms and molecules and the formation of free radicals. Besides these direct effects and primary chemical reactions chain reactions of secondary and indirect transitions take place. In systems as complex as food and for biological systems usually high in water content most primary reactive species are formed by the radiolysis of water and the pathways of further reactions largely depend on composition, temperature, dose rate and relative reactivities. Only for a few very simple single-component models have the full pathways of reactions been identified; for highly complex systems a complete picture has not yet been achieved. Nevertheless, some aspects of the picture are beginning to emerge, especially with regard to the main components, i.e. carbohydrates, lipids and proteins. The effects of radiation on micronutrients, in particular on vitamins, are complex and are also dependent on overall composition; some macronutrients may protect micronutrients from radiolysis. Minerals and trace elements are not studied because they cannot be affected by radiation processing of food. However, the toxicological and nutritional consequences are discussed in further sections of this chapter.

Biological effects include the beneficial use of irradiation for sprout inhibition, ripening delay and insect disinfestation. Microbiological effects include the use of irradiation for the suppression of pathogen microorganisms and the reduction of other, spoilage-causing microorganisms. For both procedures, the principal reaction is irreversible radiation damage to the DNA disabling essential functions of the cell. Such DNA changes are irrelevant with regard to food and nutrition. There was previous concern as to whether irradiation and recycling these irradiated microorganisms could cause mutations that were capable of survival and were more toxic or vigorous as their precursors. It has been shown that this is not the case and that 'no special microbiological problems' are introduced (World Health Organization, 1981). The storage of irradiated food is important in order to avoid growth of microorganisms or recontamination.

17.5 The safety of irradiated food

Irradiated food does not become radioactive and this is now accepted even by opponents of the procedure. The limitation of allowable isotope sources to cobalt-60 and caesium-137 and the limitation of the maximum energy of electrons to 10 MeV and of the maximum nominal energy for X-rays (bremsstrahlung or braking radiation) to 5 MeV provides adequate safeguards. Even if the nominal energy for X-rays is increased to 10 MeV the theoretically induced radioactivity would be much less than the natural activity there already is in food due mainly to the presence of potassium-40. Furthermore, it would be very difficult to measure such sparse induced activity in the presence of the natural radioactivity. It can be generally stated that the safety record of the radiation processing industry is slightly higher than that of other branches. There have been only a few accidents related to radiation exposure or radioactive contamination and the reason for all of them was a conscious violation of safety rules or non-adherence to prescribed procedures that included bridging safety circuits.

From the beginning of systematic studies in the late 1940s it was recognised that irradiated food needed careful toxicological study before the technology could be applied to food manufacturing and processing. It is useless to question why the word 'radiation' carries such a negative image and causes considerable suspicion, not only among lay persons, but also among many scientists. In such a situation, governments and food control authorities were well advised to restrict the application of the new technology. However, further results have become available and the final judgement has been stated by the World Health Organization (1981) as: 'Irradiation of any commodity . . . presents no toxicological hazard'. This means that governments and authorities are responsible for the consequences and recognise the radiation processing of food as safe and as simply one among several other technologies. There have been thorough chemical studies, leading to the principle of 'chemiclearance' and classes of food that are chemically similar have been compared. It was also standard procedure to feed the food under consideration to animals and to look for possible effects on factors such as longevity, reproductive capacity, tumour formation, growth, unusual behaviour, haematological and biochemical indices, chromosomal abnormalities and genetic defects. These studies are very numerous and difficult for the non-specialist to follow; expert reviews are available elsewhere (Diehl, 1995). There have been also several publications reporting negative effects; however, a thorough follow-up always revealed deficiencies in the experimental organisation or in the final evaluation and validation of the results. This is not the place to discuss such findings as increased polyploidy in malnourished children and the reasons why those experiments have been dismissed by expert bodies; full details and arguments can be found elsewhere (Diehl, 1995). It is sufficient to state that the validation of competent expert bodies (World Health Organization, 1981, 1994) always resulted in the 'green light' for food irradiation, and finally for any food at any dose (World Health Organization, 1999).

17.6 The nutritional adequacy of irradiated food

Most food preservation and decontamination procedures, including irradiation, cause some loss in the nutritional value of foods. Further losses generally occur during storage and during preparation for consumption (e.g. in cooking). The specific chemical changes brought about in foods by irradiation include some that alter the nutritional value, but the magnitudes of the changes are small when compared with those that result from other procedures currently in use. This has led most expert groups to conclude that reduction in the nutritional quality of foods resulting from the widespread use of irradiation is an insignificant part of the total diet as a whole (Elias and Cohln 1977; Advisory Committee on Irradiated and Novel Foods, 1986). One expert group concluded that 'irradiation of food... introduces no special nutritional problems' (World Health Organization, 1981). This conclusion emphasises the word 'special', recognising that there might be particular problems with some individual food products. Most expert groups also recommend that the nutrient content of irradiated foods should continue to be monitored while such foods are being introduced.

A problem with many of the literature reports on the effects of irradiation on food constituents is that the studies have used laboratory 'model' experiments, often with pure or relatively pure target substances and irradiated in such media as water or buffers. Whilst these studies are ideal for investigating the chemistry of the radiation-induced changes, it is very difficult to extrapolate from them to the situation in real foods. In real foods, many of the other components present, usually in large quantities, interact, quench and otherwise interfere with the reactions of the radiolysis-derived products. Consequently, the magnitude of the changes that occur in specific components in a food matrix is generally much lower than the magnitude of those observed in simpler laboratory studies (Josephson et al, 1979).

In general, the nutritional values of the macronutrients in foods (e.g. the carbohydrate, lipid and protein components) are very little affected by ionising radiation. Some of the micronutrients, including some vitamins and polyunsaturated fatty acids, are more sensitive but their sensitivity is very dependent on the nature of the food. At the 1 kGy dose level, which is in excess of insect disinfestants applications, virtually no nutrient depletion is usually measurable although there have been reports of rise and fall in ascorbic acid (vitamin C) levels made in conflicting publications. At the 10 kGy level, the vitamins ascorbic acid, thiamine (vitamin B_1) and pyridoxine (vitamin B_6) are generally the most sensitive to change but the extent varies considerably and depends on the specific food.

Certain minerals and trace elements are essential for health but their irradiation at the energies employed in food processing does not result in any change (Harris and von Loeseke, 1969).

17.7 Vitamins

Some vitamins are well known for their sensitivity to the effects of ionising radiation. Their inactivation (i.e. loss of biological activity) results predominantly from reactions with free radicals and other reactive species generated by the radiolysis of water in foods. Since these reactive molecules interact with a wide variety of food components, the exact effect of irradiation on a particular vitamin depends not only on the chemical nature of the particular vitamin, but also varies greatly with the nature of the food itself. *In vitro* studies, in which dilute solutions of vitamins have been irradiated, may indicate sensitivities that are never seen in foods, where substantial 'quenching' by competitor molecules usually occurs (Goldblith, 1955).

Reactivity of individual vitamins varies according to their chemical nature (World Health Organization, 1994). The most important with respect to food irradiation, include the water soluble vitamins: ascorbic acid (vitamin C); thiamine (vitamin B_1); riboflavin (vitamin B_2); niacin (vitamin B_5); biotin (vitamin B_{10}); folic acid (pteroylglutamic acid); pyridoxine (vitamin B_6); pantothenic acid; cyanocobalamin (vitamin B_{12}); and the fat soluble vitamins: retinol and some of its derivatives (vitamin A); calciferol and some of its derivatives (vitamin D); tocopherols (vitamin E); naphthaquinone derivatives (vitamin K).

Among the fat-soluble vitamins the ranking by decreasing sensitivity to radiation is:

$$E \gg A \gg D \gg K$$

Carotenoids have a similar sensitivity to vitamin A. However, this is no strict order as sensitivity is largely affected by the protective properties of the other main components of a particular food. For this reason, conflicting findings from the published literature are easily explained by the experimental conditions, sometimes using low concentrations of a single vitamin in a solvent which does not resemble a real food. Such findings always need expert interpretation. Among the water-soluble vitamins B_1 (thiamine) is the most sensitive. However, it is notable that radiation-sterilised pork and beef still retains more thiamine than a heat-sterilised equivalent. The most contradictory results have been obtained with vitamin C. One main explanation is whether only ascorbic acid or ascorbic and dehydroascorbic acid was determined, or whether the results are reported as 'total vitamin C'. Vitamin C is also very sensitive to storage conditions and natural variability might even mask irradiation effects. The following sections discuss particular vitamins.

17.7.1 Vitamin A (retinol)

Dry retinol and dietary precursors, such as β-carotene, are relatively radiation-tolerant, with little inactivation brought about by doses up to about 20 kGy (Lukton and MacKinney, 1956). Even doses as high as 200 kGy only reduced β-carotene levels in tomatoes by about 10 to 20% (Lukton and MacKinney, 1956), depending on whether or not oxygen was present. Irradiation of carrot purée at 20 kGy caused no more than a 5% loss. Changes in vitamin A activity in fruits given low doses for disinfestation or to delay ripening were well below this level of loss, e.g. mangoes (Thomas and Janave, 1975), papayas and strawberries (Beyers et al, 1979).

17.7.2 Vitamin B

This section discusses the following vitamins: B_1 (thiamine), B_2 (riboflavin), B_5 (niacin), B_6 (pyridoxine), B_{10} (biotin) and B_{12} (cyanocobalamin).

Irradiation of thiamine causes deamination and destruction of the pyrimidine ring (Groninger and Tappel, 1957) with loss of biological activity (Ziporin et al, 1957). Thiamine is relatively radiation sensitive in some foods.

Low disinfestation doses of 0.25–0.35 kGy, delivered to cereal grains resulted in losses of thiamine of 20–40% (Diehl, 1975). In cooked pork chops, irradiated at 0.3 and 1.0 kGy (the dose range proposed for *Trichina* control), losses were 5.6 and 17.6% (Fox et al, 1989). It is calculated that loss of thiamine in the American diet, due to irradiation of pork chops and roasts, would be 1.5% at 1 kGy.

When radiation doses as high as 25 kGy were used, raw fish retained nearly 40% of total thiamine (Brooke et al, 1966), and treatment of clams, at 45 kGy, led to no detectable loss of thiamine (Brooke et al, 1964). Following a major US study of the potential nutritional and toxicological effects of radiation sterilisation on chicken breasts, Black et al (1983) concluded that γ-irradiation, at doses of 45–68 kGy, reduced thiamine levels to a similar level as that produced by heat sterilisation.

As a consequence of its relative chemical inertness, riboflavin is the vitamin most resistant to irradiation in the majority of foodstuffs. Sometimes levels of riboflavin in foods have been found to rise following irradiation, most probably due to release from binding to proteins, e.g. in pork meat (Fox et al, 1989) and onions (Le Clerk, 1963).

Although slightly less stable to irradiation than is riboflavin in simple aqueous solution, niacin has substantial radiation tolerance in foods. As has been observed with riboflavin, niacin levels in some foods rise on radiation, e.g. in pork and chicken (Fox et al, 1989) and in bread made from irradiated flour (Diehl, 1980).

In general, radiation-induced losses of pyridoxine in foods have been found to be small, similar to or slightly greater than losses of thiamine. Losses induced by radiation sterilisation of poultry and liver, at doses up to 55 kGy, were less than those induced by sterilisation by heat (Richardson et al, 1961). The converse was true for cabbage. Most studies have found little pyridoxine loss in foods irradiated at realistic doses and little further loss on subsequent storage.

Biotin is very radiation resistant in foods. Sterilising doses of gamma and electron beam irradiation did not significantly reduce levels in poultry (Black et al, 1983), or in eggs, at doses up to 50 kGy (Kennedy, 1965). Its relative stability to irradiation is reduced in the presence of oxygen more so than that of the other vitamins (Watanabe et al, 1976).

Most studies have indicated that little or no loss of vitamin B_{12} occurs during food irradiation, e.g. in various seafoods at doses up to about 4.5 kGy (Brooke et al, 1964); in pork irradiated at doses up to about 7 kGy (Fox et al, 1989); and in poultry, in a study comparing the nutritional effects of preservation by freezing with sterilisation by heat and with sterilisation by irradiation (Thayer et al, 1987).

17.7.3 Vitamin C (ascorbic acid)

Ionising radiation initially induces oxidation of ascorbic acid to dehydroascorbic acid (Barr and King, 1956). This reaction (in which the biological activity of the vitamin is retained) has been found to occur in many studies of irradiated fruits and vegetables. Further irradiation eventually leads to losses of activity as biologically non-functional products are formed.

Low doses of γ-radiation, used to delay sprouting of potatoes, reduced ascorbic but not dehydroascorbic acid levels. However, during subsequent storage, ascorbate levels rose, so that the differences between irradiated and non-irradiated potatoes disappeared (Schrieber and Highlands, 1958). Similarly, losses of ascorbic acid in orange and lemon juices, irradiated at 16 kGy, were accompanied by neat stoichiometric increases in dehydroascorbic acid (Romani et al, 1963).

Losses of about 16% ascorbic acid occurred in 3 kGy irradiated freeze dried apples. Tomatoes lost between about 8 and 20% according to the state of ripeness of the fruit (Maxie and Sommer, 1968). In other studies, virtually no losses of vitamin C (nor of the B vitamins riboflavin, niacin or thiamine) were detected in mangoes, papayas, lychees or strawberries, irradiated at 2 kGy (Beyers et al, 1979). No vitamin C losses were detected in grapefruits irradiated at up to about 1 kGy (Moshonas and Shaw, 1984).

Overall, the most likely changes occurring in low dose irradiated fruit and vegetables seem to be the conversion of a proportion of ascorbate to dehydroascorbate, and, sometimes, a small reduction in total vitamin C level. This reduction may then be reversed in intact fruits and vegetables as metabolism continues.

17.7.4 Vitamin D (calciferol)

Although the presence of water increases sensitivity, the D vitamins are relatively stable to ionising radiation in their normal lipid-rich food environments. At doses of up to 15 kGy, cholecalciferol is more radiation resistant than is vitamin A or vitamin E. Irradiation resistance of vitamin D in fish oils was even greater than in solvents, such as iso-octane, presumably due to the presence of tocopherols and other naturally occurring antioxidants (Knapp and Tappel, 1961).

17.7.5 Vitamin E (tocopherols)
Vitamin E is the most radiation-sensitive of the fat-soluble vitamins. A sterilising dose for beef (30 kGy) reduced beta-tocopherol levels by about 60% in air, but not significantly in nitrogen. Alpha- and gamma-tocopherols decreased similarly in irradiated chicken breast (Lakritz and Thayer, 1992).

Oats irradiated at a dose of 1 kGy had lost only 5% tocopherol after 8 months storage in nitrogen, but nearly 60% when stored in air (Diehl, 1979). Diehl (1980) reported a near 20% loss following 1 kGy irradiation of hazelnuts.

17.8 Carbohydrates

Apart from water, the major constituents of most foods are carbohydrates, proteins and lipids. Irradiation of low molecular weight food carbohydrates, such as glucose, mannose, ribose and lactose results in the formation of low levels of radiolytic products mostly derived from reaction of hydroxyl radicals (OH°), generated from water, with the sugar. A predominant reaction is the oxidation of hydroxyl groups, often with loss of a neighbouring hydroxyl group. Products such as 2-deoxy-gluconolactone and gluconic acid are formed, and the pH value of simple sugar solutions falls (von Sonntag, 1980). Carbohydrates irradiated in the solid state are generally more resistant than those irradiated in solution.

Irradiation of high molecular weight carbohydrates (starch, pectin, cellulose, carrageenans, etc.) sometimes causes major changes in the physical properties of the foods that contain them. Properties such as viscosity, mechanical strength, swelling and solubility are likely to change in such a way as to reduce their functionality in a food, but sometimes change to improve their effectiveness for a particular function.

Irradiation of lignocelluloses, in woody materials, has been shown to increase their subsequent biodegradability by microorganisms such as *Flavobacterium* species (Bhatt et al, 1992). The limited breakdown that occurs increases their susceptibility to the microorganism's hydrolytic exoenzymes. The properties of gums, such as Karaya gum (Le Cerf et al, 1991) change greatly on irradiation with, for example, very large increases in solubility, falls in viscosity and loss of water-swelling properties.

17.9 Lipids

The irradiation of unsaturated fatty acids in foods predominantly results in the formation of alpha and beta unsaturated carbon compounds (Nawar, 1983).

Further reaction, and the addition of oxygen, leads to the formation of a hydroperoxyl radical.

$$\left[\begin{array}{c} R-CH=CH-CH-R^1 \\ | \\ O-O^\bullet \end{array} \right]$$

Then formation of a hydroperoxide:

$$\left[\begin{array}{c} R-CH=CH-CH-R^1 \\ | \\ O-OH \end{array} \right]$$

The hydroperoxides are generally unstable in foods and breakdown to form mainly carbonyl compounds, many of which have low odour thresholds, and contribute to the rancid notes often detected when fat-rich (and particularly unsaturated fat-rich) foods are irradiated (Hammer and Wills, 1979; Wills, 1981). For example, irradiation of whole egg and egg yolk powder resulted in the generation of lipid hydroperoxides (Katusin-Razem et al, 1992). In the absence of air, their formation was limited by available oxygen. Interestingly, destruction of carotenoids was strongly correlated with hydroperoxide formation. Irradiation in the presence of oxygen leads to accelerated autoxidation (Diehl, 1995), but the end products are similar to those found following long storage of unirradiated lipids (Urbain, 1986).

17.10 Proteins

Many studies of the nutritional effects of irradiation on proteins have been made with generally only small or insignificant changes found. For example, irradiation of fish and meat meal, eggs, wheat and wheat gluten (Kennedy and Ley, 1971) showed little change in nutritive value in feeding studies after irradiation at doses up to 10 kGy. The biggest changes were in wheat gluten (7%). At 50 kGy larger losses occurred, but were largely reversed by supplementation of the diets with methionine.

17.11 The wholesomeness of irradiated food

The definition of 'wholesomeness' (in the sense of being sound, healthy, clean and otherwise fit for human consumption) requires some elaboration as it does not occur in food laws and regulations. It was originally introduced in the 1950s in the US, expanded by the FDA and others and developed in food and inspection acts. At the same time the studies on the safety of irradiated food for consumption were begun on a large scale and in international cooperation. During the procedure the terminology of wholesomeness was unanimously accepted to mean 'safety for consumption' under any relevant aspect and comprises the following features: radiological safety, toxicological safety, microbiological safety, and nutritional adequacy.

The main contribution to the judgement of wholesomeness was made by the FAO/IAEA/WHO Joint Expert Committee on Food Irradiation (World Health Organization, 1965, 1970, 1977, 1981). At the time of the Committee's foundation in 1961 it was concluded that 'general authorization of the commercial use of radiation for the treatment of food is premature'. Based on the work of the International Project in the Field of Food Irradiation (IFIP, founded in 1970 and concluded in 1981) and on the international work coordinated through IFIP the World Health Organization concluded finally (1981) that:

> ... the irradiation of any food commodity up to an overall average dose of 10 kGy presents no toxicological hazard; hence, toxicological testing of foods so treated is no longer required.

and

> ... the irradiation of food up to an overall average dose of 10 kGy introduces no special nutritional or microbiological problems.

Several national advisory groups have endorsed those findings and many national governments that had previously banned food irradiation introduced permission legislation for irradiated food. In addition, the European Commission asked their Scientific Committee on Food for advice, the JECFI conclusions were expressedly endorsed and a list of foods for clearance was proposed. However, at the time of writing no resolution of this issue has been achieved.

17.12 Current and potential applications

Some of the benefits of food irradiation are listed in Table 17.2. Food safety will present great challenges for all involved, including governments and industry (Loaharanu, 2001; Osterholm and Potter, 1997). Globalisation brings food from previously unavailable sources to markets that were previously unreachable. Production conditions are not always acceptable and the rules and regulations that are already in place do not always accord with targets and measurements. This means that attempts at harmonisation are indispensable (Mortarjemi et al, 2001). New hazards are emerging which means that appropriate and coordinated action must be taken. Food security is still the main issue in developing areas, but in industrialised countries the problem of food safety is paramount and the main aspects are hygienic quality and, in particular, microbial contamination (Doyle, 2000). Processing of food by ionising radiation is a perfect tool (Molins et al, 2001), supplementing traditional methods and in some applications is the only

Table 17.2 Some of the benefits of food irradiation

Benefit
• improves microbiological safety • reduces chemical treatment • facilitates international trade regarding food safety and quarantine security • improves availability and quality of tropical products previously unavailable • fresh food remains fresh, raw food remains raw • can be applied to solid foods for pasteurisation • can be applied in the frozen state; there is no need for warming-up • leaves no residue • can be applied to pre-packed food

procedure available. Irradiation will not be at all effective if it displaces good practices and is most effective if used as the final critical control point in an overall HACCP-concept.

Under the SPS-agreement (Sanitary and Phytosanitary) food safety is the first aspect and quarantine for plant products is the second. Here again, radiation processing is a perfect tool to achieve quarantine and at the same time conserve the environment, thus avoiding the use of ozone-layer depleting chemicals. It contributes to occupational safety by avoiding the use of toxic fumigants. Both uses are spreading, the volume of treated goods is increasing; governments and competent international bodies are developing harmonised protocols. The potential of such applications in the future is high despite the fact that at present world-wide only about 250 000 tonne per annum are irradiated (Loaharanu, 2001).

17.13 Consumer attitudes and government regulations

It is widely said that consumers reject food irradiation and any irradiated product on the market will be turned down. Table 17.3 lists common objections to irradiation. In most countries, however, irradiated food products are not on the market and the consumer has no decision left to buy or to abstain and so it appears that there is no consumer demand. On the other hand, the food industry is reluctant to bring irradiated products on the market or to be identified with food irradiation. There have even been advertising campaigns of consumer activists publishing names of companies who guarantee that their products are not treated by ionising radiation.

This is a vicious circle which can only be broken by strong arguments which has occurred in the US where a number of people, in particular children, died because they ate undercooked, 'raw' hamburgers. The reason is a nearly unavoidable infection of raw, minced meat by *Escherichia coli*, including type O157:H7 (also called EHEC). *E. coli* microorganisms are deadly and can spread despite tight hygienic measures; an effective safety measure is radiation processing to

Table 17.3 Some arguments against food irradiation

Argument
• allows lax food hygiene
• does not remove toxins
• spores are not killed
• causes loss of nutrients
• freshness is apparent rather than real
• spoilage may flourish without warning signs
• impairs sensory quality
• increases costs
• harms the environment
• endangers personnel
• needs restructuring of the total logistics

fight any residual risk. 'Red meat' irradiation has been legal in USA since 1999 and has been applied on a commercial scale since the middle of the year 2000. An increasing number of food suppliers now rely on hamburger patties for domestic use and for institutional catering which should be stamped with the words: 'irradiated for your safety – serve with confidence'.

The consumer appreciates the availability of such products and the choice between irradiated products and those which are not irradiated. The indications are that the well-informed consumer will respond favourably to the irradiated product once it becomes available to the market as well as being open-minded and ready for pertinent, trustworthy information. Scientific and sociological studies back these observations. Activists against food irradiation play guardians for an 'under-age population'.

There have been other studies on the market place, for instance on the sale of irradiated fruit from the Hawaiian islands in mainland USA where strict quarantine regulations against Mediterranean fruit fly are in place. Consumers responded favourably to such tests and now the product is on the commercial market; in Hawaii a facility dedicated to fruit irradiation has been established.

From this it can be inferred that alleged consumer resistance to irradiated food either does not exist or that it can be overcome (anon, 1998). Such resistance is created by certain opponents and is taken over by a timid food industry. In the history of food irradiation there have been many ill-founded claims, misunderstandings, half-truths, and intentional distortions. Much controversial information has been published and the discussions contain more emotion than fact. However, the professional view is that the benefits by far outweigh any potential, still unidentified, risk.

From this position of alleged consumer resistance, reinforced by the loud voices of consumer activists, politicians and governments are very cautious when it comes to regulating food irradiation. The Codex Alimentarius (1984) in its standard on food irradiation does not restrict by individual food, nor by groups or

Table 17.4 Legislation concerning food irradiation

European Union clearances
only for 'dried aromatic herbs, spices and vegetable seasonings': Austria, Denmark, Finland, Germany, Greece, Ireland, Luxembourg, Portugal, Spain, Sweden
'dried aromatic herbs, spices and vegetable seasonings' and other specified items: Belgium, France, Italy, Netherlands, United Kingdom
Non-EU countries in Europe
Clearance: Croatia, Czech Republic, Hungary, Norway, Poland, Russian Federation, Switzerland, Turkey, Ukraine, Former Yugoslavia
Other countries with clearances
Asia/Pacific: Australia, Bangladesh, China, China, Republic of (Taiwan), Indonesia, India, Iran, Japan, Korea, Pakistan, Republic of, Philippines, Thailand, Vietnam
Africa (including Middle East): Egypt, Ghana, Israel, South Africa, Syrian Arab Republic
Latin America (Middle and South): Argentina, Brazil, Chile, Costa Rica, Cuba, Mexico, Uruguay
North America: Canada, United States of America

classes, most countries have preferred to regulate by this approach (Table 17.4). A very few have adopted Codex Alimentarius completely (namely Brazil, which has removed any upper dose limit, Ghana, Mexico, Pakistan, Turkey and ASEAN member states). On the other hand, the USA prefers 'permit as petitioned' and requires documentation in addition to Codex Alimentarius and WHO evidence (the US regulatory system is explained in much detail elsewhere (Looney at al, 2001)).

At present, some 53 countries have regulations on food irradiation; this varies widely and conflicts with international trade. The International Consultative Group on Food Irradiation (ICGFI) holds an inventory of regulations by country and by item (http://www.iaea.org/icgfi) and provides other useful information. In some cases, the minimum or the maximum dose or both are regulated; in other cases an 'average' is regulated. Under the aspects of food irradiation technology only the upper and the lower dose limits are of interest because they are related to the effectiveness of the treatment. An average dose is of interest under rather rare circumstances: a liquid being stirred after irradiation.

The idea of 'overall average dose' originated from toxicological considerations (World Health Organization, 1981), a concept which is totally unsuitable for regulatory purposes. Regulating the average requires the food inspector to execute a certain integration over a prescribed extent of the sample. This problem has been resolved by more recent regulations in the Netherlands and in the United Kingdom: the regulated reference value is the average of the 'batch' and the minimum and the maximum dose values are strictly bound to this set value. However, the common regulation for all EU-members falls back to crude average limits. As such details vary widely and are sometimes contradictory, international trade is severely hampered. For this reason regional harmonisation efforts have been undertaken (1993/1999 Asia/Pacific; 1996 Africa; 1997 Latin America and Caribbean; 1998 near east) and are now being implemented by ASEAN-members. Imports and exports are permitted in most regulations; the mutual conditions, however, are not coordinated. In particular, the European Union requires that the irradiation facility in the exporting country must be registered with and inspected by the EU authorities.

17.14 World Trade Organization, Codex Alimentarius and international trade

The World Trade Organization (WTO) agreement has replaced the former GATT and the standards of Codex Alimentarius have become the indisputable reference for trade in food. Most countries have adopted the rules of WTO and disputes between signatories must be settled in a WTO conciliation procedure. Such disputes have already arisen in the European Union because of its regulations on 'hormone beef' and on 'dollar bananas'. Irradiated food might become the next case. The specifications in the Codex Alimentarius Standard on Irradiated Food and its associated Code of Practice (1984) are not restricted to any class or group of food. Such specifications are presently under revision, and the upper dose limit will be removed in order to follow the latest development (World Health Organization, 1999).

The Joint FAO/WHO Codex Alimentarius Commission (CAC) was created in 1962 with the intention to facilitate international trade in food by world-wide harmonisation and the Codex Alimentarius has become a collection of accepted and internationally recognised standards. With the emergence of WTO these standards have become the only technical reference; there are particular references under the agreements on Technical Barriers to Trade (TBT) and on Sanitary and Phytosanitary (SPS) measures which are an integral part of WTO. In this situation, even the existence of any regulation that does not cover all food but restricts permission to a particular list may be considered as a TBT and a violation of the WTO rules. The SPS agreement explicitly refers to processing by ionising radiation as one of the generally acceptable tools for achieving sanitary and phytosanitary purposes. Only a few countries have initiated the legal procedures to convert to the new framework (as described for Brazil in section 17.13). The European Union in particular has issued directives on food irradiation that are at variance with the rules of WTO underwritten by all EU-Member States. For instance, Germany is bound by a parliamentary vote to object to and block any clearance of food irradiation beyond spices: 'We strictly object to any expansion of the (EU) "positive list" [which presently only contains spices] because we deem irradiation of any further products as unnecessary.'

As can be seen from the possible applications and from reports from many countries on their food safety and food security needs it is obvious that there is a technological need for processing food by ionising radiation. Negating such needs lacks arguments founded on sound science which is a prerequisite for regulations under WTO. Or as WHO worded it, the countries which need the new technology most would also suffer most from the resistance of developed countries. There are provisions in national regulations for imports from third countries. However, when using such rules administrative obstacles must still be overcome. The US is preparing to accept imports of irradiated fruits from its southern partners; ASEAN member states are harmonising their national regulations; many countries are joining forces to develop the standards of the Codex Alimentarius to the present state of the art. The parties to the Montreal Protocol of 1997 agreed to a phase out (2005 and 2015 for advanced and developing countries, respectively) of several fumigants, with radiation processing being the technology that will take its place. Other fumigants such as ethylene oxide are already banned in several areas because of their toxicological properties and radiation processing has been demonstrated as an effective replacement for such fumigants. The International Plant Protection Organization (IPPO) has decided that radiation processing is the broad spectrum quarantine treatment that has no specific requirements regarding insect species or host commodities. Regional organisations such as the North American Plant Protection Organization (NAPPO), the European and Mediterranean Plant Protection Organization (EPPO) and the Asian and the Pacific Plant Protection Commission (APPPC) have endorsed this alternative technology. Furthermore, under such competent bodies certification systems have been developed to facilitate international trade in commodities carrying a phytosanitary risk. Similar efforts have not yet been undertaken for sanitary purposes.

17.15 Future trends

Industrialised countries increasingly face the problem of providing their populations with safe food. As the tip of the iceberg, *Escherichia coli* type O157:H7 (EHEC) has become a major threat to the US food industry. The arrival of 'electronically pasteurised hamburgers' on the US market, i.e. treated with high-energy electrons as ionising radiation and their acceptance by the consumer mark a new era; the change in the public opinion occurred when consumers realised the deadly risk of foodborne pathogen microorganisms. It would be too simple an argument to state that only the diversion of the US food industry from natural production to industrial mass production is the cause of this new challenge. The increase in world population and the concentration of population in centres of economic activity and wealth is unavoidable, and there is no way to return to the days of our ancestors. Even under strict hygienic control and at the best level of Good Manufacturing Practices there always remains a residual hazard. Radiation processing of food can help ease this problem, to improve hygienic quality of the food available, to save human lives, to save costs to the society and its social system and to contribute to the wellbeing of everyone. Ionising radiation is one tool among many; it has specific limitations and advantages but is superior to traditional means in its hygienic applications.

Less industrialised and developing countries in particular face the problem to secure the food supply; the growing population can 'eat up' any increase in food production and 20 to 40% (estimation by FAO) of the harvest can be lost during distribution and storage. Ionising radiation is a tool here but must be combined with substantial improvement of the logistics of the food production and distribution system. The usual improvement of Good Agricultural Practices and Good Manufacturing Practices alone cannot alleviate the problem.

Furthermore, the application of ionising radiation can replace traditional chemical treatments that are becoming more and more suspect. Fumigants which were an upholder of agricultural production are likely to become unavailable in the near future; several developed countries have banned their use because of the toxicity to workers of some and of the ozone-depleting properties of others (as detailed in the Montreal Agreement). Most advanced countries have even banned the imports of raw materials produced using such chemicals and their long-term availability is questionable because production is already dramatically reduced. Because developing countries achieve a considerable part of their gross net income from exports of food and agricultural raw materials this development is a threat to their economies. Insect infestation is a major cause of such loss of food exports, followed by spoilage through moulds, yeasts and other bacteria. Once the harvest is stored in insect-tight silos and transported in insect-tight sacks, re-infestation can be avoided and the contents are preserved for human consumption, the insects can be prevented from proliferation by irradiation. When the storage of grain, cocoa and coffee beans is under controlled humidity conditions, the outgrowth of pathogen bacteria is retarded and the formation of mycotoxins excluded.

Consequently, food irradiation is a tool that supplements traditional methods of food preservation; it has already found its niche application. The total volume of goods treated is still small, estimated at about 200 000 tonne per annum, one half of which is spices and dry seasonings. Official statistics are unavailable for other methods such as canning, cooling and freezing. As the development in the US clearly demonstrates, the industrial implementation of radiation processing and its acceptance by the consumer come at the time when awareness for such needs has been established and the product is clearly labelled. This means that a slow but steady growth of the amount of irradiated food is to be expected.

17.16 Sources of further information and advice

At present, 45 governments are members of the International Consultative Group on Food Irradiation (ICGFI) with a secretariat at Vienna, Austria (c/o IAEA, P.O. box 100, A-1400 Vienna, Austria; http://www.iaea.org/icgfi). ICGFI has developed technical guidelines and Codes of Practice for radiation processing of food. It is an international group of experts designated by Governments to evaluate and advise on global activities of food irradiation. A few very general and introductory publications are available (Satin, 1996; Murano, 1995; World Health Organization, 1991); renowned and competent organisation have published 'position papers' (Olson, 1998; anon, 2000; anon 1999); full details of the technology are covered in multipage compendia (Josephson and Peterson, 1983; Elias and Cohen, 1977; Elias and Cohen, 1983). The crucial question of the safety of irradiated food is covered in full detail by Diehl (1995) and WHO has published the results of expert evaluations (World Health Organization, 1981, 1994 and 1999). The actual status of the technology can be determined from the proceedings of recent conferences (Loaharanu and Thomas, 1999) and from textbooks (Molins, 2001). Nor must it be forgotten that in many countries national, competent bodies have published positive judgements of the technology. Through national and international consumer organisations more information is available to the general public and it completes the picture by analysing the technology from different aspects.

17.17 References

Advisory Committee on Irradiated and Novel Foods (1986), *The Safety and Wholesomeness of Irradiated Foods*, ACINF, London, HMSA

ANON (1998), 'A round table on food irradiation: identifying, addressing and overcoming consumer concerns', *World Food Regulation Review* **7** (12), 23–30

ANON (1999), 'IFST position statement: The use of irradiation for food quality and safety', *Food Sci. Technology Today* **13**, 32–6

ANON (2000), 'Position of the American Dietetic Association: Food irradiation', *Journal of the American Dietetic Association*, **100**, 246–53

APPLEBY J and BANKS A J (1905), *Improvements in or relating to treatment of foodstuffs, more specially cereals and their products*, British Patent No. 1609 (26 Jan 1905)

BARR N F and KING C G (1956), 'The γ-ray induced oxidation of ascorbic acid and ferrous ion', *Journal of the American Chemical Society*, **78**, 303–5

BEYERS M, THOMAS A C and VAN TONDER A J (1979), 'γ-Irradiation of sub-tropical fruits, 1. Compositional tables of mango, papaya, strawberry and litchi fruit at the edible-ripe stage', *Journal of Agriculture and Food Chemistry*, **27**, 37–42

BHATT A K, BHALLA T C and OM-AGRAWAL H (1992), 'Enhanced degradation of gamma-irradiated lignocelluloses by a new xylanolytic *Flavobacterium* species isolated from soil', *Letters in Applied Biology*, **15**, 1–4

BLACK C M, CHRISTOPHER J P, CUCA G C, DAHLGREN R R, ISRAELSON E L, MIRANTI R H, MONTI K L, REUTZEL L F, RONNING D C and TROUP C M (1983), 'A chronic toxicity, oncogenicity and multi-generation reproductive study using CD-1 mice to evaluate frozen, thermally sterilized, cobalt-60 irradiated and 10 MeV electron irradiated chicken meat', Vols 1–14, Springfield VA, National Technical Information Service

BROOKE R O, RAVESI E M, GADBOIS D M and STEINBERG M A (1964), 'Preservation of fresh unfrozen fishery products by low level radiation, 3. The effects of radiation pasteurization on amino acids and vitamins in clams', *Food Technology*, **18**, 1060–4

BROOKE R O, RAVESI E M, GADBOIS D M and STEINBERG M A (1966), 'Preservation of fresh unfrozen fishery products by low level radiation, 5. The effects of radiation pasteurization on amino acids and vitamins in haddock fillets', *Food Technology*, **20**, 1479–82

CODEX ALIMENTARIUS COMMISSION (1984), Codex General Standard for Irradiated Foods and Recommended International Code of Practice for the Operation of Radiation Facilities for the Treatment of Foods, in *Codex Alimentarius*, Rome, Codex Alimentarius

Commission, Food and Agriculture Organization of the United Nations, vol. XV (under revision)

DIEHL J F (1975), 'Thiamine in bestrahlten Lebensmitteln, 1. Einfluss verschiedener Bestrahlungsbedingungen und des Zeitablaufs nach der Bestrahlung', *Zeitschrift Lebensmittel Untersuchung Forschung*, **157**, 317–21

DIEHL J F (1979), 'Einfluss verschiedener Bestrahlungs-Bedingungen und der Lagerungen auf strahlenindu zierte Vitamin E Verluste in Lebensmitteln', *Chemica Microbiologica Technologie Lebensmittel*, **6**, 65–70

DIEHL J F (1980), 'Effects of combination processes on the nutritive value of food', in *Combination Processes in Food Irradiation*, Vienna, International Atomic Energy Agency, 349–66

DIEHL J F (1995), *'The Safety of Irradiated Foods'*, New York, Marcel Dekker

DOYLE M P (2000), 'Reducing foodborne disease: what are the priorities?', *Nutrition* **16**, 647–9

ELIAS P S and COHEN A J (eds) (1977), *Radiation Chemistry of Major Food Components, its Relevance to the Assessment of the Wholesomeness of Irradiated Foods*, Amsterdam, Elsevier Biomedical Press

ELIAS P S and COHEN A J (eds) (1983), *Recent Advances in Food Irradiation*, Amsterdam, Elsevier

FOX J B, THAYER D W, JENKINS R K, PHILLIPS J G, ACKERMAN S A, BEECHER G R, HOLDEN J M, MORROW F D and QUIRBACH D M (1989), 'Effect of gamma irradiation on the B vitamins of pork chops and chicken breasts', *International Journal of Radiation Biology*, **55**(4), 689–703

GILLETT DC, *Apparatus for preserving organic materials by the use of X-rays*, United States Patent No. 1 275 417 (13 Aug 1918)

GOLDBLITH S A (1955), 'Preservation of foods by ionizing radiations', *Journal of the American Dietetic Association*, **31**, 243–9

GRONINGER H S and TAPPEL A L (1957), 'The destruction of thiamine in meats and in aqueous solution by gamma radiation', *Food Research*, **22**, 519–23

HAMMER C T and WILLS E D (1979), 'The effect of ionising radiation on the fatty acid composition of natural fats and oil lipid peroxide formation', *International Journal of Radiation Biology*, **35**(4), 323–32

HARRIS R S and VON LOESEKE H (1969), *Nutritional Evaluation of Food Processing*, New York, Wiley

JOSEPHSON E S and PETERSON M S (eds) (1983), *Preservation of Food by Ionizing Radiation*, Boca Raton, CRC Press, vols. I–III

JOSEPHSON E S, THOMAS M H and CALHOUN W K (1979), 'Nutritional aspects of food irradiation: an overview', *Journal of Food Processing and Preservation,* **2**, 299–314

KATUSIN-RAZEM B, MIHALJEVIC B and RAZEM D (1992), 'Radiation-induced oxidative chemical changes in dehydrated egg products', *Journal of Agricultural and Food Chemistry*, **40**, 662–8

KENNEDY T S (1965), 'Studies on the nutritional value of foods treated with γ-radiation. 1. Effects on some B-complex vitamins in egg and wheat', *Journal of the Science of Food and Agriculture*, **16**, 81–4

KENNEDY T S and LEY F J (1971), 'Studies on the combined effect of gamma radiation and cooking on the nutritional value of food', *Journal of the Science of Food and Agriculture*, **22**, 146–8

LAKRITZ L and THAYER D W (1992), 'Effect of ionizing radiation on unesterified tocopherols in fresh chicken breast muscle', *Meat Science*, **32**, 257–65

LE CERF D, IRIENI F and MILLER G (1991), 'The effect of gamma-irradiation on the water-swelling properties of Karaya gum', *Food Hydrocolloids*, **5**, 155–7

LE CLERK A M (1963), 'Effets des radiation ionisantes sur la teneur en vitamines de quelques produits alimentaires', *Annales Nutrition et Alimentation*, **17**, B449–B461

LOAHARANU P (2001), 'Rising calls for food safety: radiation technology becomes a timely answer', *IAEA Bulletin* **43**(2), 37–42
LOAHARANU P and THOMAS P (eds) (1999), *Irradiation for Food Safety and Quality*, Technomic, Lancaster
LOONEY J W, CRANDALL P G and POOLE A K (2001), 'The matrix of food safety regulations', *Food Technol.* **55**(4), 60–76
LUKTON A and MACKINNEY G (1956), 'Effect of ionizing radiations on carotenoid stability', *Food Technology* **10**, 630–2
MAXIE E C and SOMMER N F (1968), 'Changes in some chemical constituents in irradiated fruits and vegetables', in *Preservation of Fruits and Vegetables by Radiation*, Vienna, International Atomic Energy Agency, 39–56
MOLINS R (ed) (2001), *Food Irradiation – Principles and Applications*, New York, Wiley-Interscience
MOLINS R A, MOTARJEMI Y and KÄFERSTEIN F K (2001), 'Irradiation: a critical control point in ensuring the microbiological safety of raw food', *Food Control* **12**, 347–56
MOTARJEMI Y, VAN SCHOTHORST M and KÄFERSTEIN F (2001), 'Future challenges in global harmonization of food safety legislation', *Food Control* **12**, 339–46
MOSHONAS M G and SHAW P E (1984), 'Effects of low dose γ-irradiation on grapefruit products', *Journal of Agricultural and Food Chemistry*, **32**, 1098–101
MURANO E A (ed) (1995), *Food Irradiation – A Sourcebook*, Ames, Iowa State Press
NAWAR W W (1983), 'Reaction mechanisms in the radiolysis of fats: a review', *Journal of Agricultural and Food Chemistry*, **26**, 21–5
OLSON D G (1998), 'Irradiation of food. Scientific status summary by the Institute of Food Technologists' Expert Panel on Food Safety and Nutrition', *Food Technol.* **52**(1) 56–62
OSTERHOLM M T and POTTER M E (1997), 'Irradiation pasteurization of solid foods: taking food safety to the next level', *Emerging Infectious Diseases* **3**, 575–7
RICHARDSON L R, WILKES S and RITCHEY S J (1961), 'Comparative vitamin B_6 activity in frozen, irradiated and heat-processed foods', *Journal of Nutrition*, **73**, 363–8
ROMANI R J, VAN KODY J, LIM L and BOWERS B (1963), 'Radiation physiology of fruit ascorbic acid, sulphydryl and soluble nitrogen content in irradiated citrus', *Radiation Botany*, **3**, 363–9
SATIN M (1996), *Food Irradiation – A Guidebook*, Lancaster, Technomic
SCHRIEBER J S and HIGHLANDS M E (1958), 'A study of the biochemistry or irradiated potatoes stored under commercial conditions', *Food Research*, **23**, 464–77
THAYER D W, CHRISTOPHER J P, CAMPBELL L A, RONNING D C, DAHLGREN R R, THOMPSON G M and WIERBICKI E (1987), 'Toxicology studies or irradiation-sterilized chicken', *Journal of Food Protection*, **50**, 278–88
THOMAS P and JANAVE M T (1975), 'Effects of gamma irradiation and storage temperature on carotenoids and ascorbic acid content of mangoes on ripening, *Journal of the Science of Food and Agriculture* **26**, 1503–12
URBAIN W M (1986), *Food Irradiation*, Academic Press, London
VON SONNTAG C (1980), 'Free radical reactions of carbohydrates as studied by radiation techniques', *Advances in Carbohydrate Chemistry and Biochemistry*, **37**, 7–11
WATANABE H, AOKI S and SATO T (1976), 'Gamma ray inactivation of biotin in dilute aqueous solution', *Agricultural and Biological Chemistry*, **40**, 915
WILLS E D (1980), 'Studies of lipid peroxide formation in irradiation of synthetic diets and the effects of storage after irradiation', *International Journal of Radiation Biology*, **37**(4), 383–401
WORLD HEALTH ORGANIZATION (1965), *The Technical Basis for Legislation on Irradiated Food*, Geneva, Technical Report Series 316, World Health Organization
WORLD HEALTH ORGANIZATION (1970), *Wholesomeness of Irradiated Food with Special Reference to Wheat, Potatoes and Onions*, Technical Report Series 451, Geneva, World Health Organization

WORLD HEALTH ORGANIZATION (1977), *Wholesomeness of Irradiated Food*, Technical Report Series 604, Geneva, World Health Organization

WORLD HEALTH ORGANIZATION (1981), *Wholesomeness of Irradiated Food*, Technical Report Series 659, Geneva, World Health Organization

WORLD HEALTH ORGANIZATION (1991), *Food Irradiation: A technique for preserving and improving the safety of food*, Geneva, World Health Organization

WORLD HEALTH ORGANIZATION (1994), *Safety and Nutritional Adequacy of Irradiated Food*, Geneva, World Health Organization

WORLD HEALTH ORGANIZATION (1999), *High-dose Irradiation: Wholesomeness of Food Irradiated with Doses above 10 kGy*, Technical Report Series 890, Geneva, World Health Organization

ZIPORIN Z Z, KRAYBILL H F and THACH H J (1957), 'Vitamin content of foods exposed to ionizing radiations', *Journal of Nutrition*, **63**, 201–9

18

Microwave processing

D. A. E. Ehlermann, Federal Research Centre for Nutrition, Germany

18.1 Introduction

Generally, the effects of microwave energy can be classified as either 'macroscopic' or 'microscopic'. When the energy is used for heating food the effect is macroscopic and results in a specific heating pattern. However, the causes of certain features are due to microscopic effects, i.e. to physics at the atomic level. The advantages of the technology are quick and uniform heating and the reduction of water usage.

Food is a complex system that contains many components such as biological molecules, water and microorganisms. Its structure is determined by such structures as cells, membranes, polymers, proteins and lipids. There has always been a suspicion that microwaves might have 'athermal' properties that influence unexpected changes in microorganisms, nutrients and living cells but at the time of writing the allegations are unproven and the reported effects could always be attributed to particular heating patterns and insufficient temperature control in the experiments. Representatives of mainstream science have therefore concluded that microwave heating is a safe method of food processing and can be usefully applied both in the domestic household and in the food industry. Various aspects are discussed in several of the sections that follow.

Electromagnetic waves in the frequency range of 300 MHz to 300 GHz are usually called 'microwaves'; this terminology is inappropriate but popular. The prefix 'micro' would lead one to expect that the wavelength is in the micrometer range but in free space the wavelength ranges from decimetre to millimetre and therefore is in agreement with the dimensions of articles of daily use. For example, in radar systems microwaves provide reasonable spatial resolution and considerable radius of action and can be compared with optical imaging systems using electromagnetic waves in the frequency range of THz (10^{12} Hz), equivalent to a wavelength of µm (micrometre). Photons of microwaves correspond to an energy range of 1 µeV to 1 meV and are incapable of ionisation (binding energies of electrons to the atom are 4 eV or above). Applications of microwaves are mostly in radiocommunication, radar and heating.

Electromagnetic radiation was discovered by Rudolf Hertz in 1888 who did not believe in its practical value nor in any possibilities for its industrial exploitation (Hermann, 1988) but today nearly every household uses the microwave oven or the cellular phone. In order not to disturb other uses of microwaves, the application of microwave heating is limited by the International Telecommunication Unions (ITU) to a number of frequency bands (Fig. 18.1). For practical purposes only the following frequency bands are exploited:

- 2450 MHz in domestic ovens and industry.
- 970 MHz, 915 MHz and 897 MHz in some countries for industrial applications.
- 22 125 MHz, reserved bands for future use.

The most relevant application to food is that of heating, both in the household and in the food industry. In industry, a range of practical applications exploit the particular heating patterns achievable by microwaves, which are superior to conventional heating in the given circumstances. The aim of microwave processing in general is to deliver more homogeneous heating at a faster rate and in particular for pasteurisation and sterilisation. It is therefore necessary to understand the physical principles and to achieve an insight into the limitations of potential systems in this respect. For general information the reader is referred to

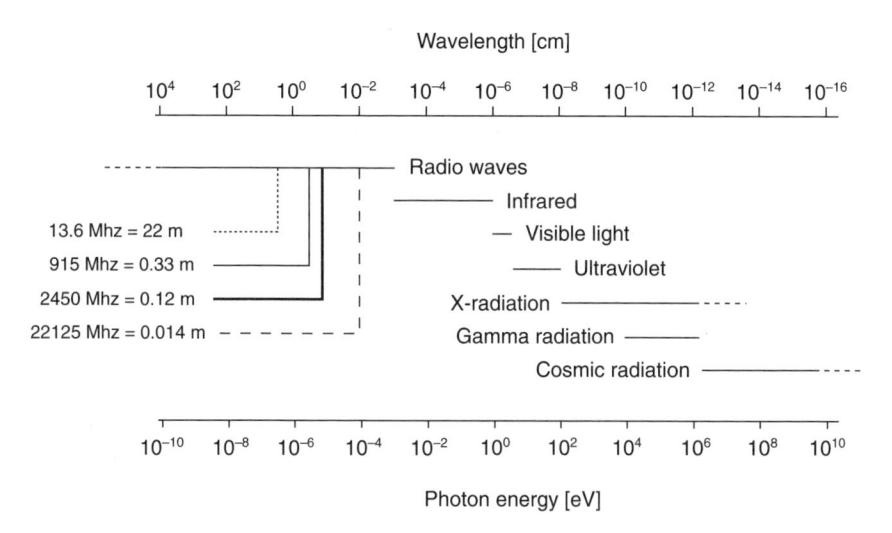

Fig. 18.1 Range of energies (electromagnetic spectrum): the range of frequencies useful for microwave heating is marked.

textbooks and reviews or survey articles (Rosenthal, 1972; Dehne, 1999; Harris and Von Loeseke, 1960; Decareau, 1985; Mullin, 1995).

18.2 The principles of microwave heating

Microwave processing is simply heating by radiation (Kaatze, 1995). As such it is similar to infrared heating; the energy transfer is by radiation and not by convection or conduction. However, there are significant differences: in infrared heating the penetration of the radiation into the substance is marginal and the main portion is heated by conduction from the surface into the centre, in microwave processing microwaves penetrate throughout the volume of the substance and the 'heat-sources' are dissipated inside it. This can contribute to a more uniform heating of the substance. However, the penetration of microwaves is limited and this must be taken into consideration both industrially and domestically. Microwaves are reflected by metals but transmitted by materials such as glass, plastics, paper and ceramics. Microwaves are produced by a vacuum tube device called a magnetron and the power in household ovens ranges from 600 to 1500 W while industrial installations use up to 50 kW. Energy conversion efficiency by magnetrons is around 50% and the remaining heat is usually dissipated by air cooling.

In order to understand the physical principles behind the radiation energy transfer, it is necessary to understand that electromagnetic energy comes in portions called 'photons' or 'quanta' that are discrete but very small quantities. An impinging photon must match exactly the energy difference between several allowed atomic energy states of the electrons in the treated material; otherwise, no energy is absorbed and the object is 'transparent' to the electromagnetic wave. This is the reason that food, which is mainly water with regard to microwave heating, can be heated, but glass or plastic containers remain cold. (A mother heating a baby's bottle in a microwave oven and testing the temperature by sensing its surface temperature with her cheek may not realise that the milk is boiling inside.) In addition, the 'heat capacity' of the substance must be considered. It determines the heating effect: some food components such as fat do not absorb the microwave energy as efficiently as water does; but their heat capacity is much lower than that of water and despite the lower absorbance they are heated much faster. (A piece of meat containing massive fat portions, being cooked in the microwave oven will appear evenly cooked and ready to eat but when cutting it the hot, liquid fat will spurt from inside!)

On the atomic level the following effects determine the energy transfer from the radiation to the food (Fig. 18.2). When an electric field, whether static or alternating, is applied the product undergoes polarisation. Polar molecules that carry locally separated charges will orient in the direction of the actual electric field, and water is such a polar molecule. Once oriented the electrical field will stretch the molecule. Other molecules that are normally neutral and nonpolar will become polarised as the electrons are moved to opposite ends of the molecule by

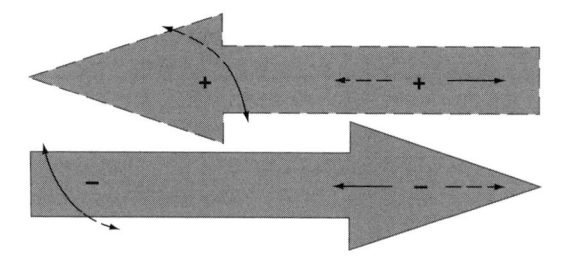

Fig. 18.2 Dipole rotation and ion oscillation or orientation polarisation versus space charge polarisation: the horizontal arrows symbolise the alternating electrical field; the ellipsoid (left) symbolises a polar molecule with the alternating rotation indicated by arrows; the circles (right) with the charge marked symbolise ions with the linear oscillation indicated by arrows.

the external field. As soon as this is complete the effects of rotation and stretching will also occur for these particular molecules. In addition, aqueous solutions may contain components such as salts that easily dissociate and form electrically charged ions and in the presence of an electrical field such ions move. The microwaves are not static but oscillate regularly; i.e. these effects of polarisation, rotation, stretching and migration repeat at the rate of oscillation and are ideally synchronised. However, in practice there is a frictional effect i.e. interaction with the electrical field of neighbouring molecules. This retards oscillation of the polarised molecules, the molecules always follow the microwave that drives them and heat energy is transferred to the medium. This means that at very low electromagnetic frequencies no energy is imparted because the water molecules can rotate and reorientate themselves quickly enough to follow the field of the microwave and at very high frequencies (approaching 1000 GHz) no energy is imparted because the molecules are too inert to follow the field of the microwave. Furthermore, ions in an aqueous solution cannot follow the oscillation of the electrical field and cannot move over significant distances so energy is consumed in keeping such ions oscillating and this also contributes to heat formation in the medium. From this discussion the complexity of the physics of microwave heating is evident. This is true even when cooking a simple item such as mashed potatoes with table salt; the salt content may affect the heating pattern.

Because microwave heating of food (Ponne and Bartels, 1995) is dominated by the physical properties of water it is informative to take a closer look. As long as water molecules are well separated, such as in the gaseous phase, there is only marginal coupling between neighbouring molecules and only a very small number of allowed rotational and vibrational transitions exist. This means that water vapour is transparent to microwaves except for photons of very distinct frequencies which are absorbed. When the water condenses to a liquid, hydrogen bonds between the molecules prevail and the allowable transitions are converted (widened) to a range (or bands) of photon energies. Hence, liquid water can be heated by a range of microwave frequencies. Quite dramatically, when water

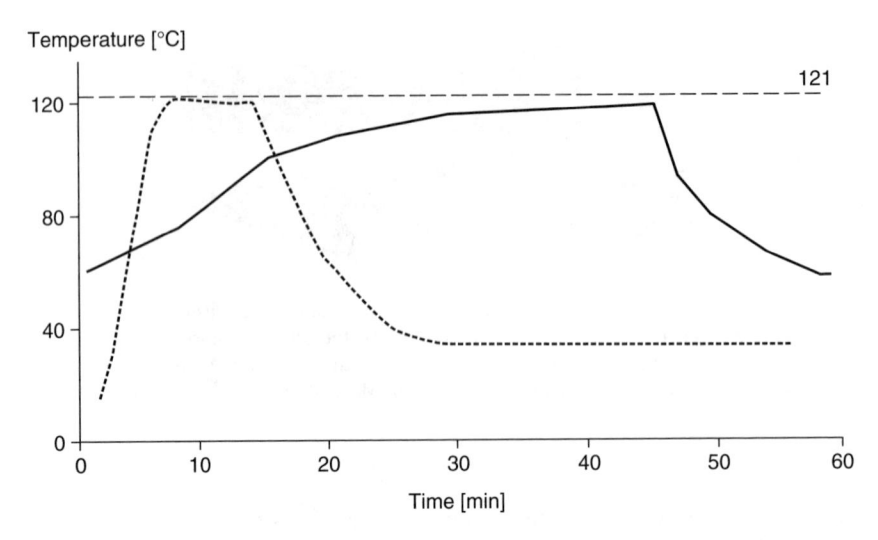

Fig. 18.3 Comparison of heating curves: broken line: microwaves can cause a short warming up period, the targeted holding temperature of 121 °C is perfectly reached for the desired and shorter period of time; solid line: conventional heating, the warming up period is rather long, the targeted holding temperature is reached only after prolonged periods. Cooling behaviour is nearly identical in both cases.

becomes solid, that is it freezes to ice, rotation of the water molecules becomes impossible and only small vibrations within the crystalline structure are still possible and so ice becomes nearly transparent for microwaves. This effect is the limiting factor in thawing frozen food by microwaves; but there is a practical solution that is discussed below.

As a practical consequence, the time-course of heating patterns is most beneficial for microwaves compared to conventional methods (Fig. 18.3). The warming up time is much shorter and results in the protection of nutrients from excessive heat damage and leaching. The target temperature (in this example 121 °C to achieve sterility) is reached nearly instantaneously and held for a well-defined period of time; whereas in conventional heat-sterilisation the central temperature only approaches the target value asymptotically. Unfortunately, fast and direct cooling is not possible and the cooling behaviour of the product is identical for any sterilisation method.

The other practical consequence concerns the freezing point (Fig. 18.4). Distilled water clearly shows the heat absorption behaviour theoretically expected and, for food such as raw meat, behaviour is similar at the freezing point of water due to the physical properties of water at this temperature. However, with increasing temperatures behaviour differs from that of distilled water and is due to substances such as salts dissolved in the cell contents.

In practice, microwave heating is controlled by a multitude of interwoven factors such as the radiation source, the volume and design of the oven, the composition of the food (e.g. proportions of water, salts, fats) and its bulk density as

Relative absorption

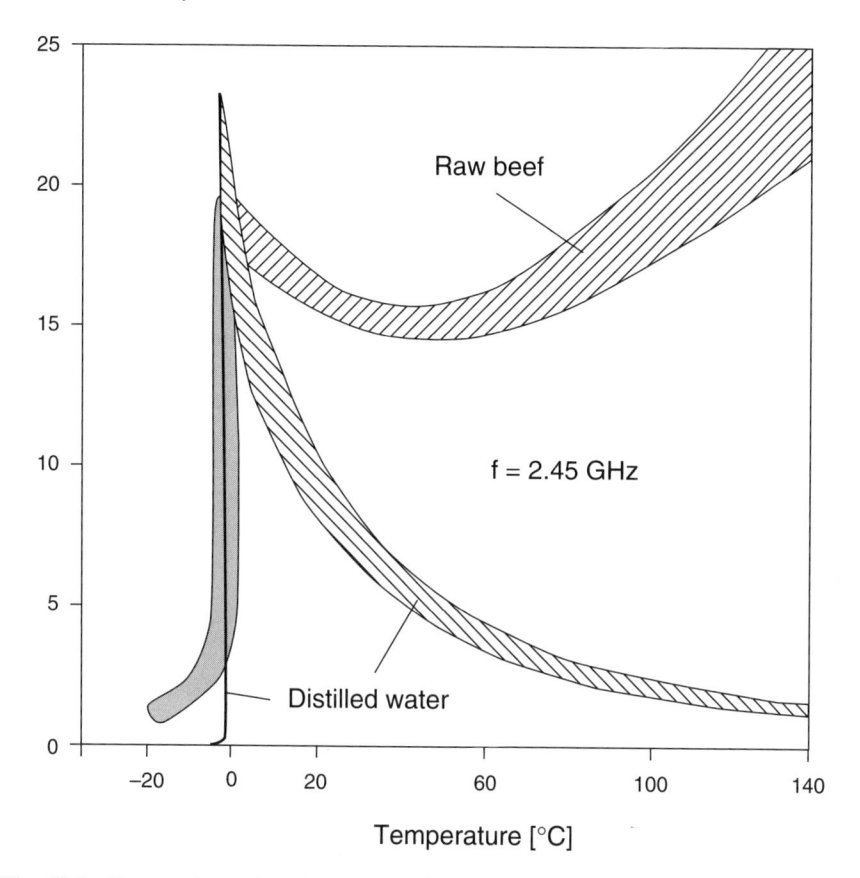

Fig. 18.4 Energy absorption, water vs. beef in relation to temperature. Distilled water and beef are mainly determined by the course of the dielectric properties of water below the freezing point; around the freezing point energy absorption reaches a maximum; at higher temperatures the energy absorption efficiency decreases continuously for water; for raw beef there is an initial decrease and a later increase because of the mobility of ions in aqueous solution within the meat.

well as such related parameters as dielectric properties, electrical conductivity, heat capacity and thermal conductivity. Packaging formats may introduce another difficulty because increased field strength at corners and edges can lead to local over-heating that leaves other portions under-treated.

18.3 The effects of microwave radiation on food

It is common practice to classify the effects of microwave energy on a medium as 'thermal' or 'non-thermal'. However, this terminology is incorrect. The interaction of matter with the electromagnetic field always results in an energy transfer and therefore in a temperature change. However, some effects are specific to the interaction with electromagnetic energy and cannot be achieved by conventional heating. Other effects are identical to interaction with thermal energy i.e. by conventional conductive or convective heating. For microwaves, the optical and geometrical effects during exposure of matter can result in locally high and low power levels and therefore in hot spots and cold spots. In many cases, researchers were unaware of such phenomena and therefore their conclusions on microwave-specific effects were incorrect. The objects exposed to microwaves can be considered as antennae: if they are geometrically separated and are small compared to the wavelength(s) they will not be 'seen' by microwaves, in the same way as a radio or TV antenna must be of correct size for optimal reception. As a consequence, many reported observations about biological effects in living cells must be carefully compared to and separated from possible heating effects. Literature in this field includes that of many different subjects, and the studies have been carried out from the viewpoint of various disciplines and are mostly inconsistent in terminology. The direct effects on such substances as nutrients, enzymes, proteins, microorganisms and cell membranes are of interest when considering the quality of microwaved food.

'There is no substantiated mechanism of interaction of microwaves with atoms, molecules, organisms and microorganisms other than volumetric heating' (Ponne and Bartels, 1995; Mudgett, 1989).

Over the past few decades there has been a heated debate that resurfaced during recent years due to concerns about mobile phones, electrical power lines and electro-smog. It has been shown that temperature control in most of these experiments was not possible to the level that was necessary. Several papers and patents claimed beneficial 'athermal' effects, but it could be shown that identical effects could be reached in conventional heating by simulating the heating patterns expected to occur in microwave heating. Kinetic laws lead to a variety of hypotheses: if an intermediate reactant has a long transition life time, electric fields can increase the probability of molecular collision; if the reactant has a short life time, the electric field can re-orient the molecules to more favourable positions for further reaction. Another hypothesis assumes extremely high temperatures at locations of atomic or molecular dimensions. All those theories still need experimental verification. The principal difficulty for such experiments can be understood by recognising that 'temperature' is defined at the macroscopic level by the average of the molecular oscillations in the volume under consideration and this does not apply for a point at the atomic level. How could the temperature of an atom or inside a microorganism be measured experimentally?

From the viewpoint of the food technologist it is possible to conclude that the strong electric and magnetic fields have an effect on cell membranes. These effects result in a change of permeability, in functional disturbances and even in rupture, but do not change the nutritional value and do not affect the technology of microwave heating. Some theories also predict a direct effect of microwaves on enzymatic activity, but there is not yet any experimental proof. The effect of microwave chemistry on reaction rate and specificity of reaction needs to be investigated.

In conclusion, the microwave heating of food only confers properties to food that are conferred through conventional heating. Lethal effects to microorganisms, parasites and other organisms are exclusively due to heat. Speed and homogeneity of heating are influenced by the composition of the food and the mass in relation to power of the oven, as well as by the technical features of the appliance. Because cold spots may occur care must be taken when anticipating the reduction of microorganisms. Pathogen microorganisms might survive in one area of the food while other parts show elevated temperatures. Standing time after cooking may be used to achieve more even temperatures by heat exchange through conduction.

18.4 The safety of microwave-heated food

Unknown hazards and mysterious phenomena in microwave heating are intimidating to most people and, in contrast to conventional heating, there is no visible heat source. Inside the oven the food is heated up to cooking temperature so the obvious query is whether radiation leaking from the device can heat anyone standing close to it. For this reason, the permissible energy density at the surface of any microwave facility is limited to $10\,mW/cm^2$ for an unlimited length of time of exposure in the USA and European countries. In some eastern European countries and the former Soviet Union the upper limit for long-term exposure to microwaves has even been set to $10\,\mu W/cm^2$. This very low limit was justified because of supposed non-thermal effects attributed to interaction of microwaves with living organisms. The alleged health problems included nervousness, hormonal imbalance, malformations and anomalous brain activity. The experimental evidence, however, for such phenomena is unsubstantiated (Foster, 1992; Hileman, 1993).

The practical and achievable limit of $10\,mW/cm^2$ is justified because the microwaves that are used are identical with those used in therapy. (For therapeutic effects the energy density must be well above a level of $100\,mW/cm^2$.) There are numerous studies to determine damage thresholds and it has been observed that no permanent effects occur at levels below $100\,mW/cm^2$. For a critical organ, the eye, it was observed that cataract formation may occur at $150\,mW/cm^2$ when the microwaves are applied for more than 90 minutes. Within certain limits the body can absorb energy including microwaves and compensate for the temperature increase easily by removing excessive heat by means of blood flow. There are certain avascular structures in the body that may have a relatively poor heat exchange; this is possibly true for testicles and temporary sterility has been reported after microwave exposure. The energy flow from the sun may be considered for comparison: on a sunny day in summer the infrared portion of the spectrum may carry as much as $100\,mW/cm^2$, which is not responsible for sunburn. Hence, introducing a safety factor of 10 is considered sufficient and the limiting energy density of 10 mW/cm² is widely accepted. However, in recognising concerns about cell phones, broadcast antennas and satellites a lowering of this limit by another factor of 10 is being considered.

To enhance radiological safety of microwave appliances several features are implemented. Safety latches cut off the power as soon as the door is opened and the user is not exposed to spurious radiation. Further chokes and absorbing strips are attached to the doors as seals to eliminate any leakage of microwave radiation to the outside. Industrial facilities are equipped with energy trapping devices at the conveyor and system openings for product entry and exit. Such facilities for continuous treatment have to be operated 'open door', whereas the household oven is used batchwise and the door must always be closed. The majority of household appliances and industrial facilities that are built and installed today are well shielded. At the time of purchase, for a domestic appliance the energy leakage is usually considerably less than 1 mW/cm² at 5 cm from the door as presently regulated in most countries. Microwave appliances have been regularly used in households for several years and no major accident has been reported. Survey studies have confirmed the radiological safety of the appliances that are on the market. However, there have been certain consumer demands regarding larger door openings and bigger transparent windows at the front that have led the industry to be more rigorous regarding the regulated leakage limits of 1 mW/cm² at 5 cm. The statistics from such surveys have shown that an increasing number of appliances is manufactured as close as possible to the limits but this should not cause concern because the energy limits already include a reasonable safety factor.

The presence of metallic conductors in the human body, especially if they are heart pacemakers, can lead to complex effects and locally high electrical currents as does a piece of metal left in food while being heated in a microwave oven. This may lead to unforeseen interactions and so a particular note of caution must be given to people with pacemakers. Experiments with volunteers have shown that the most critical frequency is around 9 GHz which is used in radar facilities; at those frequencies commonly used for heating purposes, 2450 MHz, only small changes of the heart rhythm have been observed (the maximum energy density in such experiments was limited to 25 mW/cm²). However, such warnings are irrelevant in the case of household appliances as the regulated leakage limit is usually 1 mW/cm² at 5 cm distance. Some precautions may be advisable where microwave facilities are installed on a food production line in industry. However, radiological safety at open-door facilities has also been generally established.

Prejudice and lack of technical understanding are causes of unfounded allegations that food heated by microwave might become toxic and exotic chemical compounds could be formed. However, microwave radiation cannot break chemical bonds and cannot cause ionisation nor create free radicals. Here there is an essential difference from ionising radiation which has a quantum or photon energy that is larger by several orders of magnitude. For this reason the possibility of induced chemical reactions other than thermal ones is nonexistent. This has been confirmed by many studies and it has been possible to attribute any particular chemical effect to uncontrolled heating patterns in various experiments. Microwave heating is newer than traditional methods such as broiling, roasting, frying, smoking and barbecuing so it is less understood and accepted by the public. However, in practice, microwave ovens are used in a large and increasing number of households with no concerns.

Variations in food shape, size or composition can also result in underdone products, and this is another risk in microwave cooking. Lack of understanding has resulted in illness from surviving pathogen microorganisms or the formation of microbial toxins; however, this is no different from undercooking food by traditional methods. In the same way, local overcooking can lead to the formation of unacceptable chemical changes as it does in traditional heating methods. Because there are no substantiated, special mechanisms of the interaction of microwaves with atoms, molecules, organisms and microorganisms the toxicological concerns regarding the consumption of food that is heated by microwave have no foundation in reality.

18.5 The nutritional adequacy of microwave heated food

Since the discussion above has shown that chemical, biological, microbiological, radiological and toxicological implications for microwave heated food give no cause for concern, it should be expected that there are no particular nutritional problems associated with the procedure. Any difference in the nutritional value of microwaved food compared with food treated by conventional means must be attributed to the different heating regimes. Microwaves bring the advantage of fast heating throughout the food with a lower temperature burden because of reduced cooking time. As a consequence, the loss in heat-sensitive vitamins is minimised. In addition, the extent of chemical reactions, such as the Maillard reaction, may be reduced and the retention of nutrients be enhanced. In microwave heating, less water is needed so that less extraction of valuable nutrients including minerals occurs. The quantification of such advantageous effects is largely dependent on the way the appliance or industrial facility is set up. However, in industrial applications the amount of water may be tailored to achieve the optimal effect between heating, microorganism reduction and retention of nutrients.

18.6 Future trends

Because of its ease and convenience microwave cooking has been established considerably more in the domestic situation than it has in the food industry. Many homes today have a microwave oven and have done since the beginning of the 1970s and it may be expected that the food industry will now learn about the advantages. Even the formulation of complex recipes and composite dishes can be adapted to technical needs of microwave heating and some conventional recipes are easy to tailor (George, 1993, Ramaswamy and van de Voort, 1990).

Uncritical enthusiasm about the potential of microwave processing should not disguise the facts and technological conditions. Discerning scientists and engineers point to technical difficulties which still exist and to potential problems of unknown dimensions in large-scale industrial exploitation of the technology. Some present techniques and operational designs may be inadequate in dealing with microwave technology and future requirements. Any limitations should be recognised and be compared with the achievable advantages, otherwise elevated expectations may be deflated by realities. However, it is hoped that scientists and engineers will find solutions to the problems associated with microwave applications as they have done with other problems in the past.

One aspect of such future developments is the choice of appropriate containers and the development of more suitable materials with which to make them. Intensive research and development efforts have already led to new materials adapted for unique features in microwave heating because the container is an active component for a microwavable product; the browning pan is an example. Fractions of the microwave energy are absorbed in the wall material, or reflected and transmitted to the product in the container.

18.7 References

DECAREAU R V (1985), *Microwaves in the Food Industry*, Orlando, Academic Press

DEHNE L I (1999), *Bibliography on Microwave Heating of Food*, BgVV-Hefte 04/1999, Berlin, Bundesinstitut für gesundheitlichen Verbraucherschutz und Veterinärmedizin

FOSTER K R (1992), 'Health effects of low-level electromagnetic fields: phantom or not-so-phantom risk?', *Health Phys.* **62**, 429–35

GEORGE R M (1993), 'Recent progress in product, package and process design for microwavable foods', *Trends Food Sci. Technol.* **4**, 390–4

HARRIS R S and VON LOESECKE H (1960), *Nutritional Evaluation of Food Processing*, New York, Wiley

HERMANN A (1988), 'Heinrich Hertz und seine große Entdeckung' (Heinrich Hertz and his great discovery), *Naturwissenschaften* **75**, 219–24

HILEMAN B (1993), 'Health effects of electromagnetic fields remain unresolved', *C&EN* (Nov. 8, 1993), 15–29

KAATZE U (1995), 'Fundamentals of microwaves', *Radiat. Phys. Chem.* **45**, 539–48

MUDGETT R E (1989), 'Microwave food processing. Scientific status summary by the Institute of Food Technologists' Expert Panel on Food Safety and Nutrition', *Food Technol.* **43**(1), 117–26

MULLIN J (1995), 'Microwave processing' in Gould G W (ed.) *New Methods of Food Preservation*, London, Blackie Academic & Professional

PONNE C T and BARTELS P V (1995), 'Interaction of electromagnetic energy with biological material – relation to food processing', *Radiat. Phys. Chem.* **45**, 591–607

RAMASWAMY H and VAN DE VOORT F R (1990), 'Microwave applications in food processing', *Can. Inst. Food Sci. Technol.* **33**(1), 17–21

ROSENTHAL I (1972), *Electromagnetic Radiations in Food Science* (Advanced Series in Agricultural Sciences 19), Berlin, Springer

19

Ohmic heating

R. Ruan, X. Ye and P. Chen, University of Minnesota; and
C. Doona and I. Taub, US Army Natick Soldier Center

19.1 Introduction

Preventing the loss of vitamins and nutrients in foods is a paramount concern at all stages of food processing involving heating. One example of the critical need for retaining vitamins is to nourish hospital patients who require vitamins to recover from the stress of illness or surgery.[1] This issue has invoked recent studies comparing cook/chill and cook/hot-hold foodservice practices in hospitals in an effort to minimise the loss of vitamins and nutrients that occurs when foods are heated.[2] Thermal processing is the most widely used method for destroying microorganisms and imparting foods with a lasting shelf-life.[3] Despite its many significant advantages, this mode of food preservation unavoidably degrades the vitamin and nutrient levels to some extent. As an alternative thermal method, ohmic heating ensures the benefits of conventional thermal processing (food safety and preservation) while offering the potential for improvements in the retention of vitamins and nutrients.

This chapter starts with a brief introduction to ohmic heating followed by descriptions of its unique heating characteristics that can attenuate the thermal destruction of nutrients. The effects of ohmic heating on nutrients will be discussed under three headings: (1) thermal destruction of nutrients and functional compounds, (2) nutrient loss through diffusion, and (3) electrolysis and contamination. Future trends and need for research are also discussed.

19.2 The principles of ohmic heating

Ohmic heating is a thermal process in which heat is internally generated by the passage of alternating electrical current (AC) through a body such as a food

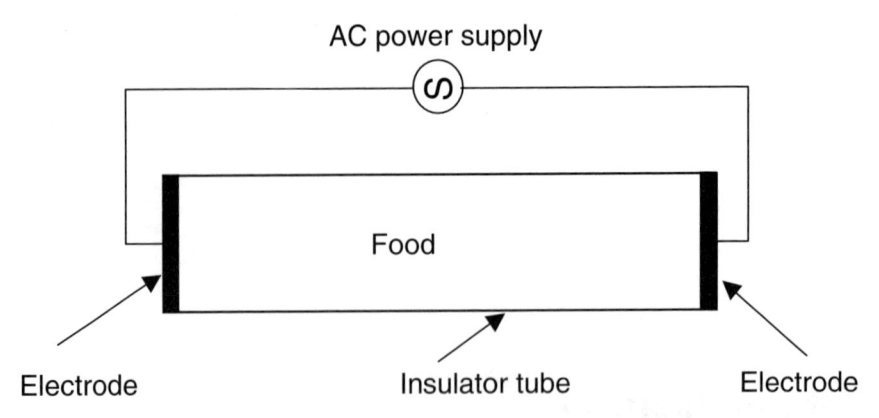

Fig. 19.1 A schematic diagram of an ohmic heating device.

system that serves as an electrical resistance. Ohmic heating is alternatively called resistance heating or direct resistance heating. The principles of ohmic heating are very simple, and a schematic diagram of an ohmic heating device is shown in Fig. 19.1. During ohmic heating, AC voltage is applied to the electrodes at both ends of the product body. The rate of heating is directly proportional to the square of the electric field strength, the electrical conductivity, and the type of food being heated. The electric field strength can be controlled by adjusting the electrode gap or the applied voltage, while the electrical conductivities of foods vary greatly, but can be adjusted by the addition of electrolytes.

Sufficient heat is generated to pasteurise or sterilise foods.[3] Generally, pasteurisation involves heating high-acid (pH < 4.5) foods to 90–95°C for 30–90 seconds to inactivate spoilage enzymes and microorganisms (vegetative bacteria, yeasts, molds, and lactobacillus organisms). Low-acid (pH > 4.5) foods can support *Clostridum botulinum* growth, and depending on the actual pH and other properties of the food, require heating to 121°C for a minimum of 3 minutes (lethality F_o = 3 min) to achieve sterility (12D colony reduction).

Within the past two decades, new and improved materials and designs for ohmic heating have become available. The Electricity Council of Great Britain has patented a continuous-flow ohmic heater and licensed the technology to APV Baker.[4] The particular interest in this technology stems from the food industry's ongoing interest in aseptic processing of low-acid liquid-particulate foods. In the case of particulates suspended in viscous liquids, conventional heating transfers heat from the carrier medium to the particulates, and the time required to heat sufficiently the center of the largest particulate (the designated 'cold-spot') results in overprocessing.[5] In contrast, ohmic heating is volumetric and heats both phases simultaneously. Ohmic heating is a high-temperature short-time method (HTST) that can heat an 80% solids food product from room temperature to 129°C in about 90 seconds,[6] allowing the possibility to decrease the extent of high temperature overprocessing. A stark contrast between ohmic heating and conventional heating is that ohmic can heat particulates faster than the carrier liquid, called the heating inversion,[7] which is not possible by traditional, conductive heating.[5]

19.3 The advantages of ohmic heating

Ohmic heating has unique characteristics with associated advantages, which will certainly have significant impact on the nutritional values of ohmically heated products. Briefly, these characteristics and advantages are:[4,8]

1. Heating food materials volumetrically by internal heat generation without the limitations of conventional heat transfer or the non-uniformities commonly associated with microwave heating due to dielectric penetration limit.
2. Particulate temperatures similar to or higher than liquid temperatures can be achieved, which is impossible for conventional heating.
3. Reducing risks of fouling on heat transfer surface and burning of the food product, resulting in minimal mechanical damage and better nutrients and vitamin retention.
4. High energy efficiency because 90% of the electrical energy is converted into heat.
5. Optimisation of capital investment and product safety as a result of high solids loading capacity.
6. Ease of process control with instant switch-on and shut-down.

Microbiological and chemical tests demonstrated the characteristics and benefits of ohmic heating as an HTST thermal processing method for particulate-liquid mixtures.[7,9] Conventionally heating a mixture of carrot and beef cubes in a viscous liquid to attain a lethality in the liquid phase of $F_o = 32$ min would have produced[7] an F_o value at the particulate center of 0.2 min. Ohmically heating the same mixture containing alginate analogs of beef and carrot cubes inoculated with spores of *Bacillus stearothermophilus* produced $F_o = 28.1$–38.5 for the carrots and $F_o = 23.5$–30.5 for the beef.[7] Additionally, the intra-particulate distribution of F_o values showed that the periphery and center had experienced similar temperature–time profiles (for carrots $F_o = 23.1$–44.0 and the center $F_o = 30.8$–40.2; for beef $F_o = 28.0$–38.5 and the center $F_o = 34.0$–36.5). Particulates were heated by electrical resistance and not simply by conductive heat transfer from the carrier liquid.

Other tests with a commercial facility demonstrated[6] that after ohmic heating the particulates transferred sufficient heat to the liquid to increase the liquid temperature eight degrees in the third holding tube. Accordingly, microbiological measurements and intrinsic chemical analysis verified that the particulate center experienced a higher temperature–time profile than the particulate surface.[7] In a bench-top ohmic heating set-up, configuring whey protein gels samples to mimic equivalent electrical circuits and manipulating the relative electrical conductivity of each phase by the addition of electrolytes also demonstrated the capacity to heat the food solids faster than the liquid phase.[10] Heating the particulates faster than the liquid can ensure greater lethality in the solids, which means that the carrier liquid can serve as a convenient monitor of sterility for regulatory purposes, although it is recommended that validation be carried out with each type of food product in order to establish the correct temperature–time profile and ensure a safe, stable product.

19.3.1 Effect of electrical conductivity on heating rate

Ohmic heating is considered very suitable for thermal processing of particulates-in-liquid foods because the particulates heated simultaneously at similar or faster rates than the liquid.[11-15] However, a number of critical factors affect the heating of mixtures of particulates and liquids. For commercial ohmic heating facilities, the control factors are[16] flow rate, temperature, heating rate, and holding time of the process. The factors influencing the heating in the food are the size ($2.54\,cm^3$), shape (cubes, spheres, discs, rods, rectangles, twists), orientation, specific heat capacity, density (20–80%), and thermal and electrical conductivity for the particle, and the viscosity, addition of electrolytes, thermal and electrical conductivity, and specific heat capacity of the carrier medium. The electrical conductivity and its temperature dependence are very significant factors in ohmic heating for determining the heating rate of the product.

Generally, samples with higher conductivities show higher heating rates, with variations in heating rates in different materials most probably caused by differences in specific heat.[16] When the product has more than one phase, such as in the case of a mixture of particulates and liquid, the respective electrical conductivity of all the phases must be considered. The solid particulates usually have smaller electrical conductivities than the carrier liquid. Interestingly, the heating patterns are not a simple function of the relative electrical conductivities of the particulates and liquids. When a single particulate with an electrical conductivity much lower than the carrying liquid is undergoing ohmic heating, the liquid is heated faster than the particulate. However, when the density of the particulates in the mixture is increased, the heating rate for the particulates will increase, and even exceed that for the liquid.[17]

The electrical conductivity of particulates or liquids increases linearly with temperature.[18,19] Differences in the electrical resistance (and its temperature dependence) between the two phases can make the heating characteristics of the system even more complicated. Furthermore, the orientation of particulates in the carrier liquid has a very strong effect on the heating rates of the particulate phase and liquid phase.[17,20-23] Since electrical conductivity is influenced by ionic content, it is possible to adjust the electrical conductivity of the product (both phases) with ion (e.g., salts) levels to achieve balanced ohmic heating and avoid overprocessing.[15,24,25]

Ohmic heating 411

It should be noted that although the conductivity of each component plays a role in how the total product heats, knowing the total electrical conductivity of a food product is insufficient to characterise how individual particulates heat. For instance, fats and syrups are electrical insulators, and strong brines, pickles, and acidic solutions have high conductivities. Heating might not be uniform because the conductivity of the individual types of particulates may vary (meats, vegetables, pastas, fruits) or because a particulate might be heterogeneous (meat interspersed with fat). Non-uniform heating patterns could potentially create cold spots that promote the growth of vegetative pathogenic microorganisms such as *Salmonella, Listeria, Clostridia,* and *Campylobacter.* Since microbial destruction occurs in response to heating irrespective of its mode of generation (thermal, ohmic, or microwave),[26] generating an average temperature of a food product that surpasses minimal lethal requirements does not ensure the complete sterility of that product. The temperature-time profile for all regions of the food product undergoing thermal treatment must surpass sterility to ensure sterilisation of the entire food product.[27] In particular, the actual temperature–time history experienced by the coldest spot must experience sufficient heat treatment, and validation with each type of food product to establish correct temperature–time conditions to ensure a safe, stable product is therefore recommended.

19.3.2 Temperature distribution in ohmically heated foods

A heating method as complex as ohmic heating requires the development of more innovative techniques to validate its efficacy, and noninvasive MRI methods are suitable for mapping temperature distributions in samples containing water or fat. To demonstrate the unique heating patterns of the ohmic process, Fig. 19.2 shows several magnetic resonance images of a whey gel–salt solution model. These temperature maps, showing the levels and distribution of temperature were obtained using a special magnetic resonance imaging (MRI) technique called 'proton resonance frequency shift (PRF)'. The sample preparation and experiment procedures are as follows: whey gels composed of 20% Alacen whey protein powder (New Zealand Milk Products) and 80% distilled deionised water, and NaCl solution were used as models of particulate–liquid mixtures. Two samples of the model system were prepared. The sample consisted of a 305 mm long hollow cylinder of whey gel containing 1.5% NaCl and a 0.01% NaCl solution. A PVC thermal/electrical barrier was inserted into the hollow whey gel to form an isolated passage in the centre of the gel cylinder. The configuration of the model system resembled a parallel electrical circuit, which was ohmically heated by the application of an AC power supply with a constant voltage of 143 V and frequency of 50 Hz.

An experimental ohmic heating device was constructed of Plexiglas. It consisted of a Plexiglas vessel with a 43 mm inner diameter and a nylon stopper at each end. A 35 mm diameter stainless steel electrode was fixed to each of the stoppers and connected to the power supply. The distance between the two

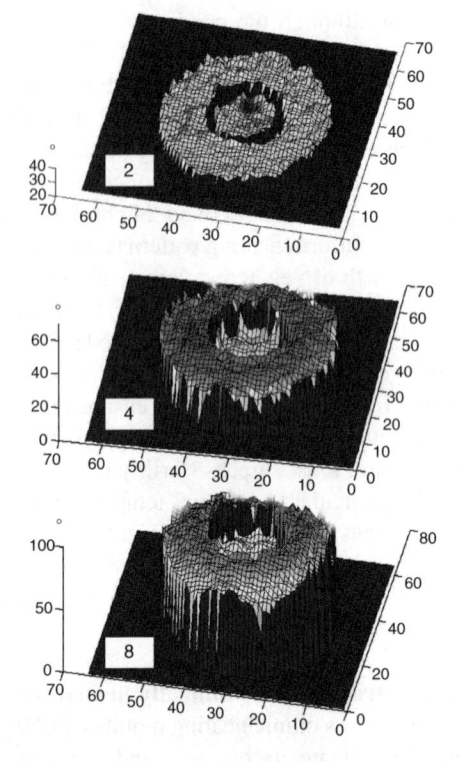

Fig. 19.2 Temperature maps of whey gel during ohmic heating (2, 4, and 8 min).

electrodes was 305 mm. A small hole was drilled in one of the stoppers of the Plexiglas vessel to allow the release of pressure build-up during heating. Two fluorescent fiber-optic temperature sensors were inserted through the holes into the whey gel and the solution at the same cross-sectional location that would be scanned to monitor the temperature for calibration. The absolute accuracy of the fiber-optic measurements was ±0.2°C. The use of these non-metal temperature sensors eliminated MR susceptibility artifacts.

The temperature maps shown in Fig. 19.2 were obtained at 2, 4 and 8 minutes during heating. The spatial resolution and temporal resolution were 0.94 mm and 0.64 sec respectively. PRF shift was linearly and reversibly proportional to the temperature change. The temperature uncertainties determined were about ±1°C for the whey gel and about ±2°C for the NaCl solution. The temperature maps show that there existed a gradient in the radial direction. The existence of this gradient is due to the internal heat generation of the ohmic heating process and the radiation heat transfer from particle surface through the vessel wall to the ambient. Therefore, the cold spots of the particle should be the surfaces and corners.

19.4 The effect of ohmic heating on nutrient loss: thermal destruction

Since systematic research on ohmic heating has a much shorter history than has conventional heating, food scientists and technologists might look to microwave heating for information on nutrient changes. In general, many improvements in nutritional quality were found using microwaves (cooking in a minimum of water retained more K, vitamin B_{12}, and vitamin C, and the absence of surface browning retained more amino acid availability, especially lysine), and microwave heating induces no significant effects different to those induced by conventional heating.[11]

The benefit of attaining food safety with less nutrient degradation using HTST processes such as ohmic heating or microwave heating is based on differences in the kinetics parameters (k, z, Ea) for bacterial spores compared to those for biochemical reactions.[28] First, rate constants for microbial destruction are usually much larger than those for the chemical reactions responsible for nutrient degradation, and second, rate constants for microbial destruction are usually more sensitive to temperature increases (z(thiamin) = 48, z(peroxidase) = 36.1, and z(*C. botulinum*) = 10°C).[29] Methods for rapidly reaching the target temperatures therefore tend to destroy microorganisms while giving less time to compromise the nutrient content and other quality attributes.[26,30] In fact, the slow heating rate associated with conventional retorting can activate protease to degrade myofibrillar proteins before the protease is eventually heat-inactivated.[31] Tests for conventional heating showed[9] that heating large (25 mm) particulates in a liquid medium at 135°C to achieve F_o = 5 at the particulate center required extensive overprocessing of the liquid phase (F_o = 150 for the liquid). For this reason, the common process conditions for scraped surface heat exchangers are maximum particulate sizes of 15 mm and sterilisation temperatures of 125–130°C (producing liquid F_o = 25) while limiting particulates to 30–40% so that there is enough hot liquid available to heat particulates. For ohmic heating, direct heating sterilisation temperatures can reach 140°C (the temperature limit of plastics in the machinery) without grossly overheating the liquid phase and can support greater particulate loading suspended in highly viscous carrier liquids. For comparative purposes, conventional heating at 130°C to produce a lethality of F_o = 8 produced a cook value Co (based on thiamin degradation) of Co = 8, whereas ohmic heating at 140°C produced F_o = 24 and Co = 4.

Vitamin losses in foods are determined by the temperature and the moisture of the applied heating method. Vitamin C is particularly temperature sensitive and destroyed at relatively low temperatures,[32] so heating foods must be for as short a time as possible to retain the vitamin C. Thiamin and riboflavin are unstable at higher temperatures such as those used in rapid grilling.[3] Vitamin C is also water soluble and can be lost when cooking with moist heat or by autooxidation with dissolved oxygen in the food or cooking water. This reaction is catalysed by adventitious iron and copper ions. By comparison, thiamin is the most water soluble vitamin, and vitamin A and vitamin D are water insoluble. Unfortunately, studies on food nutrients affected by ohmic heating are sparse in the literature. Ohmic heating is an effective method to pasteurise milk (220V, 15kW AC, C electrodes-70 C for 15 seconds) and has been used successfully to produce quality viscous products and to foods containing various combinations of particulates such as meat, vegetables, pastas, or fruits in a viscous medium,[33] including a wide variety of high acid (ratatouille, pasta sauce and vegetables, vegetables Provençale, fruit compote, strawberries, apple sauce, sliced kiwi fruit) and low acid (tortelline in tomato sauce, cappaletti in basil sauce, tagliatelle a la crème, beef bourguignonne, Beijing lamb, beef and vegetable stew, lamb Wala Gosht, vegetable curry, minestrone soup concentrate) food products. Sensory evaluations of ohmically heated food dishes such as carbonara sauce, California Beijing beef, winter soup, mushroom à la Greque, ratatouille, and cappaletti in tomato sauce produced good to very good ratings.[34]

Recent published data[35] compared the application of conventional and ohmic heating on the kinetics of ascorbic acid degradation in pasteurised orange juice exposed to identical temperature–time profiles in each case. The reaction followed pseudo-first-order kinetics and the kinetics parameters obtained from the Arrhenius plot in each case are similar. The data also indicate that ascorbic acid degrades as a result of thermal treatment and that the electric field contributed no additional influence on the degradation of the vitamin. Yongsawatdigul and co-workers[36,37] in their studies on gel functionality of Pacific whiting surimi found that ohmic heating can rapidly inactivate protease to avoid the enzymatic degradation of myofibrillar proteins, and hence increases the gel functionality of Pacific whiting surimi without the addition of enzyme inhibitors. Ohmic heating has been found to inactivate other enzymes.[38,39] Enzyme inactivation should help prevent or reduce enzymatic degradation of nutrients. However, more studies are warranted.

There are several reports on relationships between ohmic heating and changes in properties of carbohydrates and fats. These studies did not directly address the nutrition issues of ohmically heated foods, although the physical changes that occur during ohmic heating affect the heating characteristics of the solids and liquids, which may have impact on thermal destruction of nutrients. Halden et al[40] suggested that changes in starch transition, melting of fats and cell structure changes of the food material were responsible for changes in electrical conductivity that influenced the heating rate in foods such as potato during ohmic heating. In conventional thermal processes, starch gelatinisation was found to cause rheological and structural changes, and similar changes were observed for ohmic heating. Wang and Sastry[41] indicated that ohmic heating caused significant changes in physical properties including viscosity, heat capacity, thermal and electrical conductivity. They found that conductivity decreased with degree of gelatinisation. When we design ohmic heating processes, we must take changes in electrical conductivity caused by physical property changes of major compounds such as starch, fats and proteins into account so that no significant undercooking of solids or over-cooking occurs.

19.5 The effect of ohmic heating on nutrient loss: diffusion

Studies[40,42] have shown that compared with conventional heating, ohmic heating enhanced diffusion of charged species between solid particles and the surrounding liquid, which could have some impact on loss of nutrients from solid particles to carrier liquid. This becomes undesirable only if the carrier liquid is not to be consumed together with the solid particles.

Figure 19.3 shows that the transfer of betanin dye between beetroot and the surrounding fluid increases linearly with applied electric fields. One explanation for the differences in this phenomenon between the ohmic heating and conventional heating is 'electroosmosis,'[43] which results in increased transport through the cell membrane.

Another mechanism, 'electroporation', may also be responsible for enhanced diffusion between plant tissues and the surrounding liquid. When an electric field is applied across a membrane, it causes an induced membrane potential. When the induced membrane potential reaches a critical level, membrane ruptures occur, resulting in the formation of pores in the cell membrane,[44,45] and consequently increased permeability.

On the other hand, ohmic heating is superior over conventional heating in the case of blanching of plant tissues such as vegetables.[46] The loss of soluble solids in water blanching of vegetables affects both the quality and nutrition of the products. In addition, blanching water containing a large amount of soluble solids

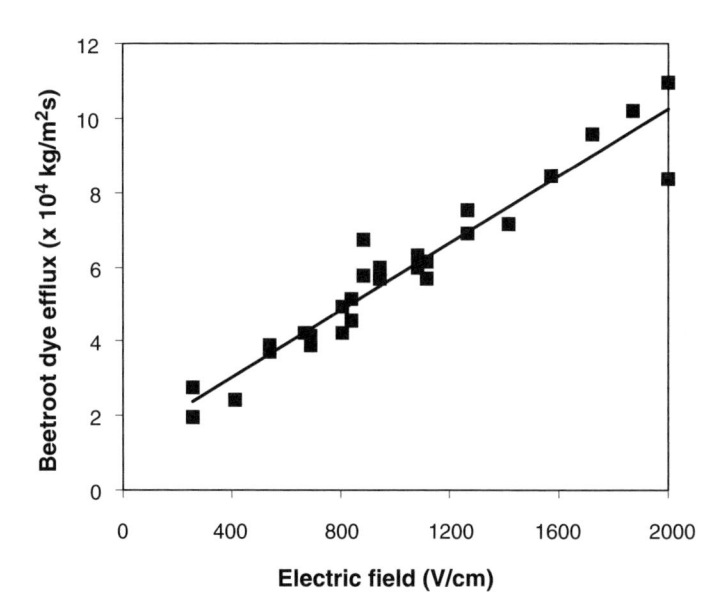

Fig. 19.3 Diffusion of betanin dye between solid beetroot and surrounding fluid as a function of applied electric field.[42]

cannot be discharged without proper treatment. Mizrahi[46] compared hot water blanching and ohmic heating blanching. Hot water blanching was carried out by placing sliced or diced beet into boiling water and taking water samples every 30 seconds; blanching by ohmic heating was done by immersing whole, sliced or diced beets in an aqueous salt solution and passing an AC voltage through the medium. Betanine and betalamic acid concentration in the samples were determined. Solute leaching with both methods followed a similar pattern, and was proportional to the surface to volume ratio and the square root of the process time. By removing the need for dicing and shortening the process time, ohmic heating blanching considerably reduced by one order of magnitude the loss of solutes during blanching of vegetables.

19.6 Electrolysis and contamination

Another factor we must consider is electrolysis, particularly the dissolution of metallic (stainless steel) electrodes at 50–60 Hz, which could contaminate the finished products, and/or contribute to undesirable chemical reactions. Several measures have been taken to circumvent this problem. For example, commercial facilities using frequencies above 100 kHz showed no apparent indications of metal hydrolysis after 3 years (the industry safety standard). Low frequencies such as 50 or 60 Hz power can be used with inert carbon or coated electrodes without causing noticeable dissolution. Some new plastic materials with suitable electrical and mechanical properties can be used for housing the electrodes and for lining the stainless steel pipes through which food products flow.

19.7 Future trends

We have demonstrated that ohmic heating is a very unique thermal process. Ohmic heating is considered a 'minimal process' besides the 'HTST' process. Potential uses of ohmic heating include:[15,47–50]

1. Cooking.
2. Sterilisation and pasteurisation.
3. Blanching.
4. Thawing.
5. Baking.
6. Enhanced diffusion.

However, as mentioned earlier, there has been only limited research quantifying the potential benefits of ohmic heating processes in terms of nutrition preservation. More research is needed to realize the advantages of ohmic heating and to promote the commercialisation of the process.

There are other major challenges hindering the commercialisation of the ohmic heating process. They are: (1) lack of temperature monitoring techniques for locating cold/hot spots in continuous throughput systems, (2) differences in electrical conductivity between the liquid and solid phases, and their dynamic responses to temperature changes, which cause irregular heating patterns and complexity and difficulty in predicting or modeling heating characteristics of particulates in carrier medium, and (3) a lack of data concerning the critical factors affecting heating (residence time distribution, particulate orientation, ratio of electrical conductivity, loading rates, etc.).

These problems must be addressed before the process can be fully commercialised and gain approval from FDA. Below are listed some areas identified as research priorities for ohmic heating processing.

19.7.1 Quantification of effect of ohmic heating on major nutrients

As mentioned earlier, there is serious lack of data demonstrating the changes in major nutrients in food products and quantifying the advantages of ohmic heating over conventional heating in terms of nutrition retention. Kinetic studies are desirable to provide information that will be useful for process and product design. Occasionally, improvements in product throughput 'accidentally' result in better nutrient retention and sensory quality attributes, and directed studies on optimising critical process factors to achieve food safety and improve nutrition retention with ohmic heating are highly recommended.

19.7.2 Reliable modeling and prediction of ohmic heating patterns

Predicting the heating patterns of ohmic heating is a very difficult task because of its unique heating characteristics. The heating rate is critically dependent on parameters such as the electrical conductivity, temperature dependence of electrical conductivity, and volumetric specific heat. Furthermore, possible heat channeling, causing hot spots and cold spots, complex coupling between temperature and electrical field distributions, and sensitivity to process parameters, e.g. residence time distribution, particle shape and orientation, etc., all contribute to the complexity of the process. To ensure sterilisation, the heating behavior of the food must be known. Without the information, process validation – an actual demonstration of the accuracy reliability, and safety of the process – is impossible.

Mathematical modeling allows insight into the heating behavior of the process. Spatial and temporal temperature distribution obtained from a reliable mathematical model which incorporates the critical factors can provide information for the calculation of lethality and cook value. It will also save time and money for validation experiments, process and product design. Modeling of a continuous ohmic heating process is extremely difficult due to a number of different physical phenomena occuring during the heating process. De Alwis, Fryer, Sastry, Palaniappan, and their co-workers are pioneers in modeling the ohmic heating process. Their published models have been used to predict the temperature within particles for very specific heating conditions. The models are of limited usefulness in establishing the heating characteristics of a commercial product because of their inability to model a multicomponent system undergoing a continuous process. The verification of the models is also limited in selected regions within the system. Another limitation is the lack of understanding about some interactions within the system. For example, limited information is available for the temperature dependence of the electrical conductivity, and a reliable method does not exist to measure the convective heat transfer coefficient at the liquid–particle interface. These types of limitations require that actual physical measurements of the temperature of the product and its constituents be conducted when establishing a process. Some of these limitations can be compensated for by using appropriate conservative assumptions at the expense of the product quality. A more accurate and reliable model is needed.

19.7.3 Well-defined product specifications and process parameters

Product specification includes information that defines the product and its physical/chemical aspects that play important roles in determining how much lethal treatment is delivered during the process. Critical factors may include particle size and shape, liquid viscosity, pH, specific heat, thermal conductivity, solid liquid ratio, and electrical conductivity. It is also important to know how these factors interact and how they are influenced by the process, for which only limited information is available.

Particulates are the centerpiece around which an ohmic heating formulation is built. Contrary to conventional heating where we would expect no difference due to the change in particle orientation, the heating pattern of an ohmically heated food system would be greatly affected by particle orientation. De Alwis and Fryer[51] showed the heating of identically-shaped potato particles parallel and perpendicular to the electrical field. The particle heating rate changed considerably as a result of the change in orientation. De Alwis and Fryer[51] explained that this uniqueness is due to the fact that the orientation of the particles changed the electrical field and thus the heating rate.

Though there seems no limit to the particle size which can be processed in an electrically uniform mixture, cooling of particulates will always be controlled by thermal conduction and the cooling rates possible may impose an upper limit on the particle size. This is important in HTST processes, since rapid cooling is desired. The center of large particles may cool too slowly and thus become overprocessed during prolonged cooling. Unlike conventional heating where the outside may be overcooked, here the inside might be. Particulate size is typically limited to $2.54\,cm^3$. Fundamental particulate considerations include size, shape, concentration, density, conductivity, and specific heat capacity. The fluid phase cannot be neglected. Liquid viscosity should be determined at various temperatures to assure adequate suspension of particulates. Moreover, the liquid viscosity may affect the liquid/particle interface heat transfer and thus the heating and cooling rates and process control. More research is needed to address and understand the many aspects of the product and process design and their effects on the product quality.

Ohmic heating 419

19.7.4 Reliable real-time temperature monitoring techniques for locating cold/hot spots

Pioneers of ohmic heating researches have documented that a particle does not heat uniformly during an ohmic heating process because of the non-uniform nature of the electric field and the food materials within the ohmic system.[52] As in other thermal processes, it is important to have information on the temperature–time history of the coldest point within the liquid–particulate system undergoing ohmic heating.

It is assumed that the agitation of a continuous system minimises these variations in temperature profiles. However, there is insufficient published evidence to indicate what the temperature is within a particle, let alone how the temperature profile changes during a continuous process. It does appear that for a particle with a homogeneous electrical conductivity, if the particle heats faster than the liquid phase, the particle's coldest spot is at its surface.[53] There is little published information for particles with heterogeneous electrical conductivity (i.e., fatty meat). The location of the coldest spot is especially important because that is the place where the thermal lethality must be ensured and this is the key factor in determining the processing time. Conventional tools such as thermocouple and optic fiber are apparently invasive when used to measure the ohmic heated food system. A non-destructive and non-invasive technique which can be used to monitor the spatial distribution of temperature is important for understanding and control of ohmic heating technology. In addition, a non-destructive and non-invasive temperature mapping technique is essential for the model development and the validation of this novel process. MRI seems to be a valid approach to this problem. There is a need to improve the technique further, to collect more data under various product specifications and processing conditions with the technique, and to use this technique to validate mathematical models.

19.8 Sources of further information and advice

Specific information can be found in the cited references provided in section 19.9. The following research institutes have major research programs on ohmic heating:

(1) Department of Food, Agricultural, and Biological Engineering, The Ohio State University, expertise: ohmic heating in general, and mathematical modeling, contact: Professor S.K. Sastry
(2) Department of Chemical Engineering, University of Birmingham, Birmingham, UK, expertise: general and mathematical modeling, contact: Professor P. Fryer
(3) US Army Soldier Command, Natick RD&E Center, expertise: general and temperature mapping, contact: Dr. Irwin Taub, Dr. Christopher Doona
(4) Department of Biosystems and Agricultural Engineering and Department of Food Science and Nutrition, University of Minnesota, expertise: MRI temperature mapping and mathematical modeling, contact: Professor R. Ruan

19.9 References

1. DONELAN A and DOBSON D (2001), 'Vitamin retention in prepared meal services', *Food Service Technol*, **1**, 123–4
2. WILLIAMS P (1996), 'Vitamin retention in cook/chill and cook/hot-hold hospital foodservices', *Journal of the American Dietetic Assoc*, **96**, 490–8
3. RANESH M N (1999), 'Food preservation by heat treatment', in *Handbook of Food Preservation*, R S Rahman (ed), New York, Marcel Dekker, 95–172
4. SKUDDER P J (1988), 'Ohmic heating: new alternative for aseptic processing of viscous foods', *Food Engineering*, **60**(1), 99–101
5. NOTT K P and HALL L D (1999), 'Advances in temperature validation of foods', *Trends in Food Science and Technology*, **10**, 366–74
6. ZUBER F (1997), 'Ohmic heating: a new technology for stabilising ready-made dishes', *Viandes et Produits Carnes*, **18**(2), 91–5
7. KIM H-J, CHOI Y-M, YANG T C S, TAUB I A, TEMPEST P, SKUDDER P, TUCKER G and PARROTT D (1996), 'Validation of ohmic heating for quality enhancement of food products', *Food Technology*, 253–61
8. KIM H J, CHOI Y M, YANG A P P, YANG T C S, TAUB I A, GILES J, DITUSA C, CHALL S and ZOLTAI P (1996), 'Microbiological and chemical investigation of ohmic heating of particulate foods using a 5kW ohmic system', *Journal of Food Processing and Preservation*, **20**(1), 41–58
9. TEMPEST P (1992), *Experience with Ohmic Heating and Aseptic Packaging of Particulate Foods*. Technical Report. No. PT/FBD1368. Crawley, UK: APV Baker Ltd., Automation Process Division
10. DOONA C J, TAUB I A, KANDLIKAR S, RUAN R and YE X (2001), *Mapping Temperature Distribution in Ohmically Heated Whey Protein Gels 'Electrical Circuits'* in IFT Annual Meeting, New Orleans, LA, June 20–5, Chicago, Ill, Institute of Food Technologists
11. ANON (1988), 'Ohmic heating: a breakthrough in profitable food manufacture', *Food Review*, **15**(5), 27
12. KIM H J, CHOI Y M, HESKITT B, SASTRY S K and LI Q (1995), *Chemical and Microbiological Investigation of Ohmic Heating of Particulate Foods Using a Static Ohmic Heater* in IFT Annual Meeting
13. RUAN R, CHEN P, CHANG K, KIM H J and TAUB I A (1999), 'Rapid food particle temperature mapping during ohmic heating using FLASH MRI', *Journal of Food Science*, **64**(6), 1024–6
14. ZITOUN K B (1997), 'Continuous flow of solid-liquid food mixtures during ohmic heating: fluid interstitial velocities, solid area fraction, orientation and rotation', *Dissertation Abstracts International, B*, **57**(7)
15. ZOLTAI P and SWEARINGEN P (1996), 'Product development considerations for ohmic processing', *Food Technol*, **50**(5), 263–6
16. PALANIAPPAN S and SASTRY S K (1991), 'Electrical conductivities of selected solid foods during ohmic heating', *Journal of Food Process Engineering*, **14**(3), 221–36
17. SASTRY S K and PALANIAPPAN S (1992), 'Mathematical modeling and experimental studies on ohmic heating of liquid-particle mixtures in a static heater', *Journal of Food Process Engineering*, **15**(4), 241–61
18. WANG W C and SASTRY S K (1997), 'Changes in electrical conductivity of selected vegetables during multiple thermal treatments', *Journal of Food Process Engineering*, **20**(6), 499–516
19. DE ALWIS A A P and FRYER P J (1992), 'Operability of the ohmic heating process: electrical conductivity effects', *Journal of Food Engineering*, **15**(1), 21–48
20. SASTRY S K and PALANIAPPAN S (1992), 'Influence of particle orientation on the effective electrical resistance and ohmic heating rate of a liquid-particle mixture', *Journal of Food Process Engineering*, **15**(3), 213–27

21 ZITOUN K B and SASTRY S K (1996), 'Study on solid-liquid flow food mixture during ohmic heating', *Journal of Food Science*, **46**, 1082–236
22 FRYER P J, DE ALWIS A A P, KOURY E, STAPLEY A G F and ZHANG L (1993), 'Ohmic processing of solid-liquid mixtures: heat generation and convection effects', *Journal of Food Engineering*, **18**(2), 101–25
23 FRYER P and ZHANG L (1993), 'Electrical resistance heating of foods', *Trends in Food Science and Technology*, **4**(11), 364–9
24 WANG W C and SASTRY S K (1993), 'Salt diffusion into vegetable tissue as a pretreatment for ohmic heating: electrical conductivity profiles and vacuum infusion studies', *Journal of Food Engineering*, **20**(4), 299–309
25 WANG W C and SASTRY S K (1993), 'Salt diffusion into vegetable tissue as a pretreatment for ohmic heating: determination of parameters and mathematical model verification', *Journal of Food Engineering*, **20**(4), 311–23
26 OHLSSON T and BENGTSSON N (2001), 'Microwave technology and foods', in *Advances in Food and Nutrition Research*, S L Taylor (ed), San Diego, Academic Press, 65–140
27 LARKIN J W and SPINAK S H (1996), 'Safety consideration for ohmically heated, aseptically processed, multiphase low-acid food products', *Food Technology*, 242–5
28 CHANDARANA D I and GAVIN A (1989), 'Establishing thermal processes for heterogeneous foods to be processed aseptically: a theoretical comparison of process development methods', *Journal of Food Science*, **54**(1), 198–204
29 KIM H-J and TAUB I A (1993), 'Intrinsic chemical markers for aseptic processing of particulate foods', *Food Technology*, **47**(1), 91–7
30 WATANABE F, ABE K, FUJITA T, GOTO M, HIEMORI M and NAKANO Y (1998), 'Effects of microwave heating on the loss of vitamin B_{12} in foods', *Journal of Agricultural Food Chemistry*, **46**, 206–10
31 RAHMAN M S (1999), 'Preserving foods with electricity: ohmic heating', in *Handbook of Food Preservation*, M S Rahman (ed), New York, Marcel Dekker, 528–32
32 HENSHALL J D (1981), 'Ascorbic acid in fruit juices and beverages', in *Vitamin C (ascorbic acid)*, J N Counsell and D H Hornig (eds), Englewood, Applied Science Publishers, Chapter 8
33 ZOLTAI P and SWEARINGEN P (1996), 'Product development considerations for ohmic processing', *Food Technology*, 263–6
34 YANG T C S, COHEN J S, KLUTER R, TEMPEST P, MANVEL C, BLACKMORE S and ADAMS S (1997), 'Microbiological and sensory evaluation of six ohmicaly heated slew type foods', *J of Food Quality*, **20**, 303–13
35 LIMA M, HESKITT B F, BURIANEK L L, NOKES S E and SASTRY S K (1999), 'Ascorbic acid degradation kinetics during conventional and ohmic heating', *Journal of Food Processing and Preservation*, **23**(5), 421–34
36 YONGSAWATDIGUL J, PARK J W, KOLBE E, ABU DAGGA Y and MORRISSEY M T (1995), 'Ohmic heating maximizes gel functionality of Pacific whiting surimi', *Journal of Food Science*, **60**(1), 10–14
37 YONGSAWATDIGUL J, PARK J W and KOLBE E (1996), 'Kinetics of myosin heavy chain degradation of Pacific whiting surimi', *Journal of Food Science*, **144**, 1082–236
38 PALANIAPPAN S, SASTRY S K and RICHTER E R (1990), 'Effects of electricity on microorganisms: a review', *Journal of Food Process Preservation*, Oct, 393–414
39 MIZRAHI S, KOPELMAN I J and PERLMAN J (1975), 'Blanching by electro-conductive heating', *Journal of Food Technology*, **10**(3), 281–8
40 HALDEN K, DE ALWIS A A P and FRYER P J (1990), 'Changes in the electrical conductivity of foods during ohmic heating', *International Journal of Food Science and Technology*, **25**(1), 9–25
41 WANG W C and SASTRY S K (1997), 'Starch gelatinization in ohmic heating', *Journal of Food Engineering*, **34**(3), 225–42
42 SCHREIER P J R, REID D G and FRYER P J (1993), 'Enhanced diffusion during electrical heating of foods', *International Journal of Food Science and Technology*, **28**, 249

43 BARRY P H and HOPE A B (1969), 'Electroosmosis in membranes: effect of unstirred layers and transport numbers', *Biophysics Journal*, **9**, 700
44 KINOSHITA M, HIBINO M and ITOH H (1992), 'Events of membrane electroporation visualization on a time scale from microsecond to seconds', in *Guide to Electroporation and Electrofusion*, D C Chang, B M Chassy, J A Saunders and A E Sowers (eds), New York, Academic Press, 24
45 SOWERS A E (1992), 'Mechanisms for electroporation and electrofusion', in *Guide to Electroporation and Electrofusion*, D C Chang, B M Chassy, J A Saunders and A E Sowers (eds), New York, Academic Press, 119
46 MIZRAHI S (1996), 'Leaching of soluble solids during blanching of vegetables by ohmic heating', *Journal of Food Engineering*, **29**(2), 153–66
47 DE ALWIS A A P and FRYER P J (1990), 'The use of direct resistance heating in the food industry', *Journal of Food Engineering*, **11**, 3–27
48 PARROTT D L (1992), 'Use of ohmic heating for aseptic processing of food particulates', *Food Technology*, **46**(12), 68–72
49 ANJU B and JOSHI V K (1998), 'Ohmic processing of foods, the concept, application, present status and future outlook', *Alimentaria*, No. **83–88**, 32
50 SASTRY S K (1992), 'Application of ohmic heating to continuous sterilization of food', *Indian Food Industry*, **11**(4), 28–30
51 DE ALWIS A A P and FRYER P J (1990), 'A finite element analysis of heat generation and transfer during ohmic heating of foods', *Chemical Engineering Science*, **45**(2), 1547–59
52 FRYER P J, DE ALWIS A A P, KOURY E, STAPLEY A G F and ZHANG L (1993), 'Ohmic processing of solid-liquid mixtures: heat generation and convection effects', *Journal of Food Engineering*, **18**(2), 101–25
53 SASTRY S K and PALANIAPPAN S (1992), 'Ohmic heating of liquid-particle mixtures', *Food Technology*, **46**(12), 64–7

20
Infrared processing
C. Skjöldebrand, ABB and Lund University, Sweden

20.1 Introduction: the principles of infrared heating

Sir William Herschel discovered infrared – or heat radiation – in the 1800s when he was attempting to determine the part of the visible spectrum with the minimum associated heat in connection with the astronomical observations he was making. In 1847 AHL Fizeau and JBL Foucault showed that infrared radiation has the same properties as visible light. It was being reflected, refracted and was capable of forming an interference pattern (Encyclopedia Internet, 2000). There are many applications of infrared radiation. A number of these are analogous to the use of visible light. Thus, the spectrum of a substance in the infrared range can be used in chemical analysis much as the visible spectrum is used. Radiation at discrete wavelengths in the infrared range is characteristic of many molecules. The temperature of a distant object can also be determined by analysis of the infrared radiation from the object.

Medical uses of infrared radiation range from the simple heat lamp to the technique of thermal imaging, or thermographs. It has also been used for drying dye and lacquer for cars, glue for wallpaper, paper in paper machines, and dye to plastic details, as well as shrinkage of plastics and activation of glue in the plastic industry, etc.

The electromagnetic spectra within infrared wavelengths can be divided into 3 parts; long waves (4 μm to 1 mm), medium waves (2–4 μm) and short waves (0.7–2 μm). The short waves appear when temperatures are above 1000°C, the long waves appear below 400°C and the medium waves appear between these temperatures. The electromagnetic spectrum is shown in Fig. 20.1 (Anon, *The Infrared Handbook*). For food the technique has been used in many applications, as the long waves are one of the main heat transfer mechanisms in ordinary ovens or other heating equipment. Short waves are new for the food industry.

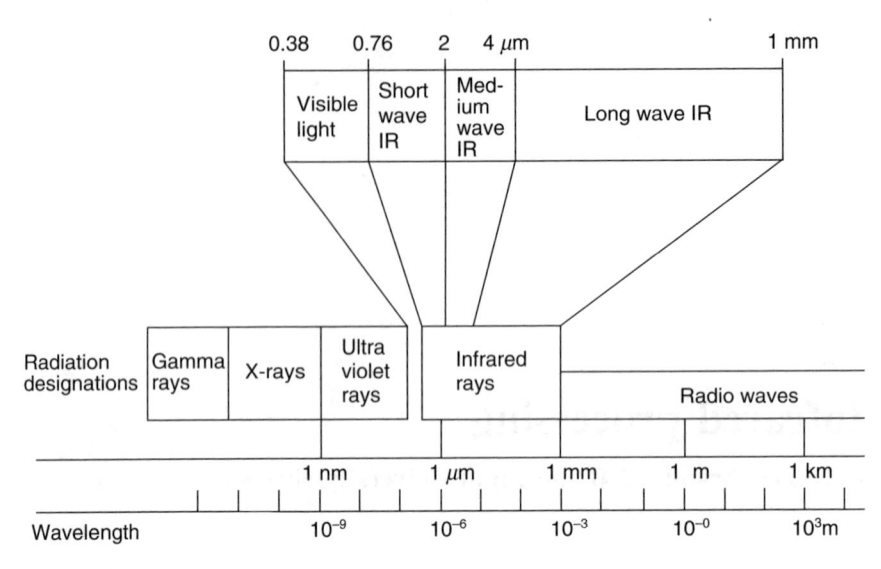

Fig. 20.1 The electromagnetic spectrum (Anon, *The Infrared Handbook*).

In the USSR in the 1950s AV Lykow and others reported the results of their theoretical and experimental studies of infrared drying (Ginzburg, 1969). In the 1960s W Jubitz carried out substantial work on infrared heating in East Germany and in France M Dáribéré and J Leconte did some work on different applications of infrared irradiation in various industries. During this time IS Pavlov in the Soviet Union carried out a lot of work on infrared heating and food. Long wave radiation was already used in the United States during the 1950s in many industrial food processes.

During the early 1970s there were many discussions concerning finding new methods for industrial frying/cooking meat products (Skjöldebrand, 1986). Deep fat frying, the process most often used in industrial frying, was criticised because of the fat and flavour exchange and surface appearance. Also, environmental and nutritional aspects had to be considered. The consumer also wanted products more like the ones cooked at home. One of the new techniques discussed was near infrared heating (NIR) or short wave infrared heating. This technique is used in the car industry for drying coatings, as well as the paper and textile industries. Thus, like many other processes in the food industry, infrared heating was transferred from other industries. Therefore, why has short wave infrared radiation not been used before? The answer is that there was a lack of knowledge about many of the factors concerning this process. The radiators, the reflectors and the different systems for cassettes were developed during the 1960s but there was not very much knowledge about the optical properties of the foodstuffs and how these develop during processing. The problems then were also braking the radiators and cleaning the equipment.

During the 1970s and 1980s most of the research work on food was carried out in Sweden at the Swedish Institute for Food and Biotechnology (SIK) (Dagerskog and Österström, 1979; Skjöldebrand, 1986; Skjöldebrand and Andersson, 1989).

In this chapter the application of infrared processing in the food industry will cover the following areas:

- Examples of applications in the food industry;
- The infrared process and its impact on quality;
- The infrared process and its impact on nutrition;
- Future outlook.

20.2 Infrared processing in the food industry

The basic concepts of infrared radiation are:

- High heat transfer capacity;
- Heat penetration directly into the product;
- Fast regulation response;
- Good possibilities for process control;
- No heating of surrounding air.

These qualities indicate that infrared radiation should be an ideal source of energy for heating purposes (Skjöldebrand, 1986).

Distinguished from microwave heating, the penetration properties of infrared radiation are such that a suitable balance for surface and body heating can be reached, which is necessary for an optimal heating result. Some empirical work in this field can be found in the literature by Ginzburg for example (Ginzburg, 1969). The penetration properties are important for optimising the system. The penetration depth is defined as 37% of the unabsorbed radiation energy. For short waves, the penetration ability is ten times higher than for long waves. The direct penetration ability of infrared radiation makes it possible to increase the energy flux without burning the surface and thus reduces the necessary heating time that conventional heating methods require. This is especially true for thin products.

In a special study, a method was developed to determine optical properties of bread at different degrees of baking (Skjöldebrand et al, 1988). The results showed that the transmission by the crust was less than in the crumb. Even the thinnest dough sample did not transmit any radiation.

Reflection curves for crust and dough are very similar while reflection for the crumb is about 10–15% less. Table 20.1 shows calculated penetration depths for crust and crumb for radiators used in baking ovens. Measurements have been carried out for other foods and Table 20.2 shows some examples (Dagerskog and Österström, 1979).

In infrared (IR) heating, heat is transferred by radiation, the wavelength of which is determined by the temperature of the body – the higher the temperature, the shorter the wavelength. Present interest in industrial heating applications centres on short wave IR (wavelengths around 1 μm) and intermediate IR (around

Table 20.1 The calculated penetration depths for crust and crumb for radiators used in baking ovens (Skjöldebrand et al, 1988)

Power level (%)	Maximum energy wavelength	Spectral range (nm)	Penetration depth	
			Crumb	Crust
100	1300	800–1250	3.8	2.5
		1250–2500	1.4	0.6
		800–2500	1.9	1.2
75	1320	800–1250	3.8	2.5
		1250–2500	1.4	0.6
		800–2500	1.9	1.1
50	1410	800–1250	3.8	2.5
		1250–2500	1.4	0.6
		800–2500	1.8	1.1

Table 20.2 Measured penetration depths for some foods (Dagerskog and Österström, 1979)

Product	Radiation source $\lambda_{max}(\mu m)$	Penetration depth		
		Wavelength range (μm)		
		$\lambda < 1.25$	$1.25 < \lambda < 1.51$	$\lambda > 1.51$
Potato	1.12	4.76	0.48	0.33
Potato	1.24	4.17	0.47	0.31
Pork	1.12	2.38	0.28	
Bread	1.12	6.25	1.52	

10 µm), since these wavelengths make it possible to start up and reach working temperatures in seconds, while also offering rapid transfer of high amounts of energy and excellent process control. In some food materials, short wave IR demonstrate penetration depths of up to 5 mm.

The most popular industrial applications (for non-food uses) are in the rapid drying of automobile paint and drying in the paper and pulp industry. For paper drying IR has superseded microwaves because it offers superior process control and economy. IR technology has long been underestimated in the food field, despite its great potential. Most applications of IR within the area of food came during the 1950s to 1970s from the USA, the USSR and the eastern European countries. During the 1970s and 1980s SIK did a lot of basic work applying this technique within the area of food. In later years work was carried out in Japan, Taiwan and other countries.

The main part of this work is still of an experimental nature. Applications are mainly in the following areas:

- Drying vegetables and fish;
- Drying pasta and rice;

- Heating flour;
- Frying meat;
- Roasting cereals;
- Roasting coffee;
- Roasting cocoa;
- Baking pizza, biscuits and bread.

The technique has also been used for thawing, surface pasteurisation of bread and surface pasteurisation of packaging materials.

The main commercial applications of IR heating are drying low moisture foods (for example breadcrumbs, cocoa, flours, grains, malt, pasta products and tea). The technique is often used at the start of the whole process to speed up the first increase in surface temperature. Such processes are frying, baking and drying. The effect of radiation intensity (0.125, 0.250, 0.375 and 0.500 W/cm^2) and slab thickness (2.5, 6.5 and 10.5 mm) on the moisture diffusion coefficient of potatoes during far IR drying have been investigated by Afzal and Abe in 1998 in Japan. They found that the diffusivity increased with increasing radiation intensity and with slab thickness. In contrast, activation energy for moisture desorption decreased with increasing slab thickness and resulted in higher drying rates for slabs of greater thicknesses. Some more specific examples will be described below.

20.2.1 Baking

When baking with infrared radiation it seems that short wave radiators should be used. The short wave infrared radiation may be combined with convection for drying the surface with good results.

Ginzburg divided the baking process using infrared radiation into three periods:

1. The first phase is characterised by an increase in the surface temperature (1–2°C) to 100°C. Very little weight loss occurs during this period.
2. The second period is characterised by the start of mass transfer. An evaporation zone forms, which moves towards the central parts. Energy is used to evaporate water and to heat the dough.
3. In the third and final period the central parts have reached 90°C. The temperature increases by a further 8°C at the end of baking. The duration of this period amounts to about 25% of the total time of baking.

When comparing time–temperature relations between infrared radiation and conventional baking it is clear that IR radiation is more efficient both at the surface parts and the central sections. The following results were achieved using short wave infrared heating in the baking oven at SIK (Skjöldebrand et al, 1994):

- The baking time was 25–50% shorter compared to an ordinary baking oven. The thickness of the product determined the time saving.
- Energy consumption was comparable to ordinary baking.

- Weight losses were 10–15% lower.
- Quality was comparable.

These results show that infrared heating for bakery products is very promising compared to other heating techniques.

Further studies at SIK have shown that baking bread using the short wave infrared heating technique is a very interesting alternative to traditional baking (Skjöldebrand and Andersson, 1987). The baking time can be reduced by 25% and in some cases 50%, depending on the thickness of the product. This is due to penetration of the waves into the product. Depending on the radiators in the oven and their wavelength distribution, the penetration properties of the bread change during baking. At the start they are almost zero, with the crust having poorer penetration depth than the porous water-rich crumb. The baking time reduction is also due to the more effective heat transfer to the surface than occurs in convection or conduction heating. Using short wave infrared radiation may reduce weight losses. In some of the experiments it was found that the water content in the centre had increased during baking, causing a better and longer storage.

20.2.2 Frying meat

Several studies on frying meat by infrared radiation have been carried out by researchers in the former Soviet Union. There have also been studies carried out in Sweden. These studies have shown that maximum transmission falls in the region of the electromagnetic spectrum of $1.2\,\mu m$. For wavelengths over $2.5\,\mu m$ the transmission capacity was negligible (Bolshakov et al, 1976). Consequently it was necessary to use sources with maximum radiation falling in the region of maximum transmission to achieve deep heating of pork. For heat treatment of the product surface, radiators in the region of maximum transmission and reflectance ($\lambda > 2.3\,\mu m$) had to be used. It was recommended to design a two-stage frying process. In the first stage surface heat treatment was achieved by radiant flux with λ at maximum $1.04\,\mu m$ providing deep heat to the product. The studies showed that the final moisture content and sensory quality of the product were higher when heated by the two-stage process than by conventional methods.

20.3 Infrared processing and food quality

The improvements in bread quality from using the baking oven at SIK mentioned earlier were achieved using short wave infrared heating (Skjöldebrand et al, 1994). Suggestions have been made that radiant heating elements should be operated at temperatures between 1200 and 1800°C as only wavelengths longer than $2\,\mu m$ are effective in developing colour in particular. Successful results have also been reported for several frying applications (Dagerskog, 1978).

Four different frying methods were compared in work carried out by researchers at Lund University and at SIK. The product studied was a meat patty

(Dagerskog and Sörenfors, 1979). They studied convection, deep fat frying, contact and long wave IR, and found that from pure heat transfer considerations the four techniques gave almost equivalent results if appropriate frying conditions were used. The surface crust of the meat was, however, rather different for the four methods, influencing the sensorial experience. For IR and convection frying the crust was similar with burned areas and a skin-like surface, but the periphery of the meat patty was browned first during convection heating in contrast to IR heating, where the surface area was browned first. For flavour, no difference among the methods were found, except for deep fat frying which gave a significantly stronger 'off-flavour', probably due to the absorbed fat. The juiciness of the IR fried meat patties was rated by the panel because of the exceptionally long frying times needed, which in turn was due to the recipe. The results also showed that it was very important to have the recipe tailor-made for the technique used. In this study it was also reported that, as expected, the surface crust became darker as intensity levels grew higher. However, the total impression scores indicate an optimum at intermediate levels. The optimum levels often coincided for both texture, flavour and brightness.

When parboiling at a similar degree of heat treatment as compared with conventional technology, the infrared treatment required a shorter time (83%) with lower weight losses (50%). The flavour, colour and texture of the infrared braised meat were claimed to be far superior (Asselberg et al, 1960).

Researchers testing a baking oven in a Swedish bakery during the 1980s found that the colour for ordinary wheat bread was very good and acceptable but the evenness could be better. This was due to the fact that radiation cannot be distributed evenly to all bread sides in an optimal way. The volume and the porosity were very good and comparable to ordinary baked bread (Skjöldebrand et al, 1988). The products tested were sweet rolls, buns, baguettes, white bread loaves and rye bread loaves. It is, however, difficult to use steam in a baking oven when using NIR as the water molecules absorb the waves. Weight losses for some of the baked products are about the same when baking in an NIR oven as in a conventional oven. However, the baking times are reduced by 25–30% when using short wave infrared radiation as a heating technique. The reduction depends on geometry and thickness of the product. In general it was found that volume increased in bread baked in an infrared oven compared to bread baked in a conventional oven.

Colour is comparable if flat bread is baked. It was found that as energy levels reach 100% white spots occur on the bread surface, due to ungelatinised starch. Also, big pores or even holes in the crumb can occur when too high energy levels are used in a baking oven based on infrared heating. However, as there is a fast response when changing energy levels, the heat transfer may be controlled to get an optimised colour on the surface.

An industrial process for pre-cooking of bacon in a continuous infrared oven at Swift & Company has been investigated by Hlavacek (1968). Electric resistance heaters below the seamless stainless steel belt supplemented the 288 kW of infrared radiant heating from overhead quartz lamps. The frying time was 2–3 minutes and pre-cooked bacon was found to taste as good or better than freshly fried bacon. The results showed that the final moisture content and sensory quality of the product heated by the two-stage process were higher than those heated by conventional methods. In Taiwan IR has also been used for dehydration of fish. Over 90% of the far IR dried products were of a higher quality than currently marked sun dried products (Wei-Renn-Lein and Wen-Rong-Fu, 1997).

20.4 Infrared processing and nutritional quality

There are very few studies in the literature on the infrared process and its impact on food nutrients. However, some of it is reported here. Comparisons between conventional heating techniques and infrared heating give some hints as to their effect on the nutritional value of heated products.

Recent studies of intense IR radiation treatment on nutritional value and anti-nutritional factors of cereals (corn, rice, brown sorghum) and common beans show that digestibility and energy values were not altered significantly but protein quality decreased (Keya-EL and Sherman U, 1997). No anti-nutritional factors were found in rice. Tannin in sorghum was denatured extensively by IR treatment. Small amounts of aflatoxins in corn and sorghum trypsin inhibitors in common beans were destroyed.

Mackerel were dried in IR radiation at 180°C for 40 minutes and the results revealed better nutritional values than after conventional treatment (Shyue-Bin-Ho, En-Chie-Lin, Fu-Jin-Wang and Sheu-Der-Wu, 1996). The Maillard reaction in the crust of bread or meat can be better controlled when using NIR heating than using grilling or frying or in an ordinary baking oven. This is due to the fast response when changing the energy levels of radiators. However, too high energy transfer at the start of the process may give white spots of ungelatinised starch.

As the IR heating technique in most applications shows shorter drying, frying or heating times for food nutrition, spoilage is less than that of most conventional techniques. The spoilage can also be controlled in a better way. Knowing the kinetics of the chemical reaction of different nutritional components and using mathematical models based on knowledge about the IR heating temperature and mass transfer is one way to optimise the nutritional value of the ready-made product (Skjöldebrand, 2000).

20.5 Future trends

The infrared technique of heating foods shows a lot of advantages compared to conventional techniques. These cover both process aspects as well as nutritional and quality aspects. However, the technique is not widely used in the industry.

- More knowledge about the interaction between processes and products needs to be gained. The relationship between raw material properties and how these are affected by the process to obtain the desired properties in the end product

Infrared processing 431

should be studied. These are necessary for the success of using new techniques like NIR or short wave infrared heating equipment.
- IR heating should be particularly useful for continuous baking, drying and grilling as well as for surface pasteurisation.
- All different heating techniques have their own limitations concerning application areas and possibilities. Good background knowledge may combine the techniques in the most optimal way. More knowledge is important for the success of the heating technique.
- The use of IR technology in the food industry is quite limited today, and the available equipment is not optimised for the various heating operations along the processing lines for baking, drying, etc. Its application is certain to grow as food equipment manufacturers begin to realise its full potential.
- Along with the development of process control and information technology the IR technique will show its full potential with fast regulation of radiators and rapid heat transfer.
- IR heating will certainly fulfil its role in the requirements of flexible production units.
- With the development of new products the heating technique will be important and used. New flavour can be created via both the recipe and the heating technique.

The combination of different heating techniques is probably a meaningful road to examine for heating of food in the most optimal way (Wählby, 2002). There are already several types of combination ovens available on the market; essentially these types of ovens are based on microwave technology with conventional technology added. From a food quality point of view this is an interesting field – how to optimise combinations of heating technologies. The IR technology should probably be used at the start of the heating procedure or a stepwise combination of different power levels should be designed. In drying the NIR technology should be used and with a stepwise change from high to low power levels.

The behaviour of food has been explored quite a bit, but the introduction of new sensing techniques (e.g. gas sensing, IR, radio and microwave) shows that there are several areas of research to be continued. By using the new sensing technologies, it may be possible to let food control the process on-line. To be able to do this, a good relationship between these sensor outputs and food quality is necessary. When this is known the quality and the nutritional value of food can be controlled better and the correct heating technique can be selected.

20.6 References

AFZAL T M and ABE T (1998), 'Diffusion in potatoes during far infrared radiation drying', *Journal of Food Engineering* **37**(4), 353–65
ANON, *The Infrared Handbook*, Philips
ASSELBERG E A, MOHR W P and KEMP J G (1960), *Food Technology* **14**, 449

BOLSHAKOV A S, BOUSKOV V G, KASULIN G N, ROGOV F A, SKRYABIN U P and ZHUKOV N N (1976), *Effects of Infrared radiation rates and conditions of preliminary processing of quality index on baked products*, 22nd European meeting of meat research workers, Malmö, Sweden

DAGERSKOG M (1978), Stekning av livsmedel pHD thesis, Gothenburg (In Swedish)

DAGERSKOG M and ÖSTERSTRÖM L (1979), *Infrared radiation for food processing. A study of the fundamental properties of infrared radiation*. Lebensmittel Wissenschaft u. Technologie **12**, 237–42

FELLOWS P (1988), *Food Processing Technology Principles and Practice* Ellis Horwood, Chichester, England and VCH, Weinheim, Germany

GINZBURG A S (1969), *Application of Infrared Radiation in Food Processing* Leonard Hill, London

HALLSTRÖM B, TRÄGÅRDH C and SKJÖLDEBRAND C (1988), *Heat transfer and food products* Elsevier Science, London

HLAVACEK R G (1968), *Food Proc.* **28**, 51

KEYA-EL and SHERMAN U (1997), 'Effects of a brief, intense infrared radiation treatment on the nutritional quality of maize, rice, sorghum and beans', *Food and Nutrition Bulletin* **18**(4), 382–7

SHYUE-BIN-HO, EN-CHIE-LIN, FU-JIN-WANG and SHEU-DER-WU (1996), 'The study on processing smoked mackerel slices by far infrared heating'. *Food Science – Taiwan* (In Chinese) **23**(6), 801–8

SKJÖLDEBRAND C (2000), 'Infrared heating' in *Thermal technologies in food processing*. Chapter 9 (Ed Philip Richardsson) p 208–28 Woodhead Publishing Ltd, Cambridge, England

SKJÖLDEBRAND C (1986), *Cooking by Infrared Radiation* In Proceedings from Progress in Food Preparation processes, p 157–73

SKJÖLDEBRAND C and ANDERSSON C G (1989), 'A comparison of infrared bread baking and conventional baking' *Journal of Microwave Power and Electromagnetic energy* **24**, 91–101

SKJÖLDEBRAND C and ANDERSSON C G (1987), *Baking using short wave infrared radiation*. Proceedings from Cereals in a European Context, First European Conference on Food Science and Technology. Chapter 7.6 (Ed ID Morton) Ellis Horwood, Chichester, UK, p 364–76

SKJÖLDEBRAND C and FALK C (1990), *Development of a simulation programme for IR heating*. Engineering and Food **Vol 1** Physical properties and process control. (Eds Spiess WEL and Schubert H) Proceedings of the Fifth International Congress on Engineering and Food 28 May–3 June 1989, Cologne Federal Republic of Germany London p 869–86

SKJÖLDEBRAND C and SCHMIDT M (1985), Kortare bakningstider med ny teknik. Bröd konditorn 11.22. (In Swedish)

SKJÖLDEBRAND C, ELLBJÄR C, ANDERSSON C G and ERIKSSON T (1988), 'Optical properties of Bread in the Near Infrared Range' *Journal of Food Engineering* **8**, 129–39

SKJÖLDEBRAND C, VAN DEN HARK S, JANESTAD H and ANDERSSON C G (1994), *Radiative and convective heat transfer when baking dough products*, Proceedings from the Fourth Bath Food Engineering Conference, University of Bath, UK 19–21 September

WEI-RENN-LEIN and WEN-RONG-FU (1997), 'Small fish dehydration by far infrared heating'. *Food Science Taiwan* **24**(3), 348–56 (In Chinese)

WÄHLBY U (2002), *Heat and Mass Transfer in Impingement Cooking – Aspects of Food Quality*. PH D thesis, Gothenburg, Sweden

21

High pressure processing

Indrawati, A. Van Loey and M. Hendrickx,
Katholieke Universiteit, Leuven

21.1 Introduction

Food quality, including colour, texture, flavour and nutritional value, is of key importance in the context of food preservation and processing. Colour, texture and flavour refer to consumption quality, purchase and product acceptability whereas the nutritive values (i.e. vitamin content, nutrients, minerals, health-related food components) refer to hidden quality aspects. In conventional thermal processing, process optimisation consists of reducing the severity of the thermal process in terms of food quality destruction without compromising food safety. Due to the consumer demand for fresher, healthier and more natural food products, high pressure technology is considered as a new and alternative unit operation in food processing and preservation.

21.2 High pressure processing in relation to food quality and safety

The effect of high pressure on food microorganisms was reported for the first time by Hite in 1899, by subjecting milk to a pressure of 650 MPa and obtaining a reduction in the viable number of microbes. Some years later, the effect of high pressure on the physical properties of food was reported, e.g. egg albumin coagulation (Bridgman, 1914), solid–liquid phase diagram of water (Bridgman, 1912) and thermophysical properties of liquids under pressure (Bridgman, 1923). A more extensive exploration of high pressure as a new tool in food technology started in the late 1980s (Hayashi, 1989).

Recently, extensive research has been conducted and is in progress on possible applications of high pressure for food preservation purposes or for changing the physical and functional properties of foods. The potentials and limitations of high pressure processing in food applications have become more clear. A number of key effects of high pressure on food components have been demonstrated including (i) microorganism inactivation; (ii) modification of biopolymers including enzyme activation and inactivation, protein denaturation and gel formation; (iii) quality retention (e.g. colour, flavour, nutrition value) and (iv) modification of physicochemical properties of water (Cheftel, 1991; Knorr, 1993). One of the unique characteristics of high pressure is that it directly affects non-covalent bonds (such as hydrogen, ionic, van der Waals and hydrophobic bonds) and very often leaves covalent bonds intact (Hayashi, 1989). As a consequence, it offers the possibility of retaining food quality attributes such as vitamins (Van den Broeck et al, 1998), pigments (Van Loey et al, 1998) and flavour components, while inactivating microorganisms and food-quality related enzymes, changing the structure of food system and functionality of food proteins (Hoover et al, 1989; Knorr, 1995; Barbosa-Cànovas et al, 1997; Messens et al, 1997; Hendrickx et al, 1998). Furthermore, by taking advantage of the effect on the solid liquid phase transition of water, some potential applications in food processing such as pressure-assisted freezing (pressure shift freezing), pressure-assisted thawing (pressure shift thawing), non-frozen storage under pressure at subzero temperature and formation of different ice polymorphs can be offered while keeping other food quality properties (Kalichevsky et al, 1995). Besides, pressure can also induce increased biochemical reaction rates with effect on bioconversions and metabolite production (Tauscher, 1995). Based on these effects of high pressure on food systems, several potential applications can be identified such as high pressure pasteurisation of fruit and vegetables products (Parish, 1994; Yen and Lin, 1996), tenderisation of meat products (Elgasim and Kennick, 1980; Ohmori et al, 1991; Cheftel and Culioli, 1997), texturisation of fish proteins, applications in the dairy industry (Messens et al, 1997) and high pressure freezing/thawing (Kalichevsky et al, 1995).

With regard to food safety, the effect of combined high pressure and temperature on microorganisms has been investigated extensively (Sonoike et al, 1992; Hashizume et al, 1995; Knorr, 1995; Heinz and Knorr, 1996; Hauben, 1998; Reyns et al, 2000). The number of vegetative cells can be remarkably reduced by applying pressures up to 400 MPa combined with moderate temperatures up to 40°C for 10–30 minutes (Knorr, 1995). On the other hand, exposing the surviving fraction of vegetative cells to repeated pressure cycles can also increase their pressure resistance, e.g. *Escherichia coli* mutants resistant to high pressure inactivation were created (Hauben, 1998; Alpas et al, 1999; Benito et al, 1999). Microbial spores can be inactivated by exposure to high pressure but a pressure treatment at room temperature may not be sufficient for substantial reduction of viable spore counts. Most studies show that pressure can induce spore germination and the extent of spore inactivation can be increased by increasing pressure and temperature (Knorr, 1995; Wuytack, 1999). However, tailing phenomena for germination and inactivation curves can occur for 'super dormant' spores after long exposure times. As a consequence, to achieve sterility with minimal impact on nutrition value, flavour, texture and colour, high pressure processing using multiple high pressure pulses and achieving an end temperature above 105°C under pressure for a short time has been proposed (Meyer et al, 2000; Krebbers et al, 2001).

21.3 High pressure technology and equipment for the food industry

High pressure technology has been used in the industrial production process of ceramics, metals and composites in the last three decennia. As a result, today, high pressure equipment is available for a broad range of process conditions, i.e. pressures up to 1000 MPa, temperatures up to 2200°C, volumes up to several cubic meters and cycling times between a few seconds and several weeks.

Since high pressure technology offers advantages in retaining food quality attributes, it has recently been the subject of considerable interest in the food industry as a non-thermal unit operation. High pressure equipment with pressure levels up to 800 MPa and temperatures in the range of 5 to 90°C (on average) for times up to 30 minutes or longer is currently available to the food industry.

The actual high pressure treatment is a batch process. In practice, high pressure technology subjects liquid or solid foods, with or without packaging, to pressures between 50 and 1000 MPa. According to Pascal's principle, high pressure acts instantaneously and uniformly throughout a mass of food and is independent of the size and shape of food products. During compression, a temperature increase or adiabatic heating occurs and its extent is influenced by the rate of pressurisation, the food composition and the (thermo)physical properties of the pressure transfer medium. The temperature in the vessel tends to equilibrate towards the surrounding temperature during the holding period. During pressure release (decompression), a temperature decrease or adiabatic cooling takes place. In high pressure processing, heat cannot be transferred as instantaneously and uniformly as pressure so that temperature distribution in the vessel might become crucial. During the high pressure treatment, other process parameters such as treatment time, pressurisation/decompression rate and the number of pulses have to be considered as critical.

Two types of high pressure equipment can be used in food processing: conventional batch systems and semi-continuous systems. In the conventional batch systems, both liquid and solid pre-packed foods can be processed whereas only pumpable food products such as fruit juice can be treated in semi-continuous systems. Typical equipment for batch high pressure processing consists of a cylindrical steel vessel of high tensile strength, two end closures, a means for restraining the end closures (e.g. a closing yoke to cope with high axial forces, threads, pins), (direct or indirect) compression pumps and necessary pressure controls and instrumentation. Different types of high pressure vessels can be distinguished, i.e. (i) 'monobloc vessel' (a forged constructed in one piece); (ii) 'multi layer vessel' consisting of multiple layers where the inner layers are pre-stressed to reach higher pressure or (iii) 'wire-wound vessel' consisting of pre-stressed vessels formed by winding a rectangular spring steel wire around the vessel. The use of monobloc vessels is limited to working pressures up to 600 MPa and for high pressure application above 600 MPa, pre-stressed vessels are used. The position of high pressure vessels can be vertical, horizontal or tilting depending on the way of processing (Mertens and Deplace, 1993; Zimmerman and Bergman, 1993; Galazka and Ledward, 1995; Mertens, 1995; Knorr, 2001).

21.4 Commercial high pressure treated food products

With regard to the large-scale application of high pressure technology in the food industry, a problem still to be solved today is the improvement of the economic feasibility, i.e. the high investment cost mainly associated with the high capital cost for a commercial high pressure system. The cost of a vessel is determined by the required working pressure/temperature and volume. Furthermore, once technically and economically feasible processes have been identified, one needs to evaluate whether the unique properties of the food justify the additional cost and to what extent consumers are willing to pay a higher price for a premium quality product.

High pressure technology is unlikely to replace conventional thermal processing, because the second technique is a well-established and relatively cheap food preservation method. Currently, the reported cost range of high pressure processes is 0.1–0.2 $ per litre (Grant et al, 2000) whereas the cost for thermal treatment may be as low as 0.02–0.04 $ per litre. However, the technology offers commercially feasible alternatives for conventional heating in the case of novel food products with improved functional properties which cannot be attained by conventional heating.

Today, several commercial high pressure food products are available in Japan, Europe and the United States. A Japanese company, Meidi-Ya, introduced the first commercial pressure treated product (a fruit-based jam) on the market in April 1990, followed in 1991 by a wide variety of pressure-processed fruit yoghurts, fruit jellies, fruit sauces, savoury rice products, dessert and salad dressings (Mertens and Deplace, 1993). Recently, there were more than 10 pressure treated food products available in Japan. In Europe, fruit juice was the first commercially available high pressure product in France followed by a pressurised delicatessen style ham in Spain and pressurised orange juice in the United Kingdom. In the United States, high pressure treated guacamole has been launched on the commercial market. In addition, pressure treated oysters and hummus are commercially available. A list of commercially available pressurised food products in Japan, Europe and the United States in the last decade is summarised in Table 21.1.

21.5 Effect of high pressure on vitamins

Many authors have reported that the vitamin content of fruit and vegetable products is not significantly affected by high pressure processing. According to Bignon (1996), a high pressure treatment can maintain vitamins C, A, B_1, B_2, E and folic acid and the decrease of vitamin C in pressurised orange juice is negligible as compared to flash pasteurised juices during storage at 4°C for 40 days. Similar findings have been reported for red orange juice; high pressure (200–500 MPa/30°C/1 min) did not affect the content of several vitamins (vitamins C, B_1, B_2, B_6 and niacin) (Donsì et al, 1996).

21.5.1 Ascorbic acid

The effect of high pressure treatment on ascorbic acid has been more intensively studied than on vitamins such as A, B, D, E and K. Studies on ascorbic acid stability in various food products after high pressure treatment are available. Most authors have reported that the ascorbic acid content is not significantly affected by high pressure treatment. For example, in fruit and vegetables, about 82% of the ascorbic acid content in fresh green peas can be retained after pressure treatment at 900 MPa/20°C for 5–10 minutes (Quaglia et al, 1996). Almost 95–99% of the vitamin C content in strawberry and kiwi jam can be preserved by pressurisation between 400 and 600 MPa for 10–30 min (Kimura, 1992; Kimura et al, 1994). In freshly squeezed citrus juices, high pressures up to 600 MPa at 23°C for 10 min did not affect the initial (total and dehydro) ascorbic acid concentration (Ogawa et al, 1992). Similar findings are also reported in strawberry 'coulis' (a common sauce in French dessert) and strawberry nectar; the vitamin C content was preserved after 400 MPa/20°C/30 min (88.68% of the initial content in fresh sample) and in guava purée, high pressure (400 and 600 MPa/15 min) maintained the initial concentration of ascorbic acid (Yen and Lin, 1996). Also, ascorbic acid stability in egg yolk has been investigated, showing that high pressure treatment (200, 400, 600 MPa) at 20°C for 30 min did not significantly affect the vitamin C content (Sancho et al, 1999).

The evolution of the vitamin C content in high pressure treated food products during storage has also been investigated. Most studies show that storage at low temperature can eliminate the vitamin C degradation after high pressure treatment. For example, the quality of high pressure treated jam was unchanged for 2–3 months at 5°C but a deterioration of vitamin C was noticed during storage at 25°C (Kimura, 1992; Kimura et al, 1994). Another study on strawberry nectar showed that ascorbic acid remained practically the same during high pressure processing (500 MPa/room temperature/3 min) but decreased during storage (up to 75% of the initial concentration after storage for 60 days at 3°C) (Rovere et al, 1996). In valencia orange juice, the percentage of ascorbic acid in pressurised juice (500–700 MPa/50–60°C/60–90 s) was 20–45% higher than in heat treated juice (98°C/10 s) during storage at 4 and 8°C for 20 weeks (Parish, 1997).

Studies on guava purée showed that different high pressure processes have a

Table 21.1 Commercial pressurised food products in Japan, Europe and the United States in the last ten years (after Cheftel, 1997)

Company	Product	P/T/time combination	Role of HP
JAPAN			
Meidi-ya	Fruit based products (pH < 4.5); jams (apple, kiwi, strawberry); jellies; purées; yoghurts; sauces	400 MPa, 10–30 min, 20°C	Pasteurisation, improved gelation, faster sugar penetration; limiting residual pectinmethylesterase activity
Pokka Corp. (stopped c2000–2001)	Grapefruit juice	200 MPa, 10–15 min, 5°C	Reduced bitterness
Wakayama Food Ind.	Mandarin juice (winter season only) (only ≈20% of HP juice in final juice mix)	300–400 MPa, 2–3 min, 20°C	Reduced odor of dimethyl sulphide; reduced thermal degradation of methyl methionine sulphoxide; replace first thermal pasteurisation (after juice extraction) and final pasteurisation before packing: 90°C, 3 min
Nisshin fine foods	Sugar impregnated tropical fruits (kept at −18°C without freezing). For sorbet and ice cream	50–200 MPa	Faster sugar penetration and water removal
Fuji chiku mutterham	Raw pork ham	250 MPa, 3 hours, 20°C	Faster maturation (reduced from 2 weeks to 3 hours); faster tenderisation by internal proteases, improved water retention and shelf life
Kibun (stopped in 1995)	'Shiokara' and raw scallops	/	Microbial sanitation, tenderisation, control of autolysis by endogenous proteases
Yaizu fisheries (test market only)	Fish sausages, terrines and 'pudding'	400 MPa	Gelation, microbial sanitation, good texture of raw HP gel
Chiyonosono	'Raw' sake (rice wine)	/	Yeast inactivation, fermentation stopped without heating

Company	Product	Conditions	Effects
QP corp	Ice nucleating bacteria (for fruit juice and milk)	/	Inactivation of *Xanthomonas*, no loss of ice nucleating properties
Ehime co.	Japanese mandarin juice	/	Cold pasteurisation
Echigo seika	Moci rice cake, Yomogi fresh aromatic herbs, hypoallergenic precooked rice, convenience packs of boiled rice	400–600 MPa, 10 min, 45 or 70°C	Microbial reduction, fresh flavour and taste, enhances rice porosity and salt extraction of allergenic proteins
Takansi	Fruit juice	/	Cold pasteurisation
Pon (test market in 2000)	Orange juice	/	/
EUROPE			
Pampryl (France)	Fruit juice (orange, grape fruit, citrus, mixed fruit juice)	400 MPa, room temperature	Inactivation of micro flora (up to 10^6 CFU/g), partial inactivation of pectinmethylesterase
Espuna (Spain)	Deli-style processed meats (ham)	400–500 MPa, few minutes, room temperature	/
Orchard House Foods Ltd. (UK) (since July 2001)	Squeezed orange juice	500 MPa, room temperature	Inactivation of micro flora (especially yeast) and enzyme, keeping natural taste
THE UNITED STATES			
Avomex	Avocado paste (guacamole, chipotle sauce, salsa) and pieces	700 MPa, 10–15 min, 20°C	Microorganism inactivation, polyphenoloxidase inactivation, chilled process
Motivatit, Nisbet Oyster Co, Joey Oyster	Oysters	300–400 MPa, room temperature, 10 minutes	Microorganism inactivation, keeping raw taste and flavour, no change in shape and size
Hannah International Foods	Hummus	/	/

/ indicates no detailed information available.

different influence on the stability of vitamin C during storage. The ascorbic acid content in untreated and pressurised (400 MPa/room temperature/15 min) guava puree started to decline respectively after 10 and 20 days whereas that in heated (88–90°C/24 s) and (600 MPa/room temperature/15 min) pressurised guava purée remained constant during 30 and 40 days respectively (Yen and Lin, 1996).

Kinetics of vitamin C degradation during storage have been studied in high pressure treated strawberry coulis. Vitamin C degradation of pressurised (400 MPa/20°C/30 min) and untreated coulis are nearly identical during storage at 4°C. Moreover, it has been shown that a pressure treatment neither accelerates nor slows down the kinetic degradation of ascorbic acid during subsequent storage (Sancho et al, 1999).

The effect of oxygen on ascorbic acid stability under pressure has been studied by Taoukis and co-workers (1998). At 600 MPa and 75°C for 40 min exposed to air, ascorbic acid in buffer solution (sodium acetate buffer (0.1 M; pH 3.5–4)) degraded to 45% of its initial content while in the absence of oxygen, less vitamin loss was observed. Moreover, the addition of 10% sucrose resulted in a protective effect on ascorbic acid degradation. It was also noted that vitamin C loss was higher in fruit juice compared to that in buffer solutions. Vitamin C loss in pineapple and grapefruit juice after pressurisation (up to 600 MPa and 75°C) was max. 70% and 50% respectively. At constant pressure (600 MPa after 40 min), the pressure degradation of vitamin C in pineapple juice was temperature sensitive, e.g. loss 20–25% at 40°C, 45–50% at 60°C and 60–70% at 75°C in contrast to that in grapefruit juice.

Detailed kinetics of combined pressure and temperature stability of ascorbic acid in different buffer (pH 4, 7 and 8) systems and real products (squeezed orange and tomato juices) have been carried out by Van den Broeck and co-workers (1998). At 850 MPa and 50°C for 1 hour, no ascorbic acid loss was observed. The high pressure/thermal degradation of ascorbic acid at 850 MPa and 65–80°C followed a first order reaction. The rate of ascorbic acid degradation at 850 MPa increased with increasing temperature from 65 to 80°C indicating that pressure and temperature act synergistically. Ascorbic acid in tomato juice was more stable than in orange juice. It was also reported that temperature dependence of ascorbic acid degradation (z value) was independent of the pressure level. Based on this study, it can be concluded that ascorbic acid is unstable at high pressure (850 MPa) in combination with high temperature (65–80°C).

21.5.2 Vitamin A and carotene

The effect of high pressure treatment on carotene stability has been studied in carrots and in mixed juices. Based on the available literature data, we can conclude that high pressure treatment does not affect (or affects only slightly) the carotene content in food products. α- and β-carotene contents in carrot puree were only slightly affected by pressure exposure at 600 MPa and 75°C for 40 min (Tauscher, 1998). Similar findings have also been reported by de Ancos and co-workers (2000) showing that carotene loss in carrot homogenates and carrot paste was maximally 5% under pressure condition of 600 MPa/75°C/40 min. In orange, lemon and carrot mixed juice, high pressure (500 and 800 MPa/room temperature/5 min) did not affect or only slightly affected the carotenoid content and during storage at 4°C; the carotenoid content in the pressure treated juice remained constant for 21 days (Fernández Garcia et al, 2001).

In addition, high pressure treatment can affect the extraction yield of carotenoids. Studies on persimmon fruit purées showed that high pressure treatment could increase the extraction yield of carotenoids between 9 and 27% e.g. Rojo Brillante cultivars (50 and 300 MPa/25°C/15 min) and Sharon cultivars (50 and 400 MPa/25°C/15 min). The increase in extraction yield of carotene (40% higher) was also found in pressurised carrot homogenate (600 MPa/25°C/10 min) (de Ancos et al, 2000).

Pressure stability of retinol and vitamin A has been studied in buffer systems. In the model systems studied, pressure treatment could induce degradation of vitamin A. For example, pressures up to 400–600 MPa significantly induced retinol (in 100% ethanol solution) degradation. Degradation up to 45% was obtained after 5 minutes exposure to 600 MPa combined with temperatures at 40, 60 and 75°C. Pressure and temperature degradation of retinol followed a second order reaction. Another study on vitamin A acetate (in 100% ethanol solution) showed that degradation of vitamin A acetate was more pronounced by increasing pressure and temperature. About half of the vitamin A acetate concentration could be retained by pressure treatment at different pressure/temperature/time combinations, i.e. 650 MPa/70°C/15 minutes and 600 MPa/25°C/40 minutes. At 90°C, complete degradation was observed after 2–16 minutes (pressure up to 600 MPa). No effect of oxygen was noticed on retinol and vitamin A acetate degradation (Butz and Tauscher, 1997; Kübel et al, 1997; Tauscher, 1999).

However, findings on retinol pressure stability in real food products differ from those obtained in model systems. In egg white and egg yolk, the initial retinol content can be preserved by pressure treatment from 400 up to 1000 MPa at 25°C for 30 minutes (Hayashi et al, 1989).

21.5.3 Vitamins B, E and K

The stability of vitamins B, E and K towards pressure treatment has been studied in model systems and food products. In food model systems, high pressure (200, 400, 600 MPa) treatments at 20°C for 30 minutes have no significant effect on vitamin B_1 (thiamine) and B_6 (pyridoxal) (Sancho et al, 1999). Studies on the pressure effect on vitamin K_1 showed that small quantities of *m*- and *p*-isomeric Diels–Alder products were formed after 3 hours at 650 MPa and 70°C (Tauscher, 1999).

In cow's milk, high pressure (400 MPa/room temperature/30 minutes) did not alter the content of vitamin B_1 and B_6 (pyridoxamine and pyridoxal) (Sierra et al, 2000). The thiamine content in pork meat was not affected by high pressure (100–250 MPa/20°C/10 minutes) even after long exposure time of 18 h at 600 MPa and 20°C (Bognar et al, 1993). However, under extreme conditions of high temperature (100°C) combined with 600 MPa, almost 50% of the thiamine in pork meat was degraded within 15 min. Moreover, riboflavin in pork meat was only slightly affected (less than 20%) after pressure treatment at 600 MPa for 15 minutes combined with temperatures between 25 and 100°C (Tauscher, 1998). Heat-sensitive vitamin derivatives in egg white and/or egg yolk, i.e. riboflavin, folic acid, α-tocopherol and thiamine did not change during pressure treatment from 400 up to 1000 MPa at 25°C for 30 minutes (Hayashi et al, 1989).

It can be concluded that high pressure treatment has little effect on the vitamin content of food products. However, at extreme conditions of high pressure combined with high temperature for a long treatment time period, vitamin degradation is observed. Regarding the use of high pressure in industrial applications, an optimised pressure/temperature/time combination must be chosen to obtain limited vitamin destruction within the constraints of the target microbial inactivation. For example, a mild pressure and temperature treatment can be developed equivalent to the conventional pasteurisation processes in order to keep the vitamin content in food products while inactivating vegetative microbial cells. When spore inactivation is targeted, combined high pressure thermal treatments are needed and these treatments will affect nutrients. It is still an open question whether equivalent conventional thermal and new high pressure processes used for spore inactivation lead to improved vitamin retention. The available data suggest positive effects but more research is needed.

21.6 Effect of high pressure on lipids

The most interesting effect of high pressure on lipids in foods is the influence on the solid–liquid phase transition, e.g. a reversible shift of 16°C per 100 MPa for milk fat, coconut fat and lard (Buchheim et al, 1999). With respect to the nutritional value of lipids, the effect of high pressure on lipid oxidation and hydrolysis in food products is of importance. Lipid oxidation is a major cause of food quality deterioration, impairing both flavour and nutritional values (related to health risks, e.g. development of both coronary heart disease and cancer). Effect of high pressure on lipids has been reported by many authors and the available literature shows that pressure could induce lipid oxidation especially in fish and meat products but did not, or only slightly, affect lipid hydrolysis. For example, pressures up to 1000 MPa and 80°C did not affect the hydrolysis of tripalmitin and lecithin. Therefore, no fat/oil hydrolysis is expected to occur under conditions relevant for food processing (e.g. 600 MPa/60°C/time less than 30 minutes) (Isaacs and Thornton-Allen, 1998).

Pressure induced lipid oxidation has been studied in different model systems and food products. In model systems, pressures up to 600 MPa and temperatures up to 40°C (less than 1 hour) had no effect on the main unsaturated fatty acid in milk, i.e. oleic acid. Linoleic acid oxidation was accelerated by exposure to pressure treatments of less than one hour, but the effect was relatively small (about 10% oxidation) (Butz et al, 1999). Increasing pressure (100 up to 600 MPa and

40°C) lowered the decrease of alpha-linoleic acid indicating that pressure retarded lipid oxidation e.g. 15% decrease at 600 MPa/40°C/15 minutes and 30% decrease at 100 MPa/40°C/15 minutes. As a consequence, pressures above 600 MPa are suggested for retention of essential fatty acids, e.g. linoleic acids (Kowalski et al, 1996).

21.6.1 Vegetable oils

Pressure induced lipid oxidation of extra virgin olive and seed oil has been studied by Severini and co-workers (1997). The peroxide values, indicating the primary oxidation products, of untreated and pressure treated (700 MPa/room temperature/10 minutes) olive oil were not significantly different. In seed oil i.e. sunflower and grape-stone oil, this value was evidently increased due to pressure treatment and storage (−18°C, 1 year); such effects were not found for soybean, peanut and maize oil. The two former seed oils show the highest level of unsaturated fatty acids which probably affects lipid oxidation. The *para*-anisidine value, indicating secondary oxidation products such as aldehydes, generally increased after high pressure treatment (700 MPa/room temperature/10 minutes), e.g. olive oil (types A, B, C, D), sunflower, peanut and maize oil samples and after one year storage at −18°C, only the value in seed oil increased. The induction time (i.e. length of the initial stage of very slow oxidation) of pressure treated olive oil was generally shorter than that needed for untreated samples. Such a phenomenon was also found in the seed oils i.e. grape-stone, sunflower and peanut oils. It can be concluded that the olive oil was more pressure resistant to oxidation than was seed oil and, as a consequence, extra virgin olive oil is a better choice in high pressure processed foods.

The effect of high pressure on essential oils of spices and herbs has been reported. The essential oil content in basil can be retained by pulsed high pressure sterilisation (2 pulses of 1 minute holding time) using high pressure (≥700 MPa) combined with high temperature (≥65°C) processing while losses after conventional heat sterilisation were over 65%. It was stated that pulsed high pressure opens new perspectives in quality improvement of fresh spices and herbs (Krebbers et al, 2001).

21.6.2 Fish products

In fish products, some studies show occurrences of pressure induced lipid oxidation. The lipid oxidation rate (based on TCA (thiobarbituric acid) number) in cod muscle remarkably increased by pressurisation above 400 MPa (study up to 800 MPa) at 20°C for 20 min. EDTA (ethylenediaminetetraacetic acid) addition (1% w/w) in minced cod muscle inhibited the increased oxidation rate induced by pressure treatment. It was suggested that release of transition metal ions such as copper or iron or their complexes occurred under pressure and subsequently catalysed the oxidation reaction. Lipid oxidation in cod muscle packed under air was limited at treatments of 200 MPa and room temperature for 20 minutes (Angsupanich and Ledward, 1998).

Production of free fatty acids in red fish meat, i.e. sardine and bonito, during storage was inhibited after pressure treatment at 200 MPa and room temperature for 30 minutes. Pressures above 200 MPa resulted in lipid degradation. This observation was explained by the degradation of myoglobin and the loss of the water holding capacity increasing the contact surface layer between oxygen and fish meat. The oxidation pattern of pressurised (100 MPa/room temperature/30 minutes) sardine and bonito was almost the same for as long as 3 days of storage (5°C). Addition of antioxidants (a mixture of alpha tocopherol and rosemary) prolonged the storage for 12 days for untreated samples but only for 6 and 9 days respectively for 100 and 200 MPa pressurised samples. It could be that high pressure also affects the radical scavenger function of alpha tocopherol and rosemary (Wada, 1992; Wada and Ogawa, 1996).

21.6.3 Meat products

In meat products, the induction time of pressure treated (800 MPa/19°C/20 minutes) rendered pork fat ($a_w = 0.44$) was shorter (approximately 3 days) than that of untreated samples (c 4 days). Pressure treated samples showed a higher peroxide value than untreated samples and the effect became more pronounced with increasing pressure. Furthermore, the extent of lipid oxidation at 800 MPa for 20 min was increased by increasing the treatment temperature. High pressure treatment inhibited lipid oxidation at all water activities except $a_w = 0.44$. Since pork fat contains up to 1.5 ppm iron and 0.4 ppm copper, transition metals may be released from complexes and act as powerful pro-oxidants. In the a_w range between 0.4 and 0.55, pressure becomes catalytic to the oxidation and the catalytic effect of the released metal ions probably overrides the inhibiting effect of peroxide destruction. At higher a_w, free ions will hydrate with the available water, whereas at lower a_w such hydration may not be complete and increases the catalytic effects of the ions. It seemed that pressure treatment at higher temperature diminished the inhibiting/protective effect on lipid oxidation and high pressure application for a short time had a significant effect on stability of pork lipids during subsequent storage indicating that high pressure leads to irreversible changes (Cheah and Ledward, 1995). Addition of citric acid (0.02%) prior to pressure (650–800 MPa) treatment of rendered pork fat inhibited the increased rate of lipid oxidation while it was less effective in minced pork and washed muscle because of the pH decrease. On the other hand, the addition of EDTA was effective in inhibiting pressure induced oxidation. It indicated that releasing metal transition ions during pressure treatment was a major factor in increasing lipid oxidation in pressurised meat (Cheah and Ledward, 1997).

Kinetics of lipid oxidation during pressure treatment have been reported by Dissing and co-workers (1997). In this investigation, turkey meat has been chosen as a case study since it is rather susceptible to oxidation due to its relatively large content of membrane-associated phospholipids in combination with a low endogenous level of tocopherol. Pressure treatment (100–500 MPa/10°C/10–30 min) induced lipid oxidation in turkey thigh muscles prior to chilled storage. During storage, the increase of thiobarbituric acid reactive substances in pressurised (up to 400 MPa/10°C/10–30 min) meat was less pronounced than in heat (100°C/10 min) treated samples. The extent of lipid oxidation depends on the pressure level and treatment time. The enhancement of lipid oxidation was dependent on the pressure level applied, at least above a certain threshold pressure (i.e. 100 MPa).

The evidence of pressure induced lipid oxidation may limit high pressure application in meat/fish based products unless antioxidants or suitable product packaging are used. Metal chelators which effectively remove the metal catalysts have been proposed as the most appropriate antioxidants to prevent lipid oxidation in meat products.

21.7 Effect of high pressure on other health-related food compounds

21.7.1 Sweeteners

Synthetic dipeptide aspartame (aspartylphenylalanyl methyl ester) is widely used as a sweetener in light (low calorie) foods and diets for diabetics. The effect of high pressure on aspartame stability has been reported by Butz and co-workers (1997). Aspartame (0.5 g/L corresponding to the concentration in commercial diet cola and chocolate milk) in full cream milk (pH 6.8) lost almost 50% of active substances after pressure treatment at 600 MPa and 60°C for 3 minutes while the non-sweet compounds, i.e. aspartylphenylalanine and diketopiperazine, were formed. One of the important factors influencing the pressure stability of aspartame was the pH. It was stated that low pH foods containing aspartame could be treated by high pressure without great loss of active substances while high pressure treatment of dairy products (at neutral pH) such as chocolate milk and ice cream may create problems (possibly toxicological ones). After pressure treatment at 600 MPa and 60°C (pH 7), 1.15 mM of diketopiperazine (corresponding to 300 mg/L) could be present after 5 minutes. In this case, a human individual of 40 kg consuming 1 L of pressurised chocolate milk would ingest the upper limit of diketopiperazine (acceptable daily intake, ADI) of 7.5 mg/kg of body weight. As a consequence, it would be inadvisable to compensate the pressure related aspartame loss by adding higher aspartame doses prior to pressure treatment because it results in even higher diketopiperazine concentrations in the end-product.

21.7.2 Mineral content

Information on the effect of high pressure on the mineral content of food products is very scarce. Pressure treatment (600 MPa/room temperature/20 minutes) could increase up to 50% the soluble iron content of liver suggesting the break up of the protein coat surrounding the cluster of hydrous ferric oxide in ferritin. The soluble iron content in spinach and soya flour was unaffected by pressure treatment. In beef muscle, the soluble iron was decreased by up to 50% and 67% respectively after pressure and heat treatments. Based on this study, the evidence of increasing rate of lipid oxidation in pressure treated meats (see section 21.6) could be supported by iron complexes released from ferritin or perhaps haemosidrin (Defaye and Ledward, 1999).

21.7.3 Human anti-mutagenic and anti-carcinogenic compounds

Diets rich in fruit and vegetables are found to be associated with a low incidence of many types of human cancer. Unfortunately, most of the antimutagenic activity in fruit and vegetables is reduced by heat treatment. The effect of high pressure treatment at different temperatures on the antimutagenic activity of fruit and vegetables has been studied in detail by Butz and co-workers (1998). In strawberry and grapefruit, heat (100°C/10 min) and pressure (400–800 MPa/25–35°C/10 minutes) had no effect on the antimutagenic activity. Carrots, kohlrabi, leek, spinach and cauliflower were characterised by strong antimutagenic potencies that are sensitive to heat but not to pressure. Antimutagenic activity of tomatoes and beets was affected by pressure but extreme high pressure/temperature conditions were required (tomatoes: 600 MPa/50°C/10 min and 800 MPa/35°C/10 min; beets: 800 MPa/35°C/10 min). It can be concluded that high pressure processing of vegetable juices offers advantages compared with thermal processing regarding their antimutagenicity.

In broccoli, isothiocyanates have been shown to have cancer protective properties. Application of high pressure (600 MPa) combined with temperature (25, 40, 60 and 75°C) increased the degradation rate of both allyl and benzyl isothiocyanate up to 4 times compared with treatment under ambient pressure. In addition, the isothiocyanate degradation impaired such qualities as colour, flavour and some physiological properties. Therefore, high pressure technology may have limited application potential for food products containing isothiocyanates (Grupe et al, 1997).

21.7.4 Digestibility

In dairy and egg-based products, pressure induced conformational changes of albumin in relation to its technological and nutritional functionality were examined by determining the susceptibility of the treated protein to trypsin. High pressure treatment (600–800 MPa/25°C/5–10 min) of ovalbumin solutions in the absence of salt (NaCl) and sucrose did not modify the susceptibility of the residual soluble protein to trypsin. Pressure insolubilised ovalbumin was not digested by trypsin. Pressure treatment at neutral pH in the presence of NaCl or sucrose resulted in a pressure dependent increase of the susceptibility of ovalbumin to trypsin. The highest increase in proteolysis was observed for ovalbumin treated at 800 MPa and 25°C for 10 min in the presence of 10% sucrose (Iametti et al, 1998). Similar phenomena have been reported for purified egg albumin. The presence of sucrose in pressurised albumin (400–600 MPa/25°C/5 min) increased the susceptibility to proteolysis and the increase was more pronounced than in the presence of NaCl (Iametti et al, 1999).

Digestibility of pressurised foodstuffs has been studied *in vitro* (using digestibility tests) and *in vivo* (feeding trial in young pigs). Feeding trials (using a mixture of potatoes, carrots, meat, peas and vegetable oil) showed no changes in the digestibility of the individual nutrient fractions of pressurised foodstuffs as compared to fresh (untreated) ones. High pressure (500 MPa/20°C/10 min) did not affect the digestibility of the nitrogen free extract content, fats and crude extract fibre. The nitrogen retention in animals was only 45.4% of the nitrogen consumed when the heat treated feed was given while it was 58.6% using pressurised food and 57.9% using an untreated feed. *In vitro* studies showed no significant differences between the high pressure treated, heat treated (100 °C) and untreated pork samples on digestibility. Pressure treated soybean had a better digestibility than the untreated sample and the lowest digestibility was found in heat treated samples (100°C) (Schöberl et al, 1999).

For meat and lupin protein, the effect of high pressure on protein digestibility has been studied using *in vitro* tests. Protein digestibility of pressurised meat was higher than that of heat treated meat. The effectiveness of food processing on protein digestibility in meat could be ranged in the following order: untreated > pressure treated (500 MPa/10°C/10 min) (70% of digestibility) ≥ pressure treated (200 MPa/10°C/10 min) (67% of digestibility) > heat treated (95°C/30 min) samples (43% of digestibility). For lupin proteins, the pressure induced digestibility was more remarkable than for meat proteins and the ranking was different, i.e. pressure treated (500 MPa/10°C/10 min): digestibility up to 430% > heat treated (95°C/30 min): digestibility up to 300% > pressure treated (200 MPa/10°C/10 min): digestibility up to 140% ≥ untreated samples (de Lamballerie-Anton et al, 2001).

21.7.5 Allergens

Most foods contain both major and minor allergens. The majority of food-allergic individuals are sensitive to one or more of the major allergens present in common allergic foods. The effect of different food processing unit operations on the immunochemical stability of celery allergens has been studied in detail using *in vitro* and *in vivo* tests by Jankiewicz and co-workers (1997). High antigenic and allergenic activity in native celery was reduced by heat treatment and only mildly reduced by non-thermal processing such as high pressure (600 MPa/20°C), high voltage pulse treatment and irradiation.

In dairy and egg based products, modification of epitopic regions of ovalbumin in pressure-treated ovalbumin has been studied by Iametti and co-workers (1998 and 1999). Pressure treatment (600–800 MPa/25°C/5 min) resulted in modifications of the epitopic regions of the protein (determined by direct and non-competitive ELISA). Increasing the pressure level caused an increased loss of recognisability. Under pressure, ovalbumin in the presence of sucrose presented a lower recognisability than in the presence of NaCl. Samples treated at

600–800 MPa/25°C/5 min in the presence of NaCl showed an affinity towards antibodies that was 40% lower than that of untreated protein. When comparing with the result determined by direct competitive ELISA, it can be concluded that pressure treatment did modify epitopic regions of ovalbumin. In the presence of sucrose, increasing protein concentrations led to a decrease in the specific content of antibody recognition sites per unit mass protein while no effect was found in the presence of NaCl.

21.8 Future trends in high pressure research

Most review articles have pointed out the potential of high pressure as a non-thermal alternative for food processing and preservation allowing high retentions of food quality such as colour, flavour and nutrient value. The available information in literature is qualitative and fragmentary. Systematic quantitative data are very limited. The latter information is indispensable when providing satisfactory evidence for legislative bodies to enable the authorisation of high pressure technology in the food processing/preservation industries (e.g. EU legislation regarding 'novel food'). Therefore, quantitative studies must be carried out in order to allow the assessment of the impact of high pressure processing on food quality and safety.

In comparison with conventional thermal processing, high pressure as a novel unit operation should be able to guarantee increased overall quality, i.e. to increase functional properties within the constraints of microbial and toxicological safety. The occurrence of toxic or allergenic compounds in pressure treated food products must receive more attention in the future. The present situation requires further investigations and calls for more systematic studies. Today, high pressure treatments combined with high temperatures for short times have been proposed for food sterilisation because of their effective microbial spore inactivation. On the other hand, some articles have reported that the stability of nutrients (e.g. vitamins, lipids, health-related food compounds) and possibly chemical compounds is limited under such extreme pressure-temperature conditions. This calls for more research on these compounds under high pressure sterilisation conditions and both mechanistic and kinetic information are required.

21.9 Sources of further information and advice

High pressure research has been concentrated in Japan, Europe and the United States. Lists of academic and non-academic research centres actively involved in high pressure research in the field of bioscience, food science and chemistry are tentatively summarised in Appendices 21.1 and 21.2; they are based on their participation in European and/or Japanese High Pressure Research conferences and Annual IFT meetings in the period 1991–2001. Further information on annual meetings of high pressure research in Japan, Europe and the United States can be obtained from professional organisations such as the European High Pressure Research Group (*http://www.kuleuven.ac.be/ehprg*), the Institute of Food Technologists (IFT) Non Thermal Division (*http://www.ift.org/divisions/nonthermal/*), the UK High pressure club for food processing (*http://www.highpressure.org.uk*) and the Japanese Research Group of High Pressure. Information about general aspects of high pressure processing can be found at the Ohio State University website (*http://grad.fst.ohio-state.edu/hpp/*) and FLOW website (*http://www.fresherunderpressure.com/*).

21.10 Acknowledgements

The authors would like to thank the Fund for Scientific Research – Flanders (FWO) for their financial support.

21.11 References

ALPAS H, KALCHAYANAND N, BOZOGLU F, SIKES A, DUNNE P and RAY B (1999), 'Variation in resistance to hydrostatic pressure among strains of food-borne pathogens', *Appl Environ Microbiol*, **65**(9), 4248–51

ANGSUPANICH K and LEDWARD D A (1998), 'Effects of high pressure on lipid oxidation in fish', in Isaacs N S (ed), *High Pressure Food Science, Bioscience and Chemistry*, Cambridge, UK, The Royal Society of Chemistry, 284–7

BARBOSA-CÁNOVAS G V, POTHAKAMURY U R, PALOU E and SWANSON B G (1997), 'High pressure food processing', in Barbosa-Cánovas G V, Pothakamury U R, Palou E and Swanson B G (eds), *Nonthermal Preservation of Foods*, New York, Marcel Dekker, 9–52

BENITO A, VENTOURA G, CASADEI M, ROBINSON T and MACKEY B (1999), 'Variation in resistance of natural isolates of *Eschericia coli* O157 to high hydrostatic pressure, mild heat, and other stresses', *Appl Environ Microbiol*, **65**(4), 1564–9

BIGNON J (1996), 'Cold pasteurizers hyperbar for the stabilization of fresh fruit juices', *Fruit Processing*, **2**, 46–8

BOGNAR A, BUTZ P, KOWALSKI E, LUDWIG H and TAUSCHER B (1993), 'Stability of thiamine in pressurized model solution and pork', in Schlemmer U (ed), *Bioavalaibility '93 part II – Nutritional, Chemical and Food Processing Implications of Nutrient Availability*, Karlsruhe, Bundesforschungsanstalt für Ernährung, 352–6

BRIDGMAN P W (1912), 'Water, in the liquid and five solid forms, under pressure', *Proc Am Acad Arts Sci*, XLVII, **13**, 439–558

BRIDGMAN P W (1914), 'The coagulation of albumen by pressure', *J Biol Chem*, **19**, 511–12

BRIDGMAN P W (1923), 'The thermal conductivity of liquids under pressure', *Proc Am Acad Arts Sci*, XLVII, **59**, 141–69

BUCHHEIM W, FREDE E, WOLF M and BALDENEGGER P (1999), 'Solidification and melting of some edible fats and model lipid systems under pressure', in Ludwig H (ed), *Advances in High Pressure Bioscience and Biotechnology*, Heidelberg, Springer, 153–6

BUTZ P and TAUSCHER B (1997), 'Food chemistry under high hydrostatic pressure', in Isaacs N S (ed), *High Pressure Food Science, Bioscience and Chemistry*, Cambridge, UK, The Royal Society of Chemistry, 133–44

BUTZ P, FERNANDEZ A, FISTER H and TAUSCHER B (1997), 'Influence of high hydrostatic pressure on aspartame: instability at neutral pH', *J Agric Food Chem*, **45**, 302–3

BUTZ P, EDENHARDER R, FISTER H and TAUSCHER B (1998), 'The influence of high pressure processing on antimutagenic activities of fruit and vegetables juices', *Food Res Int*, **30**(3/4), 287–91

BUTZ P, ZIELINSKI B, LUDWIG H and TAUSCHER B (1999), 'The influence of high pressure on the autoxidation of major unsaturated fatty acid constituents of milk', in Ludwig H (ed), *Advances in High Pressure Bioscience and Biotechnology*, Heidelberg, Springer, 367–70

CHEAH P B and, LEDWARD D A (1995), 'High pressure effects on lipid oxidation', *J Am Oil Chem Soc*, **72**(9), 1059–63

CHEAH P B and LEDWARD D A (1997), 'Catalytic mechanism of lipid oxidation following high pressure treatment in pork fat and meat', *J Food Sci*, **62**(6), 1135–8; 1141

CHEFTEL J C (1991), 'Applications des hautes pressions en technologies alimentaire', *Ind Aliment Agric*, **108**, 141–53

CHEFTEL J C (1992), 'Effects of high hydrostatic pressure on food constituents: an overview', in Balny C, Hayashi R, Heremans K and Masson P (eds), *High Pressure and Biotechnology 224*, Montrouge, John Libbey Eurotext, 195–209

CHEFTEL J R (1997), 'Commercial pressurized foods in Japan', in Isaacs N S (ed), *High Pressure Food Science, Bioscience and Chemistry*, Cambridge, UK, The Royal Society of Chemistry, 506–7

CHEFTEL J R and CULIOLI J (1997), 'Effect of high pressure on meat: a review', *Meat Sci*, **46**(3), 211–36

DE ANCOS B, GONZALEZ E and PILAR CANO M (2000), 'Effect of high pressure treatment on the carotenoid composition and the radical scavenging activity of persimmon fruit purees', *J Agric Food Chem*, **48**, 3542–8

DEFAYE A B and LEDWARD D A (1999), 'Release of iron from beef, liver, soya flour and spinach on high pressure treatment', in Ludwig H (ed), *Advances in High Pressure Bioscience and Biotechnology*, Heidelberg, Springer, 417–18

DE LAMBALLERIE-ANTON M, DELÁPINE S and CHAPLEAU N (2001), 'Effect of high pressure on the digestibility of meat and lupin proteins', Oral presentation in *XXXIX European High Pressure Research Group Meeting*, Santander (Spain), 16–19 September 2001

DISSING J, BRUUN-JENSEN L and SKIBSTED L H (1997), 'Effect of high-pressure treatment on lipid oxidation in turkey thigh muscle during chill storage', *Z Lebensm Unters Forsch A*, **205**, 11–13

DONSÌ G, FERRARI G and DI MATTEO M (1996), 'High pressure stabilization of orange juice: evaluation of the effects of process conditions', *Ital J Food Sci*, **2**, 99–106

ELGASIM E A and KENNICK W H (1980), 'Effect of pressurization of pre-rigor beef muscles on protein quality', *J Food Sci*, **45**, 1122–4

FERNÁNDEZ GARCIA A, BUTZ P, BOGNÀR A and TAUSCHER B (2001), 'Antioxidative capacity, nutrient content and sensory quality of orange juice and an orange-lemon-carrot juice product after high pressure treatment and storage in different packaging', *Eur Food Res Technol*, **213**, 290–6

GALAZKA V B and LEDWARD D A (1995), 'Developments in high pressure food processing', *Food Technol Int Europe*, 123–5

GRANT S, PATTERSON M and LEDWARD D (2000), 'Food processing gets freshly squeezed', *Chemistry and Industry*, 24 January 2000, 55–8

GRUPE C, LUDWIG H and TAUSCHER B (1997), 'The effect of high pressure on the degradation of isothiocyanates', in Isaacs N S (ed), *High Pressure Food Science, Bioscience and Chemistry*, Cambridge, UK, The Royal Society of Chemistry, 125–9

HASHIZUME C, KIMURA K and HAYASHI R (1995), 'Kinetic analysis of yeast inactivation by high pressure treatment at low temperatures', *Biosci Biotech Biochem*, **59**, 1455–8

HAUBEN K (1998), *High hydrostatic pressure as a hurdle in food preservation: inactivation and sublethal injury of Escherichia coli*, Doctoral dissertation no. 375, Katholieke Universiteit Leuven, Leuven, Belgium

HAYASHI R (1989), 'Application of high pressure to food processing and preservation:

philosophy and development', in Spiess W E L and Schubert H (eds), *Engineering and Food*, London, Elsevier Applied Science, 815–26

HAYASHI R, KAWAMURA Y, NAKASA T and OKINAWA O (1989), 'Application of high pressure to food processing: pressurization of egg white and yolk, and properties of gels formed', *Agric Biol Chem*, **53**(11), 2935–9

HEINZ V and KNORR D (1996), 'High pressure inactivation kinetics of *Bacillus subtilis* cells by a three-state-model considering distributed resistance mechanisms', *Food Biotechnol*, **10**, 149–61

HENDRICKX M, LUDIKHUYZE L, VAN DEN BROECK I and WEEMAES C (1998), 'Effects of high pressure on enzymes related to food quality', *Trends Food Sci Technol*, **9**, 197–203

HITE B H (1899), 'The effect of pressure in the preservation of milk', *Bulletin*, **58**, 15–35

HOOVER D G, METRICK C, PAPINEAU A M, FARKAS D F and KNORR D (1989), 'Biological effects of high hydrostatic pressure on food microorganisms', *Food Technol*, **43**(3), 99–107

IAMETTI S, DONNIZZELLI E, VECCHIO G, ROVERE P P, GOLA S and BONOMI F (1998), 'Macroscopic and structural consequences of high-pressure treatment of ovalbumin solutions', *J Agric Food Chem*, **46**, 3521–7

IAMETTI S, DONNIZZELLI E, PITTIA P, ROVERE, P P, SQUARCINA N and BONOMI F (1999), 'Characterization of high-pressure treated egg albumen', *J Agric Food Chem*, **47**, 3611–16

ISAACS N S and THORNTON-ALLEN N (1998), 'The hydrolysis of lipids and phospholipids at atmospheric and at high pressure', in Isaacs N S (ed), *High Pressure Food Science, Bioscience and Chemistry*, Cambridge, UK, The Royal Society of Chemistry, 122–4

JANKIEWICZ A, BALTES W, BÖGL K W, DEHNE L I, JAMIN A, HOFFMANN A, HAUSTEIN D and VIETHS S (1997), 'Influence of food processing on the immunochemical stability of celery allergens', *J Sci Food Agri*, **75**, 359–70

KALICHEVSKY M T, KNORR D and LILLFORD P J (1995), 'Potential food applications of high pressure effects on ice-water transitions', *Trends Food Sci Technol*, **6**, 253–9

KIMURA K (1992), 'Development of a new fruit processing method by high hydrostatic pressure', in Balny C, Hayashi R, Heremans K and Masson P, *High Pressure and Biotechnology*, Montrouge, John Libbey Eurotext Ltd, **224**, 279–83

KIMURA K, IDA M, YOSHIDA Y, OHKI K, FUKUMOTO T and SAKUI N (1994), 'Comparison of keeping quality between pressure-processed and heat-processed jam: changes in flavour components, hue and nutritional elements during storage', *Biosci Biotechnol Biochem*, **58**, 1386–91

KNORR D (1993), 'Effects of high-hydrostatic-pressure processes on food safety and quality', *Food Technol*, **47**(6), 156–61

KNORR D (1995), 'Hydrostatic pressure treatment of food: microbiology', in Gould G W (ed), *New Methods of Food Preservation*, Glasgow, Blackie Academic and Professional, 159–75

KNORR D (2001), 'High pressure processing for preservation, modification and transformation of foods', Oral presentation in *XXXIX European High Pressure Research Group Meeting*, Santander (Spain), 16–19 September 2001

KOWALSKI E, LUDWIG H and TAUSCHER B (1996), 'Behaviour of organic compounds in food under high pressure: lipid peroxidation', in Hayashi R and Balny C (eds), *High Pressure Bioscience and Biotechnology*, Amsterdam, Elsevier Science B V, 473–8

KREBBERS B, MATSER A, KOETS M, BARTELS P and VAN DEN BERG R (2001), 'High presuretemperature processing as an alternative for preserving basil', Poster presentation in *XXXIX European High Pressure Research Group Meeting*, Santander (Spain), 16–19 September 2001

KÜBEL J, LUDWIG H and TAUSCHER B (1997), 'Influence of UHP on vitamin A', in Heremans K (ed), *High Pressure Research in the Biosciences and Biotechnology*, Leuven, Belgium, Leuven University Press, 331–4

MERTENS B (1992), 'Under pressure', *Food Manufacture*, **11**, 23–4

MERTENS B and DEPLACE G (1993), 'Engineering aspects of high pressure technology in the food industry', *Food Technol*, **47**(6), 164–9
MERTENS B (1995), 'Hydrostatic pressure treatment of food: equipment and processing', in Gould G W (ed), *New Methods of Food Preservation*, Glasgow, Blackie Academic and Professional, 135–58
MESSENS W, VAN CAMP J and HUYGEBAERT A (1997), 'The use of high pressure to modify the functionality of food proteins', *Trends Food Sci Technol*, **8**, 107–12
MEYER R S, COOPER K L, KNORR D and LELIEVELD H L M (2000), 'High-pressure sterilization of foods', *Food Technol*, **54**(11), 67–72
OGAWA H, FUKUHISA K and FUKUMOTO H (1992), 'Effect of Hydrostatic Pressure on Sterilization and Preservation of Citrus Juice', in Balny C, Hayashi K, Heremans K and Masson P (eds), *High Pressure and Biotechnology 224*, Montrouge, John Libbey Eurotext, 269–78
OHMORI T, SHIGEHISA T, TAJI S and HAYASHI R (1991), 'Effect of high pressure on the protease activities in meat', *Biol Chem*, **55**(2), 357–61
PARISH M (1994), 'Isostatic high pressure processing of orange juice', in Singh P R and Oliveira F A R (eds), *Minimal Processing of Foods and Process Optimization*, Boca Raton, CRC press, 93–102
PARISH M E (1997), 'High pressure effects on quality of chilled orange juice', in Heremans K (ed), *High Pressure Research in the Biosciences and Biotechnology*, Leuven, Leuven University Press, 443–6
QUAGLIA G B, GRAVINA R, PAPERI R and PAOLETTI F (1996), 'Effect of high pressure treatments on peroxidase activity, ascorbic acid content and texture in green peas', *Lebens Wiss U Technol*, **29**, 552–5
REYNS K M F A, SOONTJES C C F, CORNELIS K, WEEMAES C A, HENDRICKX M E and MICHIELS C W (2000), 'Kinetic analysis and modeling of combined high pressure-temperature inactivation of the yeast *Zygosaccharomyces bailii*', *Int J Food Microbiol*, **56**, 199–210
ROVERE P, CARPI G, GOLA S, DALL'AGLIO G and MAGGY A (1996), 'HPP strawberry products: an example of processing line', in Hayashi R and Balny C (eds), *High Pressure Bioscience and Biotechnology*, Amsterdam, Elsevier Science B V, 445–50
SANCHO F, LAMBERT Y, DEMAZEAU G, LARGETEAU A, BOUVIER J M and NARBONNE J F (1999), 'Effect of ultra-high hydrostatic pressure on hydrosoluble vitamins', *J Food Eng*, **39**, 247–53
SCHÖBERL H, RUß W, MEYER-PITTROFF R, ROTH F X and KIRCHGESSNER M (1999), 'Comparative Studies concerning the digestibility of raw, heated and high pressure treated foods in young pigs and *in vitro*', in Ludwig H (ed), *Advances in High Pressure Bioscience and Biotechnology*, Heidelberg, Springer, 385–8
SEVERINI C, ROMANI S, DALL'AGLIO G, ROVERE P, CONTE L and LERICI C R (1997), 'High pressure effects on oxidation of extra virgin olive oils', *It J Food Sci*, **3**(9), 183–91
SIERRA I, VIDAL-VALVERDE C and LOPEZ-FANDINO R (2000), 'Effect of high pressure on the vitamin B_1 and B_6 content of milk', *Milchwissenschaft*, **55**(7), 365–7
SONOIKE K, SETOYAMA T, KUMA Y and KOBAYASHI S (1992), 'Effect of pressure and temperature on the death rates of *Lactobacillus casei* and *Escherichia coli*', in Balny C, Hayashi R, Heremans K and Masson P (eds), *High Pressure and Biotechnology 224*, Montrouge, John Libbey Eurotext, 297–301
TAOUKIS P S, PANAGIOTIDIS P, STOFOROS N G, BUTZ P, FISTER H and TAUSCHER B (1998), 'Kinetics of vitamin C degradation under high pressure-moderate temperature processing in model systems and fruit juices', in Isaacs N S (ed), *High Pressure Food Science, Bioscience and Chemistry*, Cambridge, UK, The Royal Society of Chemistry, 310–16
TAUSCHER B (1995), 'Pasteurization of food by hydrostatic high pressure: chemical aspects', *Z Lebensm Unters Forsch*, **200**, 3–13
TAUSCHER B (1998), 'Effect of high pressure treatment to nutritive substances and natural pigments', in Autio K (ed), 'Fresh novel foods by high pressure', *VTT Symposium 186*, Espoo, Finland, Technical Research Centre of Finland, 83–95

TAUSCHER B (1999), 'Chemical Reactions of Food Components Under High Hydrostatic Pressure', in Ludwig H (ed), *Advances in High Pressure Bioscience and Biotechnology*, Heidelberg, Springer, 363–6
VAN DEN BROECK I, LUDIKHUYZE L, WEEMAES C, VAN LOEY A and HENDRICKX M (1998), 'Kinetics for isobaric-isothermal degradation of L-ascorbic acid', *J Agric Food Chem*, **46**, 2001–6
VAN LOEY A, OOMS V, WEEMAES C, VAN DEN BROECK I, LUDIKHUYZE L, INDRAWATI, DENYS S and HENDRICKX M (1998), 'Thermal and pressure-temperature degradation of chlorophyll in broccoli (*Brassica oleracea* L. italica) juice: a kinetic study', *J Agric Food Chem*, **46**(12), 2785–92
WADA S (1992), 'Quality and lipid change of sardine meat by high pressure treatment', in Balny C, Hayashi R, Heremans K and Masson P (eds), *High Pressure and Biotechnology 224*, Montrouge, John Libbey Eurotext, 235–8
WADA S and OGAWA Y (1996), 'High presure effects on lipid degradation: myoglobin change and water holding capacity', in Hayashi R and Balny C, *High Pressure Bioscience and Biotechnology*, Amsterdam, Elsevier Science B V, 351–6
WUYTACK E (1999), *Pressure-induced germination and inactivation of* Bacillus subtilis spores, Doctoral dissertation no. 404, Katholieke Universiteit Leuven, Leuven, Belgium
YEN G C and LIN H T (1996), 'Comparison of high pressure treatment and thermal pasteurisation on the quality and shelf life of guava puree', *Int J Food Sci Technol*, **31**, 205–13
ZIMMERMAN F and BERGMAN C (1993), 'Isostatic high-pressure equipment for food preservation', *Food Technol*, **47**(6), 162–3

21.12 Appendices

Appendix 21.1 Tentative list of universities actively involved in high pressure research in the last 10 years particularly in the field of bioscience, food science and chemistry

JAPAN

Department	Institution	City
/	Anan College of Technology	Anan
Department of Food Science	Rakuno Gakuen University	Ebetsu
Department of Applied Chemistry	Fukui University	Fukui
Department of Food and Nutrition	Nakamura Gakuen University	Fukuoka
Department of Nutrition Morphology	Nakamura Gakuen University	Fukuoka
Department of Applied Science	Kyushu University	Fukuoka
Laboratory of biochemistry, Department of Chemistry	Fukuoka University	Fukuoka
Department of Applied Biological Science	Hiroshima University	Higashihiroshima
Department of Applied Chemistry	Kagoshima University	Kagoshima
Department of Chemistry	Kobe University	Kobe
Department of Chemical Engineering	Kobe University	Kobe
The Graduate School of Science and Technology	Kobe University	Kobe

JAPAN *Continued*

Department	Institution	City
Department of Home Economics	Konan Women's University	Kobe
Laboratory of Biochemistry	Kobe Yamate College	Kobe
Division of Applied Life Sciences	Kyoto University	Kyoto
Institute of Chemical Research	Kyoto University	Kyoto
Department of Agricultural Chemistry (Research Institute for Food Science)	Kyoto University	Kyoto
Department of Chemistry	Kyoto University	Kyoto
Department of Molecular Engineering	Kyoto University	Kyoto
Department of Polymer Science and Engineering	Kyoto Institute of Technology	Kyoto
Department of Applied Biology	Kyoto Institute of Technology	Kyoto
Department of Chemistry	Ritsumeikan University	Kyoto
Department of Science	Kyoto University of Education	Kyoto
Department of Industrial Science	Kyoto University of Education	Kyoto
Faculty of Agriculture	Meijo University	Nagoya
Faculty of Agriculture	Nagoya University	Nagoya
Department of Food Science and Technology	Nagoya University	Nagoya
Department of Applied Biochemistry	University of Niigata	Niigata
Department of Biosystem Science	University of Niigata	Niigata
Department of Chemistry	Nagaoka University of Technology	Niigata
Electron Microscopic Laboratory	University of Niigata	Niigata
Department of Nutrition Science	Okayama Prefectural University	Okayama
Laboratory of Food Science and Nutrition	Hagoromo-Gakuen College	Sakai
Institute for Chemical Reaction Science	Tohoku University	Sendai
Department of Chemistry	Ritsumeikan University	Shiga
Department of Applied Biochemistry	Utsunomiya University	Tochigi
Department of Chemical Science and Technology	University of Tokushima	Tokushima
Department of Biological Science and Technology	University of Tokushima	Tokushima
Department of Biology	Japan Women's University	Tokyo
Department of Chemical and Biological Sciences	Japan Women's University	Tokyo
Food Science and Technology	Nihon University	Tokyo
Department of Biological Chemistry	Nihon University	Tokyo
Food Processing Centre	Tokyo University of Agriculture	Tokyo
Department of Food Science and Technology	Tokyo University of Fisheries	Tokyo
Faculty of Technology	Tokyo University of Agriculture and Technology	Tokyo

JAPAN *Continued*

Department	Institution	City
School of Human Life and Environmental Science	Ochanomizu University	Tokyo
Faculty of Home Economics	Ochanomizu University	Tokyo
Biotechnology Research Centre	Toyama Prefectural University	Toyama
Department of Applied Biochemistry	Utsunomiya University	Utsunomiya

EUROPE

Department	Institution	City	Country
Laboratory of Food Technology	Katholieke Universiteit Leuven	Leuven	Belgium
Laboratory of Food Microbiology	Katholieke Universiteit Leuven	Leuven	Belgium
Laboratory for Chemical and Biological Dynamics	Katholieke Universiteit Leuven	Leuven	Belgium
Unité de Technologie des Industries Agro-Alimentaires	Gembloux Agricultural University	Gembloux	Belgium
Department of Food Technology and Nutrition	Ghent University	Ghent	Belgium
Department of Food Preservation and Meat Technology	Czech Academy of Sciences	Prague	Czech Republic
Department of Dairy and Food Science	Royal Veterinary and Agricultural University	Frederiksberg	Denmark
Institute of Biochemistry	Odense University	Odense	Denmark
LBPA	Ecole Normale Supérieure de Cachan	Cachan	France
Laboratoire de Génie des Procédés Alimentaires et Biotechnologiques	ENSBANA – University of Bourgogne	Dijon	France
Laboratoire de Génie Protéique et Cellulaire	University of La Rochelle	La Rochelle	France
Unité de Biochimie et Technologie Alimentaires	University of Montpellier	Montpellier	France
Genie des Procedes Alimentaires (GEPEA)	École Nationale d'Ingénieurs des Techniques des Industries Agricoles et Alimentaires	Nantes	France
Laboratoire de Biochimie et Technologies des Aliments	Institut Supérieure de Technologie Alimentaires de Bordeaux	Talence	France

456 The nutrition handbook for food processors

EUROPE *Continued*

Department	Institution	City	Country
Interface Haute Pression	École Nationale Supérieure Bordeaux de Chimie et de Physique de Bordeaux	Talence – Bordeaux	France
Department of Food Biotechnology and Food Process Engineering	Technische Universität Berlin	Berlin	Germany
Department of Chemistry	University of Dortmund	Dortmund	Germany
Institute of Physiology	University of Heidelberg	Heidelberg	Germany
Institute of Pharmaceutical Technology and Biopharmacy	University of Heidelberg	Heidelberg	Germany
Institute of Inorganic Chemistry	University of Kiel	Kiel	Germany
Institute of Food Process Engineering	Technische Universität München	Freising-Weihenstephan	Germany
Lehrstuhl für Fluidmechanik und Prozessautomation	Technische Universität München	Freising	Germany
Lehrstuhl für Energie- und Umwelttechnik der Lebensmittelindustrie	Technische Universität München	Freising	Germany
Institut für Ernährungsphysiologie	Technische Universität München	Freising	Germany
Department of Molecular Biology	Max Planck Institute for Biophysical Chemistry	Göttingen	Germany
Lehrstuhl für Technische Mikrobiologie	Technische Universität München	Munchen	Germany
Laboratory for Food Chemistry and Technology	National Technical University of Athens	Athens	Greece
Department of Biophysics and Radiation Biology	Semmelweis University	Budapest	Hungary
Dipartimento di Scienze Molecolari Agroalimentari	University of Milan	Milan	Italy
Dipt. Di Fisiologia e Biochimica Generali	Università degli Studi	Milan	Italy
Istituto di Impianti Chimici	University of Padova	Padova	Italy
Instituto di Biofisica	CNR	Pisa	Italy
Dipartimento di Scienze degli Alimenti	University of Udine	Udine	Italy

High pressure processing 457

EUROPE *Continued*

Department	Institution	City	Country
Istituto Policattedra	University of Verona	Verona	Italy
Kluyver Laboratory for Biotechnology	Technische Universiteit Delft	Delft	The Netherlands
Department of Food Technology	University of Agriculture and Technology	Olsztyn	Poland
Department of Food Hygiene	Warsaw Agricultural University	Warsaw	Poland
Department of Chemistry	University of Aveiro	Aveiro	Portugal
Department of Chemistry	Moscow State University	Moscow	Russia
Faculty of Chemistry and Chemical Engineering	University of Maribor	Maribor	Slovenia
Tecnologia dels Aliments (CeRTA)	Universitat Autònoma de Barcelona	Bellaterra	Spain
Protein Engineering Laboratory	University of Girona	Girona	Spain
Laboratory of Physical Chemistry	ETH-Zentrum	Zurich	Switzerland
Institut de Chimie Minérale et Analytique (BCH)	University of Lausanne	Lausanne	Switzerland
Department of Agriculture for Northern Ireland	The Queen's University of Belfast	Belfast	UK
Department of Bioscience and Biotechnology	University of Strathclyde	Glasgow	UK
Department of Chemical Engineering and Chemical Technology	Imperial College of Science, Technology and Medicine	London	UK
School of Food Biosciences	University of Reading	Reading	UK
Department of Chemistry	University of Reading	Reading	UK
Department of Biomedical Sciences	University of Aberdeen	Scotland	UK
School of Biosciences	University of Surrey	Surrey	UK
Procter Department of Food Science	University of Leeds	Leeds	UK

REST OF THE WORLD

Department	Institution	City/States	Country
Department of Pharmacology	University of Western Australia	Nedlands	Australia
Department of Biochemistry	Federal University of Rio de Janeiro	Rio de Janeiro	Brazil

REST OF THE WORLD *Continued*

Department	Institution	City/States	Country
Department of Medical Biochemistry	Federal University of Rio de Janeiro	Rio de Janeiro	Brazil
Department of Biochemistry	State University of Campinas	Campinas (Sao Paulo)	Brazil
Department of Food Science and Agricultural Chemistry	McGill University	Montreal (Quebec)	Canada
Scientific Centre of Radiobiology and Radiation Ecology	The Georgian Academy of Sciences	Tbilisi	Republic of Georgia
Department of Chemical Engineering	University of California	Berkeley	USA
Center of Marine Biotechnology	University of Maryland Biotechnology Institute	Baltimore	USA
Department of Food Science and Technology	Oregon State University	Corvallis	USA
Department of Food Science and Technology	Ohio State University	Columbus	USA
Department of Biochemistry	UT South western Medical Centre	Dallas	USA
Food Science and Human Nutrition	University of Florida	Gainesville	USA
Centre for Marine Biotechnology and Biomedicine	University of California	La Jolla	USA
SCRIPPS, Marine Biology Research	University of California	La Jolla	USA
Citrus Research and Education Centre	University of Florida	Lake Alfred	USA
Department of Animal and Food Sciences	University of Delaware	Newark	USA
Department of Chemistry	Rutgers University	New Jersey	USA
Centre for Nonthermal Processing of Food (CNPF)	Washington State University	Pullman	USA
Department of Biological Systems Engineering	Washington State University	Pullman	USA
Department of Food Science and Human Nutrition	Washington State University	Pullman	USA
Food Science Department	North Carolina State University	Raleigh	USA
Department of Microbiology and Immunology	University of Rochester	Rochester	USA
Department of Pharmaceutical Chemistry	University of California	San Francisco	USA
Beckman Institute for Advanced Science and Technology	University of Illinois	Urbana	USA

Appendix 21.2 Tentative list of research centres, government institutions and industries actively involved in high pressure research in the last 10 years

JAPAN

Institution	City/Prefecture
Pokka Corporation	Achi
Department of Research and Development, Nihon Shokken Co. Ltd.	Ehime
Maruto Sangyo Co. Ltd.	Fukuoka
Department of Research and Development, Ichiban Foods Co. Ltd.	Fukuoka
Frozen Foods R&D Centre, Ajinomoto Frozen Foods Co. Ltd.	Gunma
Mitsubishi Heavy Industries Ltd., Hiroshima Machinery Works	Hiroshima
Hiroshima Prefectural Food Technological Research Centre	Hiroshima-shi
Research and Development Centre, Nippon Meat Packers, Inc.	Hyogo
Manufacturing Service Department, Nestlá Japan Ltd.	Hyogo
Mechanical Engineering Research Laboratory, Kobe Steel Ltd.	Hyogo
SR Structural Research Group	Hyogo
Toyo Institute of Technology	Hyogo
Biotechnology Research Laboratory, Kobe Steel Ltd.	Ibaraki
National Institute of Bioscience and Human Technology, Agency of Industrial Science and Technology	Ibaraki
Research and Development Centre, Nippon Meat Packers, Inc.	Ibaraki
Food Product Technologies, Central Research Laboratories, Ajinomoto Co. Ltd.	Kanagawa
Food and Drug Safety Centre	Kanagawa
Takanshi Milk	Kanagawa
Kato Brothers Honey Co. Ltd.	Kanagawa
Kumamoto Industrial Research Institute (KIRI)	Kumamoto
Hondamisohonten Co. Ltd.	Kyoto
Hishiroku Co. Ltd.	Kyoto
Teramecs Co. Ltd.	Kyoto
Miyazaki Food Processing R&D Centre	Miyazaki
Miyazaki Prefectural Institute for Public Health and Environment	Miyazaki
Marui Co. Ltd.	Nagano
Food Technology Research Institute of Nagano Prefecture	Nagano
Industrial Technology Centre of Nagasaki Prefecture	Nagasaki
Food Technology Research Institute of Nagano Prefecture	Nagoya
Mutter Ham Co. Ltd.	Nagoya
Mitsubishi Rayon Engineering Co. Ltd., Aichi	Nagoya
Research Institute, Echigo Seika Co. Ltd.	Niigata
Meidi-Ya Food Factory	Osaka
San-Ei Gen FFI, Inc.	Osaka
Yamamoto Suiatu Kogyosho Co. Ltd.	Osaka
Department of Sales Engineering, Yamamoto Suiatu Kogyosho Co. Ltd.	Osaka
Nitta Gelatin Inc	Osaka
Technology and Research Institute, Snow Brand Milk Products Co. Ltd.	Saitama
Packaging Research Institute, Dai Nippon Printing Co. Ltd.	Sayama
Technology Development Labs, Meiji Seika Kaisha Ltd.	Saitama
Packaging Research Laboratory, Toppan Printing Co. Ltd.	Saitama
Industrial Research Institute of Shiga prefecture	Shiga
Research Laboratory Takara Shuzo Co. Ltd.	Shiga

JAPAN Continued

Institution	City/Prefecture
Biochemical Division, Yaizu Suisan Kagaku Industry Co. Ltd.	Shizuoka
Research Laboratory, Yamamasa Co. Ltd.	Shizuoka
Research Institute Kagome Co. Ltd.	Tochigi-ken
Oriental Yeast Co. Ltd.	Tokyo
Research Institute of Q.P. Corporation	Tokyo
Central Research Lab., Nippon Suisan Kaisha Ltd.	Tokyo
The Japanese R&D Association for High Pressure Technology in Food Industry	Tokyo
Taiyo Central R&D Institute, Taiyo Fishery Co. Ltd.	Tokyo
Nippon Surio Denshi K.K. (Framatome Corp.)	Tokyo
Tetra Pak	Tokyo
Food Industrial Research Institute	Tottori
Sugino Machine Ltd.	Toyama
Toyama Food Research Institute	Toyama
National Institute for Materials and Chemical Research	Tuskuba
National Institute of Bioscience and Human Technology	Tuskuba
DEEP STAR group, Japan Marine Science and Technology Centre (JAMSTEC)	Yokosuka
National Research Institute of Fisheries Science	Yokohama
Wakayama Agricultural Processing Research Corporation	Wakayama

EUROPE

Institution	City	Country
FMC Food Machinery Corporation Europe N.V.	Sint Niklaas	Belgium
Engineered Pressure Systems International NV (EPSI)	Temse	Belgium
Biotechnology and Food Research, Technical Research Centre of Finland (VTT)	Helsinki	Finland
Hautes Pressions Technologies (until 2000)	Bar le Duc	France
EPL-AGRO (until 2000)	Bar le Duc	France
Pampryl	Guadeloupe	France
Centre Technique de la Conservation des Produits Agricoles	Dury	France
CLEXTRAL	Firminy	France
European Synchrotron Radiation Facility	Grenoble	France
Centre de Recherches du Service de Santé des Armées	La Tronche	France
Institute for Health and Medical Research (INSERM)U128	Montpellier	France
Gec ALSTHOM ACB	Nantes	France
Institute for Health and Medical Research (INSERM)U310	Paris	France
Equipe de Recherche Agroalimentaire Périgourdine (ERAP)	Périqueux	France
National Institute for Agricultural Research (INRA)	Toulouse	France
Max Delbrück Center for Molecular Medicine	Berlin	Germany
Nutronova GmbH	Frankfurt	Germany
UHDE Hochdrucktechik GmbH	Hagen	Germany

EUROPE *Continued*

Institution	City	Country
Institute of Chemistry and Biology, Federal Research Centre for Nutrition (BFE)	Karlsruhe	Germany
Federal Dairy Research Centre	Kiel	Germany
Max Planck Institute	Mainz	Germany
Experimental Station for the Food Preserving Industry	Parma	Italy
Flow Pressure Systems (former ABB Pressure Systems)	Milan	Italy
Exenia Group S.r.l	Albignasego	Italy
Agrotechnological Research Institute (ATO-DLO)	Wageningen	The Netherlands
Unilever Research Laboratorium	Vlaardingen	The Netherlands
State Scientific Centre of Russian Federation	Moscow	Russia
Flow Pressure Systems (former ABB Pressure Systems)	Vaesteraas	Sweden
Nestlé Research Centre, Nestec Ltd.	Lausanne	Switzerland
National Institute of Hygiene	Warsaw	Poland
Institute of Bioorganic Chemistry, Polish Academy of Sciences	Poznan	Poland
Institute of Agricultural and Food Biotechnology, Polish Academy of Sciences	Warsaw	Poland
High Pressure Research Centre, UNIPRESS, Polish Academy of Sciences	Warsaw	Poland
Institute of Organic Chemistry, Polish Academy of Sciences	Warsaw	Poland
Institute of Biomedical Chemistry, RAMS	Moscow	Russia
State Scientific Centre of Russian Federation	Moscow	Russia
Space Biomedical Centre for Training and Research	Moscow	Russia
Union 'PLASTPOLYMER'	St Petersburg	Russia
Institute for High Pressure Physics, Russian Academy of Sciences	Troitsk	Russia
Instituto del Frío (CSIC), Ciudad University	Madrid	Spain
Esteban Espuna	Olot	Spain
Stansted Fluid Power Ltd.	Essex	UK
Campden and Chorleywood Food Research Association (CCFRA)	Chipping Campden	UK
Institute of Food Research	Norwich	UK
Donetsk Physics and Technology Institute, National Ukrainian Academy of Sciences	Donetsk	Ukraine

UNITED STATES, CANADA AND SOUTH AMERICA

Institution	City	Country
Food Research and Development Centre	St. Hyacinthe (Quebec)	Canada
National Centre for Food Safety and Technology (NCFST)	Chicago	USA
Avomex	Keller	USA
Flow International Corporation	Washington	USA
BMA Laboratories, Inc.	Woburn	USA
BioSeq, Inc.	Woburn	USA

22
Continuous-flow heat processing

N. J. Heppell, Oxford Brookes University

22.1 Introduction: definition of the process

The continuous-flow heat process is a thermal heat-hold-cool process where the foodstuff to be treated is pumped in continuous flow through heat exchanger systems where it is heated to a desired temperature, held at that temperature for a pre-determined time, then cooled to around ambient temperature. After heat treatment, the product is then packaged in an appropriate manner. This process is different from in-container processes, such as canning or retorting, in which the product is firstly packaged and sealed, and then heat treated.

Different thermal processes can be applied, from thermisation and pasteurisation through to full sterilisation depending on the temperature and holding time employed, and packaging method selected. Terminology is difficult; for pasteurisation, the process is often called High Temperature Short Time (HTST); for sterilisation, it may be called Ultra High Temperature (UHT) or aseptic processing. The advantages of continuous-flow heat processes over in-container processes are the much faster rates of heat transfer that can be attained, which means that higher process temperatures can be applied, usually around 140 to 150°C, as opposed to a maximum of around 125°C for in-container processes. In addition, the slow heating and cooling rates in in-container processes can incur considerable thermal damage to the product before the desired process has been attained. A comparison between the time-temperature profiles for the two processes is given in Fig. 22.1.

Disadvantages of the process in comparison with in-container heat treatments include the fact that the process is less inherently safe than in-container processing as there are more points of potential contamination. Adequate sterilisation of the packaging material is essential; contamination may occur during the packag-

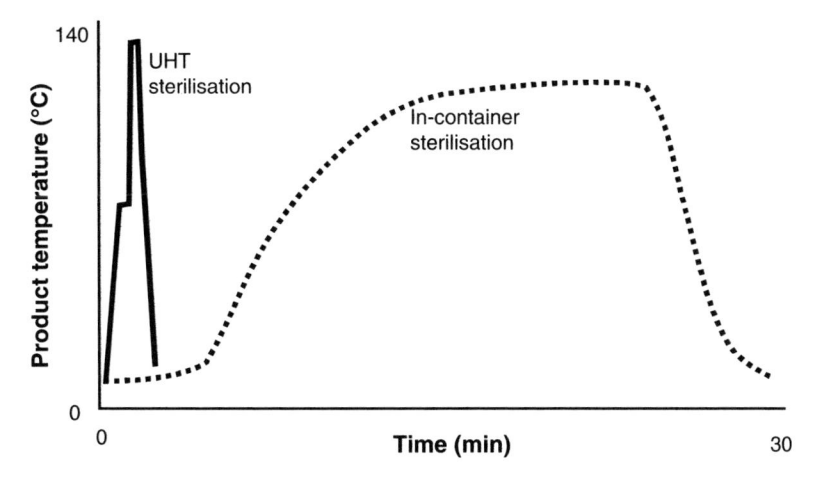

Fig. 22.1 Temperature profiles of in-container and continuous-flow heat (UHT) processes.

ing operation and all parts of process equipment after the holding section must be sterilised before processing commences. In addition, the product must be capable of being pumped and it is therefore limited to liquids: however, the product may be purely liquid or liquid with comminuted solids or fibres (e.g. milks, creams, fruit juices, tomato purée) or a liquid which contains substantial solid particulates, such as soups, stews and cook-in sauces.

22.2 Principles of thermal processing

22.2.1 Thermal degradation kinetics

Both the thermal death of microorganisms and thermal degradation of biochemical components of food have been found to obey first order chemical reaction kinetics (with a few exceptions). At constant temperature, therefore, the reaction rate is given by

$$-\frac{dN}{dt} = k.N \quad \text{and} \quad -\frac{dC}{dt} = k.C \qquad [22.1]$$

where N is number of organisms, C is concentration of biochemical, k is the reaction rate constant and t is time.

In thermal sterilisation technology, equation 22.1 can be rewritten as:

$$\frac{N}{N_0} = 10^{-t/D} \quad \text{and} \quad \frac{C}{C_0} = 10^{-t/D} \qquad [22.2]$$

where N and C are the number of microorganisms and concentration of biochemical respectively at time t, N_0 and C_0 are the initial number and concentration and D is the decimal reduction time. The decimal reduction time is the time taken to reduce the number of microorganisms or concentration of biochemical by a factor of 10 (i.e. to a value $1/10^{th}$ of that initially). This decimal reduction time is constant, i.e. for any time interval D, there will be a reduction to one-tenth.

When quantifying the effect of temperature change on the D value, there are two major models used: the traditional 'Canning' (constant-z) model and the Arrhenius model. The former is:

$$\frac{D_1}{D_2} = 10^{(\theta_2 - \theta_1)/z} \qquad [22.3]$$

where D_1 and D_2 are the decimal reduction times at θ_1 and θ_2 respectively. The z value is the temperature change required to change the decimal reduction time by a factor of 10.

The Arrhenius equation is:

$$k = A.e^{-E_a/R\theta_k} \qquad [22.4]$$

where A is a constant, the frequency factor, E_a is the activation energy, R is the gas constant and θ_k is the absolute temperature.

These two models are actually mutually exclusive but will agree within experimental error over a relatively short temperature range, which is usually the case for death of microorganisms. For larger temperature ranges, which is more usual for biochemical degradations, the Arrhenius relationship has a better theoretical basis and is generally used.

Research work which reports thermal death of different strains of microorganisms or degradation of biochemical components usually gives D and z values at a defined reference temperature (often 121.1°C) or the activation energy E_a and frequency factor, A. There are tables of data given in Holdsworth (1992, 1997) and Karmas and Harris (1988) for microorganisms and biochemical components.

22.2.2 Effect of change in temperature

An examination of the kinetics for microbial death and for degradation of biochemical components shows that the z values for the former are in the region of 10°C, while for the latter they are around 30°C. This difference is the basis of UHT processing: by increasing the temperature of a foodstuff, the microbial death rate increases much faster than biochemical degradation and, for equal levels of sterilisation, higher temperatures will give a better nutritional and organoleptic quality food than lower temperatures. One major disadvantage of this is that some enzymes may survive, especially heat-resistant proteases and lipases. It is important, therefore, that as high a process temperature be attained as is feasible and this is usually in the region of 137°C to 147°C.

22.3 Process equipment and product quality

22.3.1 Selection of heat exchangers

The selection of heat exchangers for continuous flow heat processes is dependent on the physical properties of the food to be processed, especially its viscosity, the presence of solid particulates or fibres and any tendency of the foodstuff to 'burn-on'.

Heating may be indirect, where the heating medium is kept separate from the product, or direct, where the heat transfer medium is mixed with the food product (almost exclusively steam). For indirect heat exchangers, the heating medium may be steam or pressurised hot water and cooling may be by mains water, refrigerated brine or liquid refrigerant as part of a refrigeration cycle. The process plant is based on corrugated plate, plain or corrugated tube or scraped-surface heat exchangers, a description of which, as well as applications and relative advantages and disadvantages, is given in many standard food engineering texts. Where possible, a heat recovery section (often called a regeneration section) is incorporated into the process to minimise its energy requirements. In this way, heat recovery of up to 80–90% of the total requirement may be achieved. For detailed process arrangements, see Lewis and Heppell (2000).

The rate of heating and cooling of the food product within the equipment is important, as can be seen later, and is maximised in this type of equipment in three ways:

1 By increased turbulence in the food, minimising the liquid-heating surface boundary layer and therefore increasing heat transfer. This is usually achieved by corrugating the heat transfer surface to form a convoluted channel configuration for the liquid to flow down.
2 By increasing the ratio of heating area to liquid hold-up in the equipment, i.e. by decreasing the size of the product channel.
3 By increasing the temperature difference between the food and the heating or cooling medium.

Of these, the first two can be easily accommodated, but the last often cannot be used as many food products are heat-sensitive and will increasingly form a deposit on the heating surface, increasing heat resistance and reducing heat transfer.

Direct heating takes two forms:

1 Steam injection, sometimes called steam-into-product, where steam is injected directly into the food through a steam injector nozzle and the steam bubbles condense.
2 Steam infusion, sometimes called product-into-steam, where the product is pumped into a pressurised steam chamber, forming a liquid curtain onto which the steam condenses.

Direct heating is the most rapid heating method but suffers from the disadvantages that the process is noisy and the steam must be of a culinary grade, using only permitted boiler feed water additives. In addition, during heating the condensed steam dilutes the product by adding about 10% extra water and can be handled in one of two ways:

1 The recipe for the feed to the process can be made more concentrated, so that after cooling (using a conventional indirect heat exchanger) the final product is at the correct concentration.

2   An equivalent volume of water is removed from the final product to bring the concentration back to the original value, e.g. for milk, where adulteration is illegal.

The latter may be achieved using a 'flash-cooling' process, where the foodstuff passes from the holding tube through a restriction into a cyclone under vacuum. The sudden decrease in pressure causes the excess water to vaporise (or 'flash') and simultaneously cools the product. By altering the level of vacuum in the cyclone, the same concentration of solids as in the inlet can be achieved, in the outlet stream. One disadvantage of this process, however, is that the large temperature drop in flash cooling means that heat recovery is much lower than for indirect-heating systems and the process is more expensive to operate.

22.3.2   Effect of rate of heating on product quality

The rate of heating and cooling of the foodstuff as it passes through the process gives a measurable effect on the nutritional and organoleptic quality of the product. Direct-heating systems, both injection and infusion, give the fastest rate of heating and flash evaporation gives the fastest cooling rate; both are virtually instantaneous. For indirect heating systems, on the other hand, the rate of heating is controlled by several factors:

1   The temperature difference between the foodstuff and the heating medium. The difference is limited by the heat sensitivity of the foodstuff, especially its tendency to 'burn-on' to heated surfaces.
2   The area available for heat transfer, i.e. the area of contact between the foodstuff and the heating or cooling medium. One important factor is the presence of solid particulates in the foodstuff. The channel size through the equipment must be a minimum of three times the particulate size, which reduces the ratio of heat transfer area to liquid volume in the process, severely reducing the rate of heat transfer.
3   The heat transfer coefficients either side of the heat exchanger wall. These are controlled by both the turbulence in the foodstuff or heating/cooling medium, and their thermal conductivities. In addition, the physical state of the heating medium (whether liquid or condensing steam) is important.
4   The heat recovery section. The greater the heat recovery, the cheaper the system is to operate but the larger physical size of process plant means the rate of heating is much slower.

The time–temperature profile of a continuous-flow heat process can be determined from physical measurements taken on the process. The temperature points are determined by sensing the temperature at key points in the process, e.g. at the inlet and outlet points of each heat exchanger and any holding sections. The residence time in each section is determined by measuring the volume of process plant between these temperature points and calculating the time as:

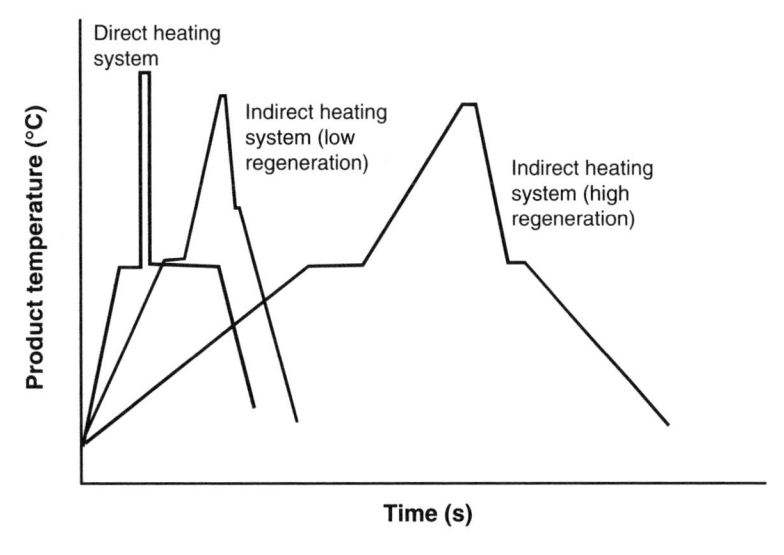

Fig. 22.2 Time–temperature profiles for direct heating, indirect heating, with low regeneration and indirect heating with high regeneration processes.

$$\text{mean residence time} = \frac{\text{volume of section}}{\text{volumetric flowrate of product through it}} \quad [22.5]$$

From this, a time–temperature profile similar to that obtained for heat penetration into a container can be constructed and used in the same way to calculate F_0 values, chemical changes etc. Typical time–temperature profiles for direct and indirect-heating processes are given in Fig. 22.2. For a further explanation of this area, the reader is directed to work by Reuter (1982) and Kessler and Horak (1981a, 1981b), who collected time–temperature profiles for a wide variety of milk UHT plants and calculated sterilisation and biochemical changes expected.

22.3.3 Effect of residence time distribution on product quality

Not all elements of the fluid food will move through the equipment at the same rate; generally, the fluid near the wall will move more slowly and that in the centre of the flow channel will move more quickly than the average flowrate. This has implications for the sterilisation of the product in that, in the holding tube, the residence time at the process temperature is lower than expected and therefore either the product will not be sterile or the holding time must be increased to compensate. This must necessarily mean that all slower-moving foodstuff will be over-processed with concomitant thermal degradation. The greater the spread of residence times, the worse the loss of thermosensitive nutrients.

The most important factor in the residence time distribution is the flow regime in the liquid; either

- Streamline flow (for slow flowrates or high viscosity fluids) where the fastest element of fluid has a velocity twice that of the average velocity.

or

- Turbulent flow (for higher velocities or low viscosity fluids) where the fastest element of fluid is about 1.3 times faster than the average velocity.

For further information relating to prediction and measurement of residence time distribution and its effect on sterilisation and quality, see Lewis and Heppell (2000).

22.4 Processing and key nutrients: proteins

The impact of any continuous-flow process on nutritional components in a food will be similar in type to the appropriate in-container process. However, as explained earlier, the difference in z values between microbiological death and biochemical degradation means that the level of that impact will generally be substantially lower. Much of the detailed work on changes to nutrients during continuous-flow heat processing concerns milk and milk products, as research in this area has been on-going since the 1950s. As the technology is more recently being applied to other products, a large body of work on further foodstuffs is progressing and will continue to do so.

In general, a variety of changes in proteins can occur at elevated temperatures, especially denaturation and its associated changes in properties such as the water-holding capacity, viscosity or whippability, development of flavours (especially sulphurous), aggregation or formation of precipitates. Proteins are known to have a maximum thermostability at their isoelectric points although at pH values on either side, thermostability decreases at different rates depending on the type of protein and its environment. The effect of inorganic salts may also be important; at low levels of salts, stability is generally lower but, at high levels, can either reduce or increase stability. Lysine and cysteine are degraded by heat; losses of the latter rarely exceed 25% during in-container processing and are generally negligible in UHT processing.

In milk, the proteins are divided into two types, caseins (in micelle form) and whey proteins. The whey proteins (α-lactalbumin, β-lactoglobulin, bovine serum albumin and immunoglobulins) are in solution and start to denature at temperatures as low as 70–90°C. Typical denaturation levels in UHT are given for pasteurised milk as 5–15%, direct heating systems as 50–75%, indirect heating systems 70–90% and in-bottle sterilised as 80–100% (Renner, 1979). However, denaturation has little or no effect on their nutritive value, biological value or true digestibility. Unfolding and denaturation of β-lactoglobulin is responsible for release of volatile sulphurous compounds and the subsequent flavour of UHT milk. Oxidisation of these compounds during storage, either by residual oxygen in the product or leakage of oxygen into the container, will reduce this cooked flavour in the first few days after production. Again, direct heating processes were found to give a lower level of volatile sulphurous compounds, partly due to removal of the compounds during flash-cooling and despite the lower residual level of oxygen also due to this.

The casein micelles are relatively heat stable and only minor changes are found. However, this reaction is important, because denatured whey proteins aggregate onto the casein and interfere with coagulation by acid or rennet, giving a looser curd. The milk is not suitable for use in cheesemaking.

Soy milk is increasing in popularity as a product in Europe and the USA but raw soybeans have been long known to have a poor nutritive value due to the high levels of trypsin inhibitors in them. It is important nutritionally to reduce these inhibitors to less than 10% of the original concentration, at which point they will not interfere with biological value of the protein. The conditions required to achieve this are quite severe, for instance the D value at 143°C is between 56 and 100s, depending on the pH. Thermal denaturation of the inhibitor has been reviewed by Kwok and Niranjan (1995).

22.5 Carbohydrates and fats

For mono- and oligosaccharides, little direct degradation occurs at temperatures typical of UHT processing but there are several reactions that occur that may affect nutritional quality. Firstly, Maillard reactions may occur, depending on the composition of the food, i.e. the presence of reducing sugars and amino acids. This is covered in Chapter 11 and will not be further discussed here. It is interesting to note that one of the intermediate compounds formed during the reactions, 5′-hydroxymethylfurfural (HMF), has been used to indicate the level of heat treatment received by milk.

Secondly, another reaction of note in milk is the formation of lactulose, an epimer of lactose formed during heating, which has also been used to distinguish between levels of heat treatment. This compound has been used in European Union legislation to distinguish between pasteurised, UHT-sterilised and in-container sterilised milks, and can also be used to distinguish between direct- and indirect-heating processes. Although lactulose has a laxative effect at around 2.5 mg/kg, milks fortunately do not reach this level, being around 2 mg/kg for in-bottle sterilised and much lower for other milks.

Native starches will gelatinise at relatively low temperatures (60 to 85°C) and have been found to break down under the high temperatures and high shear rates present in an UHT process, giving a product with a vastly reduced viscosity after heat treatment. To overcome this, it is necessary to use chemically-modified starches which have been specifically devised to be stable under these conditions. Rapaille (1995) found a highly crossbonded and hydroxypropylated waxy maize starch performed best in both plate and direct-heating UHT processes. Low crossbonded starches, however, were found to foul the process plant rapidly and gave a high viscosity during the preheating stages of the process.

22.5.1 Fats

UHT processing has not been found to cause any physical or chemical changes to fats in milk and milk products. Milk is usually homogenised during treatment, and some instability of the milk fat globule may occur due to denaturation of the proteins in the milk fat globule membrane. Because of this, homogenisation after the heat treatment section is usually preferred, especially in direct-heating systems, but has the potential to cause recontamination of the product due to leakage through the homogeniser seals and general difficulty with cleaning this area. It is important to have a well designed homogeniser with aseptic design and steam seals on the piston seals.

22.6 Vitamins

The heat stability of vitamins in foodstuffs during heating is extremely variable, depending on the foodstuff and conditions of heating, e.g. presence of oxygen. As vitamins often consist of different chemicals, all of which have vitamin activity but degrade at different rates, it is often difficult to measure vitamin loss in a mechanistic way; see the discussion on vitamin C below. Apart from straightforward denaturation, reactions between some of the vitamins may also occur, giving further losses.

The heat-sensitive vitamins are generally taken to be the fat-soluble vitamins; A (with oxygen present) D, E, and β-carotene (provitamin A); and some of the water-soluble vitamins, B_1 (thiamin), B_2 (riboflavin) (in acid environment), nicotinic acid, pantothenic acid, biotin and vitamin C (ascorbic acid). Vitamin B_{12} and folic acid are also heat labile but their destruction involves a complex series of reactions with each other. Vitamin B_6 is generally little affected by heat, but storage after heat treatment can cause high losses. Niacin and vitamin K are fairly stable to heat. As before, losses through degradation in continuous-flow heat processing will be similar to those encountered during in-container processing but at a lower level.

In milk, vitamins A, D, E, pantothenic acid, nicotinic acid, biotin, riboflavin and niacin are all stable to heat (Burton, 1988). Thiamin (B_1), B_6, B_{12} and vitamin C all degrade during sterilisation. Thiamin is the most heat labile of these and has been used as a chemical marker to define the UHT process for milk by Horak (1980) as the time–temperature combinations which produce a sterile product but have a loss of thiamin of less than 3%. The thermal degradation kinetics have been established and used to predict thiamin loss for different commercial UHT processes; again, thiamin was expected to have a better survival in direct heating processes than in indirect heating processes and, of the latter in processes with small heat recovery sections than those with large sections.

Vitamin C loss, although generally in the region of 25%, is not significant because milk is such a poor source of the vitamin in the diet. This compares well to losses of 90% of the vitamin during in-container sterilisation. The loss of the vitamin is less simple than a degradation: vitamin C exists in two forms, ascorbic acid and its oxidised form, dehydroascorbic acid. The former is relatively heat stable but the oxidised form is much more heat labile; losses of vitamin C are therefore related to the degree of oxidation of the vitamin rather than to the severity of the heat process (Burton, 1988). This is known to apply to other products, especially fruit juices (Ryley and Kadja, 1994) and vegetables.

There are some vitamin interactions which occur. In milk, vitamin B_{12} and folic acid interact with vitamin C during heat treatment so that losses of these vitamins again are not a simple function of the degree of heat treatment. Folic acid is protected by ascorbic acid, the reduced form of vitamin C, which, if oxidised, will lead to higher losses of folate. Vitamin B_{12} losses depend on the oxidative degradation of ascorbic acid, so these losses depend on the availability of oxygen and ascorbic acid, as well as on the thermal process.

Although these changes are dependent on the degree of thermal process applied to the foodstuff, the remainder of the process must also be considered when evaluating the nutritional quality of the product. Changes during storage of the product over the usual three to six month shelf-life at ambient temperatures can be considerable, even though the container is designed to exclude light and oxygen. In addition, there is usually some pre-processing during manufacture of products; for instance, soups, stews and cook-in sauces are usually cooked or fried before sterilisation. Finally, handling of the product in the home is usually out of the manufacturer's control and overheating or long standing time at warm temperatures can easily have a more severe effect on nutritional quality than any of the procedures described above.

22.7 Future trends

A relatively new technology will only succeed commercially if it offers benefits to the processor, in terms of operating costs or other means of operational efficiency, or if it offers benefits to the consumer in terms of attributes that they are prepared to pay for. In-container processing using a metal can has a poor image and appears 'old' technology, although some development with plastic trays, pouches or bottles is in evidence. Continuous flow heat processing has the advantage over in-container processing of a fresher image, because the packaging is similar to that used for fresh chilled products. The food then has an improved organoleptic quality if processed correctly but is still ambient shelf stable. The question is whether these advantages will outweigh the disadvantages of increased technical difficulty and increased unit cost, mainly due to the high cost and low filling rates of the aseptic filler. The indications are that the technology will gradually displace the in-container process to a degree; the continuous flow thermal processing of low-viscosity liquid foods such as milk, fruit juices, teas and tomato products is already well established and more, generally innovative, food products are being introduced, albeit at a fairly slow rate. This slow introduction is very useful and may even be deliberate; because the process has a high complexity a large body of processing experience needs to be built up and consumers are more likely to become accustomed to this type of product.

All difficulties in processing are multiplied when producing foodstuffs containing solid particulates. Some soups, stews and cooking sauces containing particulates up to 25 mm in size have already been developed, but the greatest potential of the process lies in this area. Technical problems still to be solved satisfactorily are:

- Pumping of the foodstuff up to approximately 500 kPa pressure at a relatively low flowrate, then releasing the pressure to atmospheric again aseptically after heating, when the solid particulates are soft and easily damaged.
- A knowledge of the residence time of the liquid and solid phases in a holding tube, to enable sufficiently long minimum holding time to be established.
- A knowledge of the heat transfer rate from the liquid (usually heated first) to the solid particulates as the solids are transported by the liquids through the heating and cooling sections and down the holding tube, to enable the solid to be sterilised throughout.
- The development of aseptic filling equipment capable of handling particulates, without them being trapped across the packaging seal and compromising sterility of the container.

There is much active research at the present into these problems and several innovative techniques have been devised to overcome or circumvent them. One technique of note is the use of time–temperature integrators to ensure that the product has been heat sterilised to the required degree. These are small particles containing some chemical or microorganism (a marker) with a known heat resistance, which may be put through the process (whether by itself or embedded at the centre of a solid particulate), recovered and the surviving marker evaluated. From a knowledge of the heat degradation kinetics of the marker, the heat treatment received can be evaluated and used to ensure sterility of the product (Maesmans et al, 1994). Research work into particle residence time distribution and liquid-solid heat transfer has been reviewed by Lewis and Heppell (2000), Lareo et al (1997) and Barigou et al (1998). Another approach is to circumvent some of the problems and to use alternative equipment. Important in this respect are ohmic heating (covered in Chapter 19) and single flow fraction specific thermal processing (FSTP), that is a method of using a device to hold back particles of different size ranges and ensure they have a minimum holding time.

22.8 Sources of further information and advice

HOLDSWORTH S D (1992), *Aseptic Processing and Packaging of Food Products*, London and New York: Elsevier Applied Science

KARMAS E and HARRIS R S (1988), *Nutritional Evaluation of Food Processing*, New York: AVI Publishing

LEWIS M J and HEPPELL N J (2000), *Continuous Thermal Processing of Foods*, Gaithersburg: Aspen Publishers

WILLHOFT E M A (1993), *Aseptic processing and packaging of particulate foods*, Glasgow: Blackie Academic & Professional

22.9 References

BARIGOU M, MANKAD S and FRYER P J (1998), 'Heat transfer in two-phase solid-liquid food flows: a review', *Transactions of the Institution of Chemical Engineers* **76**(C), 3–29

BURTON H (1988), *Ultra-high-temperature Processing of Milk and Milk Products*, London: Elsevier Applied Science

HOLDSWORTH S D (1992), *Aseptic processing and packaging of food products*, Barking, UK: Elsevier Science Publishers

HOLDSWORTH S D (1997), *Thermal processing of packaged foods*, London: Blackie Academic & Professional

HORAK P (1980), *Uber die Reaktionskinetik der Sporenabtotung und chemischer Veranderungen bei der thermischen Haltbarmachung von Milch*. Thesis, Technical University, Munich, Germany

KARMAS E and HARRIS R S (1988), *Nutritional Evaluation of Food Processing*, New York: AVI Publishing

KESSLER H G and HORAK P (1981a), 'Objective evaluation of UHT-milk-heating by standardization of bacteriological and chemical effects', *Milchwissenschaft* **36**(3), 129–33

KESSLER H G and HORAK P (1981b), 'Testing and appraisal of Type 6500 ultra-high temperature heat treatment plant', *North European Dairy Journal* **47**(9), 252–63

KWOK K C and NIRANJAN K (1995), 'Effect of thermal processing on soymilk', *International Journal of Food Science and Technology* **30**(3), 263–95

LAREO C A, FRYER P J and BARIGOU M (1997), 'The fluid mechanics of two-phase solid-liquid food flows: a review', *Transactions of the Institution of Chemical Engineers* **75**(C), 73–105

LEWIS M J and HEPPELL N J (2000), *Coutinuous Thermal Processing of foods*, Gaithersburg: Aspen Publishers

MAESMANS G J, HENDRICKX M E, DE CORDT S V and TOBBACK P (1994), 'Feasibility of the use of a time–temperature integrator and a mathematical model to determine fluid-to-particle heat transfer coefficients', *Food Research International* **27**(1), 39–51

RAPAILLE A (1995), 'Use of starches in heat processed foods', *Food Technology International Europe*, 73–6

RENNER E (1979), 'Nutritional and biochemical characteristics of UHT milk', *Proceedings of the International Conference on UHT processing and Aseptic Packaging of Milk and Milk products*, Raleigh NC Department of Food Science, North Carolina State University

REUTER H (1982), 'UHT milk from the technological viewpoint', *Kieler Milchwirtschaftliche Forschungsberichte* **34**, 347–61

RYLEY J and KADJA P (1994), 'Vitamins in thermal processing', *Food Chemistry* **49**(2), 119–29

Index

absorption
  of Amadori compounds 280
  of calcium 103
  of copper 117, 127–33
  of iron 105
  of Maillard reaction products 280–1
  of melanoidins 281
  of minerals 98–9, 103, 105, 108
  of vitamin C 62
  of zinc 108
advertising
  functional foods 310–11
  nutrition claims 147
Aeromonas species of bacteria 354, 355
alcohol consumption 9, 69
allergens 447–8
Alzheimer's disease 82
Amadori rearrangement products (ARPs) 266–9, 280
amine oxidases 119
amino acids 271, 273
  cross-linked 277–80
amino-carbalines 282–3
amino-imidazo-azaarenes (AIAs) 283
anaemia 78, 99, 106, 228
anaerobic respiration 346
analytical systems *see* functionality testing
anti-freeze peptides 339
anti-mutagenic compounds 446
antinutrients 197, 324–5

antioxidants 42, 52–4, 63–4, 281, 294
ascorbic acid 62, 258–9, 297, 322–3
  and high pressure processing 437, 440
  and irradiation 382
  see also vitamin C
Asian communities 47, 51
atherosclerosis 178

β-carbolines 283
β-carotene 35, 39–40, 42–6, 64–5, 250–1, 358–9
backcross programmes 197
bacteria 350–4, 373, 411
bakery products 427–30
beriberi 66–9
bioactivity 53, 57–9, 168–9
bioavailability of nutrients 169, 201–2
  in cereal foods 302–3
  copper 128–9
  folates 71
  iron 130, 228
  minerals 323–4
  vitamin A 38
bioefficacy of vitamin A 38–9
biogenic amines 236
biomarkers 171–2, 174–5, 181
biotin 37, 80–1, 257
  and irradiation 380, 381–2
blanching 334–5, 338, 415–16
  and vitamin loss 260–1

blood clotting 57–8, 59
blood glucose 170, 174–5
bone health
  and meat 235
  osteoporosis 50–1, 60, 103–4
  and vitamin D 50–1
  and vitamin K 58–9, 60–1

caeruloplasmin 119
calciferol 46, 48–50
  and irradiation 382–3
  see also vitamin D
calcium 50, 58–9, 98, 102–5
  absorption 103
  food sources 104
  reference nutrient intake 104
  safe intake 105
CALEUR study 21
calorific information 155
Campylobacter 373
cancer 9, 18–19, 44, 209
  and antioxidants 52
  and β-carotene 42–4
  colon cancer 51, 211–14
  and meat eating 210, 211–14
carbohydrates 154, 173–4, 175, 306–8
  and continuous-flow heat processing 469–70
  and extrusion cooking 317–19
  and irradiation 383
carbon dioxide 343–5, 346–7
cardiovascular disease (CVD) *see* heart disease
carnitine 236
carnosine 236
carotenoids
  β-carotene 35, 39–40, 42–6, 64–5, 250–1, 358–9
  and high pressure processing 440–1
  and irradiation 380
  and modified atmosphere packaging 358–9
catechol oxidase 119
cell differentiation 40
cellular growth 51
cereal foods 22, 102, 166, 185–6, 301–11
  bioavailability of nutrients 302–3
  mechanical processing 302–5
  nutritional significance 302–3
  nutritionally enhanced 308–11
  thermal processing 303, 305–8
cholesterol 198–200, 214–15, 223, 296, 320
  LDL-cholesterol oxidation 54

choline 236
Clostridium botulinum 351
cobalamins 77–80, 257
  deficiency diseases 78–9
  food sources 37, 77
  and irradiation 380, 381–2
  toxicity 80
Codex Alimentarius 388, 389–90
coeliac disease 48
cold spots 411–12, 419
colon cancer 51, 211–14
colonic bulk 181
colour of foods 276–7, 345
conjugated linoleic acid (CLA) 221–3
consumers
  food choice factors 149, 150–1, 168
  improving consumer confidence 168
  understanding of labelling 149–56
continuous-flow heat processing 462–72
  and carbohydrates 469–70
  commercialisation 471–2
  and fats 469–70
  flash-cooling 466
  food quality 466–8
  heat exchanger selection 464–6
  and proteins 468–9
  steam infusion 465
  steam injection 465
  streamline flow 468
  technical problems 472
  thermal degradation kinetics 463–4
  time-temperature profile 466–7
  turbulent flow 468
  and vitamins 470–1
copper 65, 117–35
  absorption 117, 127–33
  bioavailability 128–9
  deficiency diseases 117, 121–2
  distribution in the body 131
  in drinking water 123
  food sources 120–1
  function of cuproenzymes 118–20
  functional copper status 127
  and heart disease 122
  intake assessment 124–7
  putative indicators 125–6
  reference nutrient intake 120
  serum copper 125–6
  toxicity 117, 122–4
coronary heart disease (CHD) *see* heart disease
cross-linked amino acids 277–80

cuproenzymes 118–20
cyanocobalamin 380, 381–2
cytochrome-*c* oxidase 118

DAFNE (DAta Food NEtworking)
  project 11, 17–18
dairy products 128, 446, 447
data sources 7, 10–22
  European surveys 13–22
  food balance sheets (FBS) 10, 22
  food frequency questionnaires 13
  household budget surveys (HBS)
    11–12, 17–18
  individual dietary surveys (IDSs)
    12–13
deep frying 293, 298
dehydration, and vitamin loss 262
dephytinisation 130
diabetes 48, 172, 174–5, 178
diacylglycerols 294
diamine oxidase 119
diet
  data sources 7, 10–22
  European dietary patterns 22–8
    Mediterranean countries 25, 28–9,
      196, 213
  and health 8–10
  nutrition and the elderly 20–1
dietary reference values 34–5
digestibility of food 446–7
disease-nutrient interactions 63–5
DNA damage and repair 56
dopamine β-hydroxylase (DβM)
  119
drinking water 123
drip loss 333, 336

elderly people 20–1, 47–8
  and antioxidant vitamins 64
  immune system 55–6
electrolysis 416
electromagnetic radiation 397
electrons 374–5, 377
embryogenesis 41
end-points 171, 174, 181
energy
  information provision 155
  value calculations 146
enhanced diffusion 415–16
enhancement *see* nutritional
    enhancement
enzymes 320
  cuproenzymes 118–20
  xenobiotic enzymes 281–2

  see also Maillard reaction
equilibrium modified atmosphere
    packaging (EMAP) 347–50
Escherichia coli 373, 386, 390
Euronut-SENECA study 20–1, 28
European dietary patterns 22–8
  Mediterranean countries 25, 28–9,
    196, 213
European Prospective Investigation
    into Cancer and Nutrition
    (EPIC) 18–19, 28
European surveys 13–22
extrusion cooking 314–26
  and antinutrients 324–5
  and carbohydrates 317–19
  future trends 325–6
  and lipids 321
  Maillard reactions 320
  and minerals 323–4
  and phenolic compounds 325
  and phytohormones 325
  and proteins 320–1
  and thiamin 323
  vitamin stability 321–3
  wet extrusion 316–17

faecal bulk 171, 180–6
fats
  and continuous-flow heat processing
    469–70
  and frying 293
  information provision 153, 154
  in meat 214–23, 234
fatty acids 217–22
  and cholesterol 223
  conjugated linoleic acid (CLA)
    221–3
  monounsaturated fatty acids 218
  polyunsaturated fatty acids 219–21
  saturated fatty acids 218
  trans-fatty acids 222
ferroxidases 119
fibre 155, 166, 181–2, 309, 319
fish
  freezing 336–7
  high pressure processing 443–4
  trimethylamineoxide reduction
    345–6
flash-cooling 466
flavonoids 202
flour production 304–5
fluoride 98
folates 70–7, 202–3, 256
  bioavailability 71

and cardiovascular disease (CVD) 75–6
deficiency effects 76
food sources 37, 70–1
fortification of foods 74–5, 77
reference nutrient intake 36, 72, 74
requirements 72–5
toxicity 76–7
food balance sheets (FBS) 10, 22
food frequency questionnaires 13
food matrix properties 170
Food Standards Agency (FSA) 160–1
fortification 195, 202–3
  with folates 74–5, 77
  with minerals 102, 324
  see also nutritional enhancement
fractures see bone health
freezing 331–40
  anti-freeze peptides 339
  drip loss 333, 336
  fruit 333–6
  'glassy state' freezing 338–9
  meat and fish 336–7
  Ostwald ripening 333
  quality and nutrient loss 332–3
  vegetables and fruit 333–6
  and vitamin loss 261
fruit
  availability 24, 25
  and cancer protection 44, 65
  and cardiovascular disease 65, 75–6
  cooking methods 335–6
  high pressure processing 446
  modified atmosphere packaging 356–62
  storage after harvest 334
  washing and blanching 334–5, 338
frying 293–8
  deep frying 293, 298
  and fat consumption 293
  frying oil 294–5, 298
  impact on nutrients 296–7
  meat 428–30
  sensory characteristics 297–8
  shallow frying 293
FSA (Food Standards Agency) 160–1
functional foods
  market for 186–7
  marketing 310–11
functionality testing
  biomarkers 171–2, 174–5, 181
  data limitations 168–9, 173–4
  end-points 171, 174, 181
  extrapolation between products 167

food matrix properties 170
food processing and nutritional quality 165–7
future trends 186–8
glycaemic-glucose equivalents 174–80
indices 172–3
  faecal bulking index 180–6
  glycaemic index (GI) 173, 175–9
market for functional foods 186–7
types of tests 167
validation of tests 172
wheat bran equivalents 180–6

gamma rays 374, 375
genetic engineering 197–8, 200–1, 204–6
'glassy state' freezing 338–9
glucosinolates 325, 361–2
glutathione 236
glycaemic index (GI) 173, 175–9, 307
glycaemic-glucose equivalents 174–80
goitre 99, 111, 196
Grasbeck-Immerslund syndrome 78
Guideline Daily Amounts (GDAs) 158–9

haemorrhagic disease of the newborn (HDN) 59–60
hair colour 82
haptocorrins 78
heart disease
  cardiovascular disease 8–9, 20, 75–6, 122
  and copper deficiency 122
  coronary heart disease 9, 20, 53–5
  vascular cell dysfunction 56
  and vitamin E 53–5
heat exchangers 464–6
heat processing see thermal processing
hephaestin 131
heterocyclic amines (HAs) 282–5
high pressure processing 433–61
  and allergens 447–8
  anti-mutagenic compounds 446
  and ascorbic acid 437, 440
  and carotene 440–1
  commercial food products 436, 438–9
  dairy products 446, 447
  digestibility of food 446–7
  equipment 435–6
  fish products 443–4
  food quality 433–4

fruit 446
future trends 448
and lipids 442–5
meat products 444–5
and mineral content 445–6
and retinol 441
safety 434–5
and sweeteners 445
vegetables 446
and vitamins 437–42
histidinoalanine (HAL) 278–9, 279–80
homocysteine 72, 75–6, 80, 84–5
household budget surveys (HBS) 11–12, 17–18
Hox family genes 41
hunter-gatherer diets 227
hydroperoxides 294–5, 384
hyperglycaemia 174
hypervitaminosis A 44–5

immune system
  and elderly people 55–6
  and vitamin A 41–2, 43
  and vitamin C 65–6
  and vitamin D 51–2
  and vitamin E 55–6
  and zinc deficiency 109
Indian Childhood Cirrhosis (ICC) 124
indices 172–3
  faecal bulking index 180–6
  glycaemic index (GI) 173, 175–9
individual dietary surveys (IDSs) 12–13
infants, haemorrhagic disease of the newborn (HDN) 59–60
information panels 151–6
infrared heating 398, 423–31
  bakery products 427–30
  food industry applications 426–7
  food quality 428–30
  frying meat 428–30
  future trends 430–1
  near infrared heating (NIR) 424
  nutritional quality 430
  penetration depths 426
iodine 98, 99, 102, 111
  deficiency disorders 8, 196
ionising radiation *see* irradiation
iron 64–5, 98, 99, 105–7
  absorption 105
  bioavailability 130, 228
  deficiency diseases 228
  food sources 107
  iron/vitamin C reaction 64

in meat 228–30, 235
reference nutrient intake 106–7
safe intake 107
irradiation 371–92
  and ascorbic acid 382
  benefits 385–6
  and biotin 380, 381–2
  and calciferol 382–3
  and carbohydrates 383
  and carotenoids 380
  and cobalamins 381–2
  consumer attitudes to 386–9
  and cyanocobalamin 380, 381–2
  effect on food 377–8
  future trends 390–1
  history of 372–3
  and lipids 383–4
  and niacin 380, 381–2
  nutritional adequacy 379–80
  principles of 373–7
  and proteins 384
  and pyridoxine 380, 381–2
  regulation of 386–90
  and riboflavin 380, 381–2
  safety of 378–9, 385
  and thiamin 380, 381–2
  and tocopherols 383
  and vitamins 262, 380–3
  wholesomeness of irradiated food 384–5
isotope studies 132–3

Keshan disease 112
Korsakoff syndrome 69

labelling 142–63
  consumer understanding of 149–56
  future trends in 161–3
  Guideline Daily Amounts (GDAs) 158–9
  legibility 160
  nutrition information panels 151–6
  Nutrition Labelling Directive 144–9
  research findings 157–61
  retailer influence on 149–50
LDL-cholesterol oxidation 54
legislation *see* regulation
lipids 24–5, 297
  extrusion cooking 321
  high pressure processing 442–5
  irradiation 383–4
lipoic acid 236
Listeria monocytogenes 351–2, 373
lycopene 197

lysine 273-4
lysinoalanine (LAL) 277, 279-80

magnesium sodium 98
Maillard reaction 266-75, 280-2
  and extrusion cooking 320
manganese 129
margarines 198-200
marketing
  functional foods 310-11
  and nutrition claims 147
meat
  availability 22, 25-6
  and bone health 235
  and cancer 210, 211-14
  colour retention 345
  consumption trends 210-11
  fat components 214-23, 234
  freezing 336-7
  health-promoting components 235-6
  high pressure processing 444-5
  iron content 228-30, 235
  nutritional importance 209-10
  Palaeolithic diets 226-7
  phosphorus content 231
  protein content 223-4
  satiating powers 227
  selenium content 230-1, 235
  vitamin B content 231-2
  vitamin D content 232-3
  zinc content 230
mechanical processing 302-5
Mediterranean diets 25, 28-9, 196, 213
melanoidins 275-7, 281
menadione 57
Menkes disease 121-2, 131
methylation cycle 71, 72
methylmalonic acid (MMA) 79-80
microbial safety 350-4, 373, 411
microwave processing 396-406
  effect on food 401-3
  industrial exploitation 405-6
  nutritional adequacy of food 405
  principles 398-401
  safety 403-5
milk 250, 253, 255-7, 261, 468-9, 470
milling 302-5
  abrasive processes 303-4
  reductive processes 304
minerals 97-113
  absorption 98-9, 103, 105, 108
  bioavailability 323-4
  calcium 98, 102-5
  copper see copper

dietary sources 100-2
extrusion cooking 323-4
fluoride 98
food fortification 102, 324
frying 297
high pressure processing 445-6
iodine 98, 99, 102, 111
iron 98, 99, 105-7
magnesium sodium 98
molybdenum 98, 129
nutrition labelling 145-6
phosphorus 98
potassium 98
reference nutrient intake 97-8, 100
safe intakes 100
selenium 99, 111-13
supplements 101
zinc 99, 107-10, 129
modified atmosphere packaging
  (MAP) 342-62
  anaerobic respiration 346
  use of carbon dioxide 343-5, 346-7
  colour retention of meat products
    345
  equilibrium modified atmosphere
    packaging 347-50
  fruits 356-62
  microbial safety 350-4
  non-respiring products 346-7, 354-5
  optimal gas atmosphere 346-7
  use of oxygen 345-6
  and provitamin carotenoids 358-9
  respiring products 347-50
  trimethylamineoxide reduction
    345-6
  vegetables 356-62
  vitamin C 356-8
molybdenum 98, 129
MONICA Project 20
monoacylglycerols 294
monoamine oxidase 119
monounsaturated fatty acids 218
mutagenic heterocyclic amines (HAs)
  282-5

near infrared heating (NIR) 424
neural tube defects 70, 72-4, 203
niacin 82-3, 231, 255
  food sources 37
  and irradiation 380, 381-2
  reference nutrient intake 36
nicotinamide 82-3
nicotinic acid 82-3
night blindness 35

non-respiring products 346–7, 354–5
nuclear receptors 40
nucleotides 236
nutrition claims 147
nutrition information panels 151–6
Nutrition Labelling Directive 144–9
  declared values 146–7
  definitions 146
  energy value calculations 146
  format of information 145–6
  implementation and enforcement 148
  and nutrition claims 147
  timescales 147
nutritional enhancement 196–206
  and bioavailability 201–2
  of cereal foods 308–11
  compared to fortification 202–3
  genetic engineering 197–8, 200–1, 204–6
  pedigree selection and backcross programmes 197
  reducing antinutritional factors 197
  supplements 198
nutritional melalgia 81–2

obesity 234
ohmic heating 407–19
  advantages 409–12
  cold spots 411–12, 419
  commercialisation 416–17
  electrical conductivity and heating rate 410–11
  and electrolysis 416
  enhanced diffusion 415–16
  microbial destruction 411
  modelling heating patterns 417–18
  nutrient loss 413–16, 417
  principles 407–9
  process parameters 418
  product specifications 418
  temperature distribution 411–12, 419
1,25-OHD 48–50, 103
osteocalcin 50–1, 58
osteomalacia 233
osteoporosis 50–1, 60, 103–4
Ostwald ripening 333
oxygen 345–6

Palaeolithic diets 226–7
pantothenic acid 37, 81–2, 255
pedigree selection 197
pellagra 83

peptidyl-glycine ∝-amidating mono-oxygenase (PAM) 119
phenolic compounds 325, 359–61
phosphorus 98, 231
phytates 197
phytohormones 325
plasma homocysteine 72, 75–6, 80, 84–5
polyunsaturated fatty acids 219–21
pork lard 295
postprandial glycaemia 173–4
potassium 98
pressure treated foods see high pressure processing
product shelf life 262–3
proteins 154–5, 297
  continuous-flow heat processing 468–9
  extrusion cooking 320–1
  irradiation 384
  meat content 223–4
provitamin carotenoids see carotenoids
pyridoxine 83–5, 256–7
  and irradiation 380, 381–2
pyrolysis products 282–3

radiation processing see irradiation
radioisotopes 133, 134
receptors 60
recommended dietary allowance (RDA) 34–5
reference nutrient intake (RNI)
  calcium 104
  copper 120
  folates 36, 72, 74
  iodine 111
  iron 106–7
  minerals 97–8, 100
  niacin 36
  riboflavin 36
  selenium 112
  thiamin 36
  vitamin A 35, 36, 38
  vitamin B 36
  vitamin C 36
  vitamin D 36
  zinc 109
regulation
  of flour production 304–5
  of irradiation 386–90
  Nutrition Labelling Directive 144–9
relative glycaemic potency (RGP) 174–80
resistant starch 307–8
respiring products 347–50

retinol 35, 40–1, 44, 45, 381
    and high pressure processing 441
    see also vitamin A
retrograded starch 308
riboflavin 85–6, 231, 254–5, 255, 413
    food sources 37, 85
    and irradiation 380, 381–2
    reference nutrient intake 36
rice 200–1
rickets 47, 233

safe intakes (SI)
    calcium 105
    cobalamins 80
    copper 117, 122–4
    folates 76–7
    iodine 111
    iron 107
    minerals 100
    selenium 113
    thiamin 70
    vitamin A 44–6
    vitamin C 66
    vitamin D 52
    vitamin E 56
    vitamin K 61
    zinc 110
safety
    of high pressure processing 434–5
    of irradiation 378–9, 385
    microbial safety 350–4, 373, 411
    of microwave processing 403–5
    of thermal processing 282–5
Salmonella 373
salt 155
satiety 227
saturated fatty acids 218
scurvy 62
seasonal affective disorders (SAD) 51
selenium 99, 111–13, 230–1, 235
    reference nutrient intake 112
    safe intake 113
selenosis 99, 113
SENECA *see* Euronut-SENECA study
serum copper 125–6
shallow frying 293
shelf life of products 262–3
short-wave infrared heating 424
smokers 63–4
sodium intake 155
starches 306–8, 318, 414, 469
steam infusion 465
steam injection 465
sterilisation 463–4

Strecker degradation 269
sugars 175, 273, 317
superoxide dismutase (SOD) 119
supplements 101, 195, 198
surveys *see* data sources
sweeteners 445

thermal degradation kinetics 463–4
thermal processing 265–85, 407, 462
    of cereal foods 303, 305–8
    cross-linked amino acids formation 277–80
    Maillard reaction 266–75, 280–2
    melanoidins 275–7, 281
    molecular level reactions 265–6
    thermal degradation kinetics 463–4
    toxic compound formation 282–5
    and vitamin loss 261
    see also continuous-flow heat processing; ohmic heating
thiamin 66–70, 231, 253–4, 413
    deficiency effects 68–70
    extrusion cooking 323
    food sources 37, 67
    functions and requirements 67–8
    irradiation 380, 381–2
    reference nutrient intake 36
    toxicity 70
thioredoxin 197
tocopherols 52–3, 297, 383
    see also vitamin E
tocotrienols 52
toxicity *see* safe intakes (SI)
trans-fatty acids 222
TRANSFAIR study 21–2
triacylglycerols 294
trimethylamineoxide reduction 345–6
Tyrolean Infantile Cirrhosis (ICC) 124
tyrosinase 119

UHT milk 250, 253, 256–7, 261, 468–9

validation of tests 172
vascular cell dysfunction 56
vegetable oils 24, 26, 443
vegetables
    availability 22, 25
    and cancer protection 44, 65
    and cardiovascular disease 65, 75–6
    cooking methods 335–6
    and copper absorption 128
    freezing 333–6
    high pressure processing 446

modified atmosphere packaging 356–62
storage after harvest 334
washing and blanching 334–5, 338
vegetarians 51, 195, 224–6
vision 35, 40
night blindness 35
vitamin A 35–46, 248
bioavailability 38
bioefficacy 38–9
continuous-flow heat processing 470–1
deficiency disorders (VADD) 35, 38, 44, 196, 200
equivalence factor 39–40
food sources 37
health aspects 35, 38, 40–4
high pressure processing 440–1
hypervitaminosis A 44–5
and the immune system 41–2, 43
irradiation 380, 381
ohmic heating 413
reference nutrient intake 35, 36, 38
stability during processing 249–51
toxicity symptoms 44–5
vitamin B
cobalamins (B_{12}) 77–80, 257
continuous-flow heat processing 470–1
food sources 37
frying 297
high pressure processing 441–2
irradiation 380, 381–2
in meat 231–2
ohmic heating 413
pyridoxine (B_6) 83–5, 256–7
reference nutrient intake 36
riboflavin (B_2) 85–6, 254–5
stability during processing 253–7
thiamin (B_1) 66–70, 253–4
vitamin C 62–6
absorption 62
biochemical functions 63
continuous-flow heat processing 470–1
disease-nutrient interactions 63–5
food sources 37
health aspects 62, 63–6
high pressure processing 437, 440
and the immune system 65–6
iron/vitamin C reaction 64
irradiation 380, 382
modified atmosphere packaging (MAP) 356–8

ohmic heating 413
reference nutrient intake 36
and smokers 63–4
stability during processing 258–9
toxicity 66
vitamin D 46–52
and bone health 50–1
continuous-flow heat processing 470
food sources 37
health aspects 47–52
and the immune system 51–2
irradiation 382–3
in meat 232–3
ohmic heating 413
1,25-OHD 48–50
reference nutrient intake 36
safety 52
stability during processing 251–2
vitamin E 52–7, 247–8
bioactivity 53
continuous-flow heat processing 470
food sources 37, 52
health aspects 53–6
and heart disease 53–5
high pressure processing 441–2
and the immune system 55–6
irradiation 383
safety 56
stability during processing 251
vitamin K 57–61
biological activity 57–9
and bone health 58–9, 60–1
food sources 37, 57
health aspects 59–61
high pressure processing 441–2
ohmic heating 413
safety 61
stability during processing 252–3
vitamins
blanching 260–1
continuous-flow heat processing 470–1
and dehydration 262
extrusion cooking 321–3
freezing 261
frying 297
high pressure processing 437–42
irradiation 262, 380–3
labelling 145–6, 249
loss during processing 260–2
ohmic heating 407, 413
and product shelf life 262–3
protecting 263
stability during processing 247–59

as supplements 195
thermal processing 261, 305–6
vitamin-vitamin interactions 259–90

Wernicke-Korsakoff syndrome 69
wet extrusion 316–17
wheat bran equivalents 180–6
WHO-MONICA Project 20
wholesomeness of irradiated food 384–5
Wilson's disease 124
World Trade Organization (WTO) 389–90

X-Rays 374–5, 377, 378
xenobiotic enzymes 281–2

Yersinia enterocolitica 352–3

zinc 99, 107–10, 129
   absorption 108
   deficiency 109
   meat content 230
   reference nutrient intake 109
   safe intake 110